NEW PERSPECTIVES IN BIOSENSORS TECHNOLOGY AND APPLICATIONS

Edited by **Pier Andrea Serra**

New Perspectives in Biosensors Technology and Applications
Edited by Pier Andrea Serra

Published by InTech
Janeza Trdine 9, 51000 Rijeka, Croatia

Publishing Process Manager Mirna Cvijic

Technical Editor Teodora Smiljanic

Cover Designer InTech Design Team

Additional hard copies can be obtained from orders@intechopen.com

New Perspectives in Biosensors Technology and Applications, Edited by Pier Andrea Serra
p. cm.
ISBN 978-953-307-448-1

For EU product safety concerns:
IN TECH d.o.o., Prolaz Marije Krucifikse Kozulić 3, 51000 Rijeka, Croatia,
info@intechopen.com or visit our website at intechopen.com.

Meet the editor

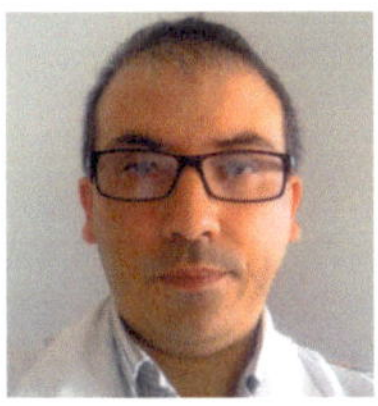

Pier Andrea Serra is associate professor of pharmacology at Medical School at University of Sassari. He received his degree of Medical Doctor at Sassari University in 1998 and studied the in vivo Neurochemistry of Parkinson's Disease using microdialysis and voltammetry under the supervision of Dr. Maddalena Miele. Prof. Serra received his PhD in Pharmacology and in 2001 and he worked as a Postdoctoral Fellow at University College of Dublin and at National University of Maynooth (Ireland) under the direction of Prof. Robert D. O'Neill and Dr. John P. Lowry. Professor Serra's research program focuses on design and application of microsensors and biosensors for electrochemical monitoring of brain signalling systems in neurodegenerative diseases.

Contents

Preface

A biosensor is defined as a detecting device that combines a transducer with a biologically sensitive and selective component. When a specific target molecule interacts with the biological component, a signal is produced, at transducer level, proportional to the concentration of the substance. Therefore biosensors can measure compounds present in the environment, chemical processes, food and human body at low cost if compared with traditional analytical techniques.

This book covers a wide range of aspects and issues related to biosensor technology, bringing together researchers from 12 different countries. The book consists of 20 chapters written by 69 authors and divided in three sections. The first section, entitled Biosensors Technology and Materials, is composed by 15 chapters and describes emerging aspects of technology applied to biosensors. The subsequent section, entitled Biosensors for Health and including three chapters, is devoted to biosensor applications in the medical field. The last section, composed by two chapters, treats of the environmental and biosecurity applications of biosensors.

I want to express my appreciation and gratitude to all authors who contributed to this book with their research results and to InTech team, in particular to the Publishing Process Manager Ms. Mirna Cvijic that accomplished its mission with professionalism and dedication.

Pier Andrea Serra
University of Sassari
Italy

Part 1

Biosensor Technology and Materials

1

FAIMS Detection Technology Based on MEMS

Fei Tang, Xiaohao Wang and Chulong Xu
Tsinghua University
Peoples Republic of China

1. Introduction

1.1 The research background of FAIMS

To build a resource-conserving and environmentally friendly society is a strategic mission in the long-term plan of a national economy and society development. Environmental protection regulation, is not only about preventing pollution and protecting ecosystem, but also includes the fast detection of environmental pollutants. Thus, analytical apparatus for the fast and effective detection of environmental pollutants is required. Besides, the real-time detection technology of the trace amounts of chemicals, drug, explosive material, etc. is also an important technical method to maintain people's health, social stability and national security.

At present, common detection methods use complex, expensive and bulky detection equipment or have complex procedures without portability, which limits their use. For example, methods like mass spectrometry, atomic fluorescence and so on need complex instruments. In contrast, titration and colorimetry only need simple equipment, but their process of operation is complex, which leads to time-consuming, low efficiency and highly demanding operations. So these kinds of methods are hard to promote.

With the increasing demand in application, portable and low power consuming micro-chemical analysis detection instruments are urgently required. Ion Mobility Spectrometry (IMS), which plays a very important role in the detection of explosive substances, poison and chemical warfare agents, etc., was developed during the 1970s. In IMS, substances are separated mainly according to differences in the mobility of ions under low electric fields in order to analyse each kind of the substance. Up until now, many kinds of commercial IMS have appeared, which have been widely used in detection of the environmental pollutants, explosive materials, drug and chemical warfare agents, etc. (West et al., 2007; Laiko et al., 2006; Borsdorf et al., 2006). The drift tube of IMS is a metal ring structure, which is adverse to miniaturisation (Miller et al., 2001). In the high-field asymmetric waveform ion mobility spectrometry (FAIMS) developed in recent years, the drift tube is a flat plate structure, which makes it easy to fabricate with Micro Electro Mechanical Systems (MEMS). It has many strengths, such as miniature size, high sensitivity, short test time, numerous test substances, low power usage, etc. So it can be used to detect substances instead of IMS. In addition, substances of same or similar ion mobility under the conditions of the low electric field which are hard to separate in IMS, can be separated by the difference in the ion mobility in the high electric field of FAIMS (Miller et al., 2000). On the other hand, FAIMS can be used together with a mass spectrograph, and can bring ion filtration and selection to the mass spectrograph, resulting in decreased background noise and improved signal to noise ratio (Barnett et al., 2002). In conclusion, wide prospects for the FAIMS sensor based on MEMS technology exist, which can bring huge social and economic benefits.

1.2 Current status and developing trend of FAIMS technology

Since the 1990s, The Canadian Institute for National Measurement Standards, New Mexico State University of the USA, Sionex company, Pacific Northwest National Laboratory, Owlstone Company of the UK, Thermo Company of the US, etc. have all developed sensors with the FAIMS principle, one after another (Guevremont et al., 1999; Eiceman et al., 2000; Nazarov et al., 2006; Shvartsburg et al., 2004; Barnett et al., 2007), in which the New Mexico State University, Sionex company and the Owlstone Company are leading the miniaturisation of the FAIMS sensors with MEMS technology (Miller et al., 2001; Eiceman et al., 2001; Shvartsburg et al., 2009).

Eiceman, etc. from the New Mexico State University developed a small ion filter based on the principle of FAIMS with MEMS technology, with which toluene with a detection limit of up to 100ppb can be measured. This device is composed by a $3\times1\times0.5cm^3$ rectangular drift tube and a set of parallel plate electrodes. The size of the whole chip is just like a coin. Figure 1 shows the chip of the FAIMS detector made by Eiceman (Miller et al., 2001).

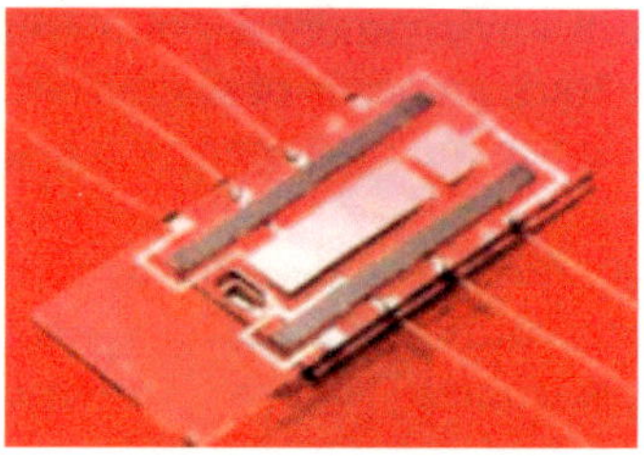

Fig. 1. Micro FAIMS detector

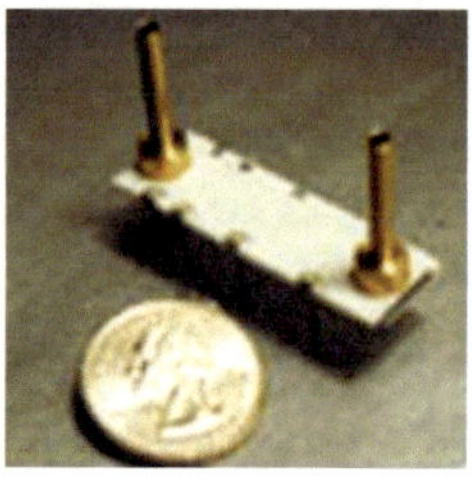

Fig. 2. MicroDMx™ chip made by Sionex

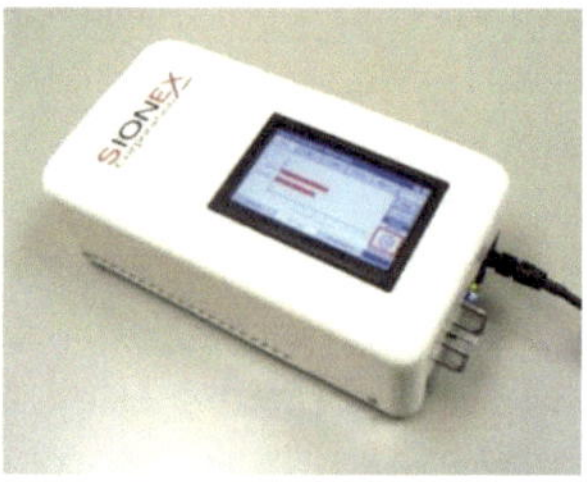

Fig. 3. Commercial FAIMS product developed by the Sionex company

The Sionex Company was founded in the USA in 2000, and is mainly engaged in the research and development of mico-FAIMS detection parts, and it is leading in the utility and commercialisation of the FAIMS technology. With the technology from the Eiceman's research group of New Mexico State University and the Charles Stark Draper Laboratory, the company has developed a micro FAIMS detector. The core of its products is the microDMx™ sensor platform, as shown in figure 2 (Miller et al., 2000).

Based on the microDMx™ chip, the Sionex company has developed a commercial product, as shown in figure 3. This product has a high detection sensitivity (up to ppb), and a short detection time (from 30 seconds to 5 minutes), which can be used in anti-terrorism, process control, environmental monitoring and medical diagnosis, etc.

The Owlstone Company in the U.K. is also engaged in the research of the micro detector based on FAIMS technology. This company plans to develop a kind of chemical sensor with the size of a coin, which can be used to detect trace amounts of explosive substances. In addition, this sensor can be used in civil applications such as family fire monitoring and early disease diagnosis, etc. In the FAIMS technology of Owlstone, one small space (10 micrometre), short path (depth of a silicon chip) and a muti-channel array type of drift tube structure is used, as shown in figure 4. Compared to the traditional FAIMS structure, the multi-channel can improve the sensitivity; the small space can decrease the radio frequency voltage amplitude needed; the short path can decrease the ion travelling time in the shift tube and increase the analytical efficiency (Shvartsburg et al., 2009).

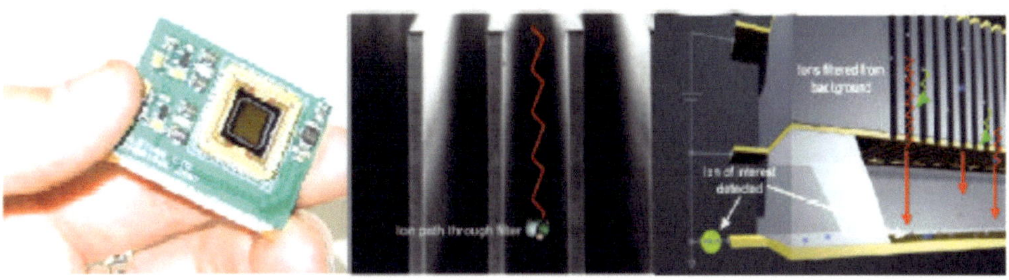

Fig. 4. FAIMS principle and chip of Owlstone Company

Based on the multi-channel FAIMS chip structure, the Owlstone Company has developed two commercial products: LONESTAR and Nexsense C, as shown in figure 5. The weight of these two products is 7.8kg and 7kg, respectively, with a built-in chargeable power supply. It can be used continuously for three hours, which is convenient for field operation.

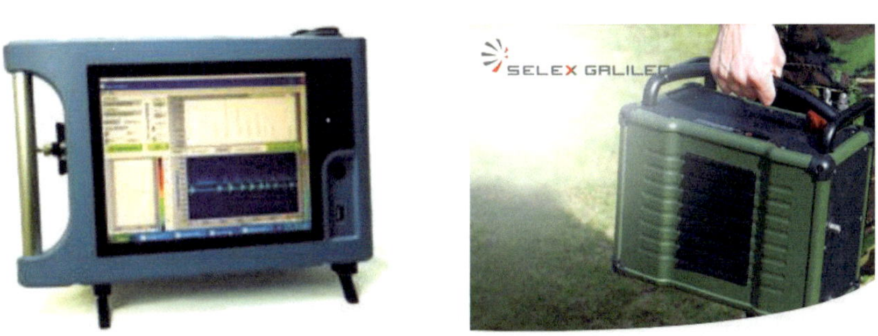

Fig. 5. FAIMS products from the Owlstone Company. Left: LONESTAR; Right: Nexsense C

2. Principle of FAIMS

FAIMS separates different kinds of compounds mainly based on the ion mobility difference under electric field changes by varying the electric field intensity. When the electric field intensity is over a certain value (over 10000V/cm), the mobility of the ion will change non-linearly with the electric field intensity, as shown in figure 6 (Buryakov et al., 1993). Here, $K = K_0(1+\alpha)$, where K is the mobility of the ion in the high electric field; K_0 is the mobility of the ion in the low electric field; α is the efficiency coefficient of the ion mobility, which is different for different kinds of ion.

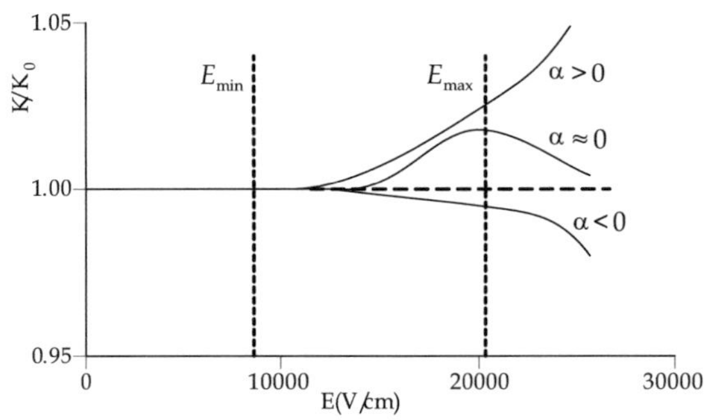

Fig. 6. Relation between ion mobility and the electric field intensity in three cases

In figure 6, we can see that the change of mobility for ions A, B and C is different in the high electric field. The mobility of ion A will increase with an increase in the electric field intensity; when the electric field intensity increases, the mobility of ion B will primarily increase and then decrease; while the mobility of ion C will decrease when the electric field intensity increases. In general, the ions with small mass-to-charge ratio m/z (m/z is less than 300) belong to the A type of ion; while ions with a large mass-to-charge ratio m/z (m/z is greater than 300) belong to the C type of ion. The change in mobility when the electric field intensity changes is related to the size of the ion, interaction between ion and molecule, and the structural rigidity of the ion.

In conclusion, when the electric field intensity is greater than 10000V/cm, the ion mobility will have a different non-linear changing trend, so that an ion with the same or similar mobility in the low electric field intensity can be separated under the influence of the high electric field intensity. The change in ion mobility under the influence of the high electric field intensity is also related to the gas concentration. The variation range of *K* with the electric field is defined by E/N, in which E is the electric field intensity and N is the gas density, namely the number of the gas molecule in unit volume. The unit of E/N is Townsend (Td). It is presumed that the electric field intensity is 1000V/cm, under the condition of one atm and 273K, the gas density N will be 2.7×10^{19}, so the value of E/N is about 3.7×10^{-17}. It is defined that 1Td is equal to 1×10^{-17}, and the value of E/N is about 3.7Td under the above conditions. When the value of E/N is about 40Td, the ion mobility begins to change when the electric field intensity increases. Under high electric field intensity, the relation between the ion mobility *K* and the electric field intensity is shown as follows (Krylov et al., 2003):

$$K = K_0[1+\alpha_1(E/N)^2+\alpha_2(E/N)^4+\ldots\ldots] \tag{1}$$

Formula (1) can be simplified or approximated into following formula:

$$K \approx K_0[1+\alpha(E)] \tag{2}$$

Where $\alpha(E)$ is the function of the electric field intensity. According to formula (2), when $\alpha(E)$ is above zero, K will increase as E increases; when $\alpha(E)$ is below zero, K will decrease as E increases; and when $\alpha(E)$ is near to zero, K will change slightly. These three cases correspond to the three kinds of ion in the high electric field intensity.
The expression of the asymmetrical waveform voltage used in the FAIMS is shown as follows:

$$U_d(t)=\begin{cases} U_d,(T-pT+mT \le t \le T+mT) \\ -\dfrac{pU_d}{1-p},(mT \le t \le T-pT+mT) \end{cases} \tag{3}$$

Where, m is an integer number, U_d is the amplitude value of the high voltage, p is the coefficient of the duty ratio, T is the cycle of the voltage signal. Thus its corresponding electric field is $E_d(t)=\dfrac{U_d(t)}{d}$, where d is the plate electrode space in the drift tube, the waveform of $E_d(t)$ is shown in figure 7. $E_d(t)$ must meet the following criteria:

$$10000\,V/cm < |E_{\max}| < 30000V\,/\,cm$$
$$|E_{\max}| >> |E_{\min}|$$
$$|E_{\max}|t_1 - |E_{\min}|t_2 = 0$$

It is supposed:

$$|E_{\max}|t_1 = |E_{\min}|t_2 = \beta \tag{4}$$

where, β is the random shadow's area in the figure 7, which is a constant value.

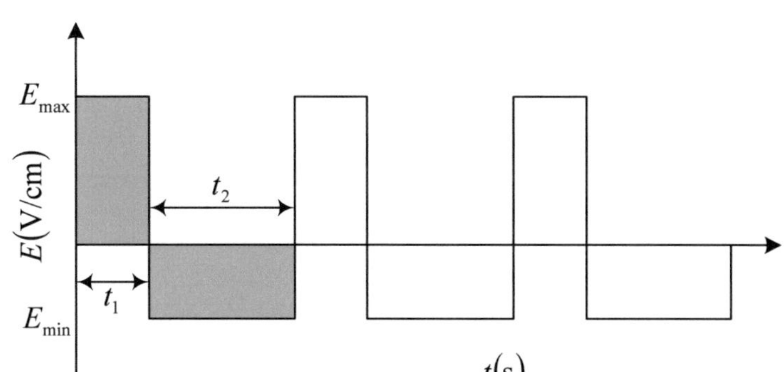

Fig. 7. Electric field of asymmetric waveform

When the high-field asymmetric waveform electric field $E_d(t)$ is applied to the narrow space formed by a pair of electrodes and the ion is brought in by the carrier gas flow, the ion will vibrate between the two plate electrodes. Taking an ion of negative electric charge into consideration, the zigzag vibration routes when $\alpha > 0$, $\alpha \approx 0$ and $\alpha < 0$ are shown in figure 8. It can be seen that in t_1 of one vibration period, corresponding with the high electric field intensity E_{max}, these three ions will move towards the upper plate of the electrode; while within t_2 of the vibration period, corresponding to the low electric field intensity E_{min}, these three ions will move towards the lower plate electrode; the vibration direction is vertical to the plate electrode.

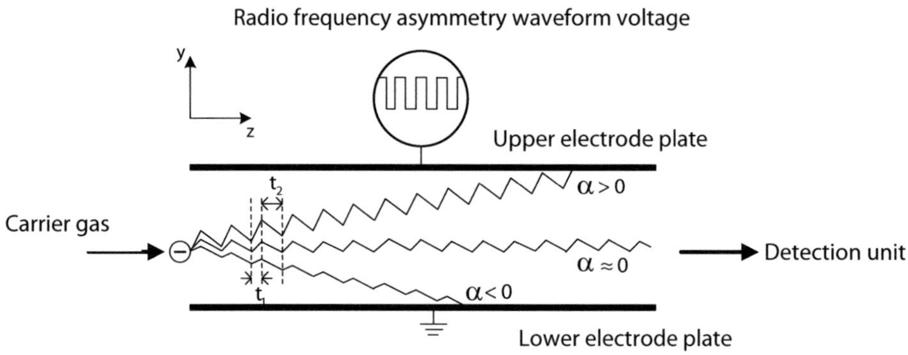

Fig. 8. Motion track of the ions in the drift tube α

During t_1 and t_2, the ion can be approximated as a uniform motion. It is supposed that the velocity of the ion during t_1 is V_1 and the velocity during t_2 is V_2. When the velocity of the ion is changed to V_2 from V_1, there is a speeding up or down, which takes time as follows (Buryakov et al., 1993):

$$\Delta t = \frac{2mV_1}{qE_{\max}} = \frac{2mK}{q} \tag{5}$$

Where, m is the mass of the ion, q is the charge of the ion, K is the mobility of the ion. The time Δt for speeding up or down of the ion is very small, so Δt can be ignored compared to the radio frequency asymmetry waveform voltage period.

The mathematical model is set up with a type A negative ion as the research object, the velocity of the ion in the Y direction is:

$$V_Y = K(E)E(t) \tag{6}$$

During t_1, the ion moves towards the upper plate electrode, the expression is as follows:

$$V_{\text{up}} = K\left|E_{\max}\right| \tag{7}$$

During t_2, the ion moves towards the lower plate electrode, the expression is as follows:

$$V_{\text{down}} = K_0\left|E_{\min}\right| \tag{8}$$

Then, the net displacement of the ion in the Y direction within a cycle:

$$\Delta Y = K\left|E_{\max}\right|t_1 - K_0\left|E_{\min}\right|t_2 \tag{9}$$

Substituting (4) into (9):

$$\Delta Y = \beta(K - K_0) = \Delta KpT \tag{10}$$

From formula (10), the net displacement ΔY of the ion in one cycle will increase when the duty ratio p or the cycle T of the asymmetry waveform radio frequency voltage increase. The average velocity of the ion within a cycle is:

$$\overline{V_Y} = \frac{\Delta Y}{t_1 + t_2} = \frac{\beta \Delta K}{T} \tag{11}$$

At the same time, the ion will move toward the detection unit along the Z direction of the drift tube driven by the carrier gas, so the total displacement in the Y direction is:

$$Y = \overline{V_Y} t_{res} \tag{12}$$

Where t_{res} is the residence time of the ion in the drift tube, which can be determined according to the following:

$$t_{res} = \frac{\mathrm{AL}}{\mathrm{Q}} \tag{13}$$

In the above formula, A is the cross sectional area of the drift tube, L is the length of the drift plate electrode, and Q is the gas flow velocity in the drift tube. So the residence time of the ion in the drift tube is proportional to the length of the drift area, and inversely proportional to the flow velocity of the gas carrier. Substitute (11) and (13) into (12), and take account of $|E_{\max}|t_1 = \beta$ in (4), if $p = \mathrm{t}_1 / T$, then:

$$Y = \frac{\Delta K E_{\max} ALp}{\mathrm{Q}} \tag{14}$$

Where Y depends on the average residence time of the ion in the drift region. It can be calculated from formula (13) that the displacement of the ion in the Y direction is in direct proportion to ΔK which is the difference in mobility between the high and low electric fields. In every cycle of the radio frequency electric field, the ion will move a net displacement towards the upper plate electrode (or the lower plate electrode). Because ΔK for different types of ions is different, there are particular motion tracks for different ions under the effect of the carrier gas and the electric field. If a DC voltage U_C acts on the electrode in the drift tube simultaneously with the RF voltage, and E_c : $|E_c| < |E_{\min}| << |E_{\max}|$, it can generate an electric field force, the direction of which is opposite to the direction of the net displacement of the ion, making the displacement of the ion in every cycle zero along the direction of the electric field and ions vibrate up and down along one right line of the Z axis. So that a specific kind of ion will be detected when it comes through the drift region between the two electrodes, instead of striking with the electrodes of the drift region. The other ions will strike the electrodes of the drift region, become neutral and then be transported out of the drift region by the carrier gas flow. Every type of ion has its specific direct current voltage, which is called compensation voltage.

From the above, it can be concluded that the drift region of the high-field asymmetric waveform ion drift spectrometer is equivalent to a filter. When the compensation voltage

U_C is set for a specific ion, only this ion can pass through, while other ions will be neutralised by the electrode and cannot pass. When U_C is swept through a certain range, all ions in the FAIMS system can be characterised, producing the FAIMS spectrogram of the ion in the carrier gas flow. In the FAIMS drift spectrogram, the longitudinal axis is the current signal intensity of the ion, and the horizontal axis is the compensation voltage.

3. Design of the ion source

3.1 Selection of the ionisation scheme

The ion source changes the neutral molecule in the sample into a charged ion, so that the substance can be detected by FAIMS. It is out of the question that the ion source is a premise for the functioning of the subsequent parts of FAIMS.

According to the operational principle and the application characteristics of FAIMS, the ion source must meet following requirements:

1. Compatibility with MEMS technology. In order to decrease the volume of the system, the FAIMS system is fabricated with MEMS technology, so the ion source should be compatible with MEMS technology.
2. Can work stably under atmospheric pressure.
3. No radioactivity.
4. Minor ion fragmenting. If one substance is ionised into many kinds of ion fragments, more ions should be filtered by the drift region, which would decrease the resolution of the system.
5. Little electromagnetic interference. If the ion source emits intense electromagnetic waves, they will affect the electric field in the drift tube, will affect the movement of ions and will interfere with the detection of the weak ion current, and finally the resolution and sensitivity of the system will also be affected.
6. Little hydration clustering. The ions will form clusters with the water molecules in the high electric field, and these clustered ions will not be stable or easy to decompose. Usually, the compensation voltages of the ion and its hydration cluster ion are different. In the drift region, the ions combine with water and then decompose repeatedly, so that the system works at improper conditions and is unable to separate ions.

The principles of corona discharge ionisation and atmospheric pressure glow discharge ionisation are similar. They are both "soft ionizing", with minor ion fragmenting effects, mainly the molecular ion peak which is consistent with the requirements of FAIMS. Gas discharge is generated through a pair of electrodes applied with a voltage, and the electrodes can be made with highly conductive silicon in MEMS technology (Khayamian et al., 2003; Tabrizchi et al., 2004; Jafari et al., 2007; Khayamian et al., 2001). The discharge can be achieved by DC voltage. This can reduce electromagnetic interference as much as possible, and reduce the effects on the drift region and detection unit.

Therefore, corona discharge ionisation and atmospheric pressure glow discharge ionisation are more suitable for the application of the FAIMS ion source.

3.2 Corona discharge ion source

Figure 9 (a) shows the traditional line - tube structure. It can be seen from the figure that the voltage is applied on the inside and outside of the electrode, and the direction of the electric field is perpendicular to the axial direction of the inner electrode. Under the effect of the electric field force, the ions generated collide with the electrode, hence cannot come out of the electrode. Even if there is a strong flow blowing the ion outwards along the direction of the inner electrode, the ions will also be lost due to the effect of the electric field, because of the frequent collisions of the ion and the carrier gas molecules, which can lead to a loss resulting from plasma chemical reactions. After making improvements based on this structure, the structure as shown in figure 9(b) is formed. In the improved structure, because of slots in the outer electrode, it is possible to make the sample pass over it. These slots can be achieved by the ICP or DRIE process. In this article, the electrode diameter in the line - tube structure is 0.16 mm, the diameter of the outer cylinder electrode is 4mm, and the outside diameter 6mm.

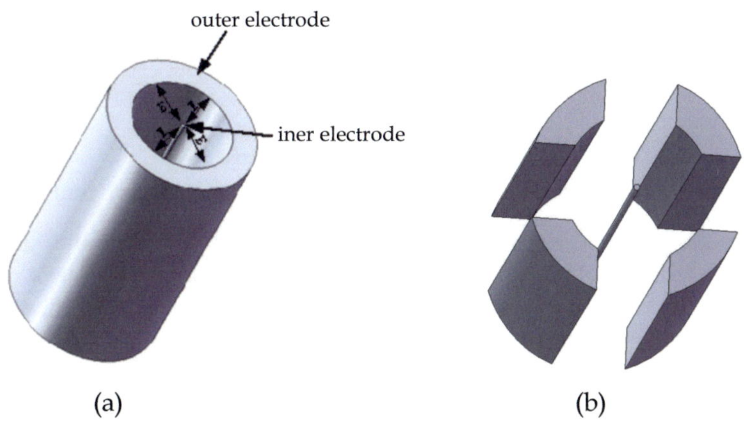

Fig. 9. Line - tube structure. (a) Traditional line - tube structure; (b) Improved line - tube structure.

3.3 Ionisation characteristics of the corona discharge ion source

In this section, at the base of the stable gas discharge, we test and analyse the performance of the corona discharge ion source through the mass spectrometry experiment.

According to the chemical characteristics, the experiment is divided into two parts: one is the positive ion experiment, and the other one is the negative ion experiment.

3.3.1 Positive ion test

Figure 10 is the circuit diagram of the mass spectrometry experiment on positive ionisation mode. When the ion source works under the environmental atmospheric pressure, the average free path of the ion is very small and the ions collide frequently during movement. In order to reduce the ion loss as much as possible, the ion should be accelerated into the mass spectrograph. The voltage on the collection cone of the mass spectrometer is 80V in positive ion mode, and the voltages of the external electrode and the pulled electrode are respectively set at 200V and 150V. The voltages of the external electrode and the pulled electrode are supplied by the power supply between 0 - 500V. After the chemical substance is carried into the ion source by the carrier gas (N_2), the high voltage direct current source is turned on. When the voltage is of about 3700V, the corona discharge starts, and the chemical substance is ionised. Then the ionised ion will fly out of the external electrode driven by the electric field force and will then enter the mass spectrometer driven by the pulling electrode.

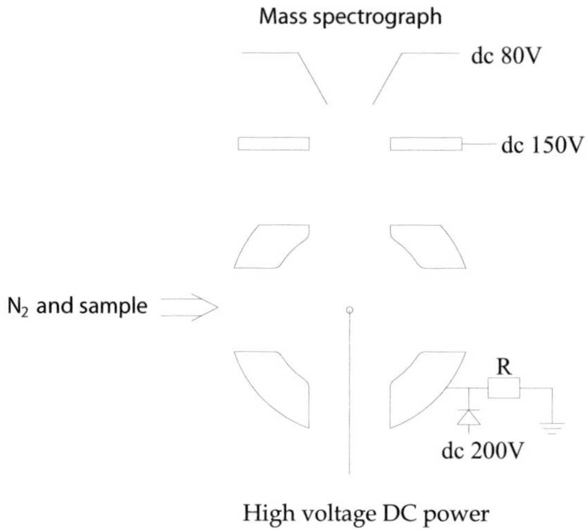

Fig. 10. Mass spectroscopic circuit diagram under the mode of positive ionisation

In this experiment, the flow velocity of the carrier gas is 100L $\cdot h^{-1}$ at room temperature and the sample is analytically pure without any preliminary treatment. We have carried out the ionisation experiment for acetone, N,N—dimethyl formamide, aniline, alcohol, ethyl acetate, dimethyl methyl phosphate (DMMP), methanol, acetonitrile, styrene. The results are shown in the figure 11.

For acetone, N,N—dimethyl formamide, aniline, alcohol, ethyl acetate, DMMP, methanol, acetonitrile and styrene, the experiment shows simple results and single ion peaks, they are mainly $[M+H]^+$ and dimeric ions $[M+M+H]^+$. However the ionisation results of benzyl alcohol, styrene are relatively complex. The ionisation of these substances possibly needs the participation of oxygen, so these ions are oxidised and dehydrated. The ionising result of benzyl alcohol is relatively simple with the main peak of m/z:91, which is possibly the result of dehydration after acquiring the proton. It can be expressed as $[M+H - H_2O]^+$. Main peaks in the ionising results of styrene are m/z:91 and m/z:103, which is possibly because the formaldehyde or water is lost after the styrene is oxidised. It can be expressed with $[M+O+H - CH_2O]^+$ and $[M+O+H - H_2O]^+$.

3.3.2 Negative ion experiment

The negative ionisation mode is the same as the positive ionisation mode, except that the voltage is negative. The voltage in the collection cone of the mass spectrometry is -80V, and the voltages of the external electrode and the pulled electrode are set at -200V and -150V, respectively. After the chemical substance is carried into the ion source by the carrier gas (N_2), the high voltage direct current source is turned on. When the voltage is up to about -3700V the corona discharge starts, and the chemical substance is ionised. Then the ionised ion will be boosted off the external electrode driven by the electric field force and then will enter the mass spectrometer driven by the pulling electrode.

In this experiment, the flow velocity of the carrier gas is 100 L $\cdot h^{-1}$ at room temperature, and the sample is analytically pure without preliminary treatment. We have carried out the ionisation experiment for formic acid, acetic acid and phenol. The results are shown in figure 12.

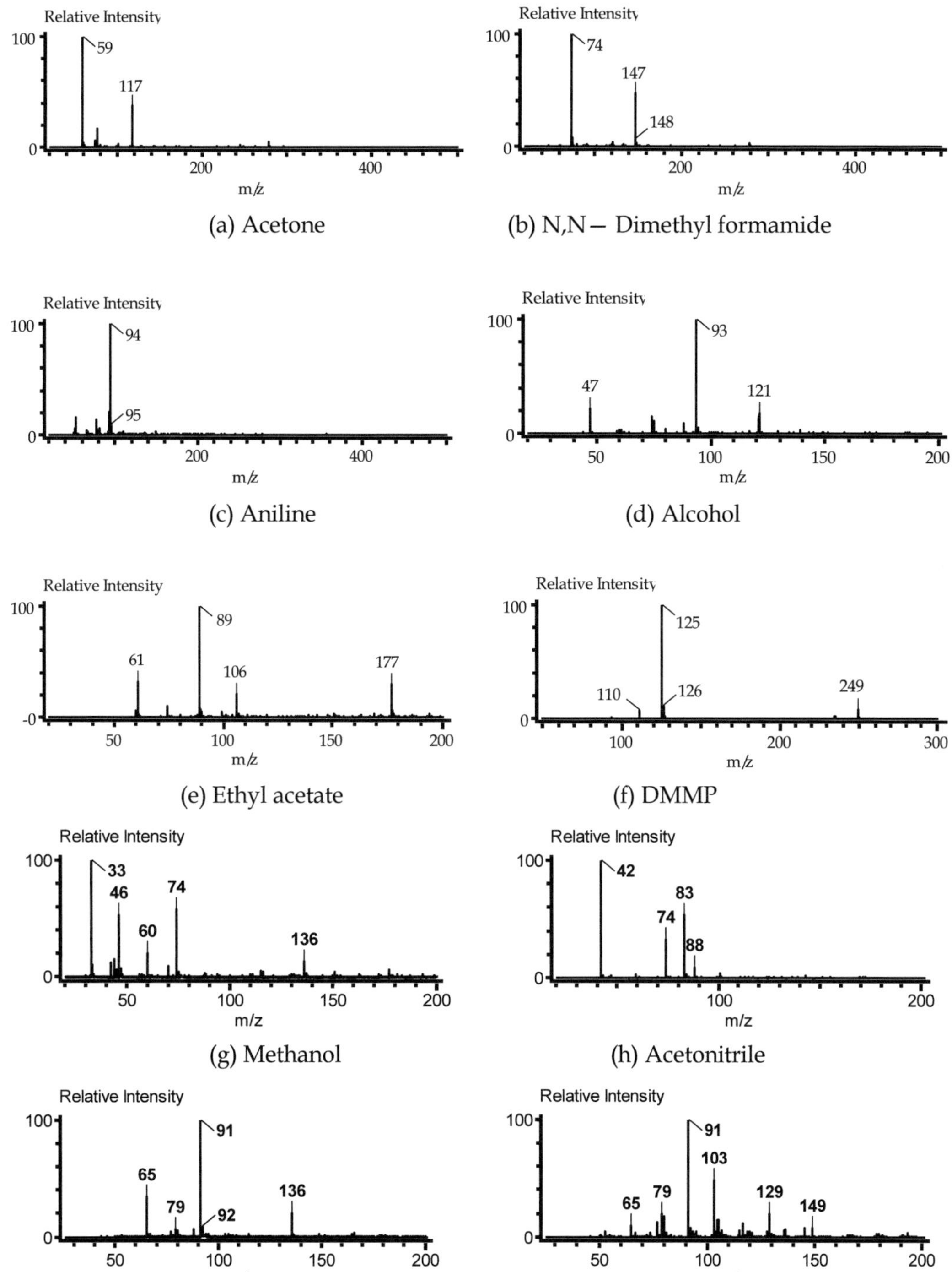

(a) Acetone
(b) N,N– Dimethyl formamide
(c) Aniline
(d) Alcohol
(e) Ethyl acetate
(f) DMMP
(g) Methanol
(h) Acetonitrile
(i) Benzyl alcohol
(j) Styrene

Fig. 11. Mass spectrum experimental results under the mode of positive ionisation

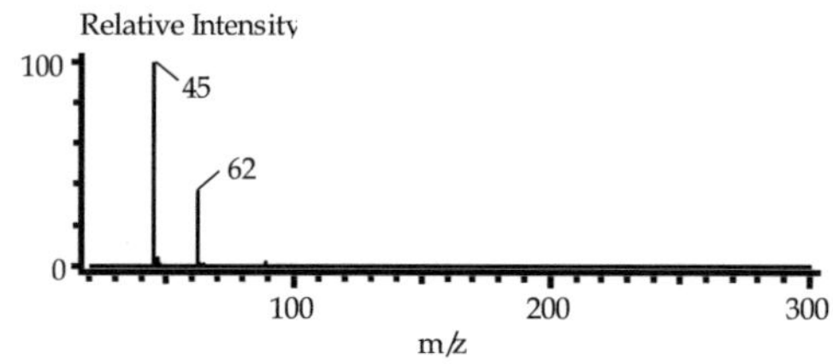

(a) Formic acid

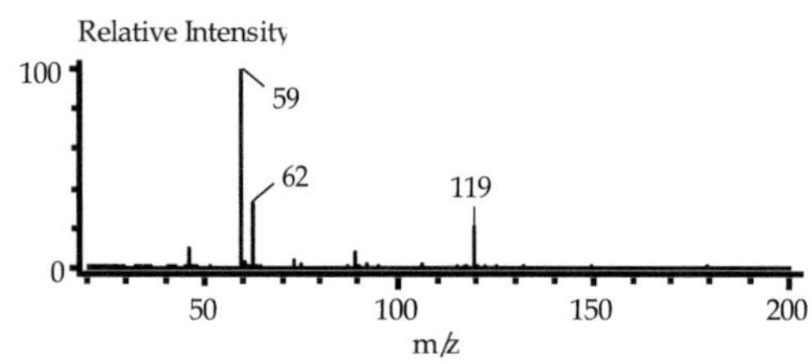

(b) Acetic acid

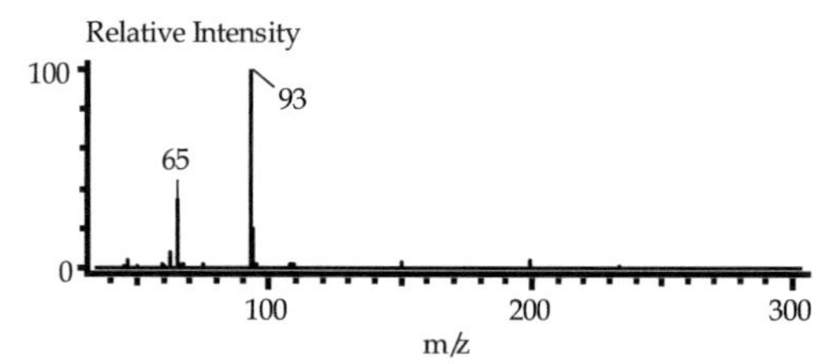

(c) Phenol

Fig. 12. Mass spectrum experimental results under the mode of negative ionisation

Under the mode of negative ionisation, the ions generated are very simple, mainly $[M\text{-}H]^-$ and $[M\text{+}M\text{-}H]^-$, besides, there will be NO_2^- (M/Z : 46) and NO_3^- (M/Z : 62) ions. This is mainly the result of the reaction between nitrogen and oxygen.

4. Design of the high voltage high frequency asymmetric waveform power supply

4.1 Impulse source system based on the power MOSFET

In view of the requirement of the FAIMS system, the FAIMS high-field asymmetric square wave power system is composed of six parts: (1) Signal generator, (2) High speed switch, (3) High voltage direct power supply, (4) High pass filter, (5) Automatic scan and collection of the compensation voltage and (6) Computer. The operation principle block diagram of the high-field asymmetric square wave radio frequency power supply system in FAIMS design is shown in figure 13.

Through electrical isolation and power level conversion, the frequency of output, duty ratio and PWM signal with variable dead band of the signal generator controls the high speed switch of the inverter circuit to generate the high voltage and high frequency square wave impulse output. Controlled by the signal generator, the high voltage direct current power supply provides the high voltage direct current signal for the high speed switch, through which the high voltage and high frequency square wave impulse output are generated. After the square wave impulse output is filtered through the high pass filter, the asymmetry waveform voltage signal output with the same positive and negative area is realised.

In the automatic scan of the compensation voltage, the signal generator is used to control the digital to analog conversion of DAC, and magnify the signal, realising the automatic scan of the compensation voltage of the saw tooth wave. In view of that the radio frequency high voltage side on the electrode plate of the drift region interferes with the low voltage side of the compensation voltage, we realise the electrical isolation between high voltage and low voltage with the inductance and resistance network, when superposing the compensation voltage onto the drift region. Through voltage attenuation and analog-digital conversion, the influence of the radio frequency can be reduced and accurate collection and detection of the compensation voltage signal can be achieved.

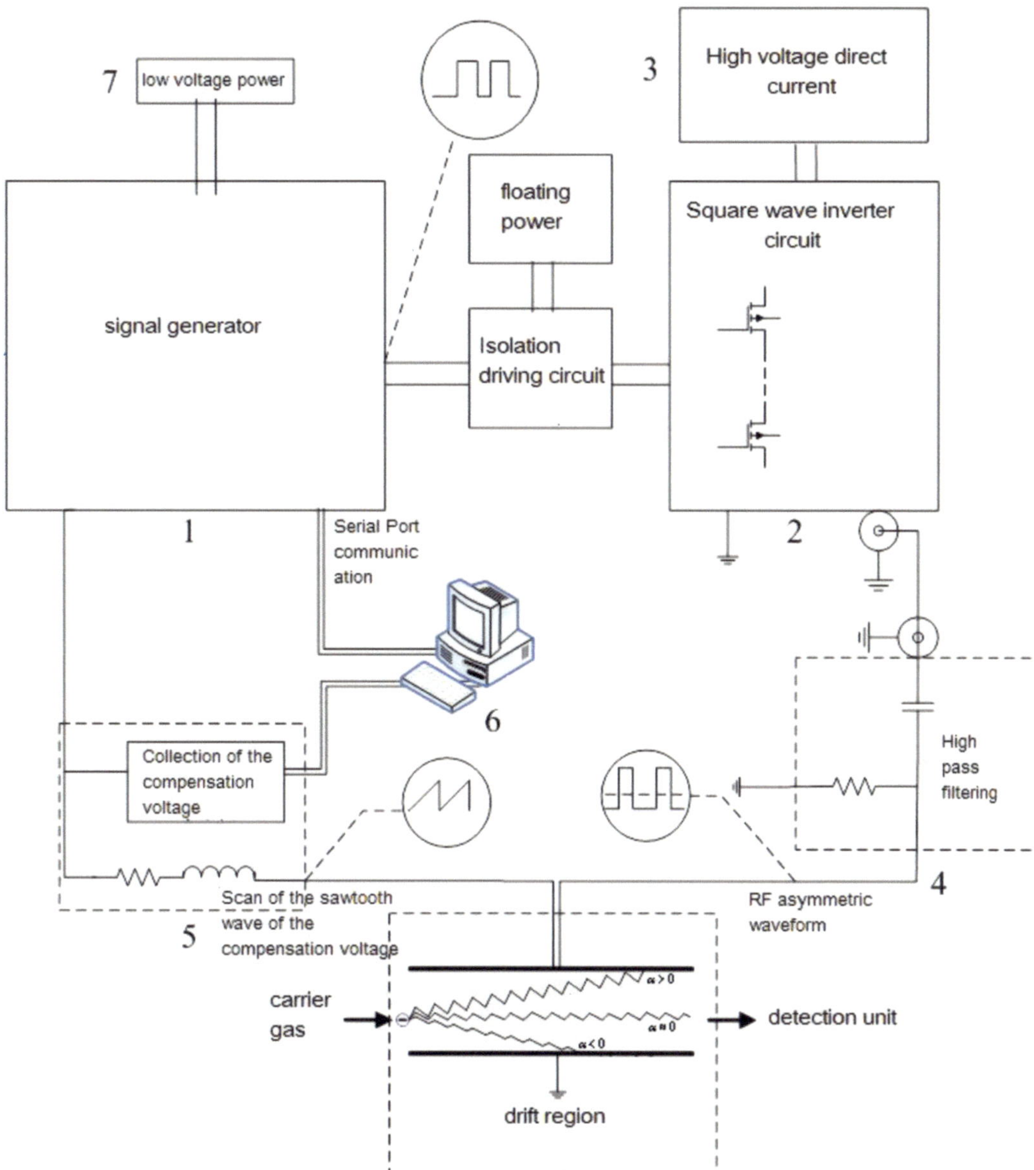

Fig. 13. Square wave RF power supply system block diagram for FAIMS detector

The signal generator is the main control section. It can communicate with the computer through a serial port to adjust the frequency, duty ratio, dead band time and scanning cycle of the compensation voltage on-line.

4.2 Design of each unit circuit in the impulse source system

4.2.1 Realisation of the automatic scanning signal of the compensation voltage

The scanning range for the compensation voltage should be -25V ~ 25V. In this circuit, a TI OPA547 high voltage amplifier is used to magnify signals, which is a precise high voltage large current operational amplifier with a wide dynamic voltage range, a high voltage slew rate of 6V/us and a low quiescent current. When it is provided with a single power supply, the maximum working voltage is 60V. When it works with a double power supply, the working voltage range is ±30V. In the mode of double power supply, the maximum voltage of the maximum input and output signal is ±27V.

4.2.2 Research and design of collection of the compensation voltage

(1) Requirements for collection of the compensation voltage

In order to get the synchronous values of the compensation voltage with the micro current collected by a Faraday Cup, the minimum step of the compensation voltage must be 0.1V. The compensation voltage should be collected at high precision because the amplitude of the compensation voltage is wide: -25V ~ 25V, and the usual collection circuit is CMOS or TTL, which requires collection of the voltage after voltage attenuation. The minimum precision should be 0.4%. Besides, there is high frequency interference and noise from the high voltage and high frequency signal in the drift region, so the interference and noise must be blocked to ensure the accuracy of collecting the compensation voltage. The connection method of the compensation voltage in the actual experiment is shown in figure 14.

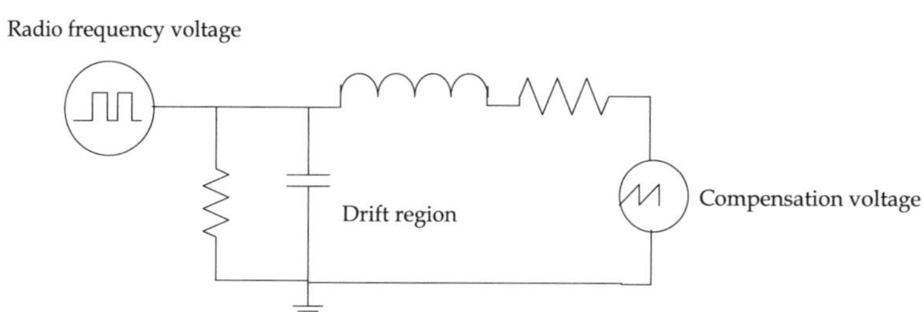

Fig. 14. Compensation voltage connection diagram

(2) Design of the compensation voltage collection

The following two methods are used to control noise: isolation and filter.

1. Isolate the ground of the drift region and the ground of the collection circuit with a bead or Zero Ohm Resistor, to avoid the influence of the noise generated by the high speed switch in the drift region of the collection circuit.
2. Convert the attenuated signal from analog to digital with a high-precision, low noise and low drift double-integral A/D converter, in which an integrator and voltage comparator are used. A double-integral A/D converter has a strong noise control with a mean value of Zero and a high stability, which is a good method to block interference and noise. The results show that when the radio frequency voltage is greater than 300V, the maximum relative error voltages of the compensation voltage will not exceed 4mV, and the measuring accuracy is 0.16%. It shows that in the second plan the compensation voltage can be accurately collected under the interference of the radio frequency, which meets the requirements of the system.

4.2.3 Structure optimisation of the half bridge inverter circuit

To solve the problems in the half-bridge inverter circuit, the circuit structure has been optimised. Figure 15 shows the basic principle diagram of the optimised half bridge inverter circuit. The working principle of the circuit is that: under the control of the driving circuit, the S1 and S2 switches take turns to turn on and generate a high voltage square signal, and then the asymmetric waveform is produced through the C3 and R3 network.

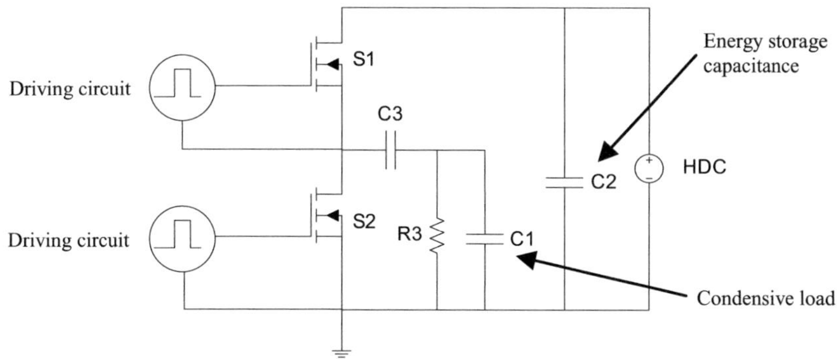

Fig. 15. Basic principle block diagram of the optimised half bridge inverter circuit

Compared with the structure of the half bridge inverter, the following parts have been optimised:

1. To realise a high frequency steep pulse square-wave output. When the frequency of the switch increases, the pulse wave form quality will always change. So we chose a new MOSFET with a low stray parameter, high switching frequency and a short time for rising and falling for wider application.
2. As for the problems of the series MOSFET switches with incomplete synchronisation, we have replaced the two MOSFET with single MOSFET with higher bearing voltage and heat dissipation as the single arm series switching power devices.
3. As for the problems in adjustment of the compensation voltage, we have analysed the generation principle of the square wave, and achieve automatic generation of the asymmetric waveform. The FAIMS asymmetric square waveform is shown in figure 7, in which it can be considered that the average value of the wave in one cycle is zero. Writing the square into a Fourier series expansion:

$$\begin{aligned} f(t) = A_{\max}\{\alpha + \frac{2}{\pi}[2\sin(\alpha\pi)\cdot\cos(\omega_1 t) \\ + \frac{1}{2}\sin(2\alpha\pi)\cdot\cos(2\omega_1 t) \\ + \frac{1}{2}\sin(3\alpha\pi)\cdot\cos(3\omega_1 t) + \cdots\} \\ = \alpha A_{\max} + \frac{1}{\pi}A_{\max}\sum_{n=1}^{\infty}\sin(n\alpha\pi)\cdot\cos(n\omega_1 t) \end{aligned} \tag{15}$$

Where α is the duty ratio of the square wave, $\alpha A_{\max}$ is its direct current component, and the other sine and cosine parts are the components of the alternating current.

The average value of the square wave in one cycle is:

$$A_{av} = \frac{1}{T}\int_0^T f(t) = \alpha A_{\max} \quad (16)$$

We can see from the above formula that the average value of the square wave is the component of its direct current. So after filtering out the DC component in the square wave, we can obtain the asymmetric positive and negative square waves with the same area.

It is required by the FAIMS system that the power consumption and the volume is small. In view of the above advantages and disadvantages of the inverter circuit, we select the half-bridge structure as the inverter circuit, and optimise the half-bridge inverter circuit to achieve a high frequency of non-symmetric square wave outputs.

5. Ion detection

5.1 Design of the micro Faraday cup

MEMS Faraday cup has got a glass - silicon - glass layer structure (as shown in figure 16). The gas route of the Faraday cup is formed with upper glass, lower glass and silicon chips. The middle layer adopts the low resistivity silicon material, the resistance of which is 0.0001 ~ 0.0009Ω·m, to achieve good conductive properties. When the ions collide with the surface of the low resistivity silicon, the ions are neutralised to achieve the drift of the charge to the low resistivity silicon. Through the current collected from low resistivity silicon, the ion beam intensity can be measured. The sensitive electrode of the Faraday cup is composed of dozens of silicon columns. The array arrangement has formed a number of fine gas routes in the sensitive electrodes. When the ions go into the Faraday cup, driven by the carrier gas, they will collide many times with the silicon column in complex micro-channels, and eventually be captured by the sensitive array. The ion signal captured will be educed by the electrode on the glass and read out from the sensitive ammeter.

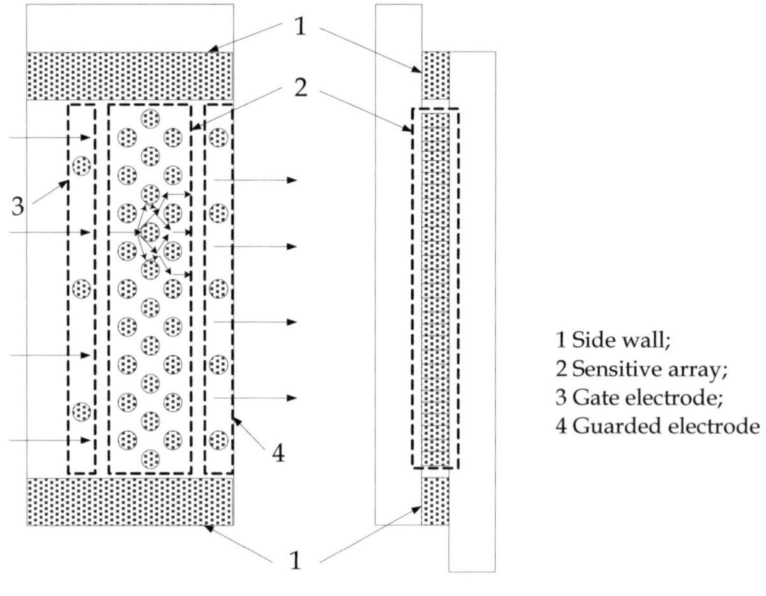

Fig. 16. Structure of the MEMS Faraday cup

For the current signal to be detected, the requirement of the system on the contact resistance characteristics of the silicon and the metal wire is not very high, and it reduces the requirement on the processing of the chips. A gate electrode is set on the front of the sensitive array gas route. The gate electrode is composed of several silicon columns of diameter 200 μm. The gate electrode of low-resistivity silicon is used with a certain voltage. The presence of the gate electrode will bring about a loss of ion signal, resulting in a decrease of sensitivity of the chip, but it can reduce the induced signal before ions reach the sensitive array.

Compared with the traditional Faraday cup, there are advantages in this micro Faraday cup array:

1. The sensitive electrode adopts the array design:
   a) To expand the contact area of the gas with the sensitive electrode
   b) As lots of micro gas flow channels are formed, it is in favour of the disturbance of the stable flow field after the gas goes into the sensitive array, making the ions in the gas more easily collide with the sensitive electrode, reducing the loss of the ion signal
   c) Due to the presence of the micro-flow channel, the carrier gas can carry ions through the sensitive electrodes to achieve ion signal collection. Compared to the electric field drive method, the gas drive approach eliminates the driving electrode and associated power supply so that the structure of the Faraday cup is simpler.
2. The gate electrode, the shielding electrode and conductive shielding wall can provide good shielding for the sensitive electrode, improving the detection limit of the Faraday cup.

5.2 Simulation of a micro Faraday cup

In the FAIMS system, the ion signal is very weak (pA level), and it is easily influenced by human body static electricity and electromagnetic waves in the environment, which brings a critical requirement on the shielding performance for the Faraday cup. The drift region will be applied on the radio frequency voltage, which is a great noise for the detection environment of the Faraday cup. The coupling capacitance of the drift region and the sensitive electrode of the Faraday cup can be used to measure the level of the noise of the electric field on the sensitive electrode of the Faraday cup. We have analysed the coupling capacitance of different structures of the MEMS Faraday cup from an ANSYS simulation, and done the theoretical calculation at the condition whether there is a side wall grounded.

Modelling: When modelling, the MEMS Faraday cup has been simplified. The sensitive electrode of the Faraday cup can be simplified as a rectangular solid conducting block, and the shielding electrode can be simplified as a rectangular solid bar. The air boundary of the Faraday cup is simulated as the outermost shield shell, which is grounded.

Network partitioning: The tetrahedron is divided with smartsize 1 and amesh.

Material and unit: There is only air for dielectric materials, with a relative dielectric constant of 1. The unit adopts the solid122 electromagnetic field solid unit.

Simulation results: Through simulating the coupling capacitance of the sensitive electrode and the drift region in the MEMS Faraday cup, it can be found that the side wall of the MEMS Faraday cup and the shielding electrode are very useful in reducing the radio frequency noise in the drift region. It can be found that through comparing the results of the models c and d, the coupling capacitance will fall a little when the back shielding electrode is added, but the total effect remains the same. In the experiment, the shielding case of the MEMS Faraday cup should be as close as possible to the Faraday cup.

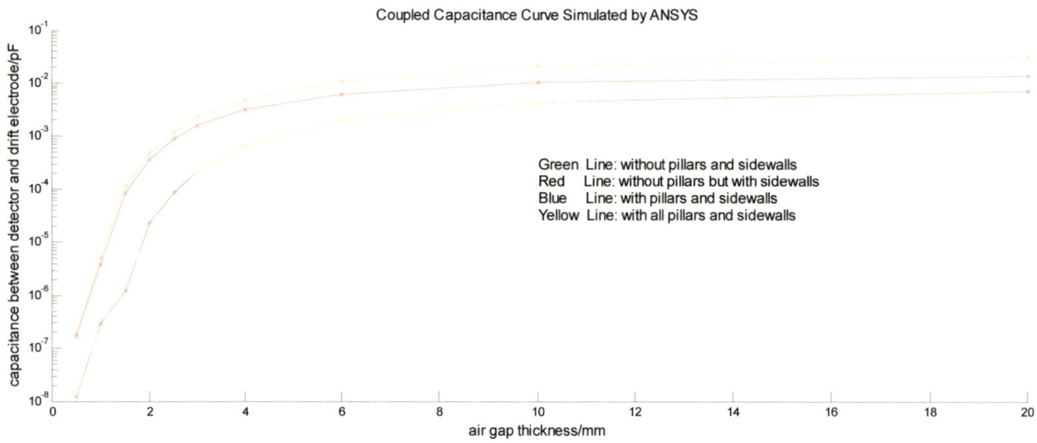

Fig. 17. Coupled capacitance of the drift region and the Faraday sensitive electrode under different conditions. Note: The air gap refers to the distance of the drift region away from the outer edge of the model, that is the space of the MEMS Faraday cup away from extra shield case.

When the sidewall is not grounded, the noise led into the detection circuit through the coupling capacitance between the drift tube and the sensitive electrode is very low. The noise is mainly led into the detection circuit through the sidewall. The equivalent noise generation circuit is shown in figure 18.

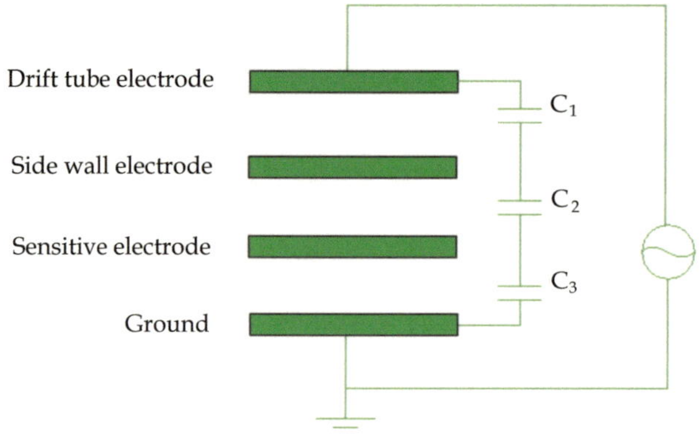

Fig. 18. Circuit model simplified with the side wall non-grounded

The noise voltage on the sensitive electrode is

$$U_d = \frac{1/C_3}{1/C_3 + 1/C_2 + 1/C_1} U \tag{17}$$

When the airgap thickness is 2 mm, $C_1 = 0.2pF$, $C_2 = 0.205pF$ and $C_3 = 0.84pF$ are obtained from the ANSYS simulation result of model c, so

$$U_d = \frac{1/C_3}{1/C_1 + 1/C_2 + 1/C_3} U = \frac{1/0.84}{1/0.2 + 1/0.205 + 1/0.84} U = 0.107U$$

where U_d is the noise voltage on the sensitive electrode, U is the noise source in the drift tube, C_1 is the capacitance between drift tube and the sidewall, C_2 is the capacitance between the sidewall and the sensitive electrode, C_3 is the capacitance between the sensitive electrode and the ground.

When the sidewall is grounded, the noise in the drift tube is mainly led into the detection circuit by electromagnetic field coupling through the coupling capacitance between the drift tube and the sensitive electrode. The equivalent noise generation circuit is shown as figure 19. The noise voltage on the sensitive electrode is

$$U_d = \frac{1/C_3}{1/C_3 + 1/C_4} U = \frac{C_4}{C_4 + C_3} U \tag{18}$$

When the airgap thickness was 2 mm, $C_4 = 0.21 \times 10^{-4} pF$ was obtained from the ANSYS simulation result of model c, so

$$U_d = \frac{C_4}{C_4 + C_3} U = \frac{0.21 \times 10^{-4}}{0.21 \times 10^{-4} + 0.84} U = 2.5 \times 10^{-5} U$$

where C_4 is the coupling capacitance between drift tube and the sensitive electrode, C_5 is the capacitance between drift tube and the ground.

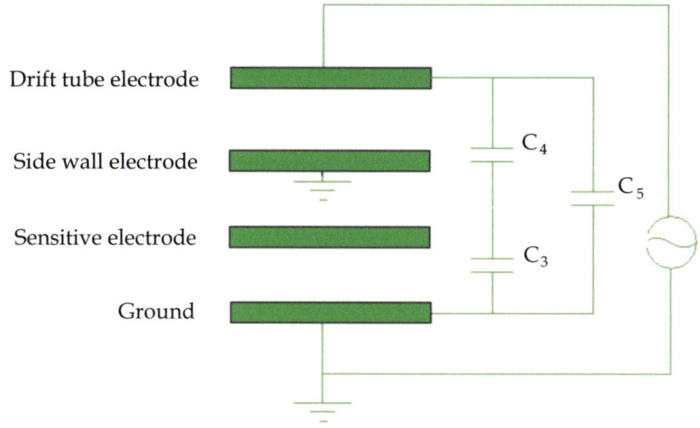

Fig. 19. Circuit model when the side wall is grounded

By comparing the both results, the sidewall grounding can greatly decrease the interference from drift tube on the sensitive electrode.

5.3 Micro Faraday cup technology

The design of the MEMS Faraday cup is shown in figure 16. We have designed the MEMS process and the latter welding process of the MEMS Faraday cup according to the structure of the MEMS Faraday cup and the technological characteristic of the MEMS production line. The thickness of the silicon chip is 200μm, which is n type of 3 inch disk with a specific resistance of 0.0001~0.0009Ω·m, the glass plate is a 3 inch disk, the thickness of which is 500μm. The MEMS Faraday cup chip fabricated is shown as figure 20.

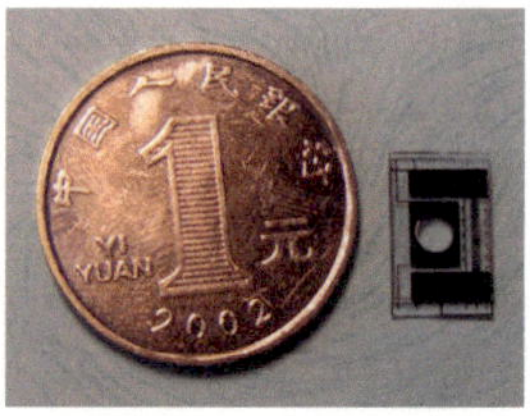

Fig. 20. Photo of the MEMS Faraday cup

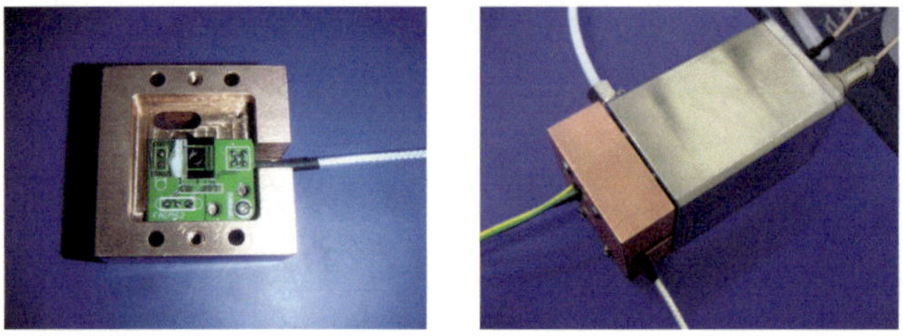

Fig. 21. Photos of the MEMS Faraday cup packaged

5.4 Testing of the micro Faraday cup

For the MEMS Faraday cup chip packaged with PCB, a base should be fabricated to realise a reliable connection between the MEMS Faraday cup and the ion source. The base is made of red copper, which can effectively shield the noise from the environment. The photos of the red copper shielding base, assembled MEMS Faraday cup and the ion source are shown in figure 21.

In order to test the performance of the MEMS Faraday cup, the chip is tested with KEITHLEY237. In this experiment, the carrier gas is nitrogen gas and the sample is acetone, the concentration of which is about 100ppm. The experimental system is shown in figure 22.

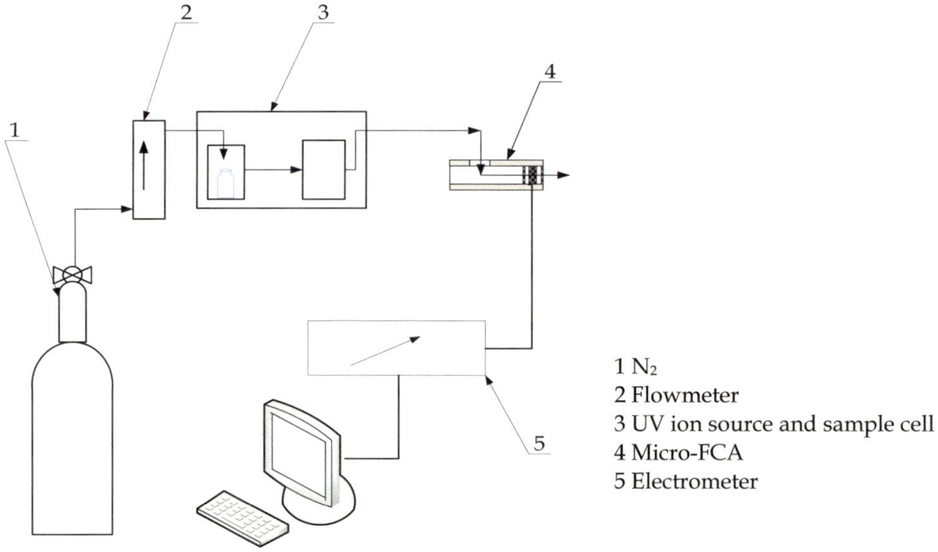

Fig. 22. Experimental apparatus of the MEMS Faraday cup

(1) Ion collection experiment with the MEMS Faraday cup

In the experimental system of figure 22, the carrier gas flow is adjusted to 100L/h. We make the comparison of the ion collection results among the chips of the MEMS Faraday cup with different structural parameters. Through comparison of the signal, the absorption efficiency of the MEMS Faraday cup with different structural parameters is evaluated.
Figure 23 shows a typical ion signal curve collected by the MEMS Faraday cup. This means that the signal of the MEMS Faraday cup is stable, which can work in the atmospheric environment, and is completely capable of detect ion.

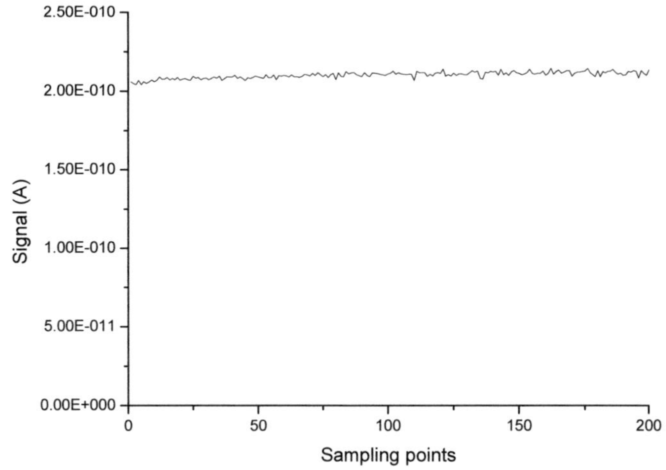

Fig. 23. Ion signal curve received by the MEMS Faraday cup

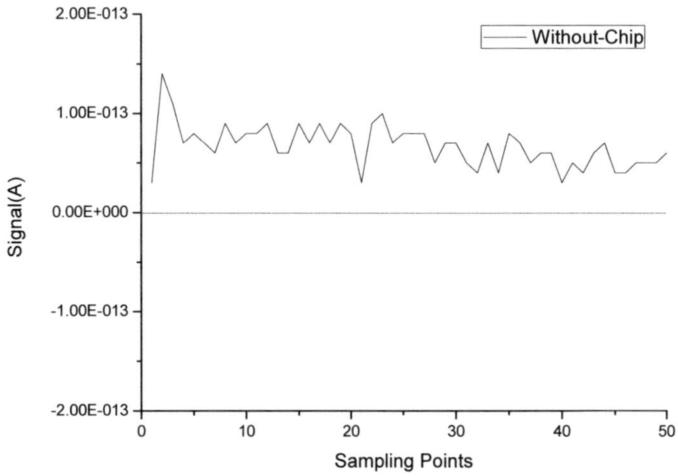

Fig. 24. Noise in the body of KEITHLEY

(2) Anti-interference experiment

Shut off the carrier gas and apply the radio frequency voltage (the maximum is 300V and the frequency is 200kHz) between the upper and lower electrodes in the front of the micro

Faraday cup. We test the influence of different shielding methods and different chip structures on the ability of anti-interference.
First of all, in the case without the chip, we tested the background noise of the system with KEITHLEY current testing module, as shown in figure 24. The average value of the noise curve is 67.2fA. The offset current may be from the interference source in the environment or the offset of the instruments. We have found biased data always from 40 to 80 fA in many measurements. In the following data treatment, the biased current should be subtracted from the original data.

1) The influence of RF electric field on the noise under different connection ways

The experimental results are shown in figure 25. In this experimental system, we found the influence of the RF electric field and the copper shielding base on the noise of the chip is not obvious. The level of the noise is about 0.1pA. It means that under this experimental system setup there is no influence of different connections on the noise of the chip.

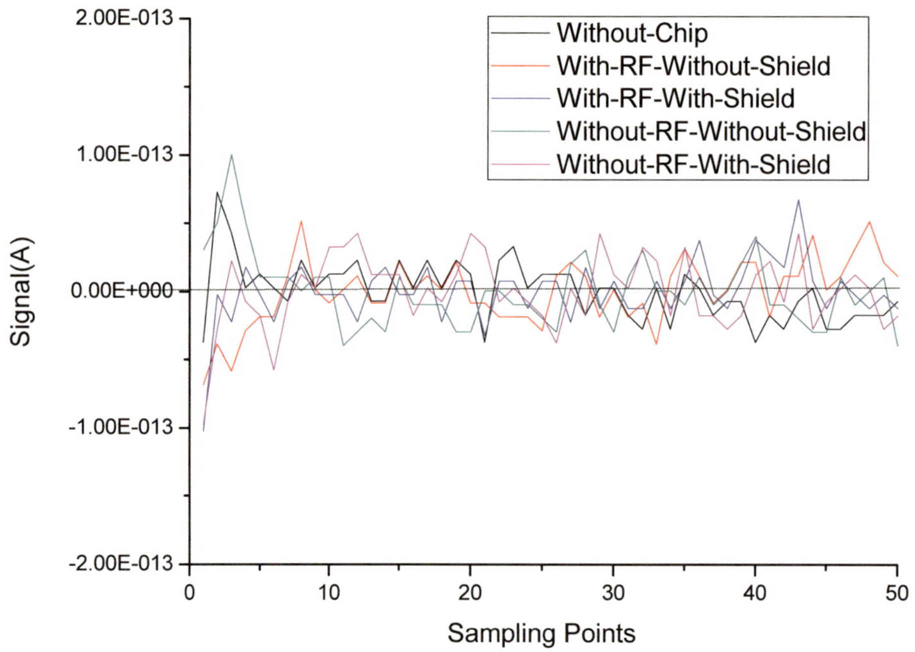

Fig. 25. The noise level of the same chip under different connections. Note: corresponding biased current has been subtracted in each curve.

2) Influence of different chip structures on the noise

Connecting ways and RF electric fields have no influence on the noise, so we have conducted the noise test for the chip with different structural parameters, without the copper shielding base and RF electric field.
It can be seen from the figure 26 that in this experimental system, whether or not the gate electrode in the chips exists or the side wall of the drift regions and the side of the Faraday cup are separated has no influence on the noise.

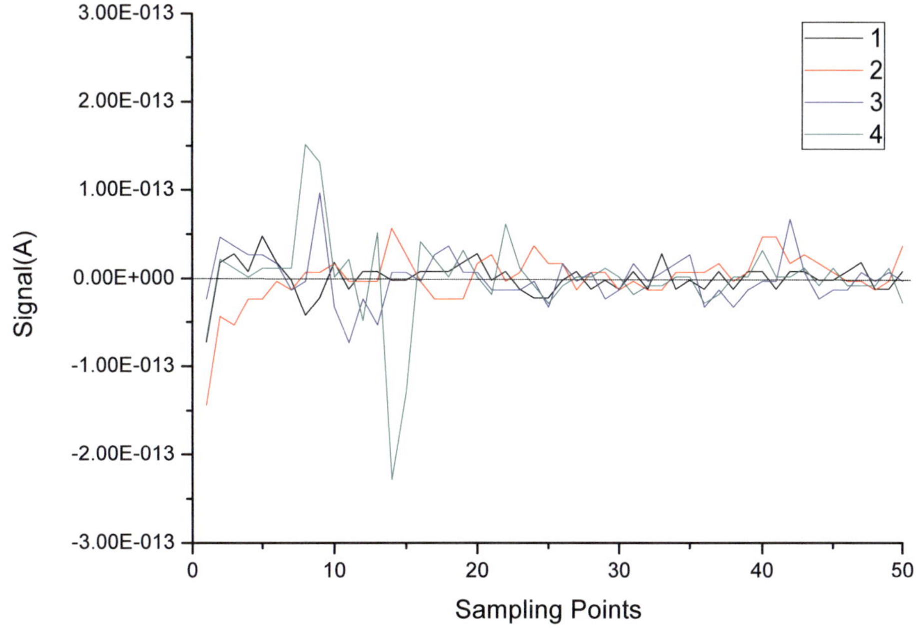

Fig. 26. Noise level with different chip structures. Note: 1) corresponding biased current has been subtracted in each curve 2) Structure1: no gate electrode, the side wall of the drift region is separated with the silicon side wall of the Faraday cup 3) Structure2: gate electrode with three silicon columns, the side wall of the drift region is separated with the silicon side wall of the Faraday cup 4) Structure3: gate electrode with five silicon columns, the side wall of the drift region is separated with the silicon side wall of the Faraday cup 5) Structure4: gate electrode with five silicon columns, the side wall of the drift region is connected with the silicon side wall of the Faraday cup

6. Sample analytical experiment

6.1 Experimental system of FAIMS chip

The experimental system of FAIMS is composed of a sample injection unit, ion source, FAIMS chip, square wave radio frequency power, and data collection unit, as shown in figure 27. The sample injection unit contains the nitrogen tank, flowmeter and sample cell. The ion source is composed of the ion source power and a 10.6eV ultraviolet lamp. The data collection unit contains amperometer, compensation voltage data collection card and computer.

6.2 Influence of the changing of the square wave radio frequency voltage amplitude on the sensitivity of FAIMS

We take absolute ethyl alcohol as the sample in this experiment. The flow velocity of the carrier gas is 0.8L/min in this experiment, the square wave radio frequency voltage frequency is 2MHz, and the duty ratio is maintained at about 30%. The amplitude of the square wave radio frequency voltage is increased to 380V from 220V, at 20V intervals. When the compensation voltage automatically scans in the scope of +10V~-10V, the FAIMS spectrogram of alcohol is shown in figure 28. In figure 28, the ion peak near the compensation voltage 0V is the background noise signal, which will be ignored in the following analysis.

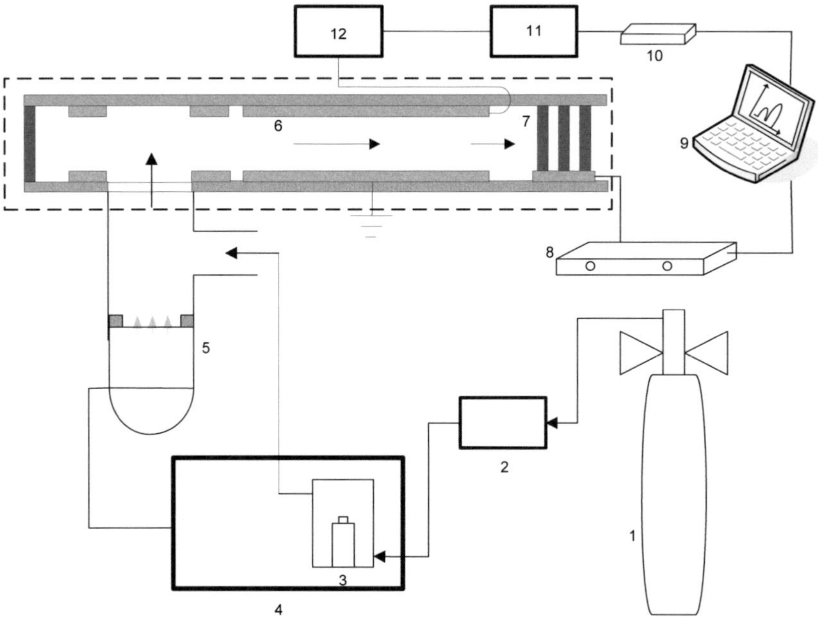

1 Nitrogen tank, 2 Flowmeter, 3 Sample cell, 4 Ion source power, 5 Ultraviolet lamp, 6 Drift region, 7 Column array micro Faraday cup, 8 Amperometer, 9 Computer, 10 Collection card, 11 Compensation voltage, 12 Square wave radio frequency voltage

Fig. 27. FAIMS chip experimental system block diagram

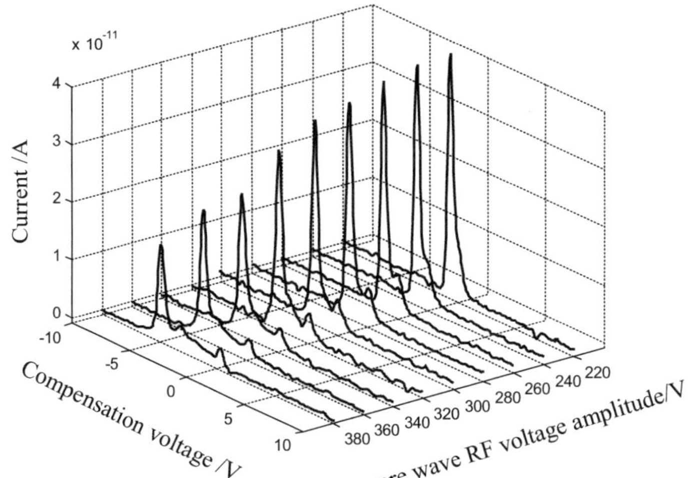

Fig. 28. The FAIMS spectrogram of alcohol corresponding with different radio frequency voltage amplitude

It can be seen from figure 28 that in the FAIMS system when the amplitude of the radio frequency voltage increases, the intensity of the ion peak signal detected will be lower. This is oppose to the influence of the voltage amplitude on the intensity of the ion peak in the

IMS system. The relation between the square wave radio frequency voltage amplitude and the ion peak signal current is shown in figure 29. With an increase of the voltage amplitude, the current will gradually decrease to 16.1pA at 380V from 41.7pA at 220V.

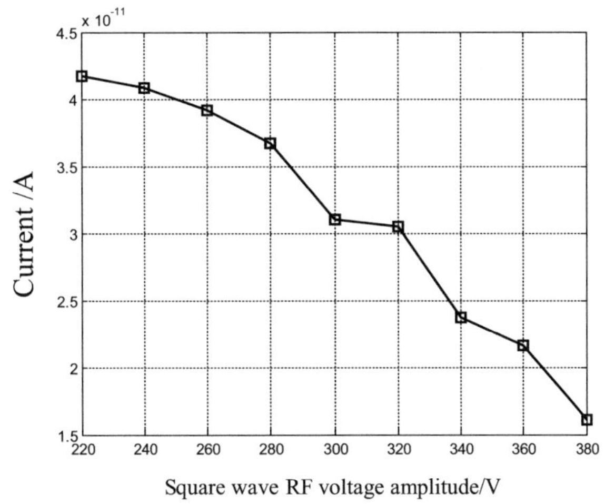

Fig. 29. Influence of the amplitude of the square wave RF voltage on the peak of the ethanol

For substances with small molecules such as ethanol, the ion mobility K will increase when the amplitude of the voltage V_H increases. $\alpha(E/N)$ will also increase when the amplitude of voltage V_H increases, and so will the compensation voltage V_{cv} and resolution R. Figure 30 and figure 31 show the curve of compensation voltage and the resolution of the ethanol with the radio frequency voltage, respectively. It can be seen from the figures that the compensation voltage and the resolution are increased to -4.86V and 6.57 at 380V from -0.64V and 1.12 at 220V, respectively. The changing trend fits closely with the theoretical analysis.

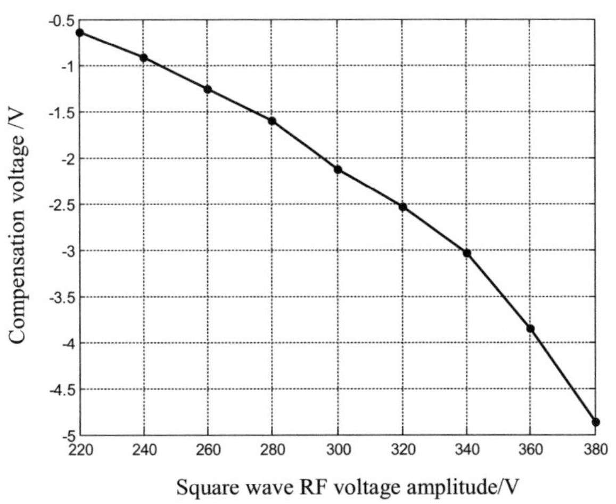

Fig. 30. Relation curve between the compensation voltage and the amplitude of the square wave radio frequency voltage

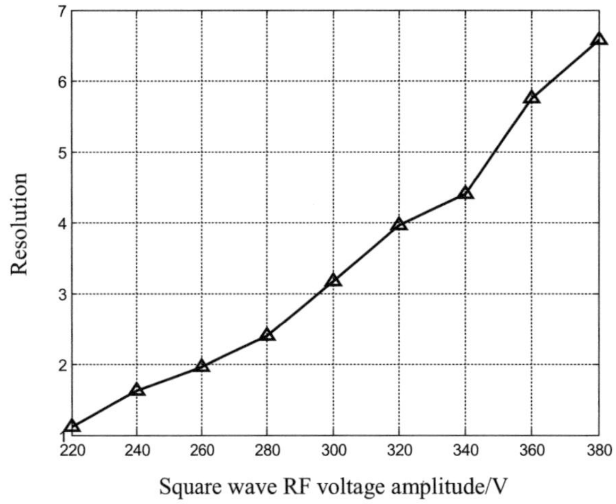

Fig. 31. Relation curve between the resolution and the amplitude of the square wave radio frequency voltage

6.3 Influence of the radio frequency voltage amplitude, frequency and flow velocity of the carrier gas on the FAIMS detection result of 2- pentane

(1) Influence of the amplitude of the voltage

If the flow velocity of the carrier gas is kept at 1L/min, the square wave RF voltage frequency is 2MHz, and the duty ratio is 30%, when the amplitude of the square wave radio frequency voltage increases from 220V to 320V at 20V intervals we can obtain the FAIMS spectrogram as shown in figure 32. We can see from figure 32 that with an increase in the amplitude of the square wave radio frequency voltage, the compensation voltage value (absolute value, same as below) will increase and the ion signal intensity will fall.

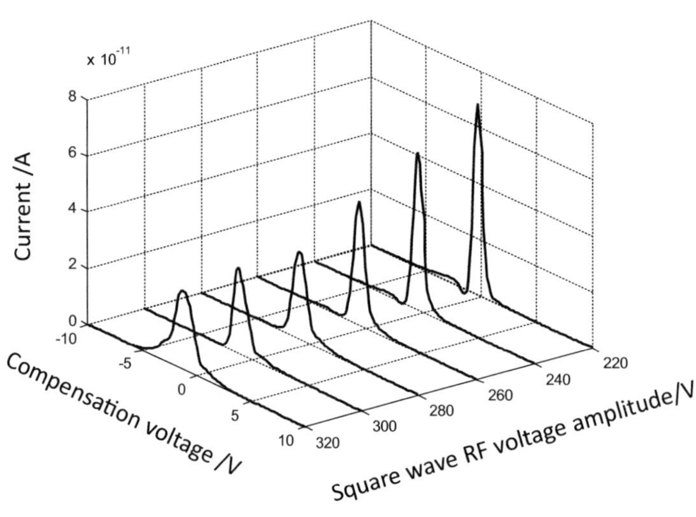

Fig. 32. The FAIMS spectrogram of 2- pentane corresponding to different square wave RF voltage amplitudes

The ion mobility of the 2-pentane will increase with increasing electric field intensity (Papanastasiou et al., 2008). So with increasing voltage amplitude, the amplitude of the ion will increase under the effect of the high electric field, the net displacement in one cycle will increase, and the compensation voltage for reverse compensation on the net displacement will also increase. On the other hand, the diffusion coefficient of the ion will increase with increasing ion mobility, so the ion loss caused by diffusion will increase while the ion signal intensity falls.

(2) Influence of the frequency

The frequency of the square wave radio frequency voltage is an important parameter of FAIMS, the value of which has directly affected the passing efficiency of ions in the drift region. Under the condition that the square wave radio frequency voltage amplitude is 320V, the duty ratio is 30% and the flow velocity of the carrier gas is kept at 1L/min, the FAIMS spectrogram of 2-pentane when the frequency is 2MHz, 1.75MHz, 1.5MHz and 1.25MHz is as shown in figure 33. We can see from figure 33 that the ion signal intensity will decrease with decreasing frequency. It drops from 28pA at 2MHz to 9.43pA at 1.25MHz, while the compensation voltage *Vc* stays the same at -1.33V. At the same time, the FAIMS spectrogram will become narrower as the frequency decreases, namely the resolution increases. The reason is that the decreasing frequency will increase the cycle, which increases the amplitude of ions, making the effective width smaller. In this way the ion loss due to collisions with the electrode becomes larger, and the ion signal intensity decreases, thus the resolution increases. It was shown from theoretical formula that the frequency change does not affect the value of compensation voltage (Papanastasiou et al., 2008).

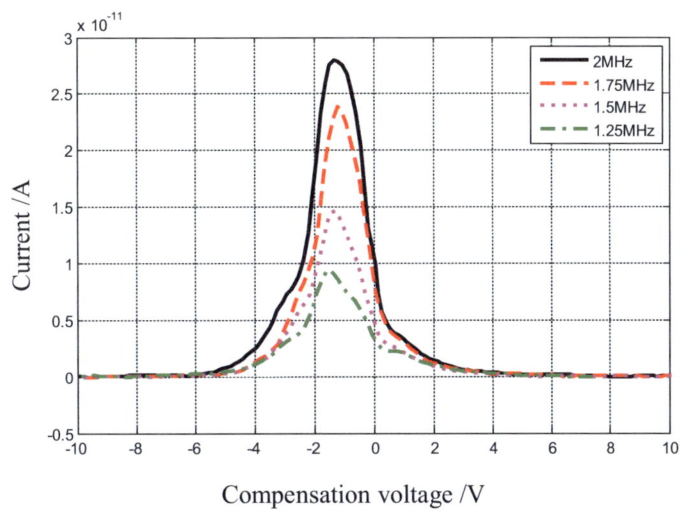

Fig. 33. The FAIMS spectrogram of 2-pentane corresponding with different square wave radio frequency voltages

(3) Influence of the flow velocity of the carrier gas

When the square wave radio frequency voltage amplitude is 320V, the duty ratio is 30%, and the frequency is 2MHz, the flow velocity of the carrier gas increases from 0.6L/min to 1.4L/min. It can be identified from figure 34 that when the flow velocity of the carrier gas increases, the signal intensity of the ion will increase, while the compensation voltage value *Vc* stays the same at -1.33V. When the flow velocity increases, the FAIMS spectrogram will broaden, namely the resolution is reduced. The increase of the carrier gas velocity makes the time the ion takes to travel through the drift region shorter and the number of movement cycles in the drift region is reduced, so the ion loss due to ion diffusion and neutralisation of the positive and negative ions becomes smaller. But the net displacement in one cycle stays the same so the ion signal intensity is improved, the compensation voltage stays the same, and the resolution is reduced.

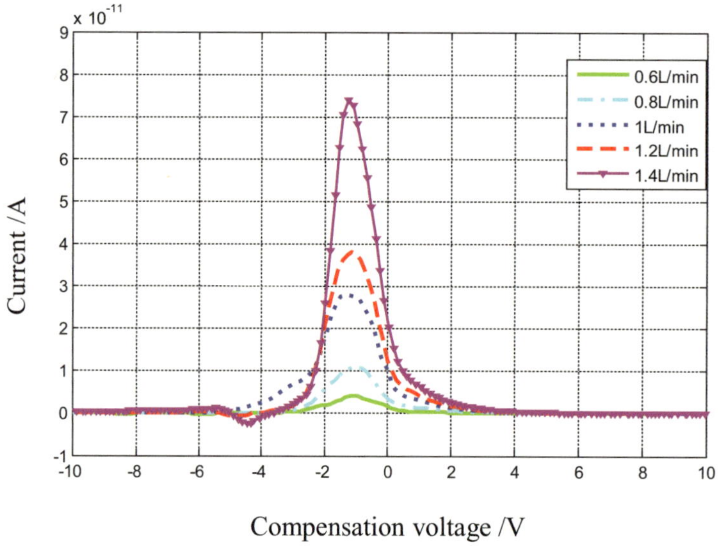

Fig. 34. Influence of the flow velocity of the carrier gas on FAIMS spectrogram

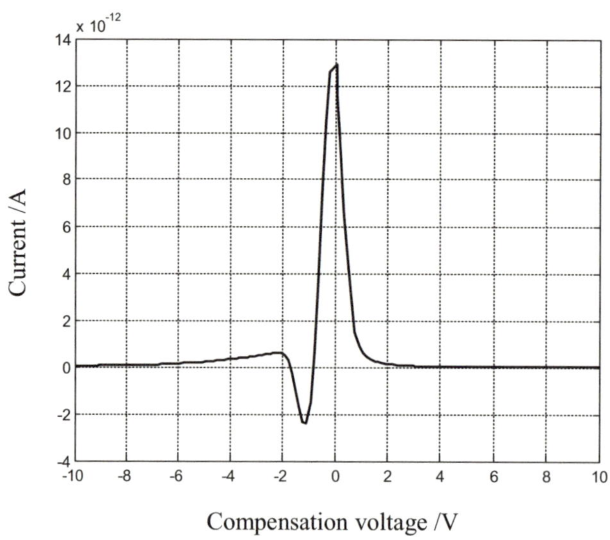

Fig. 35. FAIMS Spectrogram of 0.1ppm acetic acid

6.4 FAIMS chip detection limit experiment

The experimental sample is acetic acid. The sample bottle is sealed with a film with a 160μm diameter hole at its centre, to reduce volatilisation of the sample and acquire a sample of lower concentration. The carrier gas is high purity nitrogen (99.999%), the flow of which is 100L/h. The concentration of the acetic acid is about 0.1ppm through acid base titration with NaOH of known concentration.

The parameter setting in this experiment is as follows: the square wave radio frequency voltage amplitude is 220V, the frequency is 2MHz, and the duty ratio is 30%, the polarisation voltage of the ultraviolet lamp is -150V, the FAIMS Spectrogram of the acetic acid is shown in figure 35.

It can be concluded from figure 35 that a -2.4pA current signal can be obtained with 0.1ppm acetic acid through the FAIMS chip test. It means that the detection sensitivity of the FAIMS chip is high, with which a 0.1ppm acetic acid sample signal can be detected.

7. References

West, C.; Baron, B. & Minet, J. J. (2007). Detection of gunpowder stabilizers with ion mobility spectrometry. *Forensic Science International*, Vol.166, No.2, (March 2007), pp. 91-101, ISSN 0379-0738

Laiko, V. V. (2006). Orthogonal extraction ion mobility spectrometry. *J Am Soc Mass Spectrom*, Vol.17, No.4, (April 2006), pp. 500-507, ISSN 1044-0305

Borsdorf, H.; Nazarov, E. G.; Miller, R. A. (2006). Atmospheric-pressure ionization studies and field dependence of ion mobilities of isomeric hydrocarbons using a miniature differential mobility spectrometer. *Analytica Chimica Acta*, Vol.575, No.1, (August 2006), pp. 76-88, ISSN 0003-2670

Miller, R. A.; Nazarov, E. G. & Eiceman, G. A. (2001). A MEMS radio-frequency ion mobility spectrometer for chemical vapor detection. *Sens Actu A*, Vol.91, No.3, (July 2001), pp. 301-312, ISSN 0924-4247

Miller, R. A.; Eiceman, G. A. & Nazarov, E. G. (2000). A novel micromachined high-field asymmetric waveform-ion mobility spectrometer. *Sens Actu B*, Vol.67, No.3, (September 2000), pp. 300-306, ISSN 0925-4005

Barnett, D. A.; Ells, B. & Guevremont, R. (2002). Application of ESI-FAIMS-MS to the analysis of tryptic peptides. *J Am Soc Mass Spectrom*, Vol.13, No.11, (November 2002), pp. 1282–1291, ISSN 1044-0305

Shvartsburg, A. A.; Smith, R. D. & Wilks, S. A. (2009). Ultrafast differential ion mobility spectrometry at extreme electric fields in multichannel microchips. *Anal Chem*, Vol.81, No.15, (July 2009), pp. 6489-6495, ISSN 0003-2700

Eiceman, G. A.; Nazarov, E. G. & Miller, R. A. (2000). A micro-machined ion mobility spectrometer-mass spectrometer. *Int J Ion Mobil Spec*, Vol.3, No.1, (January 2000), pp. 15-27, ISSN 1435-6163

Guevremont, R.; Purves, R. W. (1999). Atmospheric pressure ion focusing in a high-field asymmetric waveform ion mobility spectrometer. *Rev. Sci. Instrum.*, Vol.70, No.2, (February 1999), pp. 1370-1383, ISSN 0003-46748

Nazarov, E. G.; Miller, R. A.; Eiceman, G. A.; Stone, John A. (2006). Miniature differential mobility spectrometry using atmospheric pressure photoionization. *Analytical Chemistry*, Vol.78, No.13, (July 2006), pp. 4553-4563, ISSN 0003-2700

Shvartsburg, A. A.; Tang, K. & Smith, R. D. (2004). Modeling the resolution and sensitivity of FAIMS analyses. *J Am Soc Mass Spectrom*, Vol.15, No.10, (October 2004), pp. 1487-1498, ISSN 1044-0305

Barnett, D. A.; Belford, M.; Dunyach, J. J.; Purves, R. W. (2007). Characterization of a Temperature-Controlled FAIMS System. *J Am Soc Mass Spectrom*, Vol.18, No.9, (September 2007), pp. 1653-1663, ISSN 1044-0305

Eiceman, G. A.; Tadjikov, B.; Krylov, E.; Nazarov, E. G.; Miller, R. A.; Westbrook, J.; Funk, P. (2001). Miniature radio-frequency mobility analyzer as a gas chromatographic detector for oxygen-containing volatile organic compounds, pheromones and other insect attractants. *Journal of Chromatography A*, Vol.917, No.1-2, (May 2001), pp. 205-217, ISSN 0021-9673

Buryakov, I. A.; Krylov, E. V.; Nazarov, E. G.; Rasulev, U. K. (1993). A new method of separation of multi-atomic ions by mobility at atmospheric pressure using a high-frequency amplitude-asymmetric strong electric field. *Int J Mass Spectrom Ion Processes*, Vol.128, No.3, (October 1993), pp. 143-148, ISSN 0168-1176

Krylov, E. V. (2003). Comparison of the planar and coaxial field asymmetrical waveform ion mobility spectrometer. *Int J Mass Spectrom*, Vol.225, No.1, (February 2003), pp. 39-51, ISSN 1387-3806

Khayamian, T.; Tabrizchi, M.; Jafari, M. T. (2003). Analysis of 2,4,6-trinitrotoluene, pentaerythritol tetranitrate and cyclo-1,3,5-trimethylene-2,4,6-trinitramine using negative corona discharge ion mobility spectrometry. *Talanta*, Vol.59, No.2, (February 2003), pp. 327-333, ISSN 0039-9140

Tabrizchi, M.; Rouholahnejad, F. (2004). Corona discharge ion mobility spectrometry at reduced pressures. *Rev. Sci. Instrum.*, Vol.75, No.11, (November 2004), pp. 4656-4661, ISSN 0003-46748

Jafari, M. T.; Khayamian, T.; Shaer, V.; Zarei, N. (2007). Determination of veterinary drug residues in chicken meat using corona discharge ion mobility spectrometry. *Anal. Chim. Acta.*, Vol.581, No.1, (January 2007), pp. 147-153, ISSN 0003-2670

Khayamian, T.; Tabrizchi, M. (2001). Direct determination of ultra-trace amounts of acetone by corona-discharge ion mobility spectrometry. *Fresen. J Anal. Chem.*, Vol.370, No.8, (August 2001), pp. 1114-1116, ISSN 0937-0633

Papanastasiou, D.; Wollnik, H. & Rico, G. (2008). Differential mobility separation of ions using a rectangular asymmetric waveform. *J Phys Chem A*, Vol.112, No.16, (March 2008), pp. 3638-3645, ISSN 1089-5639

2

Intelligent Sensory Micro-Nanosystems and Networks

Vladimir M. Koleshko[1], Yauhen A. Varabei[1] and Nikita A. Khmurovich[2]
[1]*Belarusian National Technical University, Dept. of Intelligent Systems*
[2]*Belarusian State University of Informatics and Radioelectronics, Dept. of Information Technologies Software*
Minsk, Belarus

1. Introduction

The presented chapter on the theme of "Intelligent sensory micro-nanosystems and networks" is devoted to scientific research, modeling and designing of sensory systems on a chip of the types of "electronic nose" (e-nose), "electronic tongue" (e-tongue), "electronic eye" (e-eye) to recognize multidimensional information patterns in modern micro-nanosensory technology, electronics, industrial biotechnology, biochemistry, bioinformatics, medicine, ecology, precision agriculture, economy, finances, logistics, computer systems and networks, personal and social safety etc. A human biosystem has an enormous number of different micro-nanobiosensors and micro-nanoactuators which are able sensitively to perceive, to transform and to transmit any patterns changes of external matters or homeostasis, therefore all in the world can be and has to be sensory and motoric. Design of surface acoustic waves (SAW) sensors in wireless micro-nanosensory laboratories on a chip e-nose and e-tongue allows to identify physico-acoustic and electroacoustic properties (viscosity, mass, impedance, dielectric conductivity, electroconductivity and etc.), e.g., of investigated human biomatters (blood, sweat, saliva, urine, tears and etc.) and to form on their basis an information pattern. A micro-nanosensory system e-eye makes it possible to analyse quantitative concentration characteristics, molecular features and acoustooptical properties of information biomatters. At the same time, an intensive development of multicore data processing systems opens up ample possibilities for express analysis and pattern recognition.

Presented developed intelligent micro-nanodiagnostic laboratories find exceptional practical and individual applications and are a new class of self-adjusting sensory and portable mobile devices with flexible learning softwares for reliable continuous control of personal and social safety using Internet intelligent global sensory networks. They don't require special application conditions, highly skilled specialists to form fast and exactly information patterns of any diagnostic object. Using of the intelligent software for processing of registered sensory data enables to get "electronic maps" of objects, their online full information descriptions and to predict efficiently future changes.

This chapter will be useful for students, young scientists, lecturers, businessmen, information theory and telecommunications specialists, neurocomputer, neural, intelligent and sensory networkers. In addition, creative persons interested in understanding, modeling, designing of intelligent sensory systems and in development of smart devices, machines and productions can find a lot of worthy of their attention.

2. Intelligent sensory systems e-nose and e-tongue

2.1 Hardware components of SAW sensory systems

2.1.1 SAW structures

Development of intelligent system engineering is of enormous importance practically in all advanced countries at the present time. The great attention is caused owing to a possibility of intelligent systems to solve tasks of a broad spectrum of applications. It is well known that any product, object, technology can be described as information patterns. The developed biosensor intelligent system ("BIS") presents a new class of intelligent analytical devices and systems including advantages of state-of-the-art micro-nanoelectronics, biochemistry, intelligent computing and up-to-date production of express-diagnostic systems on a chip. One of the most perspective directions of intelligent micro-nanosensory systems on a chip is the application of thin-film nanostructured materials acoustic properties and the design of micro-nanosystems on SAW. Micro-nanosensory systems of e-nose and e-tongue on SAW enable to generate fast a high-resolution information pattern and are distinguished by their sensitivity, rapid responses, low power consumption and nonlinearity. Developed SAW devices can be applied in any external environment and under the influence of different strains over a long period of time. A planar structure of SAW transducers defines a simple embodiment and their including in a batch process, but light weight, high reliability and high-noise protection make possible their embedding in intelligent microprocessor-based recognition systems and remote transferring in communication and computer networks (Barkaline & Polynkova, 2002).
Functioning of any SAW sensor systems is based on the influence of physically and chemically adsorbed molecules on geometrical, electrical and acoustic properties of a SAW sensitive layer (e.g., nanostructure), on changing of elastic properties and mass loading of a piezo-active substrate surface. Labs on a chip of e-tongue and e-nose on SAW are a piezoelectric thin plate (quartz, $LiNbO_3$, $LiTaO_3$, GaAs, $Si/SiO_2/ZnO$, $Si/SiO_2/AlN$) with evaporated metal electrodes for two systems of interdigital transducers (IDTs) and reflecting matrices. As a rule IDTs are used for a SAW excitation as metal electrodes pairs on a functional surface of piesoactive waveguides. Electrodes are linked to an alternating current generator in bandwidth up to 10 GHz. The alternating voltage induces an acoustic wave spreading at a rate of about 3000 mps on surface of a piezo-active substrate. The acoustic wavelength is determined by IDTs electrodes separation. E-tongues and e-noses on SAW structures can function in some modes (resonator, delay lines) or use a differential circuit of two resonators, two delay lines, one delay line and one resonator (Koleshko, 1974, 1976, 1984, 1986, 1988, 1990), which enables to measure two mechanical (physico-acoustic) and two electrical (acoustoelectric) parameters of solid, gaseous, liquid and heterogeneous investigated matters. Figure 1 presents a sensory system of e-tongue and e-nose with two delay lines: the first delay line, e.g, Au metallized measures mechanical parameters (viscosity, mass, impedance), but the second one – capacitivity and electrical conduction of a

matter. A sensitive element is placed on delay lines representing the sensitive layer: nanotubes, DNA chains or their combination (Fig. 1d, 1e).

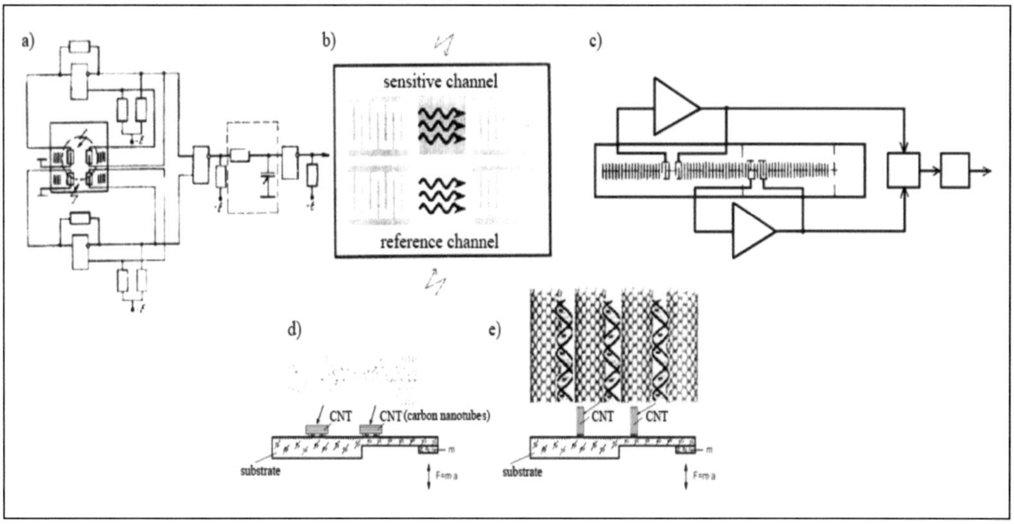

Fig. 1. SAW sensory system. (a, b, c) Sensory system of e-tongue and e-nose on SAW.
(d, e) Placements of carbon nanotubes and double DNA chains on SAW delay lines.

2.1.2 Parameters of SAW micro-nanosensors

A bandwidth of SAW transformer depends on a number of electrodes: increase of an electrodes number reduces the one, but a number of electrodes are to be minimized to decrease a device capacitance. Moreover, a number of electrodes are to be consisted of many pairs to reduce any noise, but a reduction of diffraction loss takes place in case of a wide aperture. Therefore, SAW devices are developed in which properties of input and output transducers are optimally adjusted in. Critical parameters of SAW sensors depending on materials of acoustic lines are given in the table 1.

A special circuit board contained an investigated matter is developed to control the delivery of matters, which measures 32 by 20 mm with an allocated reservoir in size 6,8 by 2,5 by 8 mm and in volume of 136 μl. A sample is placed in the centre exactly between IDTs (Fig. 2a). A new class of wireless microlabs on a chip with radio frequency identification is designed (Fig. 2b) (Polynkova, 2007).

Material of acoustic line	$LiTaO_3$	SiO_2	GaAs	$LiNbO_3$
electrodes width of IDTs, μm	17	3	2	2
velocity of SAW, mps	4212,6	3159	2604	3488
frequency synchronism, MHz	55-65	263,03	325,5	436
pairs number of IDTs electrodes	28	19	67	4
IDTs aperture, μm	30	46	4	221
SAW length, μm	7513	12	8	8

Table 1. Parameters of SAW micro-nanosensors for e-tongue and e-nose.

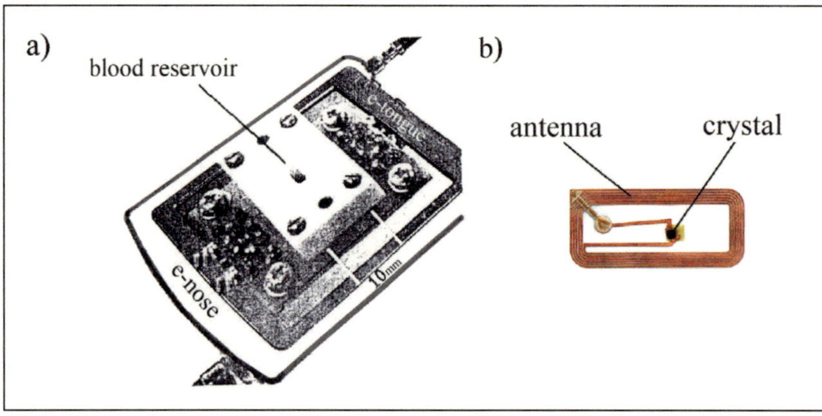

Fig. 2. Wireless multisensory system on SAW (a) with radio frequency identification (b).

Such smart labs on a chip are not expensive, don't require special operating conditions and first line maintenance men, make it possible to get biochemical information patterns, e.g., of ecological production status, technological processes, human health and to take samples promptly and on-site avoiding any delays and inaccuracies caused by data transfer in centralized expensive research labs (Fig. 3) (Gulay & Polynkova, 2010).

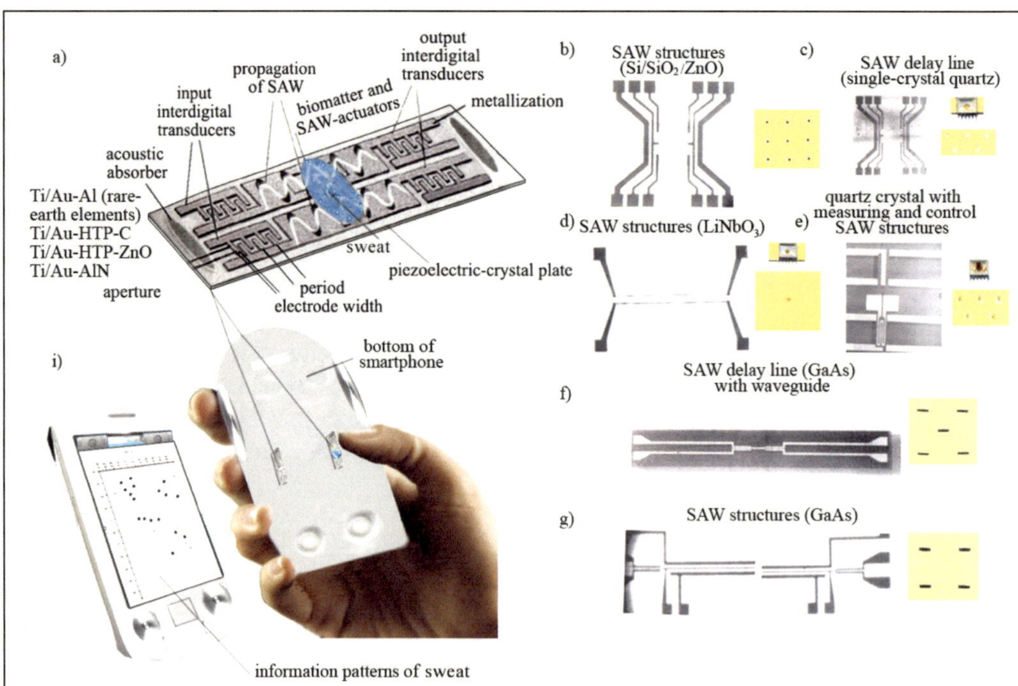

Fig. 3. Developed intelligent sensory system in smartphone. (a) Structure of SAW sensor on a chip e-tongue and e-nose. (b, c, d, e, f, g) Developed SAW structures. (i) Smartphone with sensors on SAWs and intelligent software for recognition of sweat information patterns.

2.2 Materials of intelligent sensory micro-nanosystems on SAW

2.2.1 Strain effects in SAW structures

One of the ways for developing of intelligent sensory micro-nanosystems and networks is using of new materials. This is an important factor for high-sensitivity physical quantities transducers which sensitivity values at extreme points are determined by constants of a used material. Elasticity modules of the 2nd and 3rd orders inhere in mechanical quantities transducers (pressure, acceleration, force, angular frequency etc.) on SAW. A limited influence on sensitivity of SAW transducers and substantial dependence on parameters and on a waveguide crystallographic orientation (crystal plane, SAW propagation direction) determines a profound study of SAW propagation properties depending on deformations ("strain effect") on the basis of different materials. The strain effect implies a variation in SAW propagation characteristics in a strained waveguide. Using of the strain effect in multilayer SAW structures plays a significant role in analysis and development of SAW devices. This effect also determines operating principles of precision micro-electronic mechanical transducers based on SAW structures (Koleshko, 1985, 1987).

One of the most important SAW structure parameters is a phase shift ψ_0 as SAW with a phase velocity V and a frequency f propagating between two points of the laminated structure located at a distance L from each other. Any deformation of this thin film SAW structure because of mechanical loading leads to change in a SAW phase shift due to a SAW phase velocity change dV and a concurrent length change dL. For a given method of substrate loading $d\psi/\psi_0$ can be found by determining dV/V and calculating dL/L and by means of known methods from the elasticity theory.

Analysis is carried out for a laminated structure (Fig. 4) (Koleshko, 1981, 1983, 1990) based on a semiinfinite crystal non-conducting substrate characterized by density, permittivity and the 2nd and 3rd order elastic moduli of a single-crystal silicon. SiO_2 layer is simulated by isotropic dielectric with parameters similar to those of a fused silica, but ZnO or AlN layer by 6 mm piezoelectric moduli and the 2nd order elastic moduli similar to those of ZnO or AlN single-crystal. The 3rd order elastic moduli of ZnO (AlN) are ignored because of weak bonds between crystallites in a thin polycrystalline film.

The effect of longitudinal and lateral mechanical strains on a SAW phase velocity in ZnO or AlN/ SiO_2/ Si thin film structures for {001}, {111} and {110} silicon crystal planes within the temperature range 293-673 K is studied. The obtained results enable a determination of SAW structure parameters with predetermined maximum sensitivity to a longitudinal and lateral homogeneous tension (compression) and bending as well as parameters of stable SAW structures are insensitive to mechanical loading. The Si {110}-based SAW structure with the SAW wave vector oriented in $<\bar{1}10>$ direction is shown to possess maximum operating frequency sensitivity to both longitudinal and lateral strains (Meshkov & Barkaline, 1990). ZnO or SiO_2 layer deposition on silicon increases the SAW phase velocity sensitivity to the longitudinal strain and decreases the one to the lateral strain. SAWs in waveguides from quartz single-crystal of YZ, XZ, XY orientations have equal peak responses to mass loading of a surface, but XY orientation is the least SAW responsive in the waveguide from sapphire. Using of a copper metallization appears to be more perspective as contrasted to other materials. Results of more than 60 isotropic cubic materials with different functional properties (metals, dielectrics, semiconductors, piezoelectric, magnetostrictive stuffs and superconductors) are presented in (Barkaline & Polynkova, 2002).

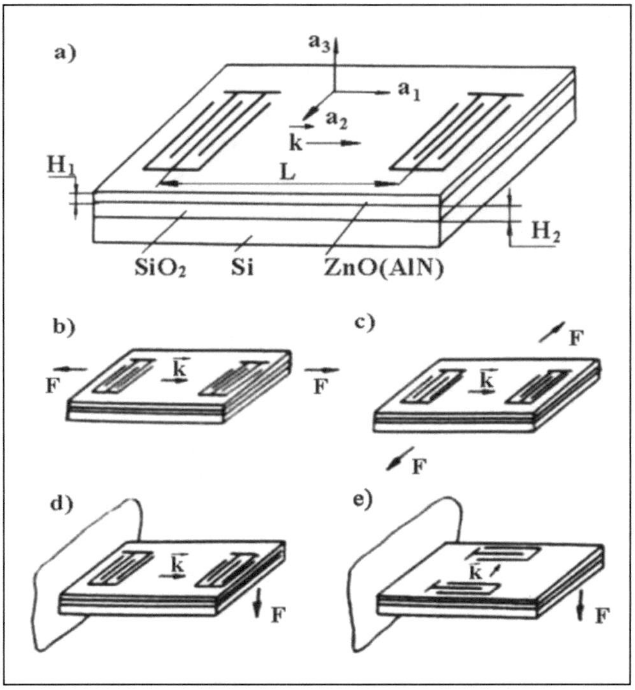

Fig. 4. Different mechanical loadings of SAW. (a) Multilayer thin film SAW structure. (b) Mechanical loading of SAW structure substrate.

2.2.2 Single-crystal silicon-based multilayer SAW structures

The strain effect is determined in cubic single-crystal SAW waveguides because of these materials have a broad variety of functional properties including semiconducting, piezoelectrical, magnetostricting and superconducting ones, the most examined constants are the simplest for analysis. Semiconducting materials (Si, GaAs and InSb) are of a particular interest in terms of developing SAW-based integrated devices with built-in information processing including sensing, executive and processor units. Piezoelectronic properties of $A^{III}B^{V}$ crystals make it possible to avoid a deposition of piezoelectric layers which are necessary for IDTs to induce SAW required by Si waveguides. Iron ittrium granatum ($Y_3Fe_5O_{15}$) or IIG has a low elastic anisotropy. High strong magnetostriction of $Y_3Fe_5O_{15}$ allows its using in devices which are based on interactions between SAWs and magnetostatic waves (spin waves).

A new approach for sensitivity coefficients definition of a SAW phase velocity to quasistatic volumetric effects on waveguide is developed on the basis of an algebraic properties research of the SAW phase velocity as a function of effective material constants. It is founded on introducing of a tensor W of SAW phase velocity partial derivatives in a crystallophysical coordinate system. Values of W component are determined by the material anisotropy factor $\eta=2\cdot C_{55}/(C_{11}-C_{12})$ and the parameter $a=C_{11}/C_{55}$. Orientation relations of the phase velocity and factors of the deformation sensitivity at longitudinal and lateral deformations for base planes of Si, InSb, GaAs, IIG, $SrTiO_3$ are investigated. These crystals can be arranged on SAW phase velocity values as $V_{InSb} < V_{GaAs} < V_{IIG} < V_{SiTiO_3} < V_{Si}$ for all investigated SAW directions. Figure 5 depicts an investigated materials distribution in the plane (a,η), but the solid line describes the limiting value a=2/η. The considered materials concentrate evidently in the range 2<a·η<7, therefore to predict characteristics of SAW devices on the basis of new materials it is important previously to know a value of partial sensitivity coefficients to different exposures. Superconducting ceramics $YBa_2Cu_3O_{7-x}$ has a record high level of deformation sensitivity because of acoustic nonlinearity large values of this material (~100).

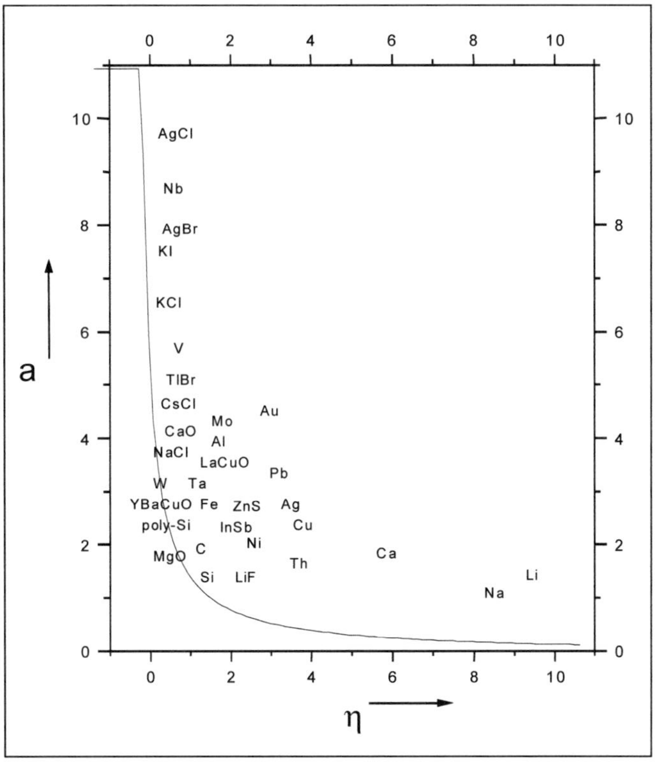

Fig. 5. Materials in plane of anisotropy factor η and calculated parameter a.

Results of a theoretical study into an orientation dependence of the SAW strain sensitivity on longitudinal and lateral deformations of Si, GaAs, InSb, $Y_3Fe_50_{15}$ (YIG), $SrTiO_3$ waveguides for {100}, {110}, {111} cuts are presented in (Barkaline & Polynkova, 2002) (Fig. 8). The wave vector direction of SAWs is characterized by an angle Θ calculated from directions <100>, $<\bar{1}10>$ and $<11\bar{2}>$. A value d is determined under longitudinal and lateral deformations of the cantilever, which is loaded at the free end by the force F (Fig. 4d, 4e) (Meshkov & Barkaline, 1990). The calculated orientation dependences of d are shown in figure 6 for {001}, {110} and {111} under longitudinal (d_{11}) and lateral ($d_{\perp}$) waveguide deformations, respectively (Koleshko, 1986, 1987, 1988, 1989, 1990).

The strain effect orientation dependencies in $SrTiO_3$ differ from each other and from corresponding dependencies for Si, GaAs and InSb which are similar. However, the strain effect is practically isotropic for the both types of materials in plane {111}. The strain effect is displayed weakly in YIG thereby indicating that it is promising for constructing stable SAW devices. At the same time, the strain effect value in $SrTiO_3$ exceeds considerably all data presented in literature on single-crystal materials indicating that it is promising as a material for highly sensitive SAW transducers of mechanical quantities and especially when superconducting metallization is used in IDTs electrodes. In addition the strain effect in semiconductors InSb and GaAs is weaker than in Si, therefore these materials are promising for single-crystal SAW transducers of mechanical quantities (Meshkov & Barkaline, 1990).

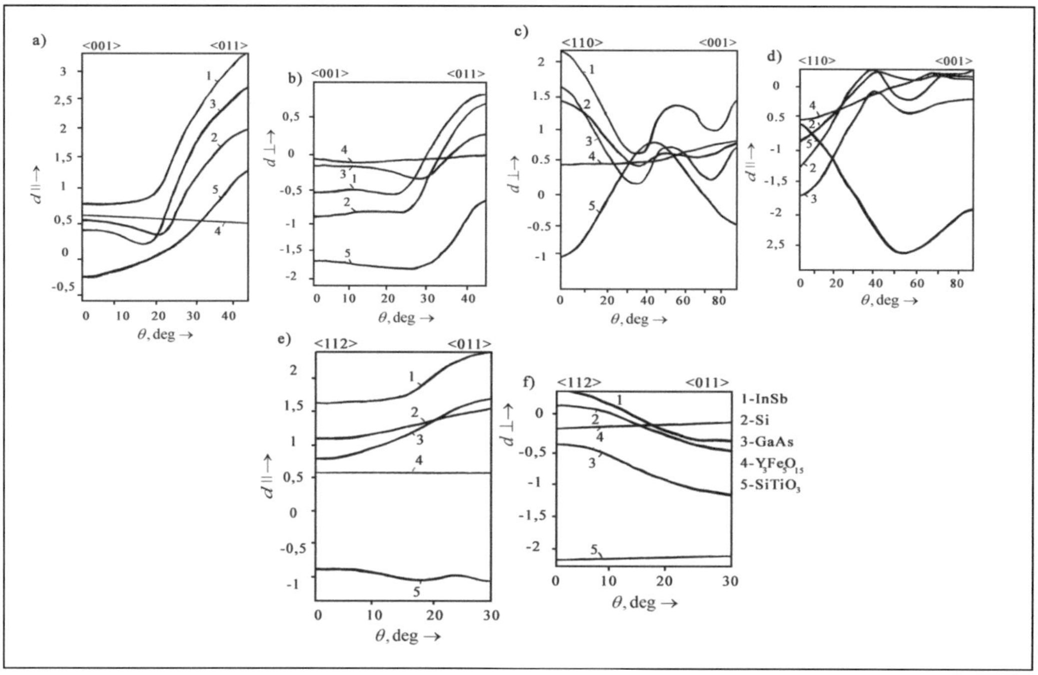

Fig. 6. Orientation dependence under longitudinal (d_{11}) and lateral ($d_{\perp}$) deformations: (a, b) $d_{\parallel}$ and $d_{\perp}$ for plane {001}, (c, d) $d_{\parallel}$ and $d_{\perp}$ for plane {110}, (e, f) $d_{\parallel}$ and $d_{\perp}$ for plane {111}.

2.2.3 High-temperature superconductors thin films-based SAW structures

SAW properties in micro-nanoelectronic structures with components based on new high-temperature superconductors (HTSC), e.g., $YBa_2Cu_3O_{7-X}$ are of interest from the point of view of a potential application of these materials in various acoustoelectronic devices as a superconducting metallization for possible reduction of a noise level in them or as a substrate. The strain effect in such SAW structures is described in the work (Koleshko, 1989). In (Meshkov & Barkaline, 1990) a non-dissipative SAW propagation is considered, for which a nonelastic contribution to the SAW phase velocity is small enough with respect to the elastic one. It means the validity of the relation $w \cdot \tau << 1$ where w is SAW angular frequency and t - relaxation time of propagation medium. For $YBa_2Cu_3O_{7-X}$ ceramic samples at a room temperature when it has semiconductor-like properties evaluations of t give $3 \cdot 10^{-10}$ sec. The data on the 3rd order elastic moduli for all materials forming a SAW propagation medium is necessary for theoretical analysis of SAW sensitivity to strains. This data for $YBa_2Cu_3O_{7-X}$ material is not presented in literature yet. To evaluate appropriate data on the 2nd order elastic moduli C_{IJ} of the ceramic $YBa_2Cu_3O_{7-X}$ pressure dependence is used. High values of dC_{IJ}/dP (P denotes pressure) are the $YBa_2Cu_3O_{7-X}$ intrinsic property not caused by ceramic nature of samples and connected with valence fluctuations of copper ions which are characteristics of copper HTSC (Meshkov & Barkaline, 1990).

2.2.4 Diamond-like carbon films-based SAW structures

Diamond-like films that reveal unique practically useful properties find a wide application nowadays in micro-nanosensory technologies due to a carbon atoms capacity to form strong chemical bonds of different character. Properties of carbon films can differ greatly from diamond and graphite varying while there is a small difference between chemical potentials of carbon phases and a high probability of transitions. In (Barkaline & Polynkova, 2002) a problem of controlled magnetron deposition of a-C:H films on various substrates in order to produce an "intelligent" carbon material for acoustoelectronic applications is studied and solved. Dispersion curves for a SAW phase velocity in a-C\ZnO\SiO_2\Si SAW-structures with different layers thicknesses for a SAW fundamental mode and ten highest modes show a possibility to realize multimode SAW propagation in such structures.

One of the most promising application areas of a-C:H films it seems to be SAW-based chemical sensors. Dominating diamond-like phase is characterized by high SAW phase velocity V and small waveguide factor F values (upper curves on fig. 7), but in case of dominating graphite-like phase this relation is inverse (lower curves). It means that SAW energy concentrates in the waveguide internal region leading to increasing of the SAW device chemical stability.

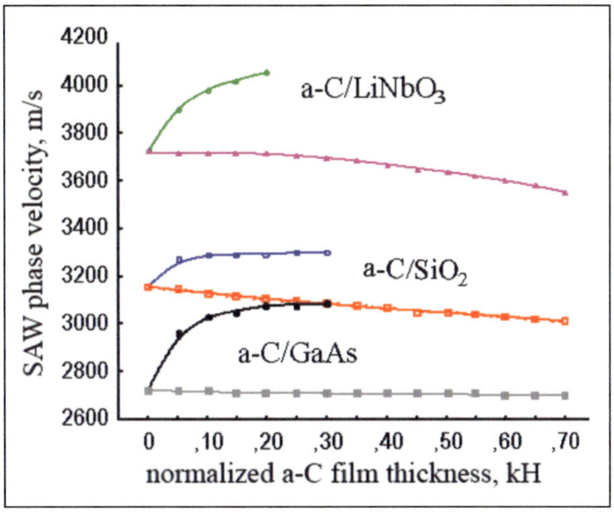

Fig. 7. Dispersion curves for SAW structures with a-C layer.

2.2.5 Dispersion relations of SAW in $LiNbO_3$/a:C structures

One of the most perspective material of a SAW substrate is a single-crystal $LiNbO_3$ with a high electromechanical coefficient and used in different passive and active acoustoelectronic devices from filters up to nonlinear circuits of memory and SAW sensors. The single crystal of $LiNbO_3$ is one of the most studied acoustic crystals, for which all material constants of the 2nd and 3rd orders are known. At the same time, the SAW deformation sensitivity in this crystal and a range of a SAW characteristics control by introducing of different functional layers in $LiNbO_3$ acoustic line are obscure. These problems can be clarified by means of a nanostructured carbon material layer containing, in particular, an ordered set of carbon nanotubes. The material parameters of the carbon material layer are determined by effective elastic medium method. The composite layer with a cylindrical form carbon nanotube in diameter 10 nm is estimated, but a composite matrix is modelled by material with parameters of amorphous carbon.

The relation of the SAW phase velocity from the carbonic layer thickness has non-linear nature. In Z-directions on X- and Y- cuts, on X- and Z-cuts a sharp reduction of the SAW velocity is evident at increasing of the carbonic layer depth. It allows to suspect sharp responses to exposures. The introducing of nanotubes in the material layer enables to execute SAW phase velocity controlling in a broad band. Thus, conducted researches show prospects of using of a nanostructured carbon material for new acoustoelectronic devices on the basis of $LiNbO_3$ (Koleshko, 1981, 1983, 1987).

2.3 Sensing elements of intelligent systems on SAW

2.3.1 Sensitivity of SAW transformers

Each piezoelectric crystal is defined by resonance oscillation frequency about 10 MHz which depends on its environment, mass and absorbed materials on a substrate. Absorption of a matter causes a change of its resonance frequency (Δf) which can be measured with the exceptional high sensitivity (500-2500 Hz/μg) and is based on sensors characterized by detection limit about some picogram. The mass change of a sensitive layer because of substance adsorption can be estimated by SAW velocity and resonance frequency:

$$\Delta f/f_0=k\cdot\Delta v/v_0=-k\cdot c_m\cdot f_0\cdot m\cdot n, \quad (1)$$

where k - SAW track length between IDTs on a piezocrystal, c_m - device mass sensitivity ($\sim 1{,}3\cdot10^{-6}$g/cm^2), n - adsorbed molecules concentration, m - adsorbed molecules mass.

In this connection, chemical sensors are the important factor of wireless monitoring and security systems which use sensible elements possessing specific reactions to environment (Meshkov & Barkaline, 1990). Carbonaceous nanotubes are structures consisting of a convoluted hexagonal lattice with carbon atoms in site. This carbon form finds a wide application along with graphite and fullerene (Deinak et al., 2009).

Sorbate molecules and radicals make possible a creation of highly sensitive devices for controlling of dangerous and hazardous substances in environment (H_2, O_2, CO etc.). Data of the SAW transformers sensitivity to NO_2, NH_3, CO_2, CO, H_2O, CH_4 with a phtalocyanme sensitive layer in 0,32 μm thickness and in 236,25 MHz SAW operating frequency is shown in the table 2. Positive values of frequency variations in relation to a light gas concentration (NH_3, CO, H_2O, CH_4) can be explained by current desorption of oxygen.

2.3.2 Molecular sieves, nanotubes and nanowhiskers

Molecular sieves can be used for different applications as adsorbents for dehumidification and cleaning of gas streams, for separation of gas mixtures depending on a molecules size. So nanotubes and nanowhiskers can be considered as sensitivity elements of SAW intelligent micro-nanosystems (Table 3). Therefore, achievements in the field of micro-nanotechnologies enable to develop "labs on a chip" for detection and analysis of different matters using multidimensional sensors.

Substrate material	Orientation	Gas concentration ΔC, one millionth					
		100	200	3500	1200	8000	400
		gases					
		NO_2	NH_3	CO_2	CO	H_2O	CH_4
quartz	ST,X	-4,900	0,800	-0,01	0,03	0,02	0,200
	Z,X	-2,97	0,49	-0,006	0,018	0,012	0,12
	Y,Z	-8,15	1,33	-0,017	0,05	0,033	0,33
sapphire	Z,X	-1,65	0,27	-0,003	0,01	0,007	0,07
	X,Z	-1,981	0,323	-0,004	0,012	0,008	0,081
	Y,Z	-1,986	0,324	-0,004	0,012	0,008	0,081
lithium niobate	Z,X	-3,235	0,528	-0,007	0,020	0,013	0,132
	Y,X	-3,467	0,566	-0,007	0,021	0,014	0,142
	X,Y	-3,213	0,525	-0,007	0,020	0,013	0,131
silicon	X,Z	-6,048	0,988	-0,012	0,037	0,025	0,247
germanium	X,Z	-4,599	0,751	-0,009	0,028	0,019	0,188
zinc oxide	Y,Z	-2,022	0,330	-0,004	0,012	0,008	0,083
	Z,X	-2,567	0,419	-0,005	0,016	0,010	0,105

Table 2. SAW transformer sensitivity of gas concentration in air $\Delta f/\Delta C$.

Nanomaterial	Original compound	Crystallization temperature, °C	Nanotubes strength σ_m kg-force/mm^2	Nanotubes length, μm
Cu	CuI, H_2	590–800	360	1-60
	CuCl, H_2	430–800	450	1-10
	CuBr, H_2	600	360	1-10
Ag	AgCl, H_2	460–925	176	1-10
Pt	$PtCl_x$, H_2	800	430	1-10
Pd	$PdCl_2$, Ar	860–1000	270	1-6
Co	$CoBr_2$, H_2	690–730	330	1-18
	$CoCl_2$, H_2	600	330	1-15
C	C_2H_2, CH_4, Ar	600–800	2450	0,1-5

Table. 3. Basic materials for creation of nanotubes and nanowhiskers.

Nanotubes bundle have better absorption of gases than graphite because of the potential well maximum value on graphite equals -2.89 kcal/mole, but on nanotubes bundle -5.18 kcal/mole in consideration of an oxygen interaction on bundle nanotubes and graphite (Fig. 8).

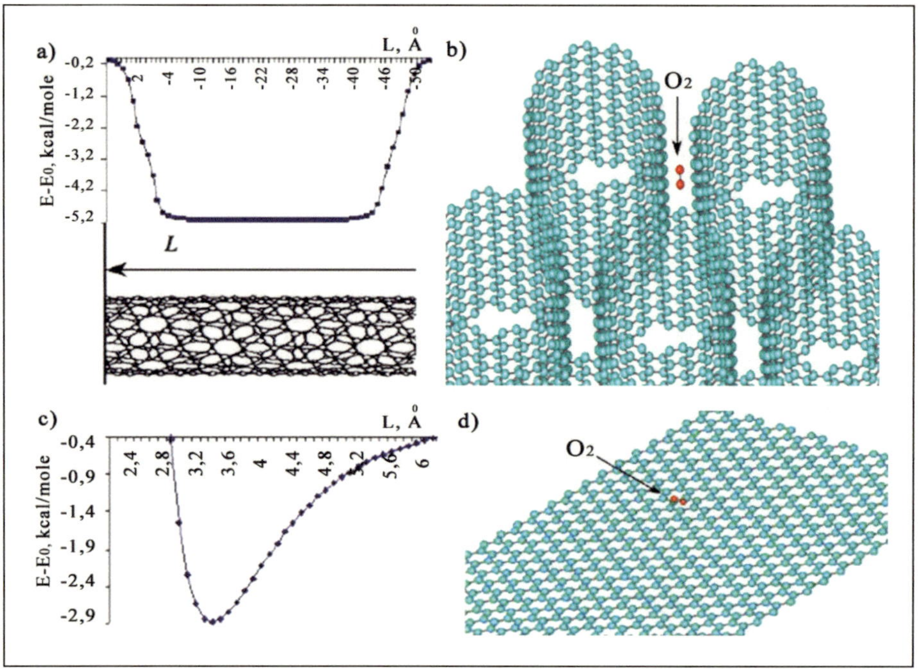

Fig. 8. Adsorption of sensitive sensor: oxygen absorption on nanotubes bundle (a, b) and on graphite film (c, d).

Modeling results of the sorption interaction of single-shell nanotubes with H_2, NO_2 and CO show the substance dependence on its binding energy. A potential well depth difference for H_2 and nanotubes bundle ($D \approx 1{,}36$nm) equals approximately -0,73 kcal/mole, $NO_2 \approx -2{,}77$ kcal/mole, CO ≈ -1,81 kcal/mole (Fig. 9) (Deinak et al., 2009).

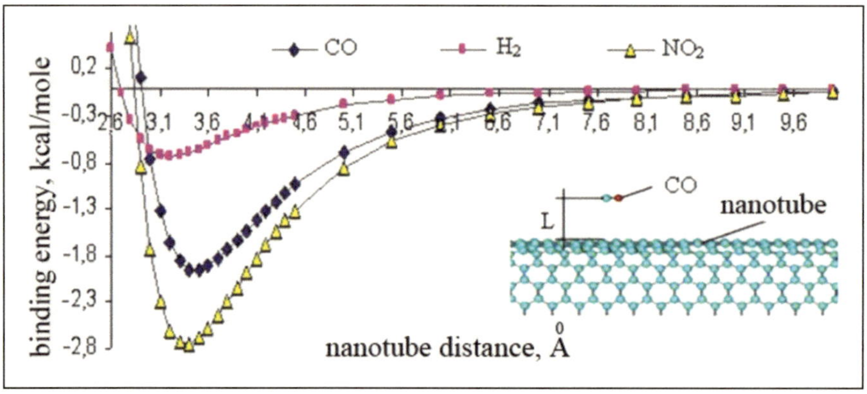

Fig. 9. Binding energy in case of adsorption in nanotubes bundle 10×10 for different gases.

The investigation results of the dangerous substance interaction with a nanotube bundle (Fig. 10) indicate that nanotubes have higher sensitivity regarding explosive materials (minimal interaction energy of a molecule ≈ 17,8 kcal/mole) and concerning RDX, TNT and NG (Barkaline & Polynkova, 2002).

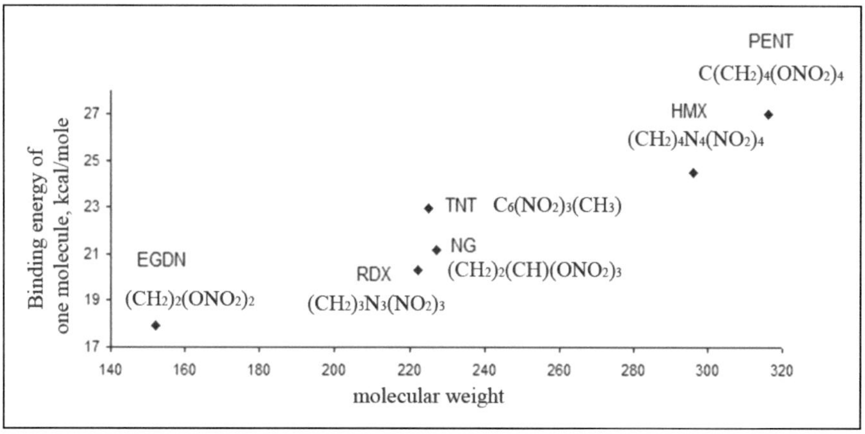

Fig. 10. Binding energy of dangerous substances.

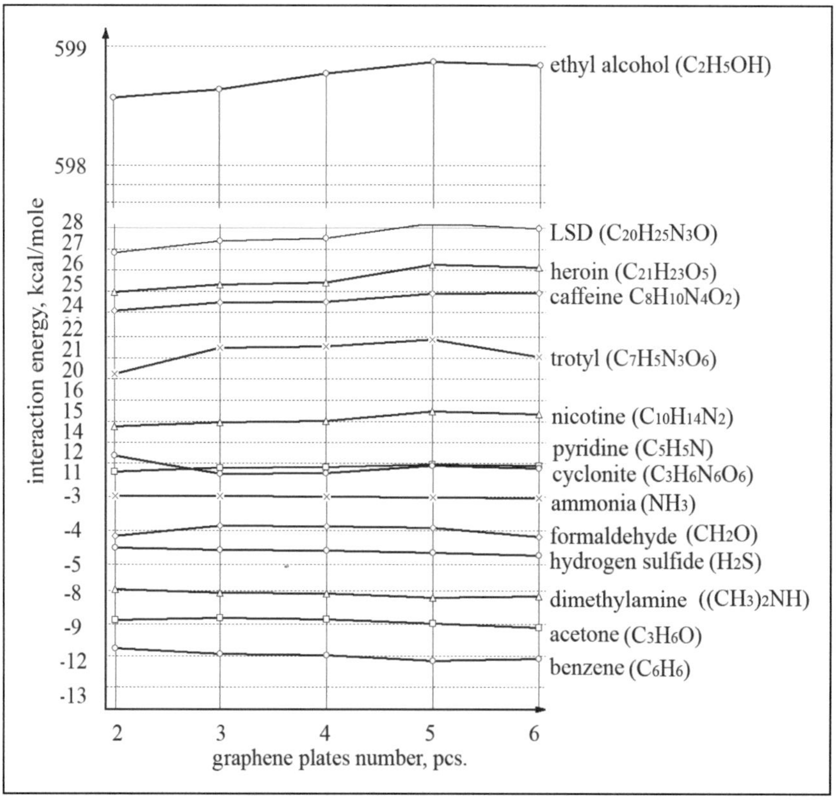

Fig. 11. Interaction energy on graphene plates for dangerous substances.

2.3.3 Multicomponent graphene structures

HypecChem can be used to analyze the absorption of biological hazardous molecules on graphene by effective potential MM+ with a single point calculation and a geometry optimization. The developed sensors on the basis of values of adsorption potential wells can be located in airports, railway stations, public transports, different institutions to ensure personal and social safety and to recognize promptly terrorists, drug addicts, alcoholic, smokers. Figure 11 presents results of interaction energy for different dangerous substances in concordance with graphene plates number which can be used for optimization of micro-nanosensory devices on SAW with a sensing element - graphene. Number of graphene plates defines adsorptivity of a specified substance and makes possible to calculate an optical structure of sensing elements because of great in magnitude values of adsorption potential wells. It means that the use of graphene structures opens new possibilities for fast detection of dangerous substances and explosives in information and communication sensory systems and networks.

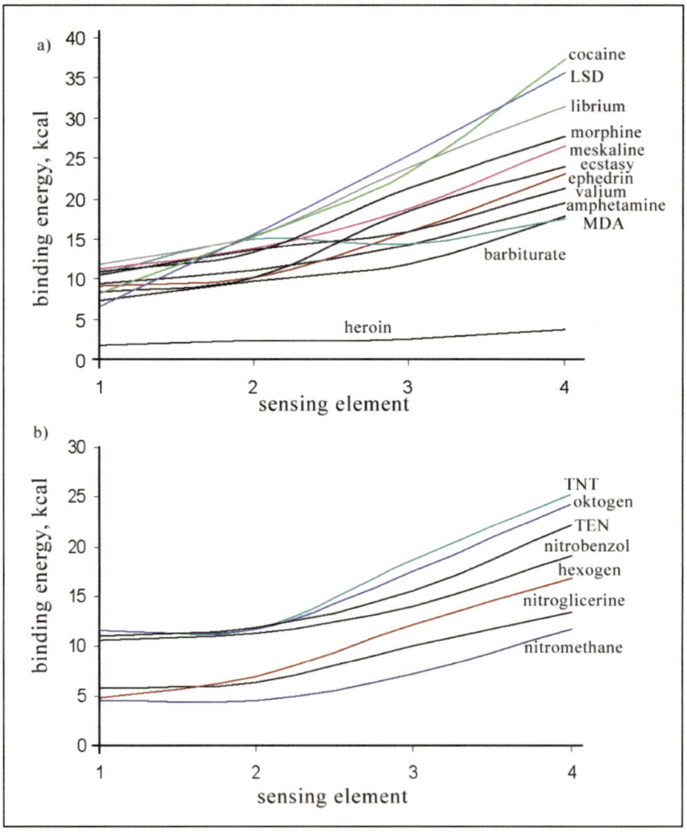

Fig. 12. Binding energy at absorption of narcotic, psychotropic matters (a) and explosives (b). Sensing element: 1 - nanotube; 2 - DNA; 3 - nanotube/6 DNA; 4 - DNA/6 nanotubes.

2.3.4 DNA sensing elements of SAW devices

E-noses and e-tongues on SAW use sensing elements in the form of nanotubes, DNA chains or their combinations. The software suite HyperChem is applied to calculate an effective potential MM+ as the most suitable for analyse of the organic molecular interaction with SAW sensing elements on the basis of atoms potential fields. Single points allow to estimate such molecular properties as a gradient of energy and a spin density which give information if the system is close to a minimum energy (Fig. 12). The system adsorption is defined by binding energy:

$$E_{BE} = E_{SE} + E_{MOL} - E_{SYS}, \quad (2)$$

where E_{SE}- total energy of a sensing element, E_{MOL}- molecule total energy of a narcotic matter and an explosive, E_{SYS}-system energy of "matter-sensing element". Thus, double DNA chains and nanotubes have practically identical absorption properties, but the optimal structure of sensing elements consists of one DNA chain and six nanotubes located in the form of the hexagonal ring round this DNA chain (Deinak et al., 2009).

A new class of unique ultraspeed genom sequenators is developed which can find applications in biological engineering, industrial micro-nanobiotechnology, biomedical technology, bioinformatics, bioengineering, information and telecommunication technologies and etc. The sensing element in the form of inorganic nanotubes (C, BeO, Si_xC_{1-x}, ZnO, BN, AlN) with nanopores is placed on the Au, Ag, Al (rare-earth metals) metallized sensitive channel. The nanotubes diameter and the nanotubes spacing are optimized for exacter control of a single DNA molecule inside of the nanotube (Fig. 13) (N.V. Khmurovich, 2010).

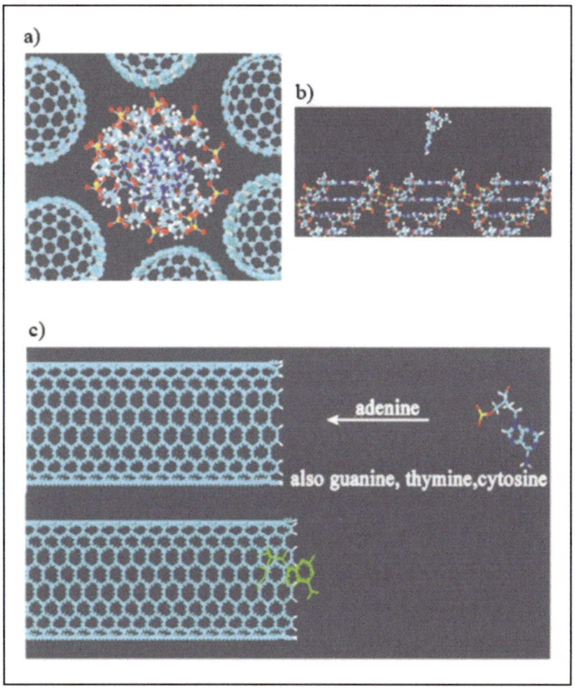

Fig. 13. Absorption of carbon nanotube DNA bases. (a) Position of DNA chain and 6 nanotubes. (b) LSD molecule over DNA chains (side view).

The SAW structure with sensing elements in the form of the nanotubes is able to pull DNA molecules through the holes of the nanotubes and between the nanotubes using acoustic wave and (or) electric field and to recognize nucleotide DNA sequences, genes, chromosomes and genome. The developed intelligent ultraspeed sensory nanosystem of genom sequencing can identify rapidly and correctly information patterns of any genotypes, detect of damaged DNA fragments and genetic changes. DNA molecules of blood, saliva, sweat, urine, tears and other investigated human biomatters can be pulled even through small nanopores of the nanotubes varying the power of acoustic wave. Analysis shows different absorption velocities of DNA nuclefotides in a nanotube depending on their molecular weights (Fig. 14). It means 60 people can be sequenced in one minute or 600 people in about 10 minutes (N.V. Khmurovich, 2010).

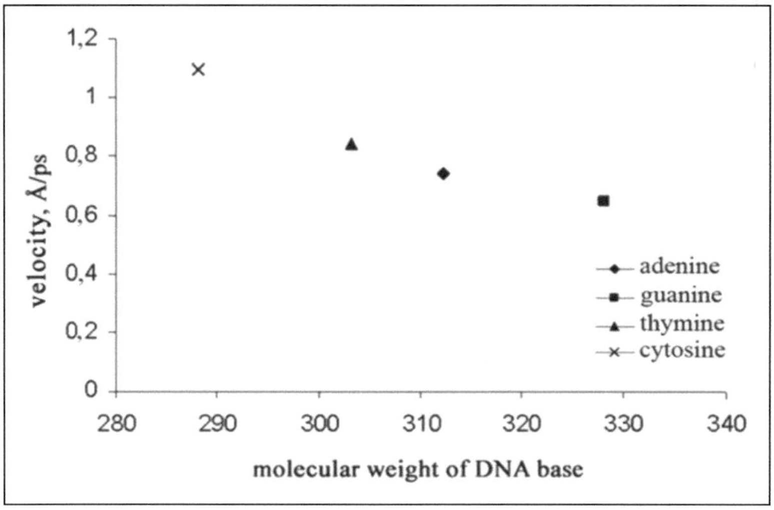

Fig. 14. Velocity changes in carbon nanotube versus molecular weight of basic DNA.

2.3.5 Biomatters sensing elements of SAW devices

The developed intelligent microlab on a chip e-tongue, e-nose is intended for rapid analysis of human individual biological components, e.g., biochemical samples of blood, saliva, urine, sweat etc. At the same time, an express-diagnosis of human blood is considered as important because values of common and biochemical blood analyses correlate not only essentially to a latent pathology of human body, but are associated closely with bioinformation patterns processing by influence on neurons. In this connection, human blood is a very sensing matter, but its information and acoustical properties are close to water (Tables 4) (N.V. Khmurovich, 2010).

Wave frequency, MHz	Attenuation coefficient, dB/cm			
	10% haemoglobin solution (t=20^0 C)	blood plasma	human blood	water
0,6	0,05	0,02	0,10	0,001
1	0,09	0,06	0,21	0,0024
10	1,14	1,55	3,13	0,21
40	9,12	10,21	9,75	3,25
100	36,22	38,54	27,63	18,29

Table 4. Changes of attenuation coefficient for different reference matters of blood.

By the way, increase in wave frequency causes marked differences of acoustic speed in a human blood and its separate biochemical components. It confirms an importance of a blood information picture for analysis of latent pathologies (Table 5). The temperature rise result an abrupt increase of acoustic speed in blood exactly as in distilled water (Table 6). Thereby, blood as well as another biomatters (saliva, lymph, sweat etc.) can reflect little changes in the functioning of human body and influence on neuroinformation metabolism in brain eventually denoting the onset of diseases (Azizov & Khudnitsky, 2009).

Wave frequency, MHz,	Acoustic speed, m/s	
	10% haemoglobin solution	human blood
0,3	1558,4	1528
1	1561,3	1529,1
5	1565,6	1530,2
8	1567,5	1531,1
9	1567,8	1531,3
10	1568	1531,5

Table 5. Acoustic speed in reference biomatters depending on wave frequency.

Temperature of matter, ^0C	Acoustic speed, m/s	
	distilled water	human blood
0	1417	1462
20	1468	1512
40	1522	1558
60	1550	1577
80	1554	1596
100	1505	1614

Table 6. Dependence of acoustic speed on temperature of reference biomatters.

In the table 7 an integrated comparative assessment of human blood characteristics for different matters is shown and a characteristic impedance is calculated depending on a consistency value of matters and an acoustic speed.

Matters	Density, kg/m^3	Acoustic speed, m/s	Characteristic impedance, $kg{\cdot}m^{-2}{\cdot}s^{-1}$
blood	1060	1530	$1{,}62{\cdot}10^{-6}$
ethyl alcohol	789	1119	$0{,}883{\cdot}10^{-6}$
water	993	1527	$1{,}516{\cdot}10^{-6}$
standard air	1,2	330	$0{,}0004{\cdot}10^{-6}$
aluminum	2700	6420	$17{,}3{\cdot}10^{-6}$

Table 7. Physical characteristics of some matters in comparison with blood.

2.3.6 Microactuators on SAW

One of the most perspective directions of micromechanics developing is a design of intelligent microelectromechanical systems and an active use in such systems of actuating devices presented as microactuators on SAW. A main principle of their functioning is based on an SAW excitation in a piezoelectric substrate (quartz, $LiNbO_3$ etc.) with 100 MHz which makes a relocatable object contacting with an acoustic line to be in motion in an opposite direction of a SAW propagation velocity vector. Mentioned waves in a substrate combine longitudinal and normal components and their resultant affects the relocatable object. The SAW excitation on the substrate is realized by IDTs connected on an alternating current generator 10-100 V. The described structure of a microactuator on SAW allows to get the following key parameters: continuous velocity of travel to 1,1 m/s, linear motion acceleration to 1000 m/s^2, output mechanical force to 3,5 N. The excitation of transmitters by means of an impulse voltage with pulse-repetition interval to 200 μs makes possible to provide the movement with step of 5 nm. Advantages of microactuators on SAW are high speed, precision and positioning simplicity of a relocatable object, the integration possibility with microsensory and microprocessor devices (Gulay & Lazapnev, 2005).

2.3.7 Recognition of biomatters information patterns

An intelligent software of a broad spectrum of applications (micro-nanotechnology, biotechnology, ecology, food industry, medicine, agriculture, personal and social safety etc.) is developed for the biosensory system of rapid blood analysis on a chip e-tongue and e-nose to recognize, e.g., state of health and implicit pathologies because of injuries, accidents and latent diseases. Moreover, early recognition is important because of biomatters patterns can considerably and fast change under the influence of different factors (Table 8).

Parameters of clinical and biochemical blood analyses	Values		
	normal	till trauma	after trauma
haemoglobin, g/l	130-160	165	148
red blood cells, l	$4{,}5\text{-}5 \cdot 10^{12}$	$4{,}5 \cdot 10^{12}$	$4{,}3 \cdot 10^{12}$
leukocytes, l	$4\text{-}9 \cdot 10^9$	$4{,}1 \cdot 10^9$	$5 \cdot 10^9$
thrombocytes, l	$160\text{-}390 \cdot 10^9$	$320 \cdot 10^9$	$280 \cdot 10^9$
band forms, %	up to 4	8	5
segmented neutrophils, %	63-67	67	65
lymphocytes, %	19-37	22	21
monocytes, %	3-11	2	6
erythrocyte sedimentation rate, mm/h	up to 8	9	14
total bilirubin, mcmole / l	5-21	10,8	13,6
blood urea, mmole / l	1,7-8,3	2,9	4,1
creatinine, mmole / l	44-106	32	48
whole protein, g/l	66-87	64	67
albumen, g/l	34-48	64	56
glucose, mmole / l	3,05-6,38	6,2	5,2
AST, E/L	4-38	49	36
ALT, E/L	3-31	30	34
potassium, mmole / l	3,84-5,12	4,2	5,8
sodium, mmole / l	130,5-174	141	147

Table 8. Blood parametric changes of suffering from internal injury.

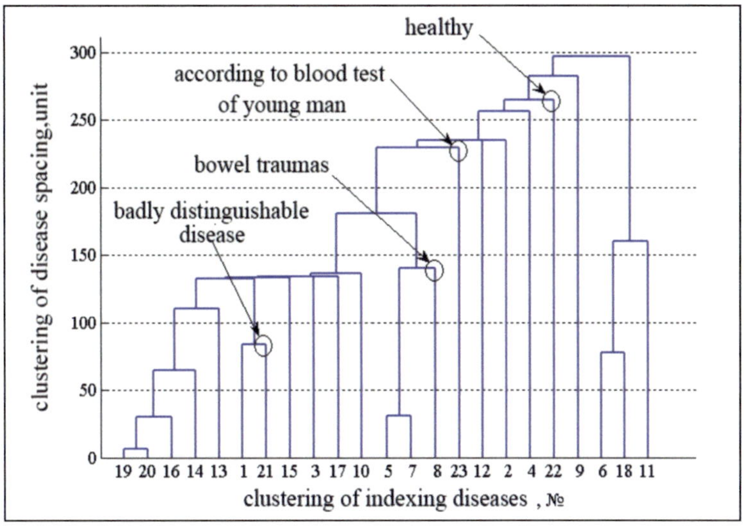

Fig. 15. Cluster analysis for recognition of bowel trauma.

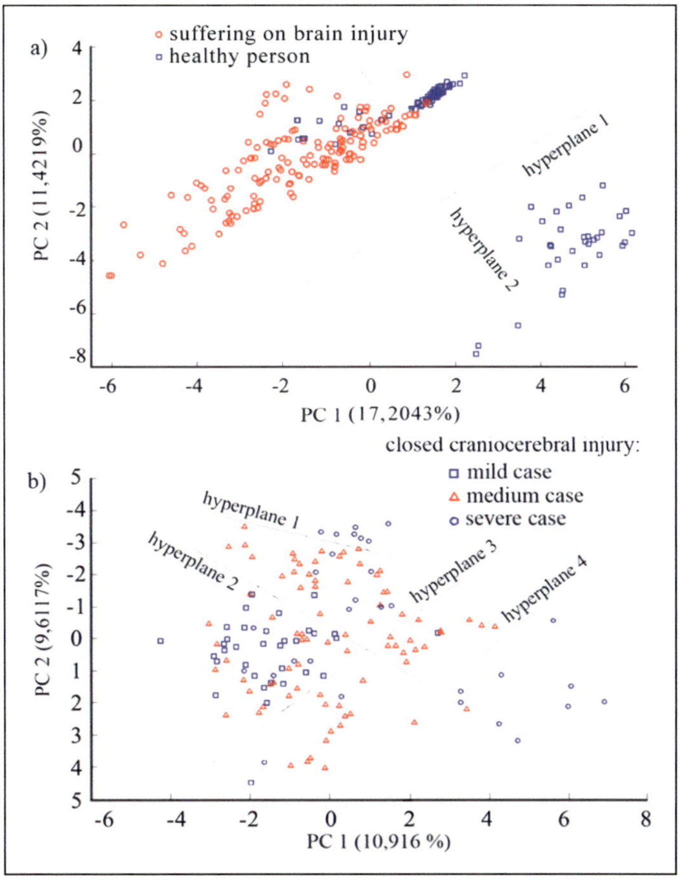

Fig. 16. Blood information patterns of closed craniocerebral injury.

The developed program carries out an analysis to detect latent pathologies, e.g., in a blood picture, but using of a matrix of symptoms in the process of diseases recognition makes it possible to achieve the highest system accuracy. Clusters algorithms rely on pattern recognition in multidimensional feature space corresponding to definitive human conditions (Fig. 15).
Figures 16, 17 and 18 show results of recognition information blood patterns before and after traumas and diseases. Therefore, it is possible to carry out rapidly a human diagnostics and to prevent the data deference in a high-cost research laboratory.

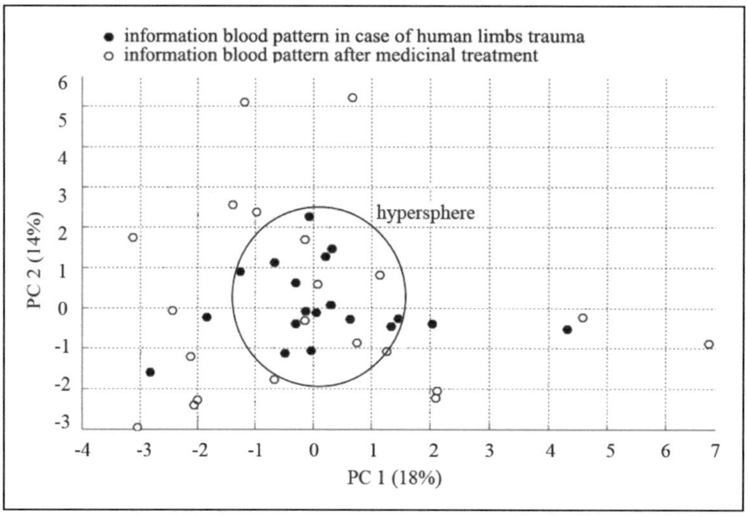

Fig. 17. Blood information patterns before/after trauma of human limbs.

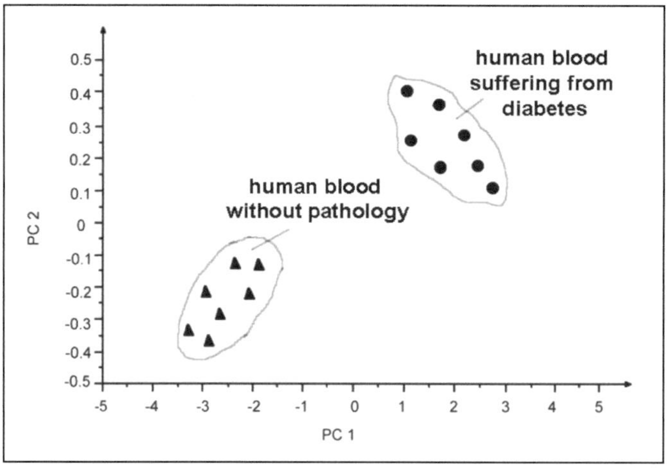

Fig. 18. Blood information patterns suffering from diabetes.

The base components of an information pattern of saliva are K^+ , Na^+ ions, protein, glucose and an acoustic coefficient equals numerically a ratio of ultrasonic waves velocity in saliva to the one in water. Figure 19 depicts information patterns of saliva in the two-dimensional space of the first two principal components for different subjects.

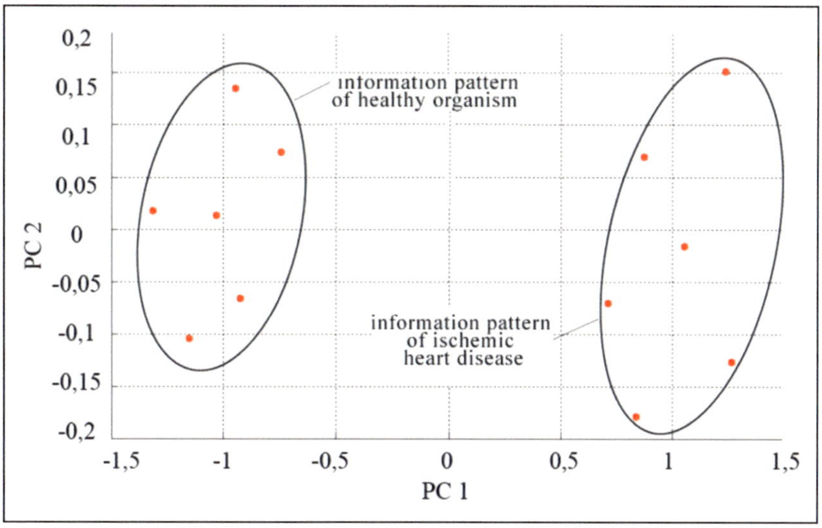

Fig. 19. Saliva information patterns suffering from ischemic heart disease.

Information pattern recognition of human urine (Table 9), e.g., in diagnostics of urolithiasis is based on a clinical urine analysis using physical-acoustic and electroacoustical properties. The developed diagnostic system allows to process data of urine analysis fast and with the high detection probability (79,07 %).

Clinical parameters of urine analysis	Values, ml		
	norm	healthy man	sick man
potassium, K	35-90	40	31
sodium, Na	150-220	175	140
calcium, Ca	2,5-7,5	3,4	2,7
chlorine, Cl	115-220	162	84
phosphorus, P	29-45	37	28
uric acid	1,2-7,1	3,6	5,2
urates	till 0,7	0,57	0,65
dielectric capacitivity, (nondimensional quantity)	less 17,5	24	15

Table 9. Information sensory pattern recognition of urine.

3. Sensory system on a chip electronic eye

Intelligent analysis systems of information optical patterns of human biomatters (blood, saliva, sweat, urine etc.) present an innovative class of smart laboratories on a chip of the type "electronic eye". The light-emitting microdiodes (LED) emit given electromagnetic waves in the frequency range 10^{11}-10^{15} Hz, but microphotodiodes register quantitative changes of a reflected radiation (absorption, refraction, light scattering coefficients etc.). It is possible to analyze different changes of optical matter properties and a hardware miniaturization of the intelligent recognition system allows to adopt it to any other systems depending on application purposes (Fig. 20) (Gulay & Polynkova, 2010).

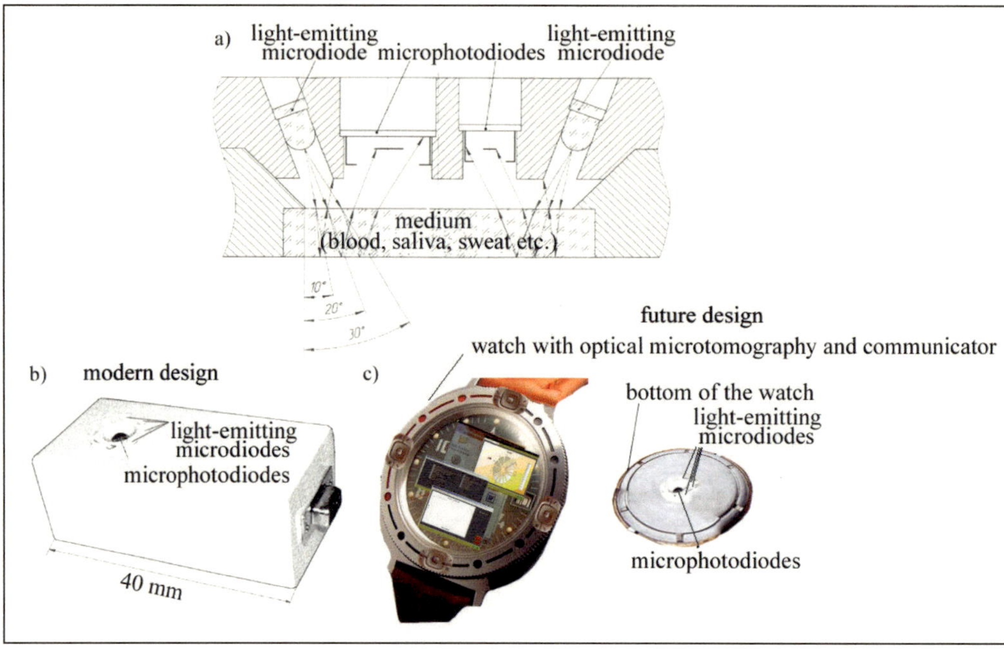

Fig. 20. Analysis of investigated matters by optical broadband microtomograph (a), general form (b) for diagnostics and in the intelligent watch (c) with optical pattern recognition.

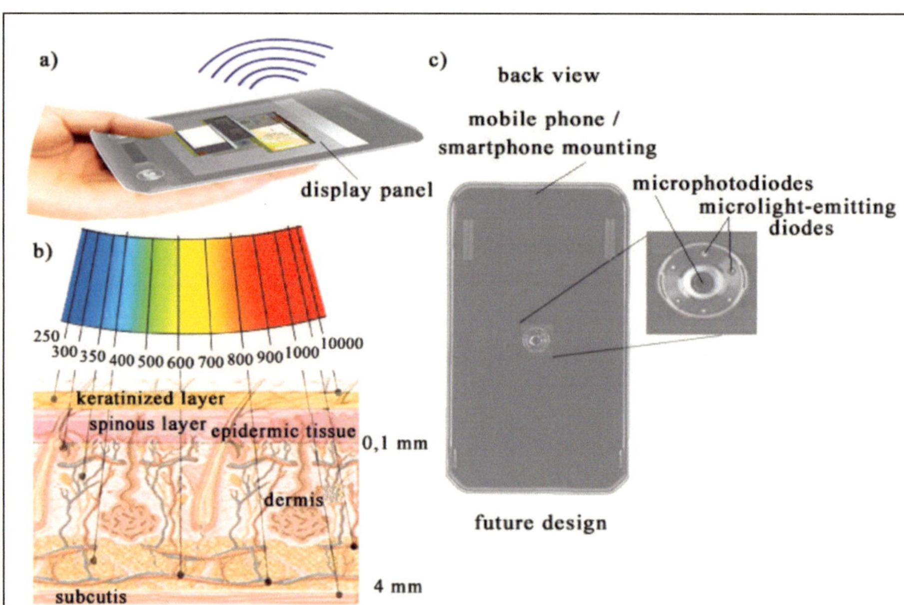

Fig. 21. E-eye sensory system in mobile devices. (a) Developed smartphone with optical recognition system e-eye. (b) Penetration of electromagnetic waves with different wavelengths in skin of user's palm holding smartphone in one's hand. (c) General view of smartphone with embedded sensory system e-eye.

Then it makes a comparison between the known information pattern and all reference models of human biomatter to determine a degree of manifestation for the given pattern and its influence on human health. Smart multiprocessing enables flexible on-line modeling of intelligent systems with a calculation of individual optimal micro-nanosensory parameters of the optical microtomography. For example, the mobile intelligent system (Fig. 21) enables to carry out an operative prediction about a health status and doesn't require special application conditions or highly skilled specialists.

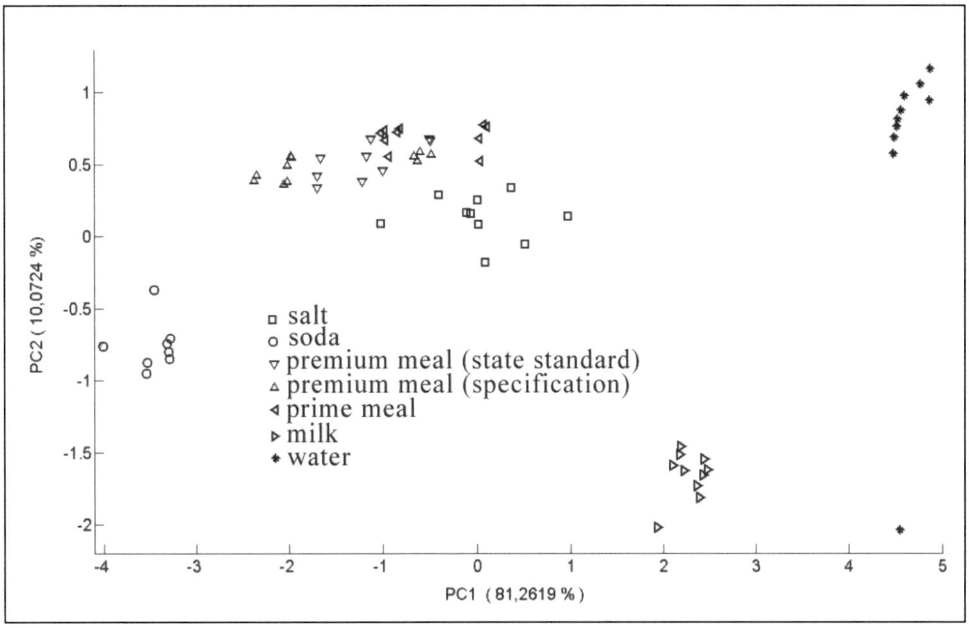

Fig. 22. Recognition of information patterns of foodstuffs.

Our developed systems find a broad spectrum of applications, e.g., for:

- toxic and biological agents, explosive hazard and narcotic searching in complex sensory systems and networks;
- rapid recognition of acute infections by the use of breathing diagnostic and early detection of latent diseases;
- monitoring of children's homes, maternity wards, old people's homes (Polynkova & N.V. Khmurovich, 1997);
- individual noninvasive monitoring of human health and continuous control of its functional state of organism due to intelligent sensory systems and networks;
- helping, e.g., medical staffs and prompting them of important decision making;
- production process monitoring (Fig. 22) in pharmaceutics, rejecting mechanism of primary goods, storage accommodation safety, drinking, nicotine and drug abuse determination;
- air analysis in industrial and agricultural enterprises, monitoring of noxious vapors, wastes;
- control of firefanging threshold in agriculture;
- analysis of soil information patterns in precise agriculture (Fig. 23) (Gulay & Polynkova, 2010);

- problem-solving of on-the-job injury rate and human-factor error accidents in modern enterprises by testing of any staff;
- ensuring of personal and social safety and safe control against terrorism and corrupt government officials.

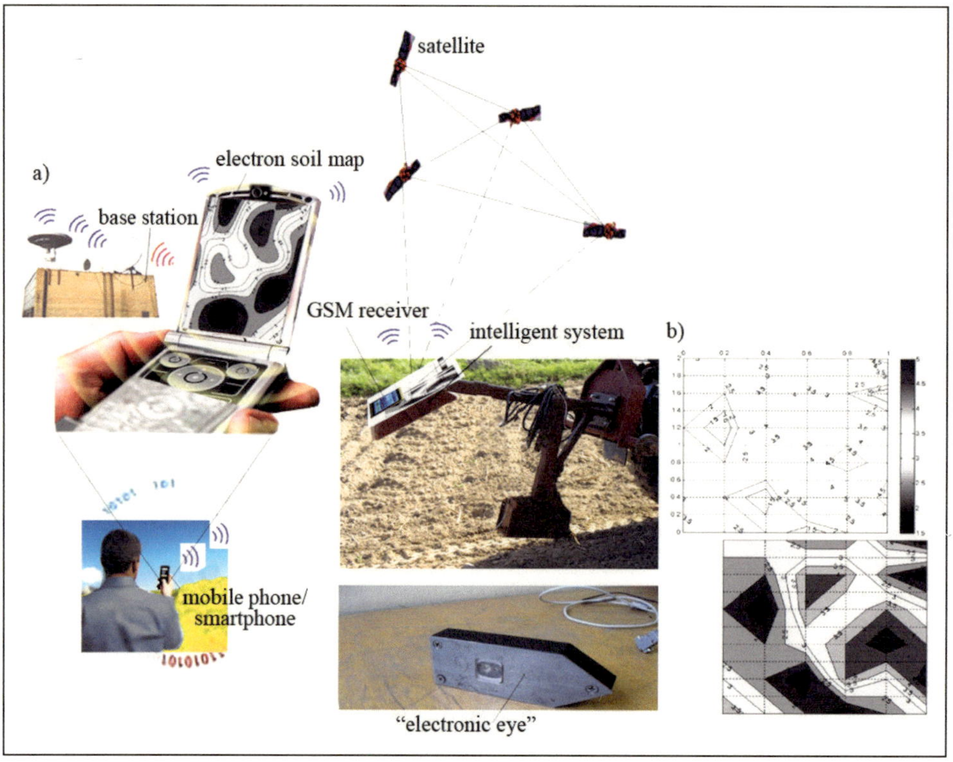

Fig. 23. Mobile soil analyser for precise agriculture (a), satellite "electronic map" of field (b).

4. Radio frequency identification systems

4.1 Remote sensing of information patterns by means of SAW sensors

Radio frequency identification (RFID) systems have been developing over recent years and find wide applications in micro-nanosensory technologies, production monitoring, ecology, security systems, transport tracking systems etc. Combining of a SAW sensor with a RFID system enables to design a new wireless micro-nanosensory device (Polunkova, 2007). A main idea of such intelligent system includes a latent placement of inexpensive SAW sensors in public gathering areas (waiting room, airport, railway terminal, cloakrooms etc.). Transducer makes a connection to an antenna in a specified operation frequency range, but SAWs are stimulated by antenna irradiation of electromagnetic signal. A substrate of SAW sensors contains IDT and many reflecting segments and metal strips reflect an electrically induced acoustic wave so that constructive interference obtains. When launching is stopped after a while, surface-mode waves goes on still and disappears in 25 μs, so next exciting acoustic wave is to be generated. The IDTs signal is transformed in SAW propagating to reflectors and backward directions and back in an electromagnetic signal. Then the generated in 5-20 μs reflected signal contains important information concerning propagation characteristics and environmental effects on acoustic lines. This one is transmitted in the antenna outside and can be successfully detected by receiver which measures its parameters and determines specific gaseous substances. The structure chart of the intelligent system for detection of odor matters is presented in figure 24.

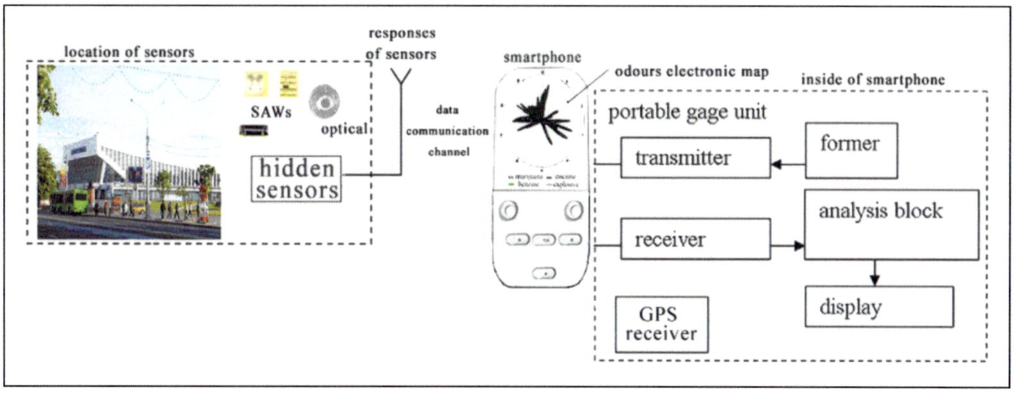

Fig. 24. Environmental intelligent monitoring system.

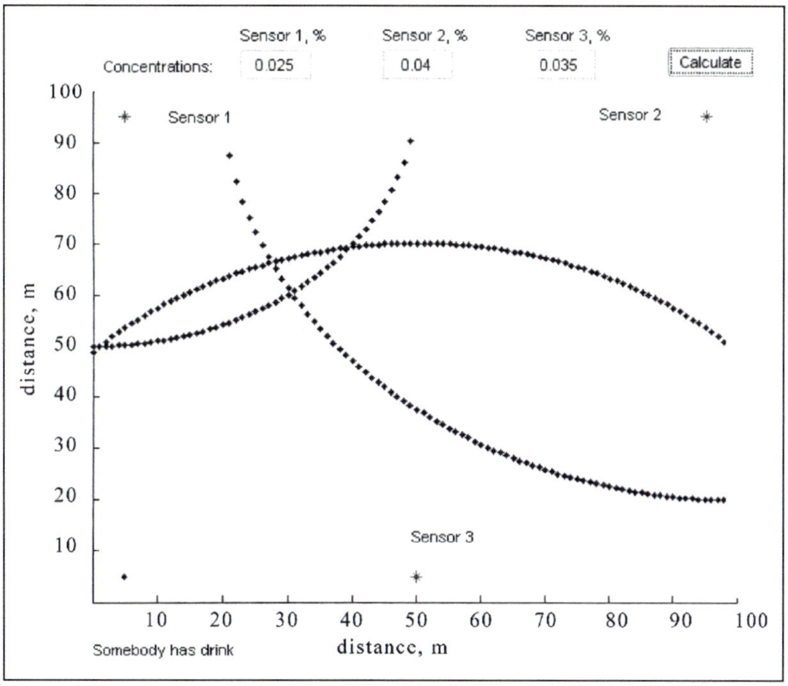

Fig. 25. Intelligent system for detection of ethyl alcohol vapors in sensory networks.

4.2 Sensory networks

A universal contactless multicore intelligent system "ISA" for control in sensory networks, e.g., of ethyl alcohol vapor in any spaces is developed which enables to define instantly drinking using not remote labs, but a distributed intellect in multidimensional space of

sensory networks to recognize of information patterns of human health status, dangerous substances and explosives etc. Vapors concentration characterises the remoteness of a source from a sensor, but radiuses of remoteness (Fig. 25) define an intersection region.
Every sensor of e-tongue and e-nose is characterized by different partial sensitivity to an analyzable taste, an odor spaces, but the combined characteristics of all sensor responses can be used to identify an information pattern in computer technologies and sensory networks. Amplitude modulation is used for information transferring on a resonance frequency of an oscillating circuit. Figure 26a presents dependence of a power propagation factor on the distance between the rider and the SAW retransmitter.

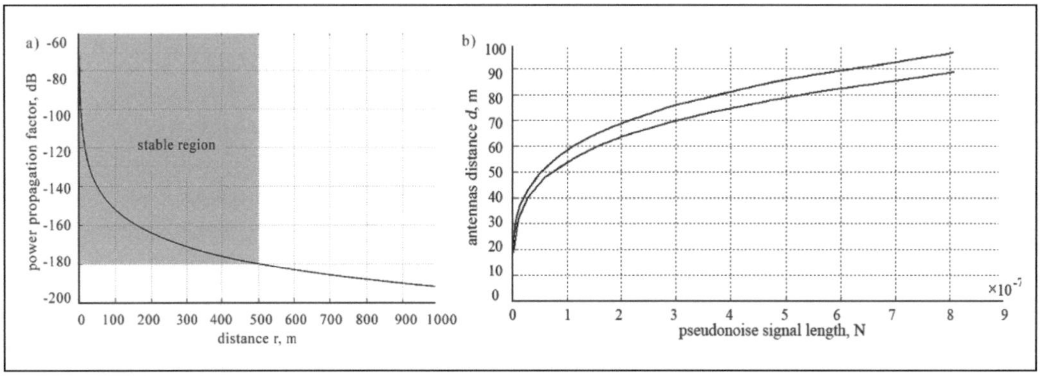

Fig. 26. Stable region of RFID system (a) and characteristics of channel reliability (b).

For example, 430 MHz sensor working in the mode of delay line or in the excitation mode has the frequency band up to 1 MHz. The receiver of this frequency range has the sensitivity $P_0=3{\cdot}10^{-15}$ W= 150 dB/W in case of the signal-to-noise ratio equals numerically 10 dB in transmission band and at the distance approximately 10 m. Using of pseudonoise signals in the length more million enables to achieve the considerable distance about 50 m for reliable functioning of remote hidden passive e-noses and e-tongues. Characteristics of channel reliability depending on used pseudonoise signals are shown in figure 26b. The maximal distance of a rider and a SAW retransmitter equals to $r_{max} \approx 500$ m, when the noise-to-signal ratio in the rider antenna makes 100. Thus, an active SAW sensory antenna makes it possible to increase the maximal distance up to r_{max}=50 km.

5. Multicore system of pattern recognition

A design of microelectronic components and a progress trend of processor throughputs are related to the development of multicore technologies with parallel architecture which are close to the functionality cerebration concerning computational powers (Table 10). An intelligent multicore recognition system of multidimensional sensory patterns is developed on the basis of SAW micro-nanosensors on a chip e-tongue, e-nose and an optical microtomography e-eye in the broadband frequency range (Gulay & Polynkova, 2010). The developed intelligent system "WIS" includes multicore and parallel processing technologies for fast self-learning and on-line recognition of information sensory patterns of blood, saliva, sweat, urine etc. Intelligent client applications in Visual Studio enable to design rapid unique softwares on different platforms by means of NET. Framework 3.5, to use a Parallel Extensions library for fast data processing depending on numbers of available cores and to

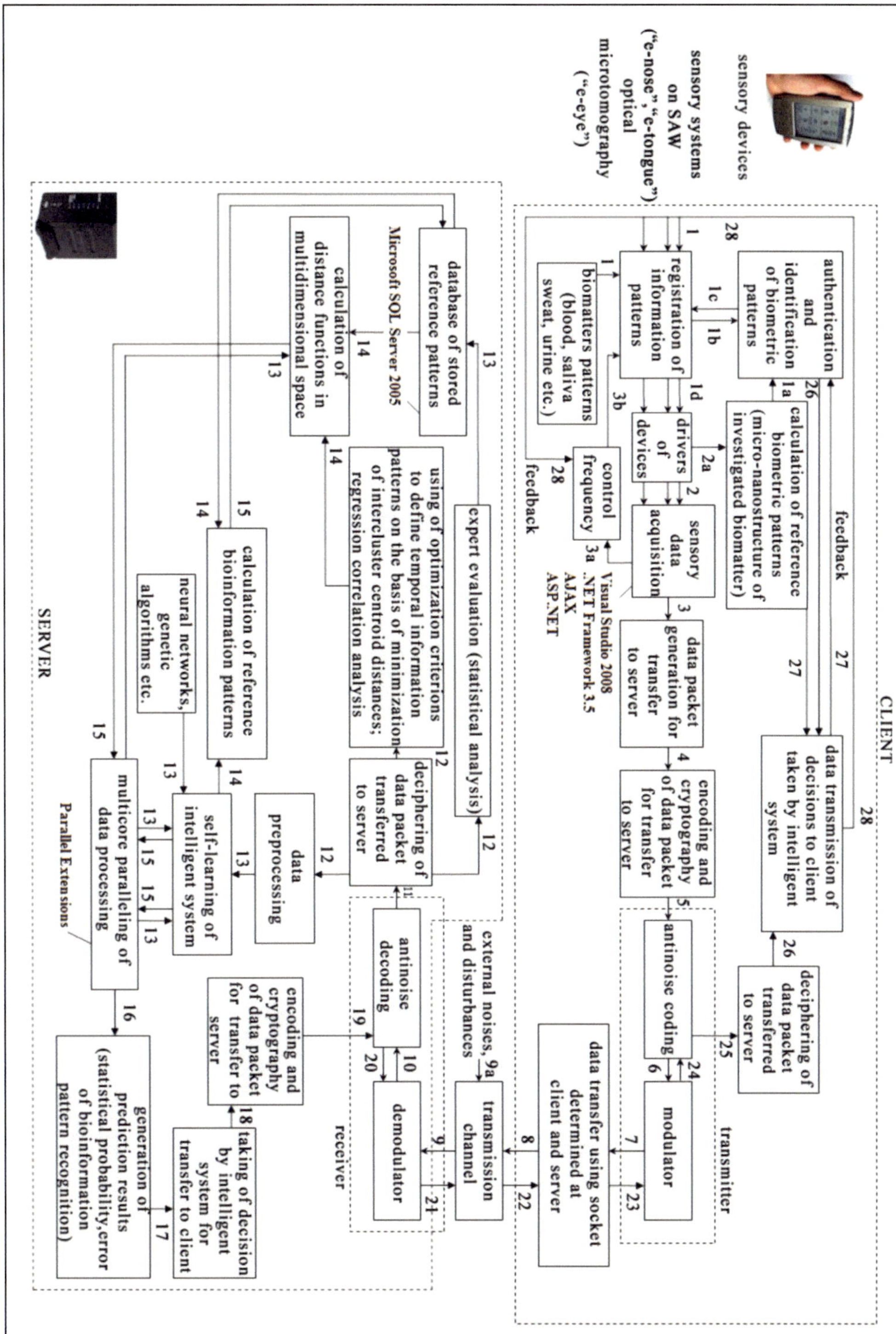

Fig. 27. Functional diagram of intelligent system "WIS".

apply practically SQL Server opening wide possibilities for Web-applications. The developed intelligent system "WIS" can be embedded, e.g., in a wristwatch or in mobile phones and smartphones for different individual applications (Fig. 27). A data packet is generated for remote wireless transferring to a server after registration of information sensory patterns of blood, saliva, sweat or foodstuffs etc. Data encoding and information encryption of sensory devices and antinoise coding are fulfilled before transmission. Information-translation process realizes using a socket determined at a client and a server to assure an entry of data to the server.

Parameters	Characteristic features	
	current systems on a chip	human brain
processor throughputs, flops	single-precision 8,942 $\cdot 10^{11}$ (supercomputer Roadrunner 1,4567$\cdot 10^{15}$)	close to 10^{16}
weight	(supercomputer Roadrunner) 226 tonnes	1,4 kg
energy consumption, W	(supercomputer Roadrunner) 3,9$\cdot 10^{6}$ (videochip AMD RV770) 150	25
clock frequency, Hz	3,33$\cdot 10^{9}$	10^{14}
heat energy, J	(switching energy of microchip) up to 10^{-13}	(energy of nerve impulse) 5$\cdot 10^{-15}$
information capacity, bit	(technical process 22 nm) 364$\cdot 10^{6}$ per cm^2	10^{23}
memory bandwidth, bit per sec	10^{12}	10^{18}
number of elements, pcs	(transistors) up to 2,9$\cdot 10^{9}$ per cm^2	(neurons) up to 4$\cdot 10^{7}$ per cm^3
linear size, m	(transistor) up to 22$\cdot 10^{-9}$	(neuron) 10^{-6}
data-processing mode	parallel-serial mode (more 80 cores)	flexible self-adjusting parallelism

Table 10. Brain and technical system.

Methods of self-learning		Execution time, sec			Root-mean-square error (RMSE)
		one-core		multicore	
		Intel Pentium 3 753 GHz	Intel Pentium 4 3 GHz	Intel Core 2 Duo T8300, 2,4 GHz	
neural networks		0,5426	0,1023	0,0409	0,3428
group method of data handling	twain	54,1732	15,3611	3,5423	0,2804
	triplet	186,8461	24,0156	12,3106	0,2093

Table 11. Information pattern recognition of urolithiasis in human urine.

Intelligent system "WIS" makes it possible to achieve high training speed, to apply advanced parallelism for the purpose of recognition of multidimensional sensory patterns of biomatters (Table 11) and for a design of effective not energy-intensive intelligent systems.

6. Intelligent information systems security

Using of traditional techniques of a biometric identification and authentication is connected with problems in relation to external influences determining a distortion of biometric information and safety features of controllable and reference objects (Azizov, 2009). Intelligent patented technology of protection against falsification, substitution, imitation of biometric parameters is developed which can be applied in different fields of human activity, in particularly, in information and communication networks. A new principle of group features on the basis of set of physicochemical and biological characteristics uses a nanostructure of traditional and prospective biometric information characteristics, their nanomechanic, electronic, gaseous, optical components (Fig. 28).

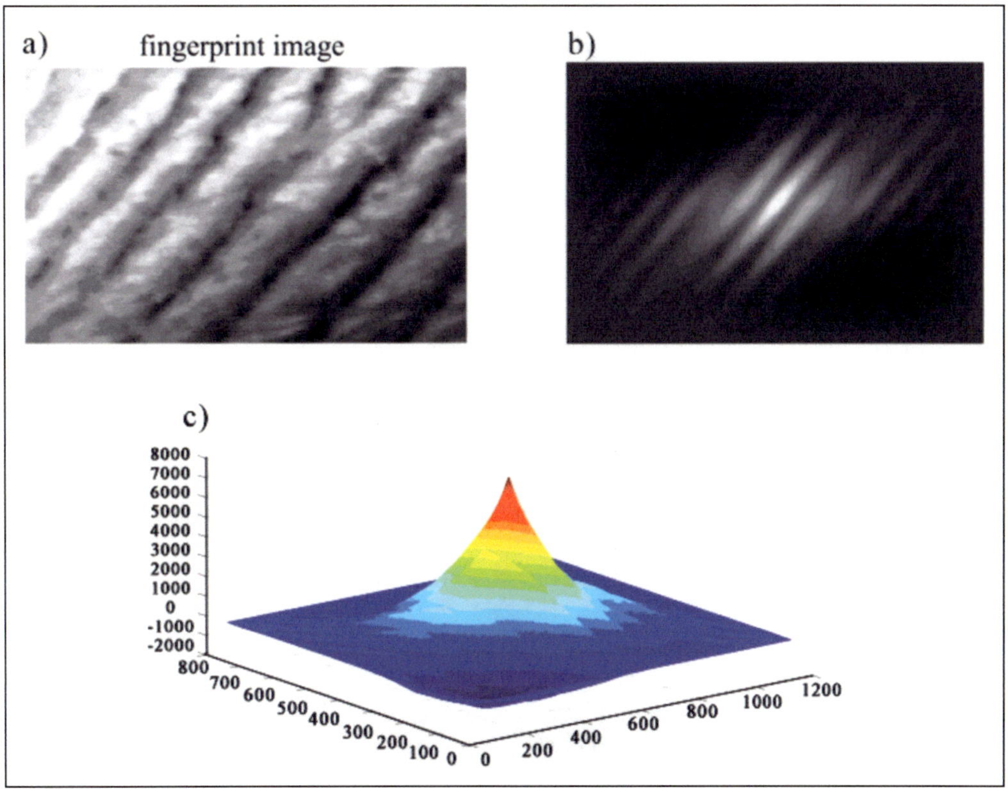

Fig. 28. Superprotection technology of biometric data: (a) information pattern of fingerprint, bivariate (b) / three-dimensional (c) cross-correlation function between fingerprint and image of reference object.

7. Conclusion

The developed intelligent sensory micro-nanosystems and networks including e-tongue, e-nose on SAW and e-eye for individual applications, recognition of information biomatters patterns (blood, saliva, sweat etc.) are shown. These multicore intelligent systems can be embedded in up-to-date mobile devices (cell phones, smartphones, communicator etc.) or in a wristwatch, can fast recognize any patterns by means of Internet global sensory networks.

8. References

Azizov, P.M. & Khudnitsky A.A. (2009). Intelligent System for Biotesting of Thoughts in Production Process. *Proceedings of the Samara Scientific Center of the Russian Academy of Sciences (Special Edition)*, pp. 254-261, Samara, Russia, April 2-3, 2009

Azizov, P.M.; Khudnitsky A.A. & Snigirev S.A. (2009). Prospective techniques of biometrical authentication and identification, *Belarusian National Technical University*, Belarus, Minsk

Barkaline, V.V. & Polynkova, E.V. (2002). Smart Materials of Sensory Microelectromechanical Systems. *Modern methods of mashines design. Computing, Engineering and Integration Technology*, Vol.3, pp. 116-121

Deinak, D.A.; Chashynski, A.S. & Khmurovich, N.V. (2009). Desing of Electronic Nose on Basis of Nanotubes and DNA, *Nano-Microsystem Technics*, Vol.9, No. 110, pp. 2-6

Gulay, A.V. & Lazapnev E.V. (2005). Analytical Modeling of the Surface Acoustic Wave Microactuators, *Perspective Technologies and Methods in MEMS Design*, pp. 14-15, Lviv-Polyana, Ukraine, May 25-28, 2005

Gulay, A.V & Polynkova, E.V (2010). Optical Sensory Recognition System of Information Patterns of Human Biomatters, *Proceedings of Medelectronics-2010 on Tools of Medical Electronics and New Medical Technologies*, pp. 42-43, Minsk, Belarus, December 6-8, 2010

Khmurovich, N.V. (2010). Intelligent Sensory Nanosystem of Genom Sequencing, *Proceedings of II International Scientific Conference on Nanostructured Materials-2010: Belarus-Russia-Ukraine (NANO-2010)*, pp. 653, Kiev, Ukraine, October 19-22, 2010

Koleshko, V.M (1974, 1976, 1981, 1983, 1984, 1985, 1986, 1987, 1988, 1989, 1990). *Certificate of USSR Authorship for Invention № 491824 ,№ 519048, № 608377, № 720693, № 843632, № 1104363, № 1105803, № 1127470, № 1138668, № 1144562, №* 1159457, *№ 1182293, № 1182939, № 1191765, № 1191817, № 1250858, № 1251661, № 1262317, № 1264013, № 1291829, № 1340521, № 1349672, № 1371176, № 1378721, № 1410642, № 1426400, № 1436831, № 1450708, № 1501867, № 1572187, № 1591724, № 1634063, № 1634069, № 1634111, № 1648234, № 1801463, № 3646150*

Meshkov, Yu.V & Barkaline, V.V. (1990). Strain Effect in Single-Crystal Silicon Based Multilayer Surface Acoustic Wave Structures, *Thin Solid Films*, Vol.190, pp. 359-372

Polynkova, E.V. & Khmurovich, N.V. (1997). *Global Monitoring and Control System of Personal and Social Safety*, BITA, Belarus, Minsk

Polynkova, E.V. (2007). Sensory Micro-Nanosystems on Surface-Acoustic-Waves with Radio-Frequency Identification, *Collection of IV Scientific and Practical Conference on Nanotechnology in Production 2007*, pp. 126-132, Frjazino, Russia, November, 2007

3

SPR Biosensor Technique Supports Development in Biomaterials Engineering

Bogdan Walkowiak et al.*
Department of Biophysics, Technical University of Lodz, Poland

1. Introduction

Various biomaterials are presently employed in the production of a very wide spectrum of medical implants. The choice of biomaterial is of course determined by the medical application for which it is intended and to date no one biomaterial has been found to be fully biocompatible and biotolerant. Furthermore, it is a well known fact that quite often implants must be removed due to tissue reactions and resultant health problems (Khan et al. 2008; Schierholz& Beuth, 2001). The key role in implant tolerance depends on a very short period of time during which the biomaterial surface first comes into contact with body fluids. During this time, water molecules come into contact with the surface of the biomaterial and the results of this reaction determine the further course of events. Water molecule interaction is generally dependent on surface nanostructure and highly dependent on its energy and hydrophobicity. The next stage of interaction, which depends on the presence of water on the biomaterial surface, is the creation of a thin protein film on this surface. A hydrophilic surface will collect a large amount of hydrophilic proteins readily available in body fluids, however these proteins are weakly adsorbed and can be easily removed or replaced by other molecules. A hydrophobic surface will adsorb proteins by their hydrophobic regions often causing changes in protein structure and biological activity. The final stage, cellular attachment, adhesion and proliferation depends on the profile of the adsorbed proteins, their accessibility and a proper spatial structure which enables expression of biologically active sites. Thus, the type of protein present on a biomaterial surface seems to be crucial for biomaterial tolerance in the human body. The most common experimental models developed to characterize protein adsorption on biomaterial surfaces involve the incubation of proteins in contact with a studied surface and the estimation of adsorbed proteins by a variety of methods including electrophoretic, enzymatic or immunoenzymatic approaches together with a number of labeling techniques. The common disadvantages of these techniques is that it is not possible to observe protein adsorption as a kinetic process and protein quantification is strongly limited by the sensitivity of the methods used, which is usually limited to nanograms per square millimeter. Surface

* Witold Szymanski[1], Jacek Szymanski[2], Marta Walczynska[1], Magdalena Walkowiak-Przybyło[1], Piotr Komorowski[1], Wiesława Okrój[1], Witold Jakubowski[1] and Marta Kaminska[1]
[1]*Department of Biophysics, Technical University of Lodz,* [2]*CoreLab of Medical University of Lodz, BioTechMed Technology Centre Lodz, Poland*

plasmon resonance (SPR) technology is a potent analytical tool for biomaterial surface study. This technology makes it possible to prepare a surface of interest (including polymers, metals, ceramics or carbon) and essentially make it the biosensor surface. Subsequently, the kinetics of molecule adsorption to the surface can be observed in real time, without the need for any labeling, together with an extremely high sensitivity of picograms per square millimeter. Moreover, this technique also allows for the identification and quantification of adsorbed molecules by use of specific antibodies. The aim of the present study was to develop conditions that enabled the measurement of plasma protein adsorption to a variety of biomaterials (including Parylene C, nanocrystalline diamond and titanium alloy) using commercially available glass plates pre-coated with gold. The preliminary results obtained regarding plasma protein adsorption were compared with blood platelets adhesion, *E. coli* and endothelial cells proliferation, as well as changes in proteome of endothelial cells grown on the surfaces of these materials.

2. SPR biosensor technique in biomaterials engineering

The SPR effect, as a convenient tool for surface investigation, was mentioned in the monograph describing usable analytical techniques for biomaterial surface study (Davies & Faulkner, 1996; Davies & Skelton, 1996). The following year a study concerning bovine serum albumin (BSA) adsorption by thiolated dextran layers present on metallic surfaces, monitored by SPR technique, was reported (Frazier et al. 1997). In subsequent years SPR sensors were used for kinetic studies of protein adsorption by polymeric surfaces (Green et al. 1997; Green et al. 1999) and degradation of polymer surface (Green et al. 2000). Papers describing SPR technique as a method of supplementing atomic force microscopy (AFM) in biomaterial studies have also been published (Vansteenkiste et al. 2000; Jung et al. 2009). Beside the most frequently studied polymeric biomaterials, SPR technique was also used to study nanocrystalline diamond surfaces and their interaction with plasma proteins (Walkowiak et al. 2002). Nevertheless, none of these reports describes the application of SPR sensors to the study of metallic biomaterials, other than substrate metals of the SPR sensor itself.

2.1 Background of SPR biosensor functioning

The first documented observation of surface plasmons was reported in 1902 (Wood, 1902). These observations concerned anomalies in the spectrum of light diffracted on a metallic diffraction grating. The first theoretical approach to these abnormalities was undertaken by Lord Rayleigh (Lord Rayleigh, 1907) and was continued by Fano (Fano, 1941), who proved that these anomalies result from excitation of electromagnetic waves on the diffraction grating. A complete explanation of this phenomenon was reported in 1968 in different studies that described excitation of surface plasmons (Otto, 1968; Kretschmann & Raether, 1968). Since that time the phenomenon of surface plasmon resonance (SPR) has found practical applications in modern optics, as a sensitive detector for monitoring molecular interactions in real time without needing to label interacting molecules. A historical overview and fundamentals of surface plasmon resonance can be found in numerous review articles and books (Tudos & Schasfoort, 2008; Kooyman, 2008; Homola, 2008). The most common geometry in which a surface plasmon can be found, is the structure of dielectric-metal interface. Analysis performed using Maxwell's equations with appropriate boundary conditions, indicates that this structure can support only a single guided mode of electromagnetic fields i.e. a surface plasmon. Several configurations of SPR devices capable of generating and detecting SPR signals can be utilized for biosensor construction. These are: a) prism coupled total internal reflection (TIR) system, b) optical fibers, c) grating coupled systems, and d) optical wave-guide systems. Of these the most frequently used is the prism-based system, which was developed for the Kretchman configuration (Kretschmann & Raether, 1968) This refers to an arrangement where a metal layer is put directly on a top of a TIR surface (prism) enabling efficient plasmon generation. The second most commonly applied configuration utilizes core optical fibers coated with a thin metallic film. When light enters the fiber at certain discrete angles, the conditions for SPR generation and signal detection are fulfilled (Kanso et al., 2008). The last two configurations are rather less important for biosensor construction, however new systems that use these techniques have aroused great interest. In a grating coupled system light penetrates a flow channel and is angle-reflected onto diffraction grating. The effective refractive index depends on the concentration of particles within a flowing sample (Hoa, et al. 2009). An optical wave-guide system is a somewhat similar to the optical fiber based configuration, here a glass plate instead of an optical fiber is used (Suzuki et al., 2005).

Most commercially available systems are working in the Kretchman configuration. Put simply this SPR method can be described as a physical process taking place when plane-polarized light, propagated in a dielectric environment, hits a metal surface under total internal reflection (TIR) conditions. Assuming that the dielectric-metal interface consists of a transparent dielectric (glass prism) and a layer of metal of suitable thickness, we can consider an evanescent p-polarized electromagnetic field (light) penetrating the metal layer, which excite plasmon surface wave propagating within the conductor surface. For a non-magnetic metal such as gold, this surface plasmon wave is also p-polarized. Because the electric field of this wave also penetrates a short distance into the external environment, usually with a lower refractive index, the conditions for SPR are sensitive to the refractive index of the media at the gold surface. When the wavevectors for the photon and plasmon are equal in magnitude and direction, the resonance condition can be fulfilled. Thus, an increased refractive index of the medium (sample) penetrated by the plasmon increases the wavevector of the plasmon wave. Varying the angle of incidence or the wavelength of light, the wavevector of the light can be attuned to the plasmon wavevector. This enables resonant absorption of energy via the plasmon excitation (SPR) causing a characteristic drop in the reflected light intensity. For a fixed wavelength of incident p-polarized light, SPR is seen as a drop in the intensity of reflected p-polarized light at a specific angle of incidence. Biomolecular interactions occurring at the sensor surface affect the solute concentration and thus the refractive index. The SPR angle is therefore altered and the resulting angle shift is measured as a response signal. In general, different biomolecules have very similar contributions to the refractive index, thus SPR provides an extremely sensitive detector of mass change on the sensor surface. Moreover, it is very important for laboratory practice that the technique requires no labeling of the interacting molecules. A linear correlation between resonance angle shift and protein surface concentration determined via a radiometric method has been reported in the literature (Stenberg et al., 1990). The sensitivity of the mass change detection on the sensor surface depends on the instrument used, more precisely the type and resolution of the refractrometer, which can vary between 50 pg/mm^2 (Stenberg et al., 1990) and 1 pg/mm^2 (our own observations).

The geometric scheme of the measurement cell used in the BiaCore X instrument is shown in Figure 1. The prism and the glass plate of the SPR sensor are made of the same high quality glass and create one piece of a transparent dielectric. The other side of glass plate is coated with a thin gold film usually carrying a dextran matrix suitable for chemical immobilization of selected biomolecules. For our experiments we used a pure gold sensor surface instead of gold coated with dextran. The gold coated side of the sensor surface completes the flow cell of a flow channel and is a place where molecular interactions can be observed. P-polarized light comes from the monochromator and passes through the prism, the glass plate and reaches the gold film, where it excites a plasmon wave. The resonance of plasmon evanescent waves and light results in the energy deficit of the reflected light, which can be detected for specific resonance angles. Binding of flowing molecules (analyte) to the immobilized molecules (ligand) results in a shift in the reflected resonance angle.

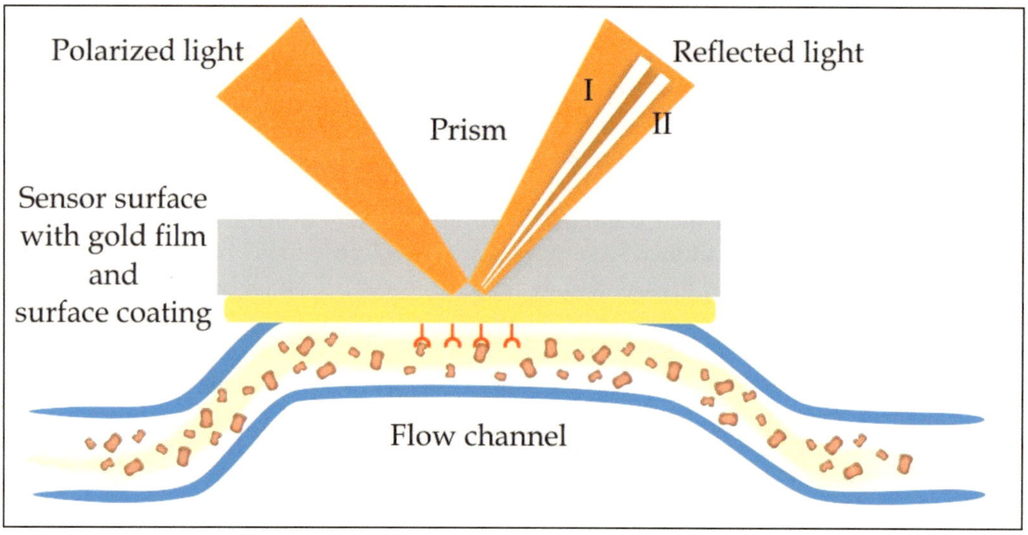

Fig. 1. The geometry scheme of the measurement cell in the BiaCore X instrument (the scheme was adopted from Surface Plasmon Resonance Technology Note 1, Biacore AB, Sweden).

A typical response produced by the SPR biosensor technique is presented in Figure 2. The response signal can be expressed as a shift in resonance angle (degree) or as a resonance unit (RU). The baseline represents the response attributed to the initial level of mass at the sensor surface. An injection of analyte over the immobilized ligand results in a two-component response. The first part, a bulk response, corresponds to the presence of a constant amount of mass flowing by the sensor surface during the injection interval. This subsequently drops to the level of the baseline when injection is finished. The second component, a binding response, corresponds to an increase in mass resulting from binding of analyte molecules, including nonspecific interactions. The response increases until binding saturation is achieved, which means an equilibrium between the number of associated and dissociated complexes is reached. This phase is considered as an association phase. When injection is stopped, the bulk response is rapidly switched off, and the dissociation phase of bound analyte is observed. The cycle can also be repeated with different analytes, for example enhancing specific antibody.

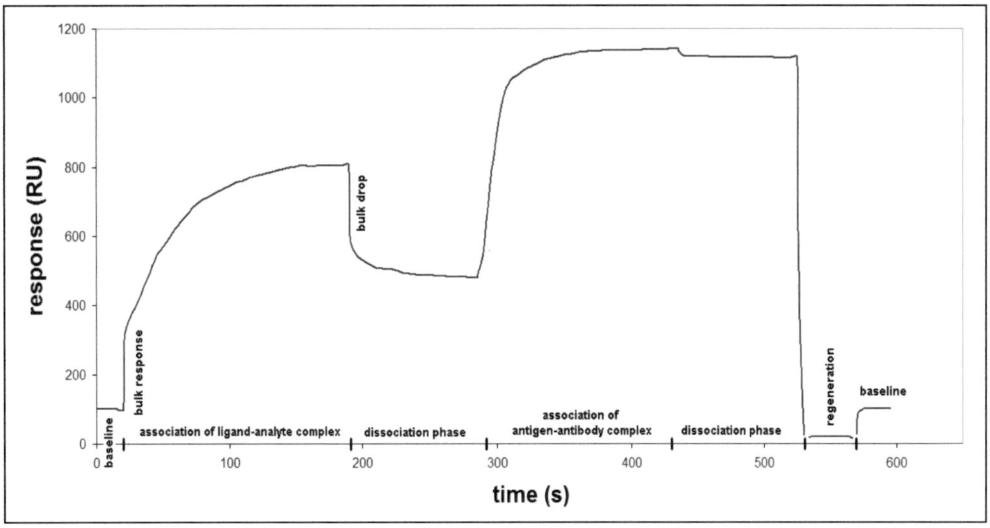

Fig. 2. Typical response produced by the SPR biosensor technique

Collected data can be used for analyte fishing and recognition, concentration estimation or kinetic analysis. Very useful surveys of literature, concerning commercially available SPR systems, containing a lot of interesting suggestions and comments, regularly updated since 1999 is accessible (Myszka, 1999; Rich & Myszka, 2010).

3. Materials and methods

Samples for the study of blood platelet adhesion, endothelial cell proliferation and bacterial biofilm formation were prepared as follows: a round bar (8 mm in diameter) of commercially available stainless steel (AISI 316 L) was cut into discs each 3 mm thick. These discs where then machined, polished and later coated with nanocrystalline diamond (NCD) or chlorinated poly(para-xylylene) (Parylene C). Titanium alloy samples were prepared as above using a Ti6Al4V round (8 mm) bar substrate. For blood plasma protein adsorption studies samples were prepared on commercially available pre-sensor glass plates precoated with gold (SIA Kit AU, BiaCore Life Sciences). A carbon layer was synthesized on the gold surface of the pre-sensor and characterized as described previously (Mitura et al. 1999; Okroj et al. 2006), with a slight modification that involved adjusting the duration of the process. The purpose of this alteration was to obtain a uniform carbon layer with a thickness of approximately 10 nm. Ten nanometer thick layer of Parylene C was deposited onto the gold surface of the pre-sensor by chemical vapour deposition (CVD) method in a manner that had been reported previously (Gazicki-Lipman 2007; Kaminska et al. 2009). Titanium alloy layer was prepared by magnetron sputtering of titanium substrate (Wendler et al. 2004) with process parameters tailored to achieve uniform and thin (10 and 20 nm) coatings. All sample surfaces were prepared at the Institute of Materials Science and Engineering, Technical University of Lodz, Poland, and were kindly provided by Prof. Stanislaw Mitura, Prof. Maciej Gazicki-Lipman and Prof. Bogdan Wendler.
Hydrophobicity of the studied surfaces was estimated by measurement of the contact angle of deionized water droplets. The values of the contact angle were determined using the commonly available software Image J.

Adsorption of blood plasma proteins on the surface of the examined samples, under flow conditions, was measured with a BIACore X system (BIACore AB, Uppsala, Sweden). The system temperature was set at 37°C. After sensor docking the system was primed with HBS-EP buffer containing 0.01 M HEPES, 0.15 M NaCl, 3 mM EDTA, 0.005% v/v surfactant P20, pH 7.4. Before any measurements were carried out, each sensor was subjected to sensitivity assessment (Kaminska et al. 2005). For this purpose 20 µl of glucose solution in increasing concentration, up to 10%, was repeatedly injected. The procedure was performed at a flow rate of 60 µl/min. When sensor sensitivity was satisfactory, small portions (10 µl) of blood plasma, diluted in HBS-EP (1:1000), were then injected and adsorption of plasma constituents on the studied surfaces was recorded for a number of flow rates starting from 10 µl/min through 25 and 50 µl/min up to 100 µl/min. The system exhibits extremely high sensitivity in determination of mass change on the sensor surface - approximately one resonance unit (RU) corresponds to one picogram per square millimetre (1 RU ~ 1 pg/mm^2). Pure gold was used as a reference surface. Monospecific polyclonal antibodies specific for human fibrinogen were produced at the Department of Molecular and Medical Biophysics, Medical University of Lodz, Poland, according to a previously published procedure (Walkowiak et al. 1994).

SPM Veeco MultiMode V atomic force microscope (Plainview, USA), equipped with NanoScope 7.3 software, working in tapping mode with a type 15 scanning probe, was used for measurement of Parylene C coat thickness. For this purpose a piece of glass plate was partially coated with an adhesive tape and treated with the same process as used for the parylene coated sensor. Next, the adhesive tape was removed and an AFM device was used to estimate the Parylene C layer thickness.

The interaction of sample surfaces with blood platelets was studied using a standard method developed in our laboratory (Okroj et al. 2006). Blood samples used for these experiments were collected from healthy volunteers and approval for this study was obtained from the Bioethical Committee of the Medical University of Lodz (RNN/46/06/KB 21.02.2006). The donors had not been treated with any antiplatelet drugs for at least two weeks prior to the examination. The investigated surfaces were immersed in whole citrated blood at 37 °C for one hour. Blood was constantly kept in motion by gentle end-to-end mixing. Thereafter, the samples were rinsed twice in 0.1 M phosphate buffer, pH 7.4. The fixing procedure was carried out with glutaraldehyde and sample dehydration was achieved with ethanol applied in increasing concentrations. Finally, the surface was sputtered with a thin layer of gold (JEE-4X, JEOL, Tokyo, Japan). Quantitative analysis of SEM (HITACHI S - 3000N, Tokyo, Japan) images, obtained from thirty randomly selected areas, was carried out for each sample.

Endothelial immortalized cell line EA.hy 926 was used for the experiment (Jerczynska et al. 2005). Cells were cultured in tissue culture plastics (TPP, Trasadingen, Switzerland) using Dulbecso's modified Eagle's medium with high glucose concentration (4,5 g/l), containing 10% FBS supplemented with HAT (100 µM hypoxanthine, 0.4 µM aminopterin and 16 µM thymidine) and antibiotics, at 37 °C in a humidified atmosphere containing 5% CO_2. The cells were applied onto the examined surfaces immersed in the above mentioned culture medium and were grown for 48 hours. For the control, cells cultured in standard conditions were used. Cell proliferation and cytotoxicity were estimated with live/dead test using calcein-AM and ethidium homodimer (Molecular Probes, Eugene, USA) and GX71 fluorescence microscope (Olympus, Center Valley, USA).

For proteome analysis 2D electrophoresis technique was carried out. Harvested cells were disintegrated with a lysis buffer containing urea (7M), tiourea (2M), CHAPS (4%), IPG buffer (2%) and DTT (40 mM), and proteins were purified with a 2D-Clean-Up Kit. IEF separation (1D) was carried out with an IPGphor integrated isoelectrofocusing system using IPG strips (11 cm, pH 4-7). The second dimension was performed with a Multiphore II system using ExcelGel SDS 2-D Homogeneous 12,5%. Finally, gels were stained with silver, scanned using ImmageScanner II and analyzed with ImageMaster 2D Platinium 6.0 software. All instruments, materials and reagents used for 2D electrophoresis were sourced from GE Healthcare (Waukesha, USA).

E. coli cells (DH5α strain, $2x10^3$ cells) were cultured on the surfaces of the examined samples. The culture was carried out for 24 h at 37°C in a medium containing NaCl (1%), bactopeptone (1%), yeast extract (0.5%) and pH 7.0. Next, the surfaces were extensively washed with deionized water and labeled by immersion in a fluorescent dye solution containing two dyes, bis-benzimide and propidium iodide, which made the visualization of both living and dead cells possible (Jakubowski et al. 2004).

Both F-Snedecor's test and unpaired Student's t-test or alternatively nonparametric ANOVA test with Bonferroni p-value correction were used for statistical analysis of the results. A value of $p < 0.05$ was considered as significant.

4. Results

4.1 Surface hydrophobicity

The measured contact angle for deionised water showed NCD and Ti6Al4V surfaces to be hydrophilic, whereas Parylene C surface was found to be hydrophobic. The differences were statistically significant. The results are shown in Table 1.

surface	contact angle (degree)	ANOVA test significance
NCD	66.34 ± 0.43	p<0.001
Parylene C	96.42 ± 0.40	
Ti6Al4V	76.28 ± 1.63	

Table 1. Hydrophobicity of examined surfaces expressed as the contact angle of water drop.

4.2 Adsorption of plasma proteins estimated with SPR biosensors

4.2.1 Sensor sensitivity

The sensitivity of sensors coated with thin layers of studied materials was assessed by sequential injection of glucose solution (20 µl) in increasing concentration (up to 10%). Figure 3 summarizes the crude results obtained for the reference (gold) sensor together with NCD, Ti6Al4V and Parylene C coated sensors. These results demonstrate, that with an increase in density of coating material the sensor response also increases, however sensitivity may decrease (see results for titanium alloy). It should be also noted that titanium alloy is a conducting material and can affect SPR phenomenon.

The responses normalized to the initial values and presented as a function of glucose concentration are shown in Figure 4. NCD and Parylene C coated sensors exhibited the same sensitivity as the reference sensor, however titanium alloy as more dense metallic material caused a decrease in the response. The thinner layer lowered sensor response by 10-15 %, whereas the thicker layer of titanium alloy diminished the response by 85-90%. The sensitivity of the last sensor was too low to be included in any further investigations.

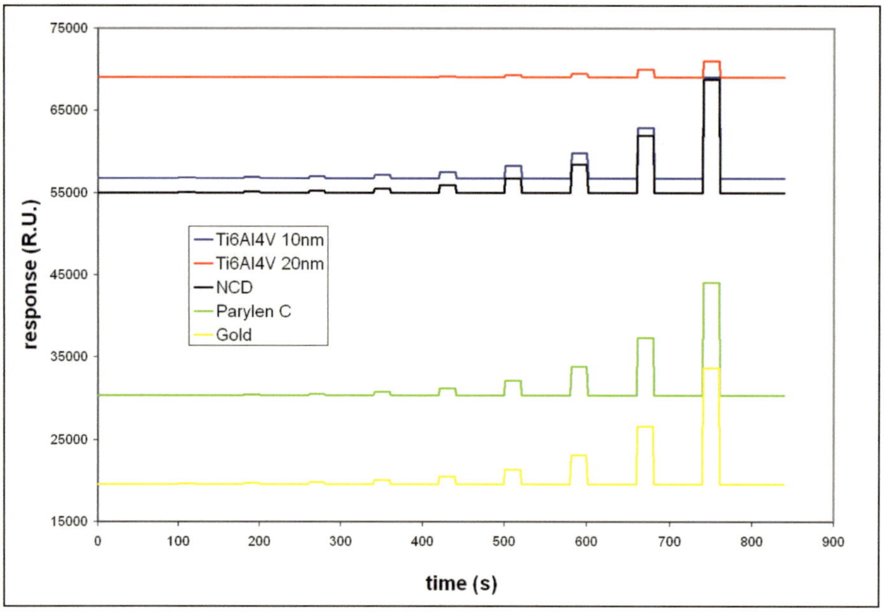

Fig. 3. Crude results of sensors response to the presence of increasing amounts of glucose. The glucose concentration varied from 0.04% up to 10%.

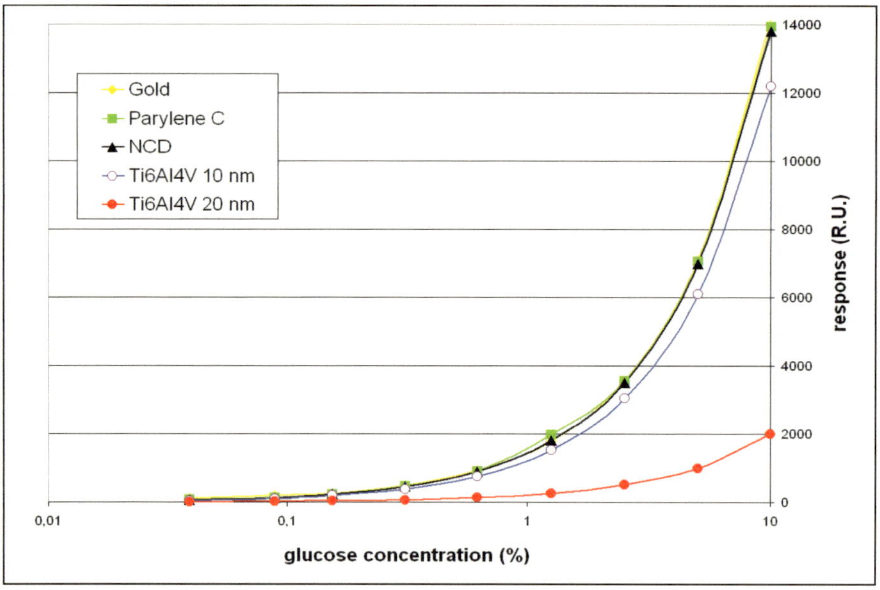

Fig. 4. Normalized to the initial values sensor responses as a function of glucose concentration.

4.2.2 Adsorption of blood plasma proteins to the sensor surface

The same volume (10 µl) of 1000 times diluted blood plasma was applied under variable flow rates starting from 10 µl/min through 25 and 50 up to 100 µl/min. It was found, that the amount of blood plasma proteins attached to the surfaces of interest strongly depends on the shear stress at the sensor surface. With higher share stress lower protein deposition was observed. En example of protein adsorption to Parylene C surface as a function of flow rate is presented in Figure 5. Figure 6 summarizes the results and shows a comparison of the amounts of adsorbed plasma proteins to different surfaces, including reference gold surface, for different levels of shear stress. It is evident, that for low shear stress, Parylene C adsorbs more proteins than other surfaces. However, with an increase in flow rate the amount of adsorbed proteins decreases and is similar to that of titanium alloy. NCD surface exhibited the highest resistance for protein adhesion for the entire range of flow rates applied.

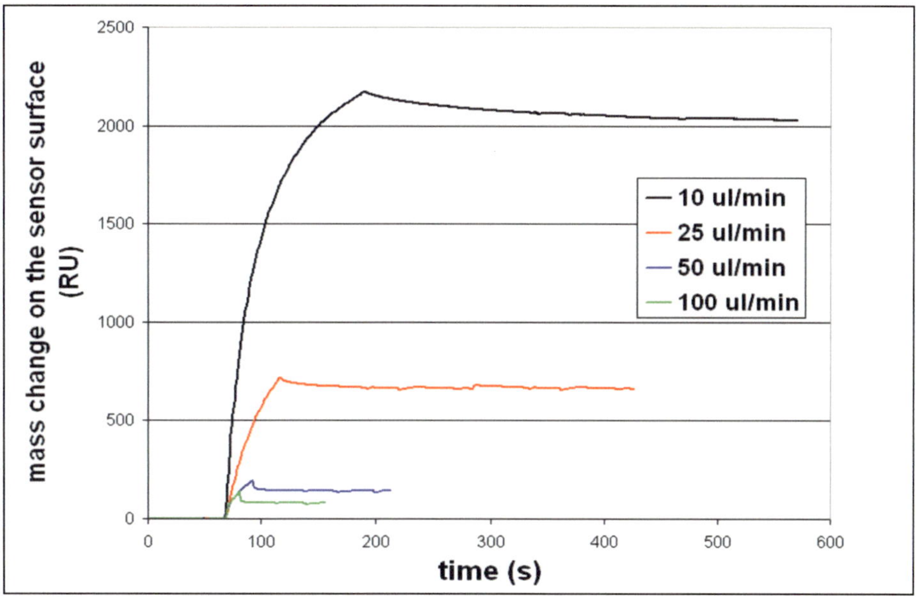

Fig. 5. Blood plasma proteins adsorption to the surface of Parylene C. Different flow rates results in different amounts of adsorbed proteins.

The following graph (Figure 7) presents example results of blood plasma protein adsorption to Parylene C and reference (gold) surfaces. In both cases curves were obtained for flow rates of 10 µl/min, and identical volumes (20 µl) of diluted plasma proteins were injected. However, the time intervals for buffer flow were twice as long for Parylene C. The arrows indicate time points of subsequent plasma protein injection. It is evident, that repeated injections initially cause an increase in the amount of adsorbed proteins, but within a short space of time the adsorption process becomes saturated. The forth injection resulted in almost no change to the mass of adsorbed proteins, moreover the desorption process was also significantly slower. The last injection, which was marked with anti-Fbg, contained rabbit anti-fibrinogen monospecific polyclonal antibodies. The observed increase in resonance signal resulted from binding of the antibodies to fibrinogen molecules present at the surface. This made it possible to quantify the amount of fibrinogen fixed to the surface. It is worth noting, that although the response for the antibody used was different, this was to a lesser degree than the recorded responses to injected plasma proteins. This may indicate that the gold surface adsorbed relatively more fibrinogen molecules than Parylene C surface.

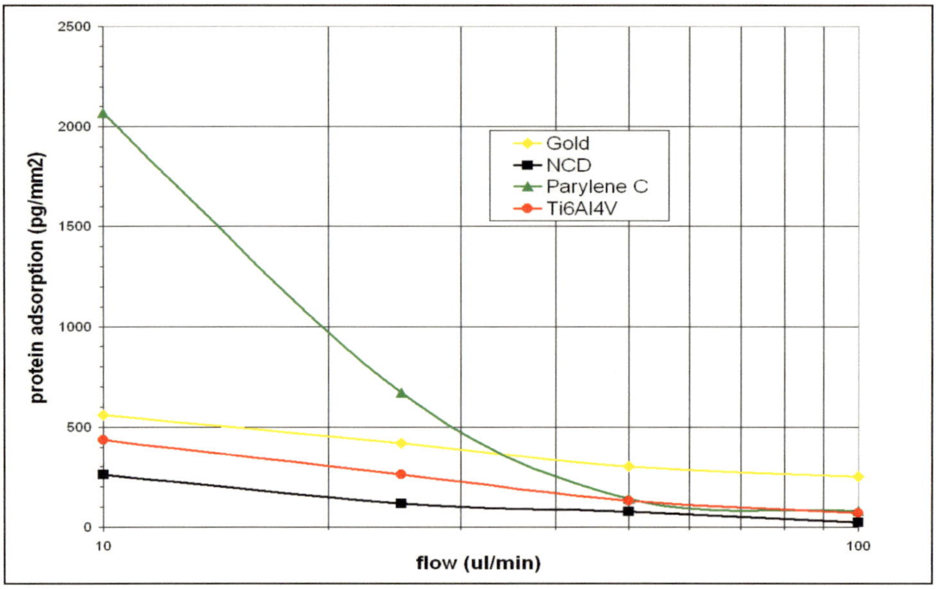

Fig. 6. Blood plasma proteins adsorption to the examined surfaces as a function of flow rate.

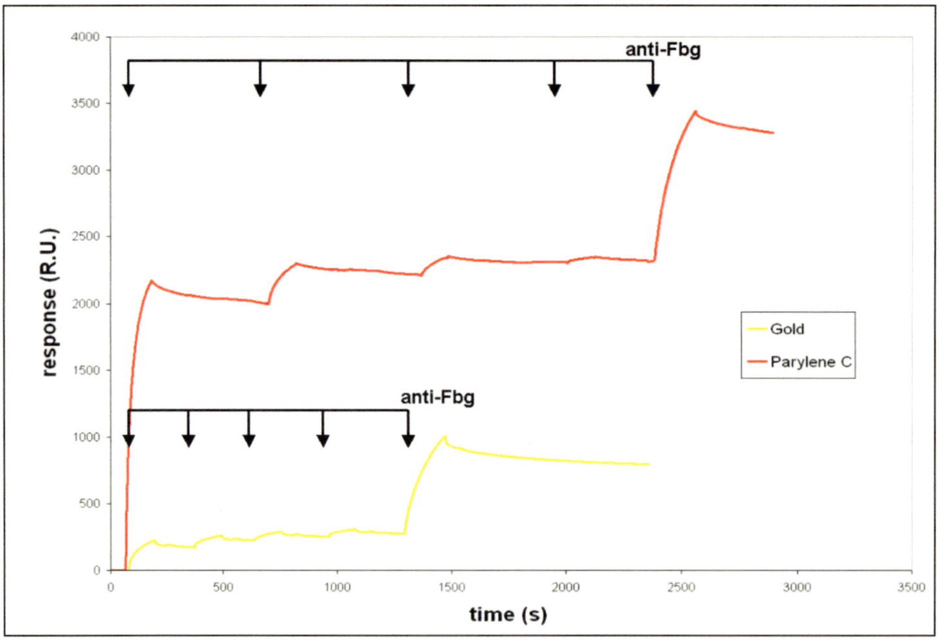

Fig. 7. An example of repetitive injection of diluted plasma proteins. The injection marked as anti-Fbg contained rabbit anti-fibrinogen monospecific polyclonal antibodies.

material	blood plasma proteins (ng/mm²)	anti-Fbg IgG (ng/mm²)	ratio IgG/plasma proteins
Parylene C	2.319	1.016	0.438
gold	0.276	0.614	2.225
ratio Parylene C/gold	8.402	1.655	

Table 2. Comparison of amounts of adsorbed proteins and IgG to the Parylene C and reference (gold) surfaces.

Table 2 summarizes the amount of plasma proteins attached to the surfaces and the amount of specific IgG molecules enhancing the signal. The ratio of IgG to plasma proteins is about 5 times higher for smooth, nonporous gold surface than for porous Parylene C surface. It also means that sticky, adhesive, large fibrillar molecules such as fibrinogen, adhere more easily to the gold surface than to the Parylene C. However, other smaller proteins must be trapped by porous Parylene C in very large amounts.

It is also important for future studies, using SPR biosensors, to know how to control the process of biosensor surface synthesis with regards to biomaterial film thickness. It must be known whether the thickness of any films of used materials correspond to the parameters we have assumed. Table 3 summarizes data of the initial responses recorded for each sensor used. If the specific density of the materials and their specific response are known, i.e. after subtracting the signal from the reference gold film signal, and assuming that 1 RU corresponds to about 1 pg/mm^2, it is possible to calculate the thickness of the films. For NCD we managed to achieve a layer that was exactly 10 nm thick. On the other hand, for Parylene C the estimated thickness was about 8,44 nm instead of the 10 nm that was assumed to present. For titanium alloy, where we assumed the layer thickness to be 10 nm, it was approximately 8.3 nm. Furthermore for the 20 nm layer it was only 11.2 nm. It is possible that for such a weak sensitivity, as was exhibited by the thicker titanium alloy, the recorded signal does not accurately represent the amount of titanium alloy on the sensor surface.

material	density (g/cm³)	response (RU)	specific response (RU)	segment mass (ng/mm²)	thickness (nm)
NCD	3.52	55 000	35 500	35.5	10.09
Parylene C	1.28	30 300	10 800	10.8	8.44
Ti6Al4V 10nm	4.42	56 000	36 500	36.5	8.26
Ti6Al4V 20nm	4.42	69 000	49 500	49.5	11.20
gold		19 500			

Table 3. Data used for estimation of thickness of the films of biomaterials. The specific response was calculated as the difference between the initial response recorded for the material of interest and the corresponding response for reference (gold) surface. The segment mass corresponds to the mass of the film falling on the flow cell surface.

Of course, it was necessary to confirm the above results with different method. For this purpose the AFM instrument was used. Figure 8 presents the surface of Parylene C film deposited on gold surface in the same process used to prepare the SPR biosensor. Prior to initiating this process, a small area of the surface was covered with adhesive tape. After the process was complete, the tape was carefully removed and AFM inspection was carried out. The resulting thickness of the Parylene C film was about 8 nm, which corresponded well with the 8,44 nm estimated from the SPR reading.

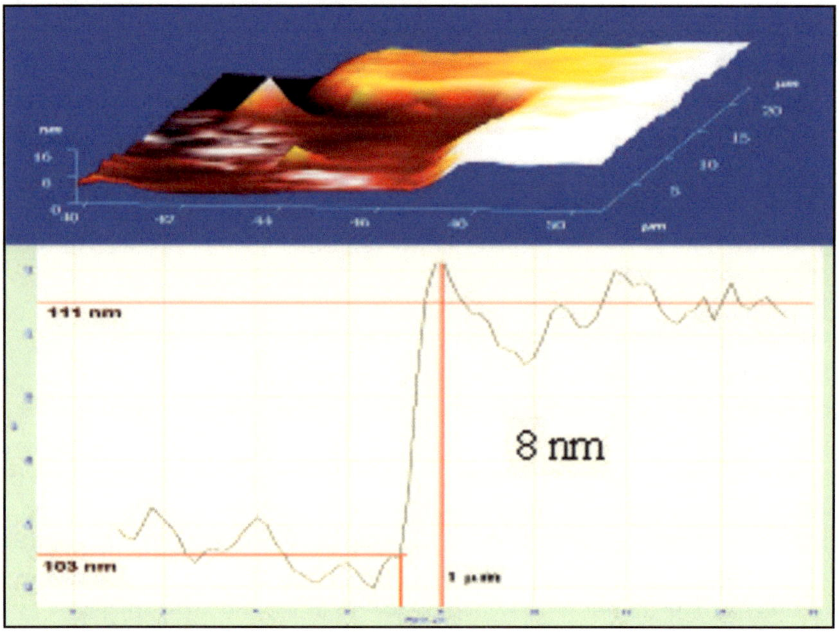

Fig. 8. Measurement of thicknes of the Parylene C film deposited on SPR sensor surface with use of AFM instrument.

4.3 Blood platelets adhesion

Blood platelet adhesion to the surface of any biomaterial strongly depends on the presence and exposure of adhesive proteins such as collagen, fibrinogen, fibronectin and others. Since plasma proteins are adsorbed by the examined surfaces, it was assumed that blood platelets would adhere to them. Figure 9 illustrates example photos of selected biomaterial surface fragments. The panels on the left side (lower magnification) were adequate for quantitative analysis, whereas the panels on the right were used to analyse the degree of activation of the adhered blood platelets. The lowest number of adhered platelets was found on the surface of NCD, a greater amount of platelets adhered to surface of titanium alloy, however the highest thrombogenic properties were exhibited by the Parylene C surface (Table 4). These differences were statistically very significant. Most platelets found on Ti6Al4V and Parylene C surfaces were in a similar dendritic-like form, but some of the platelets attached to Parylene C were also in spread form indicating a higher degree of activation. Platelets adhering to NCD were mainly in spherical form with short dendrites. This form is usually attributed to an initial level of platelet activation.

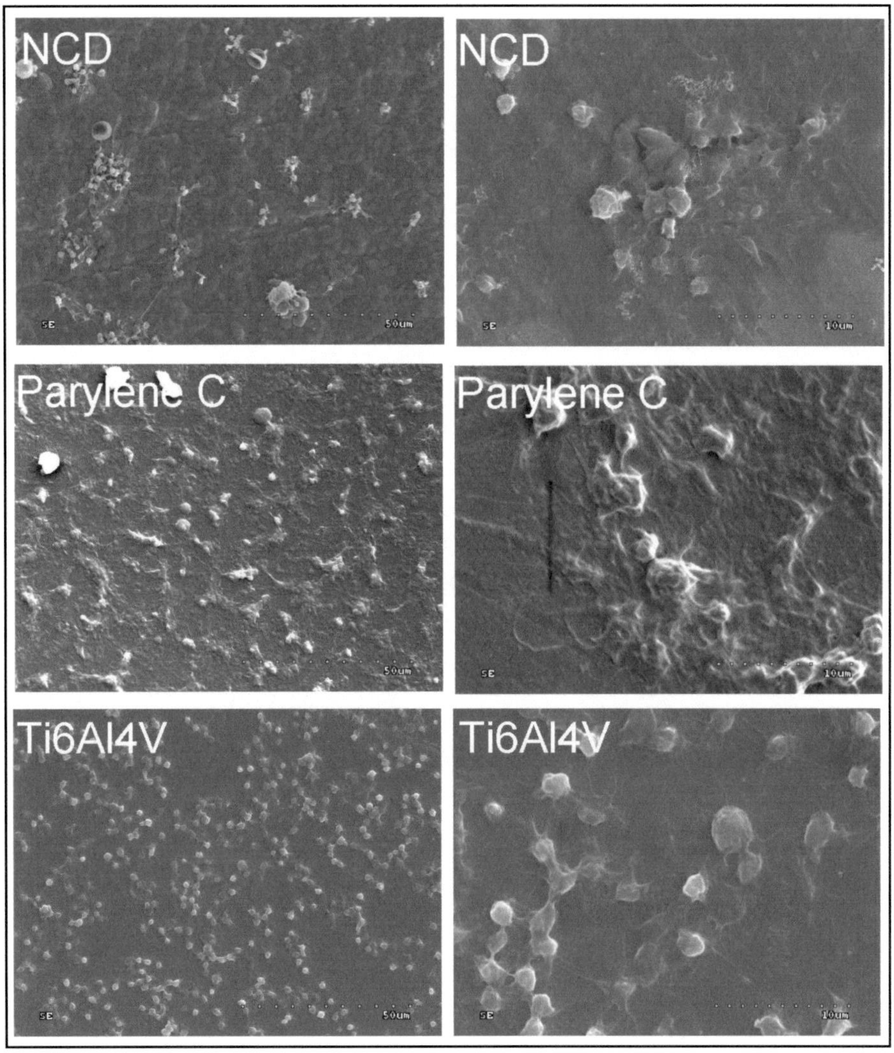

Fig. 9. Blood platelet adhesion to NCD, Parylene C and Ti6Al4V surfaces observed with SEM. Bars for left and right segments are 50 μm and 10 μm, respectively.

material	number of adhered platelets per 100 μm^2	ANOVA test (significance)
NCD	0.9 ± 0.3	
Parylene C	3.8 ± 0.2	$p<0.0001$
Ti6Al4V	1.7 ± 0.3	

Table 4. Number of blood platelets adhering to the surfaces of examined materials. Surfaces exhibited statistically relevant differences in susceptibility to blood platelet adhesion. The data were collected from at least 10 separate readings. Significance for material pairs was as follows: NCD vs. Parylene C $p<0.001$, NCD vs. Ti6Al4V $p<0.001$, Ti6Al4V vs. Parylene C $p<0.001$

4.4 Endothelial cells proliferation and proteome analysis

A thin layer of endothelial cells line the interior surface of blood vessels, forming an interface between circulating blood and the rest of the vessel wall. Endothelial cells line the entire circulatory system from the heart to the smallest capillary vessels. Thus, any implant introduced into the human body, even for a short period of time, must come in contact with endothelial cells and the cell response to this material can be crucial to the final outcome of surgery. On the other hand, cells contact and interact with the implant surface via a thin protein film created from components of body fluids immediately after implantation. In our model immortalized endothelial cell line EA.hy 926 was used to observe cell proliferation and viability on the surfaces of NCD, Parylene C and Ti6Al4V.

material	living cells (% of control)	ANOVA test (significance)	dead cells (% of living cells)
NCD	158 ± 43	$p < 0.0001$	2
Parylene C	7 ± 3		59
Ti6Al4V	145 ± 9		2

Table 5. Proliferation and mortality of EA.hy 926 cells cultured for 48 hours on the surfaces of examined materials. Data were collected from at least 10 separate readings. Significance of differences between material pairs was as follows: NCD vs. Parylene C $p<0.001$, NCD vs. Ti6Al4V ns, Ti6Al4V vs. Parylene C $p<0.001$.

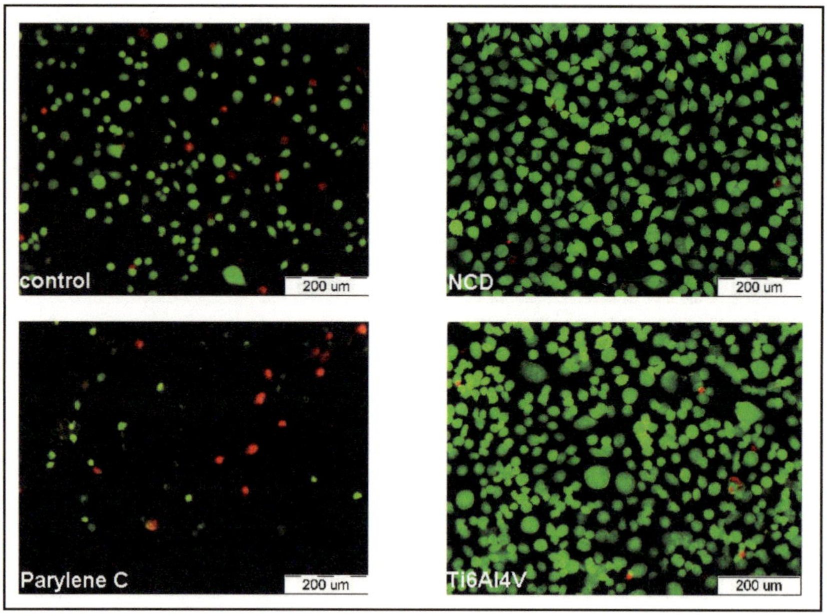

Fig. 10. EA.hy 926 cells grown (48 h) on surface of NCD, Parylene C and Ti6Al4V.

A control experiment was performed with cells grown in standard cell culture conditions described above in materials and methods. Living cells were stained green and dead cells red with calcein-AM and ethidium homodimer, respectively. It was obvious that both NCD and Ti6Al4V surfaces caused a significant increase in EA.hy 926 cell proliferation, together with a rather negligible, comparable to the control, number of dead cells (approx. 2%). In contrast to this, the Parylene C surface exhibited cytotoxic effect towards EA.hy 926 cells (about 60% dead cells).

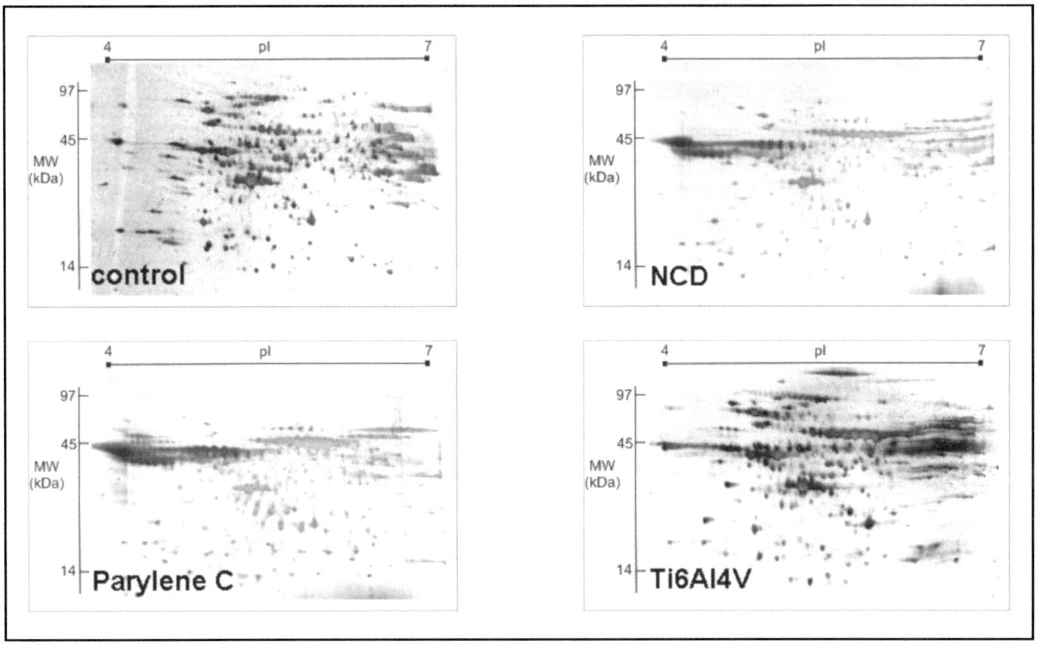

Fig. 11. Proteome analysis of EA.hy 926 cells with 2D electrophoresis.

material	detected spots (number)	matched spots (%)	up regulated matched spots (%)	down regulated matched spots (%)
control	326	100	0	
NCD	261	55.9	6.1	22.5
Parylene C	323	49.0	10.1	25.2
Ti6Al4V	256	63.2	4.9	3.8

Table 6. Quantitative analysis of EA.hy 926 cell proteome. Matched spots represent corresponding peptides present in both control and examined gels. Expression ratios higher than 1.5 or lower than 0.5, were taken as cut-off values for up or down regulated matched spots, respectively.

All the proteins extracted from the cultured cells (proteome) were separated using 2D electrophoresis (Figure 11). When compared to the control culture, the proteome pattern obtained for cells grown on all the studied materials differs significantly throughout the whole range of pI and MW. The results of simple visual inspection (Figure 11) and quantitative analysis (Table 6) indicate that Ti6Al4V titanium alloy causes the smallest changes in protein expression of endothelial cells. Although these cells expressed the lowest number of spots (peptides) in comparison with the control, the number of matched spots was the highest (63.2%). Furthermore, among the matched spots only 4.9% were up regulated and 3.8% down regulated. The proteome patterns of cells cultured on both NCD and Parylene C surfaces were similar and both materials produced lower levels of matched spots (55.9% and 49%, respectively). These materials also had the highest degree of up and down regulated matched spots (Table 6).

4.5 Biofilm of *E. coli* cells formation

Implant infection caused by opportunistic microorganisms is a frequent and difficult to cure complication after surgical implantation. Materials with a high susceptibility to microbial colonization and biofilm formation should not be used in any surgical procedures or for manufacturing implants. Otherwise, the surface of these materials will serve as an uncontrolled source of opportunistic infections that is impossible to eradicate. Thus, estimating the resistivity of biomaterials to bacterial colonization is one of the most important tasks during the process biocompatibility evaluation. As for any other cells, bacterial interaction with a material is mediated by proteins present at its surface. As shown in Figure 12 and Table 7, the NCD surface is almost entirely free from *E. coli* cells, whilst Ti6Al4V is less resistive to microbial colonization. On the other hand, Parylene C is rather susceptible to colonization, although the percent of dead cells on its surface is the highest among the studied materials.

material	number of living cells (FOV)	ANOVA test (significance)	dead cells (%of living cells)
NCD	3 ± 1		1
Parylene C	112 ± 30	$p < 0.0001$	9
Ti6Al4V	31 ± 5		1

Table 7. The number of living and dead *E. coli* cells found in the field of vision (FOV). The data were collected from at least 10 separate readings. The significance of difference between pairs of materials are as follows: NCD vs. Parylene C $p<0.001$, NCD vs. Ti6Al4V $p<0.01$, Ti6Al4V vs. Parylene C $p<0.001$.

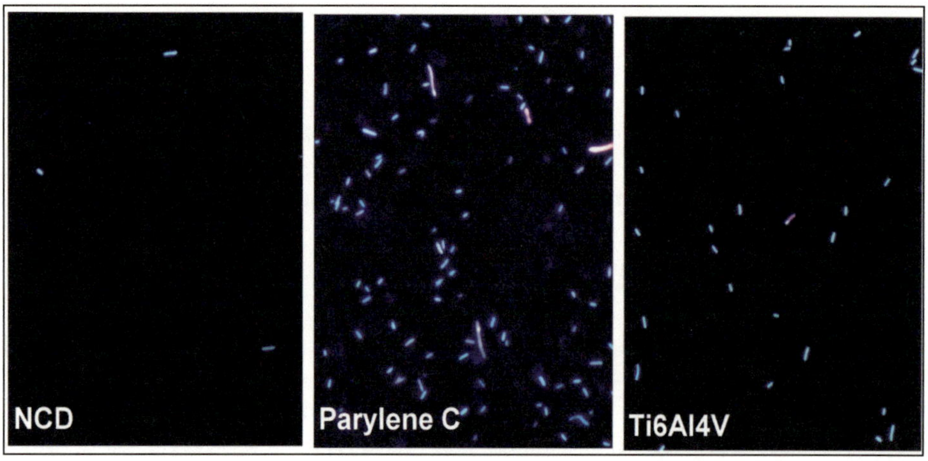

Fig. 12. *E. coli* cells detected on the surface of studied materials. The living cells (blue) were stained with bis-benzimide and the dead cells (red) were visualized with propidium iodide.

5. Conclusions

The SPR biosensor seems to be a very sensitive tool, that allows for remarkably sophisticated examination of biomolecule interactions with artificial surfaces of biomaterials. As was shown above, SPR biosensors can be used for a wide spectrum of materials, including dielectric carbon (NCD), polymers (Parylene C), and conductors (Ti6Al4V), although for the last class of materials we must be aware that the SPR effect could be disturbed by the presence of an additional layer of metallic material. Thus, a calibration procedure must be obligatory for any newly prepared biosensor surface. This strategy makes ensures that the biosensor is working properly in our experimental system. Kinetic study of biomolecule adsorption and desorption as a function of shear stress, real time observation of complex formation together with biomolecule identification without the need for any labelling, and easy experimental procedures make the SPR biosensor technique very useful and productive in numerous areas of research including biomaterials engineering. Our attempt to measure thickness of biomaterial layer indicates a possible application for assessing material aging or degradation manifested by a change of mass with time. In fact, the use of SPR phenomenon to monitor thin film deposition or removal (Woollam, 2007) and degradation of thin polymer film (Chen, et al. 1995; Green et al. 2000) has been previously reported. It is also worth noting the easy and specific recognition as well as quantitation of biomolecules adsorbed to the sensor surface. This makes it possible to monitor dynamic changes in the protein biofilm composition, which exists on the surface in contact with flowing fluid. And finally, the results obtained from SPR biosensor study correspond well with other observations. As mentioned above, cell interaction with any artificial surface is mediated by proteins attached to this surface. Our experiments showed a high amount of proteins adsorbed by Parylene C surface, and this correlates well with the elevated number of adhered blood platelets and attached *E. coli* cells to this surface. On the other hand, NCD surface gathers the lowest amount of proteins and this surface is resistant to platelet adhesion and microbial colonization. Unfortunately, this well organized arrangement is seriously disrupted by experiments with EA.hy 926 cells. Parylene C, despite very effectively adsorbing proteins, exhibits cytotoxic effects to endothelial cells. Another deviation can be seen also for NCD and Ti6Al4V alloys. Despite the limited adhesion of blood platelets and *E. coli* cells to NCD surface, which corresponds well to a low level of adsorbed proteins, endothelial cell proliferation is significantly elevated by this material. This may mean, that long term cell culture can adopt the surface to the cell needs, if this surface is not toxic to this cell. Further surprising results were obtained with 2D electrophoretic separation of EA.hy 926 cells proteome. Similarities were found between the patterns of 2D pictures obtained for NCD and Parylene C, despite the fact that NCD was able to stimulate cell proliferation and Parylene C was cytotoxic. The smallest difference was found between control cells and cells cultured on the surface of Ti6Al4V alloy. The initial impression resulting from the simple visual analysis of the gels is well supported by quantitative data from spot analysis and matching.

Summing up the above, SPR biosensor technique can significantly improve sensitivity and selectivity of tests applicable to material evaluation for biomedical use.

6. Acknowledgement

This work was supported by the Polish Artificial Heart project No. 05/WK/P01/0001/SPB-PSS/2008.

7. References

Chen, X., Shakesheff, KM., Davies, MC., Heller, J., Roberts, CJ., Tendler, SJB., Williams, PM. (1995). Degradation of a Thin Polymer Film Studied by Simultaneous *in Situ*Atomic Force Microscopy and Surface Plasmon Resonance Analysis, *J. Phys. Chem.* Vol. 99, pp. 11537-11542, ISSN 1089-5639

Davies, J. & Faulkner, I. (1996). Surface Plasmon Resonance - Theory and Experimental Considerations, In: *Surface analytical techniques for probing biomaterials process,* J. Davies, (Ed.), 67-88, CRC Press Inc., ISBN 0-8493-8352-8, Boca Raton, Florida, USA

Davies, J. & Skelton, L. (1996). Flow Cell Designe Considerations for SPR Measurements, In: *Surface analytical techniques for probing biomaterials process,* J. Davies, (Ed.), 89-104, CRC Press Inc., ISBN 0-8493-8352-8, Boca Raton, Florida, USA

Fano, U. (1941). The Theory of Anomalous Diffraction Gratings and of Quasi-Stationary Waves on Metallic Surfaces, *J. Opt. Soc. Am.,* Vol. 31, pp. 213-222.

Frazier, RA., Davies, MC., Clive, GM., Roberts, J., Schacht, E., Tasker, S. & Tendler, SJB. (1997). The Self-Assembly and Inhibition of Protein Adsorption by Thiolated Dextran Monolayer at Hydrophobic Metal Surfaces, In: *Surface modification of polymeric biomaterials,* BD. Ratner & DG. Castner, (Eds), 117-129, Springer-Verlag, ISBN 0306455129, New York, USA

Gazicki-Lipman, M. (2007). Parylene Coatings, *Encyclopedia of Chemical Processing,* S. Lee, (Ed.), Taylor & Francis eBooks, p. 13, ISBN 978-0-8247-5499-0

Green, RJ., Davies, J., Davies, MC., Roberts, CJ. & Tendler SJB. (1997). Surface Plasmon Resonance for Real Time in situ Analvsis of Protein Adsorption to Polymer Surfaces, *Biomaterials,* Vol 18, No. 5, pp. 405-413, ISSN 0142-9612

Green, RJ., Davies, MC., Roberts, CJ. & Tendler, SJB. (1999). Competitive Protein Adsorption as Observed by Surface Plasmon Resonance, *Biomaterials,* Vol. 20, pp. 385-391, ISSN 0142-9612

Green, RJ. Frazier, RA., Shakesheff, KM., Davies, MC., Roberts, CJ. & Tendler, SJB. (2000). Surface Plasmon Resonance Analysis of Dynamic Biological Interactions with Biomaterials, *Biomaterials,* Vol. 21 pp. 1823-1835, ISSN 0142-9612

Hoa, XD., Tabrizian, M. & Kirk, AG. (2009). Rigorous Coupled-Wave Analysis of Surface Plasmon Enhancement from Patterned Immobilization on Nanogratings, *Journal of Sensors,* Vol. 2009, pp. 1-7, ISSN 1687-725X

Homola, J. (2008). Surface Plasmon Resonance Sensors for Detection of Chemical and Biological Species, *Chem. Rev.,* Vol. 108, pp. 462-493, ISSN 0009-2665

Jakubowski, W., Bartosz, G., Niedzielski, P., Szymanski, W. & Walkowiak, B. (2004). Nanocrystalline Diamond Surface is Resistant to Bacterial Colonization, *Diamond and Related Materials,* Vol. 13, pp. 1761–1763, ISSN 0925-9635

Jerczynska, H., Baranska, P., Koziolkiewicz, W., Walkowiak, B. & Pawlowska, Z. (2005). Growth of Endothelial Cells on Surfaces of Selected Biomaterials, *Engineering of Biomaterials,* Vol. 43–44, pp. 21–24, ISSN 0137- 5083

Jung, M., Kim, S-U., Oh, B-K. & Choi, J-W. (2009). Immobilization of Biomaterials on Nanopatterned Surface Using Nanoporous Alumina for Biodevices, *Current Applied Physics,* Vol. 9, e111–e114, 1567-1739

Kaminska, M., Okroj, W., Szymanski, W., Jakubowski, W., Komorowski, P., Nosal, A., Szymanowski, H., Gazicki-Lipman, M., Jerczynska, H., Pawlowska, Z. &

Walkowiak, B. (2009). Interaction of Parylene C with Biological Objects, *Acta of Bioengineering and Biomechanics,* Vol. 11, No. 3, pp. 1119-25, ISSN 1509-409X

Kaminska, M., Szymanski, J. & Walkowiak, B. (2005). Preparation of Real Time SPR-Biosensors for Study of Protein Deposition at Titanium and NCD Surfaces, *Engineering of Biomaterials,* Vol. 43–44, pp. 16–20, ISSN 1429-7248

Kanso, M., Cuenot, S. & Louarn, G. (2008). Sensitivity of Optical Fiber Sensor Based on Surface Plasmon Resonance: Modeling and Experiments, *Plasmonics,* Vol. 3, pp. 49-57, ISSN 157-1955

Khan, MS., Rehman, S., Ali, MA., Sultan, B. & Sultan, S. (2008). Infection in Orthopeadic Implant Surgery, its Risk Factors and Outcome, *Journal Ayub Medical College Abbottabad,* Vol.20, No.1, pp. 23-25. Available from http://www.ayubmed.edu.pk/JAMC/PAST/20-1/Shoaib.pdf

Kooyman, RPH. (2008). Physics of Surface Plasmon Resonance, In: *Handbook of Surface Plasmon Resonance,* R.B.M. Schasfoort & A.J. Tudos, (Eds), 15-34, RSC Publishing, ISBN 978-0-85404-267-8, Cambridge, UK

Kretschmann, E. & Reather, H. (1968). Radiative Decay of Nonradiative Surface Plasmon Excited by Light, *Z. Naturf.* Vol. 23A, pp. 2135-2136

Lord Rayleigh, (1907). Dynamical Theory of the Grating, *Proc. Roy. Soc.(London),* Vol. A79. pp. 399-416

Mitura, S., Mitura, A., Niedzielski, P. & Couvrat, P. (1999). Nanocrystalline Diamond Coatingnds, *Chaos, Solitons and Fractals,* Vol. 10, No. 12, pp. 2165-2176, ISSN 0960-0779

Myszka, DG. (1999). Survey of the 1998 Optical Biosensor Literature, *J. Mol. Recognit.* Vol. 12, pp. 390-408, ISSN 0952-3499

Okroj, W. Kaminska, M., Klimek, L., Szymanski, W. & Walkowiak, B. (2006). Blood Platelets in Contact with Nanocrystalline Diamond Surfaces, *Diamond and Related Materials,* Vol. 15, pp. 1535- 1539, ISSN 0925-9635

Otto, A. (1968). Exitation of Nonradiative Surface Plasma Waves in Silver by the Method of Frustrated Total Reflection, *Z. Phys.,* Vol. 216, pp. 398-410

Rich, RL. & Myszka, DG. (2010). Grading the Commercial Optical Biosensor Literature-Class of 2008: 'The Mighty Binders', *J. Mol. Recognit.* Vol. 23, pp. 1-64, 0952-3499

Schierholz, JM. & Beuth, J. (2001). Implant Infections: a Haven for Opportunistic Bacteria, *Journal of Hospital Infection,* Vol. 49, pp. 87-93. Available from http://www.idealibrary.com

Stenberg, E., Persson, B., Roos, H. & Urbaniczky, C. (1991). Quantitative Determination of Surface Concentration of Protein with Surface Plasmon Resonance by Using Radiolabelled Proteins. *J.Colloid Interface Sci.* Vol. 143, pp. 513-526, ISSN 0021-9797

Suzuki, A., Kondoh, J., Matsui, Y., Shiokawa, S. & Suzuki, K. (2005). Development of Novel Optical Waveguide Surface Plasmon Resonance (SPR) Sensor with Dual Light Emitting Diodes, *Sensors and Actuators B,* Vol. 106, PP. 383-387, ISSN 0925-4005

Tudos, AJ. & Schasfoort, RBM. (2008). Introduction to Surface Plasmon Resonance, In: *Handbook of Surface Plasmon Resonance,* R.B.M. Schasfoort & A.J. Tudos, (Eds), 1-14, RSC Publishing, ISBN 978-0-85404-267-8, Cambridge, UK

Vansteenkiste, SO., Corneillie, SI., Schacht, EH., Chen, X., Davies, MC., Moens, M. & Van Vaeck, L. (2000). Direct Measurement of Protein Adhesion at Biomaterial Surfaces by Scanning Force Microscopy, *Langmuir,* Vol. 16, pp. 3330-3336, ISSN 0743-7463

Walkowiak, B., Kochmanska, V., Jakubowski, W., Okroj, W. & Kroliczak, V. (2002). Interaction of Body Fluids with Carbon Surfaces, *J. Wide Bandgap Materials*, Vol. 9, pp. 231-242, ISSN 1524-511X

Walkowiak, B., Michalak, E., Borkowska, E., Koziolkiewicz, W. & Cierniewski, CS. (1994). Concentration of RGDS-Containing Degradation Products in Uremic Plasma is Correlated with Progression in Renal Failure, *Thromb Res*, Vol. 76, pp. 133-145, ISSN 0049-3848

Wendler, B., Kaczmarek, Ł., Klimek, L., Rylski, A., & Jachowicz, M. (2004). Nanocrystalline γ-TiAl Based Microalloyed Coatings as Gas Corrosion Barriers, *Rev. Adv. Mater. Sci.*, Vol. 8, pp. 116-121, ISSN 1605-8127

Woollam, JA., Johs, BD., Tiwald, TE., Liphardt, MM., Welch, JD. (2007). Use of Elipsometry and Surface Plasmon Resonance in Monitorin Thin Film Deposition or Removal from a Substrate Surface. *United State Patent* US 7,283,234 B1

Wood, RW. (1902). On a Remarkable Case of Uneven Distribution of Light in a Diffraction Spectrum, *Proc. Phys. Soc. (London)*, Vol. 18, pp. 269-275

4

Highly Sensitive SPR Biosensor Based on Nanoimprinting Technology

Satoshi Fujita[1,3] and Takeo Nishikawa[2,3]
[1]*OPTOQUEST Corporation*
[2]*OMRON Corporation*
[3]*CREST, JST*
Japan

1. Introduction

Detection of biomolecular interactions is becoming more important as a technique to achieve rapid diagnoses of incipient diseases and preventive medical care. Among various detection techniques currently available (e.g., fluorometry, quartz crystal microbalance, etc.), surface plasmon resonance (SPR)-based biosensing has received much attention since it does not require any labelling of the analytes and enables high-throughput real-time sensing. The SPR technique allows very fast measurements of the order of several minutes, whereas conventional enzyme-linked immunosorbent assay (ELISA) methods are often lengthy processes. Recently, SPR-based biosensors have been extensively applied to analyses in biomedical (Vaisocherová et al., 2006), environmental (Dostálek et al., 2006), and food sciences (Ladd et al., 2006).

In conventional SPR, the evanescent field penetrates into the metal surface by as much as ~300 nm (Stenberg et al., 1991, Homola, 2003). When the target analyte binds to the metal surface, changes in the local refractive index occur, which in turn causes the SPR angle to shift. However, the sensing of target molecules suffers due to unwanted noise factors such as the instability of the temperature and the change in the refractive index of the mobile phase. Thus, the "sensing depth" of conventional SPR is significantly larger than the range required for practical use such as in clinical diagnoses. In this paper, we demonstrate that the sensing depth of SPR can be controlled by producing a pattern of periodic metal nanogrooves on the sensor surface.

2. Advantages of SPR biosensor based on nanoimprinting technology

2.1 Surface plasmon resonance (SPR)

Surface plasmon resonance (SPR) is an interactive coupling phenomenon between light (electric field) and free electrons in metal. When the wave number and the frequency of propagating light match those of the eigenmode of the free electrons, the energy of the propagating light is transferred to the oscillation of free electrons. The coupling that occurs near the surface of the metal is called surface plasmon resonance (SPR) (Homola, 2003). It is known that SPR can be roughly classified in two types; the first type is propagating SPR and the second type is localized SPR.

To generate propagating SPR, light must be translated in the evanescent field for the matching of the wavenumber and frequency of the propagating light. In general, propagating SPR is generated using a prism with a Kretschmann configuration (Kretschmann & Raether, 1968). A thin gold layer (thickness, about 50 nm) is prepared on a glass substrate, which is then attached on the prism surface with matching oil. When light enters into the prism, total internal reflection of light occurs on the glass surface as a result of the thin gold layer. By changing the incident angle or the wavelength of the incident light, propagating SPR can be generated when the coupling condition is satisfied. The generated SPR propagates along the gold surface as the collective oscillation of the free electrons near the gold surface. At that time, the reflection of the incident light is almost absorbed for SPR generation.

Localized SPR occurs on nano-metal structures such as metal nanocolloids (diameter of several tens of nanometres) (Nath & Chilkoti, 2004) and metal nanorods (Huang et al., 2011) and so on. Localized SPR does not require an evanescent field. And the propagating light can couple with the eigenmode of the free electrons in the metal nanostructure. One main difference between localized SPR and propagating SPR is that the localized SPR does not propagate along the metal surface, and that the electric field generated by the localized SPR is much smaller than that of the propagating SPR. The depth of the electric field generated by the localized SPR is several tens of nanometres in size, which means it is smaller than the diffraction limit of light.

These two types of SPR have been extensively studied in physics, and are now demonstrated for the application of practical biosensors.

2.2 SPR biosensor

One important characteristic of SPR is that its coupling condition sensitively depends on the refractive index of a dielectric material located in close proximity to the metal substrate. Therefore, we can find the binding of biomolecules whose refractive index is larger than that of water on the metal surface by detecting the change of coupling angle or wavelength of incident light. To realize a practical biosensor, we immobilize probe molecules, such as antibodies that can capture specific target molecules, on the metal surface. And after that, the sample reagent is applied on its surface. When the target molecules are included, the signal change, which can be expressed as a shift of the resonant angle or wavelength, can be observed according to the concentration of the target molecules. The strong points of the SPR biosensor are that detection can be achieved without any labelling of fluorescent molecules on the target biomolecules and that it realizes quantitative and real-time sensing. As a result, it can also provide the dissociation/association coefficients that cannot be obtained by conventional detection methods.

The biosensor based on the propagating SPR principle was first commercialized by Pharmacia Biosensor AB in 1990 (Homola et al., 1999). And the SPR biosensors are widely used in the pharmaceutical field and research field now. However, the commercialized SPR biosensors are generally very expensive. Thus, low-cost and high sensitivity SPR biosensors have been demanded for a long time.

Some researchers have already started to use localized SPR in biosensors. As mentioned above, localized SPR has very unique physical characteristics that rely on the coupling between light and free electrons that occurs without the need for an optical prism. Also, the resonant electric field, "sensing depth" is much smaller than the diffraction limit of light, which means that areas further than several tens of nanometres from the metal surface are not detected by this sensor. This provides a unique advantage for biosensors as the size of the biomolecules is generally only about ten nanometres and the background noise can be all but eliminated by localized SPR rather than propagating SPR (Fig. 1). As a result, the detection system can be much simpler and the signal-to-noise ratio can be high as a result of using localized SPR.

In recent studies, biosensors using localized SPR have been keenly studied and some groups have reported that they could detect disease related biomolecules by using localized SPR.

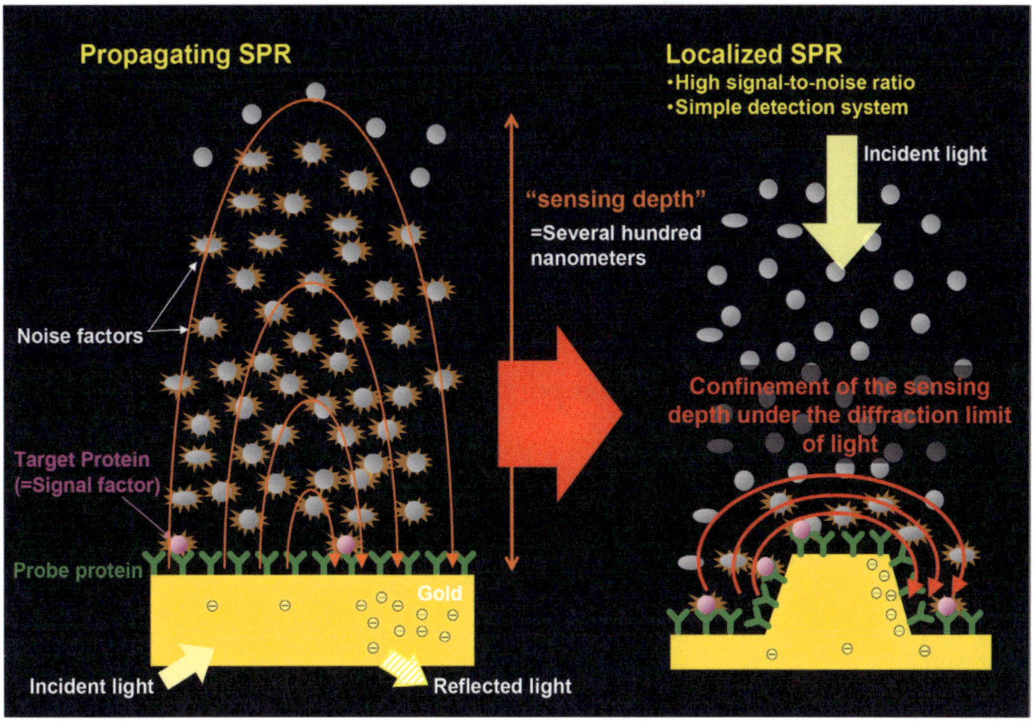

Fig. 1. Reduction of the background noise by localizing the "sensing depth" close to the surface.

2.3 SPR biosensor based on nanoimprinting technique

Localized SPR has a great potential to realize small-sized, easy operation, low-cost and high sensitivity biosensors. However, it is still challenging to fabricate uniform nanopatterns on a wide area of the metal surface. For instance, metal colloids immobilized on a substrate are commonly used as a sensor substrate. To realize a uniform quality in colloid diameter and shape, high process control in deoxidization of metal ions is necessary. In addition, the uniform immobilization of colloids on the sensor surface while avoiding aggregation and density fluctuations are still challenging in mass production. As a stable nanofabrication method, electron beam lithography is a viable candidate. However, the patterns are produced by scanning a single electron beam across a wafer, which is a time consuming and costly process. Other methods such as nano-sphere lithography etc. also have low pattern reproducibility and process throughput. To overcome these conventional problems, our group has proposed a unique way to prepare the metal nanostructures for localized SPR by using nanoimprinting technology (Table 1).

	Nanoimprint method	Metal colloidal method	Electron beam method
Structure Image	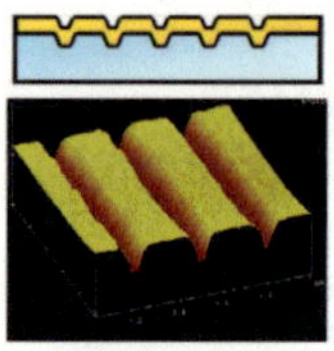	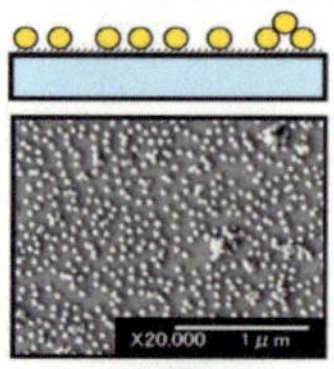	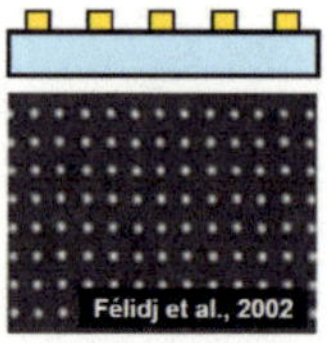
Pattern Reproducibility	Good	Not good (aggregations)	Good
Cost (Process Throughput)	Good (~several minutes)	Not good (~several hours)	Bad (~several days)
Tuning	Easy	Possible	Possible

Table 1. Advantages of Nanoimprint method compared with conventional methods.

3. Fabrication procedure of nanoimprinting SPR biosensor device

3.1 Nanoimprint method

Nanoimprinting technology was first proposed by S. Y. Chou et al. in 1995 (Chou et al., 1995). Prior to this, nanoscale patterns were fabricated using time consuming nanopatterning techniques such as X-ray lithography, electron beam lithography etc. Nanoimprinting technology basically uses the pattern transfer principle and it can foreshorten the process time. Its general process is below.

1. Prepare the master substrate with nanoscale patterns on its surface by using electron beam lithography etc.
2. Make a metal mould from the master substrate by an electroforming process.
3. Press the metal mould onto a polymer surface with heating produced during ultraviolet (UV) irradiation.
4. Peel off the metal mould from the solidified polymer.
5. Repeat steps 3) and 4) for each new polymer surface.

The preparation of the master substrate involves a conventional nano-fabrication technique, which is time consuming. However, the fabricated master substrate can be used to produce the metal mould, which can be used repeatedly. The replication process time with the metal mould is much shorter than the master fabrication process, and generally takes only several tens of seconds. It is demonstrated that nanoscale patterns as small as 5 nm can be successfully transferred by this method. By using this fabrication technology, devices with nanoscale patterns can be fabricated with very high process throughput and in low-cost.

This process is keenly focused and has been demonstrated to have wide application in various electrical (CMOS, FET, patterned media etc.), optical (anti-reflection structure etc.) and energy devices (organic solar cells, fuel cells etc.) and so on.

3.2 Nanoimprinting process for SPR biosensor device

To generate localized SPR, nanosized metal colloids and metal nano rods have been used and studied. High process reproducibility and stability are, however, demanded for the biosensor products. Furthermore, low-cost sensing devices are necessary to realise disposable usage to avoid contamination resulting from repeated use of a sensing device. These demands are not satisfied by the conventional methods as the chemical fabrication process is still unstable and of high-cost.

To overcome these conventional problems, we have proposed to make a localized SPR biosensor by using the nanoimprinting technique. The main process flow is shown in Fig. 2. As a first step, nanopatterns were created in a photoresist, ZEP520A (Nippon Zeon, Japan) coated on an 8 inch silicon wafer. The nanopatterning step typically takes around 9 hours to pattern a 45 mm^2 area. After that, the nanopatterned area was sputtered with Ni (CS-200S, ULVAC, Japan) and then electroformed with Ni (SA1m, Digital Matrix, USA) to produce a metal mould having a thickness of 250-300 μm. This metal mould is used to replicate the nanoscale patterns onto a polymer surface. Polymer resin was first deposited onto a glass substrate and then the metal mould was pressed onto the polymer surface with heating or UV irradiation. After solidification of the polymer resin, the metal mould was peeled off from the replicated polymer surface. In general, this process takes only several tens of nanometres. As a last step, a thin gold layer was sputtered onto the surface of the polymer replica. The gold nanoscale patterns generate localized SPR when exposed to incident light.

By this process, the single metal mould can be used repeatedly. As a result, nanopatterns having substantially the same dimensions can be fabricated on the surface of the replica, which is difficult to achieve by using the conventional colloid base method. And the process cost can be also very low.

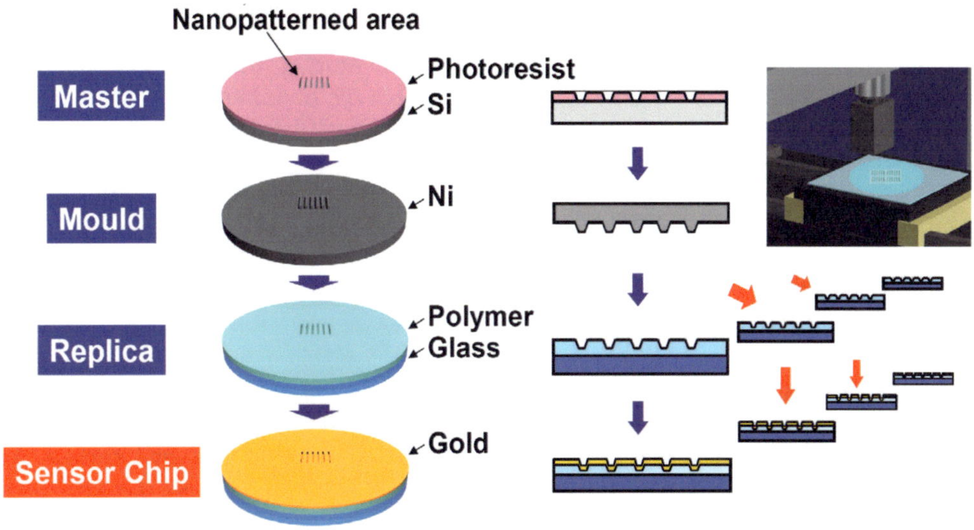

Fig. 2. Fabrication process diagram for the nanoimprint method.

Fig. 3 shows the sensor chip fabricated by the nanoimprinting technique. The nanopatterned areas are slightly red in colour, which means that green light is absorbed by the localized SPR (Fig. 3a). The nanostructures on the sensor chip surface are produced by the nanoimprint injection moulding method. The replication process takes 15 seconds. The period (300 nm) of the nano patterns and the gap size (100-140 nm) of the nanogrooves was confirmed by atomic force microscopy (AFM) image (Fig. 3b).

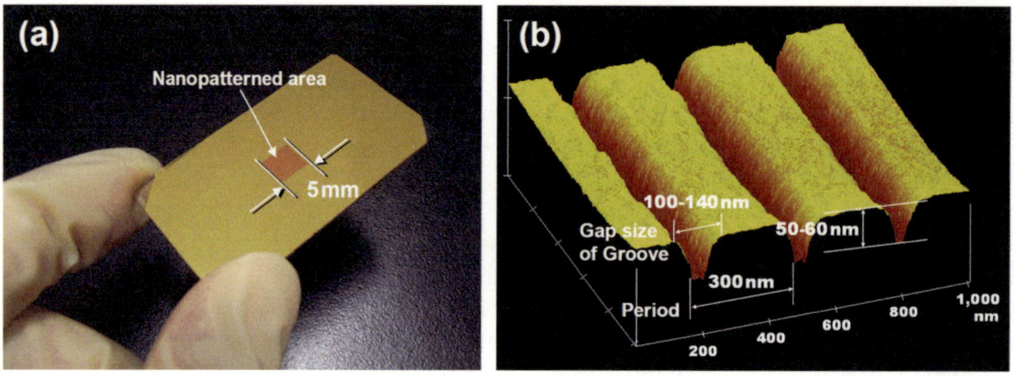

Fig. 3. The sensor chip fabricated by the nanoimprinting technique (a) and an AFM image of the nanopatterned area (b).

4. Design of nanogroove structure for SPR biosensor

4.1 Simulation methods

An analysis of the physical interaction between the metal nanostructures and the incident light (electric field) is necessary to design the shape, size, and period of the metal nanostructures. Here, we have used two simulation methods, finite-difference time-domain (FDTD) and rigorous coupled-wave analysis (RCWA) in this study.

FDTD is a major photonic analysis tool in which the space is divided into a small mesh, the so-called "Yee mesh". The electric and magnetic fields in each mesh are solved according to Maxwell's equation step by step. The dynamic behaviour of the electric field can be calculated for an arbitrary material environment by this method. However, the simulation time and memory space required for solving such complex structures are considerable. We, therefore, used the RCWA method for a static analysis. In the RCWA method, the space is transformed using the Fourier transfer method and solved. Though only the periodic structure can be analysed, the simulation time and memory required for the RCWA method are much smaller than that required for the FDTD method. We used these two methods for each purpose complementarily and optimized the metal nano structures for application in a high sensitivity biosensor.

4.2 Basic design of periodic nanogroove structure

While conducting the FDTD simulations, we found that the resonance occurs inside the metal nano-gap when the periodic nanogrooves are prepared on the metal surface. This resonance is a kind of SPR and its resonant electric field depends on the size of the nanogroove. As shown in Fig. 4, when the gap size of the nanogroove is several tens of nanometres in size, the depth of the resonant electric field is smaller than 100 nm, which overcomes the diffraction limit of light. In this simulation, the light (wavelength, 670 nm) is focused on the sensor substrate from the front side. This result means that localized SPR can occur when periodic nanogroove structures are prepared on the metal surface.

It is also proved that the resonant wavelength can be tuned by changing the structural parameters of the nanogroove. The relationship between the structural parameter and the resonant wavelength is shown in Table 2. The depth of the resonant electric field, the so-called "sensing depth", is very important for a biosensor because when the sensing depth is

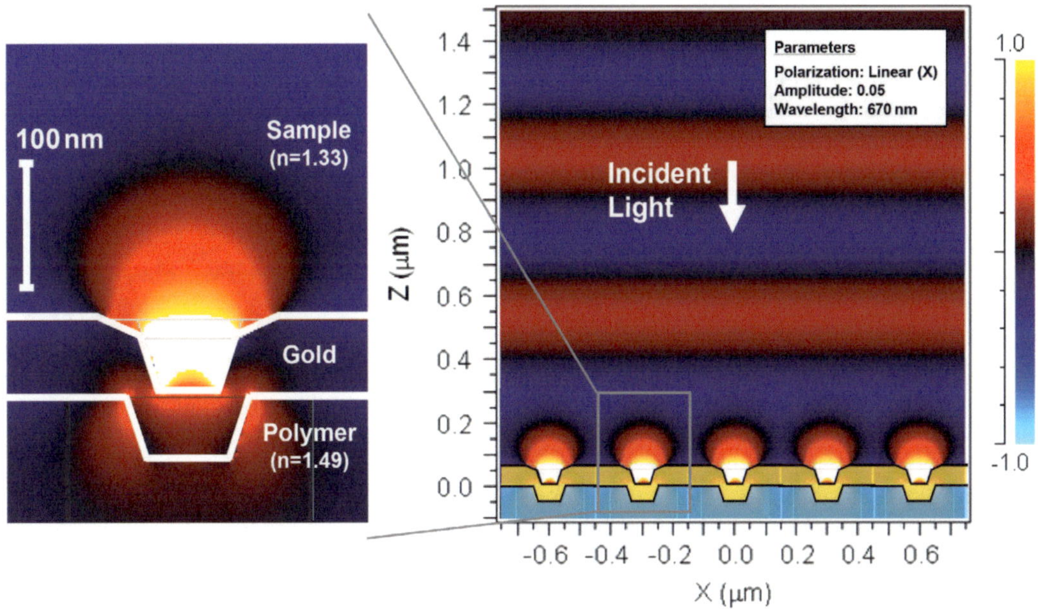

Fig. 4. FDTD simulation of the electric field generated by nanogap structures.

Structural parameter	Effects on the resonance condition
Period	The larger the period, the longer the resonant wavelength and the larger the depth of the resonant electric field.
Gap size of groove	The larger the gap size, the shorter the resonant wavelength.
Depth of groove	The deeper the groove, the longer the resonant wavelength.

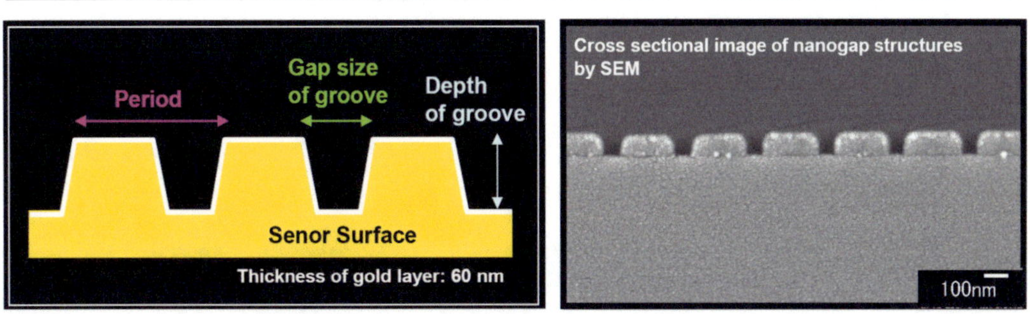

Table 2. The relationship between the structural parameter and the resonant wavelength.

too small, the target molecules are not detected. Moreover, when the sensing depth is too large, the background noise is included in the signal. The unique point of this nanogroove SPR is that the sensing depth can be easily selected by changing the structural parameters. The optimal sensing depth can be tuned according to the sizes of the probe molecule and target molecule. Furthermore, the resonant wavelength can be tuned by adjusting the gap size and the depth of the nanogroove. The wide-range tuning of the sensing depth and the resonant wavelength are not easy to accomplish in conventional localized SPR.

4.3 Experimental evaluation of periodic nano-groove structure

As a next step, we evaluated the optical characteristics of the metal nanogroove structures experimentally. Metal nanogroove structures were fabricated by the nanoimprinting process to yield structures with different period and gap sizes. The depth of the nanogrooves was found to be 50 nm, as determined by the thickness of the polymer photo-resist on the master substrate. And the gap size of the groove is varied by changing the dose energy of the electron beam on the master substrate. After making the nickel mould, the replica substrate is produced by the replication process using UV irradiation. A thin gold layer (thickness 80-100 nm) was then deposited on the replica's surface. Fig. 5 shows the optical image of the fabricated device. We can observe a reflection colour change by changing the period and gap size of the nanogrooves. When the period gets shorter, the colour changes from green to red. This result means that the absorption wavelength decreases (red to green). Also, when the gap size gets smaller (dose energy gets smaller), the pattern colour changes from red to green. This means that the resonant wavelength gets longer when the gap size gets smaller. These results are well identical to the simulation results.

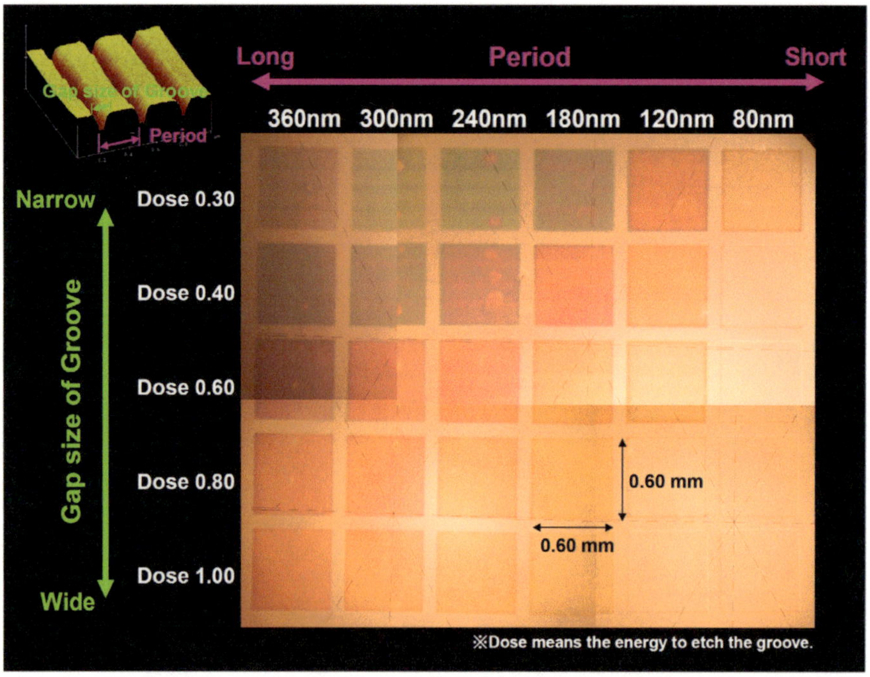

Fig. 5. The metal nanogroove structures changed their period and gap sizes by the nanoimprinting process.

5. Design of immobilization layer for an SPR biosensor

5.1 Three key factors for surface preparation

For SPR biosensing in solution, it is necessary that one interaction partner (probe molecules) is immobilized on the sensor surface to capture the target molecules. Conventional immunochemical methods such as ELISA are based on the simple physical adsorption of probe molecules onto a plastic plate. However, it is thought that a more sophisticated approach is required for surface preparation of a sensor surface for SPR biosensing. This is because the sensitivity of SPR biosensors is highly dependent on the binding capacity of the immobilized probe molecules on the sensor surface and on the resistance of the surface to nonspecific protein adsorption. The performance of the sensor surface is supported by three crucial factors (the capture agent, the surface chemistry, and the surface matrix). Fig. 6 shows a schematic diagram of an immobilization layer for SPR biosensing and the desired characteristics of the three key factors.

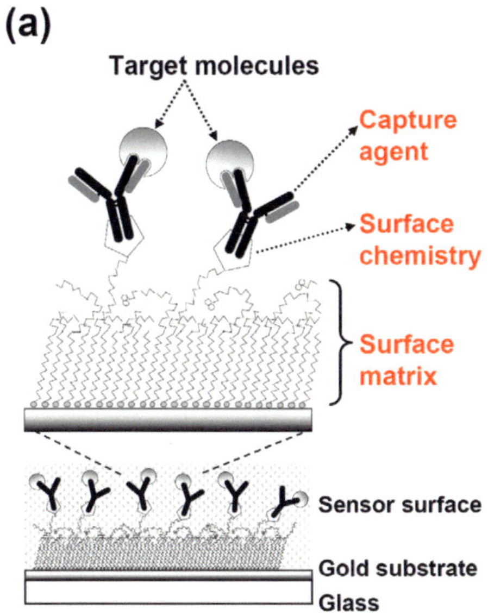

(b)

1. Desired characteristics for capture agent
    - Specificity to target molecules
    - Affinity to target molecules
    - Low nonspecificity, etc.
2. Desired characteristics for surface chemistry
    - Affinity to capture agents
    - Orientation control of capture agents
3. Desired characteristics for surface matrix
    - Low nonspecificity
    - Binding capacity of capture agents
    - Affinity to gold substrate

Fig. 6. Schematic diagram of the immobilization layer (a) and desired characteristics for the three key factors (b).

5.2 Basic design of the immobilization layer

5.2.1 Capture agent

In principle, it is difficult for SPR sensors to clearly distinguish the signal component of target molecules from the background noise factors associated with non-specific absorption. First, the capture agent must have the capability for specific recognition of the target molecules. Proteins such as immunoglobulin (IgG), which are known as immune antibodies, are frequently used as capture agents on account of their high specificity towards their target antigens (Table 3, Besselink et al., 2004, Yang et al., 2005). Second, the selection of capture agents with high affinity (equilibrium dissociation constant, in units of molar concentration; $K_D < 10^{-9}$) is necessary to achieve high sensitivity. Recently, nucleic acid aptamers and synthetic peptides have been developed as artificial antibodies with high specificity, high

Capture agent	Low affinity ←		General tendency for Affinity		→ High affinity
	Native molecules →Specificity (high)	Polyclonal antibody (not purified) =antisera	Monoclonal antibody (not purified)	Monoclonal antibody (1)(2) (purified)	Polyclonal antibody (affinity purified)
	Artificial molecules →Specificity (high-low)	Small molecule (3)	DNA/RNA aptamer (4)	Peptide/ Cyclic peptide (5)	Antibody fragment (variable region) ScFv (6) VHH (7) / Antibody fragment (Fab region, etc.) Fab, Fab'2 (8)
Surface chemistry	Random ←		Orientation		→ Site specific
	Covalent →Stability (high)	Succinimidyl ester-Amines (9)(10) Aldehyde-Amines Epoxide-Amines, Thiol group	Cutinase- (11) Phosphonate		Maleimide-Thiol group (8) Bromoacetyl-Thiol group Thioester-Cysteine at N terminus
	Non-covalent →Stability (Low)	Avidin-Biotin (12) →Stability (Middle)	Protein A/G (13) Anti-IgG antibody	Glutathione-GST (14) Maltose-MBP	Ni-NTA-His tag (15) Antibody-Peptide tag (FLAG,HA,myc, etc.)
Surface matrix	Examples of matrix and expected effects				
	Simpleness	High density	High orientation	Low nonspecificity	→Hybrid type
	Untreated (physical adsorption (3) Thiol group, etc.) (13)	Polymer (Poly-lysine etc.) (12)(16)	self-assembled monolayer (SAM) (7)(17)	phospholipid layer	SAM and EG fused layer (18)(19)
	Protein layer (BSA, etc.) (4)	Polysaccharide (2)(9) (dextran, etc.)	Protein layer (13) (Protein A/G, etc.)	Ethylene glycol (EG)	Protein and phospholipid fused layer (20)(21)
	–	–	–	Polysaccharide (2)(9) (dextran, etc.)	SAM and phospholipid fused layer (22)

(1) Besselink et al., 2004; (2) Yang et al., 2005; (3) Kim et al., 2007; (4) Polonschii et al., 2010; (5) Katz et al., 1995; (6) Torrance et al., 2006; (7) Huang et al., 2005; (8) Bonroy et al., 2006; (9) Johnsson et al., 1991; (10) Lahiri et al, 1999; (11) Kwon et al., 2004; (12) Huang et al., 2002; (13) Lee et al., 2007; (14) Ha et al., 2007; (15) Sigal et al., 1996; (16) Wazawa et al, 2006; (17) Masson et al., 2007; (18) Prime & Whitesides, 1993; (19) Sigal et al., 1998; (20) Athey et al., 2005; (21) Shah et al., 2007; (22) Ishizuka-Katsura et al., 2008

Table 3. Examples of three factors (capture agent, surface chemistry, and surface matrix) that are important in the formation of immobilization layers.

affinity, and ease of size control, using the molecular evolutionary systematic evolution of ligands by exponential enrichment (SELEX) process and phage display method. The obtained artificial antibodies have been often used as capture agents in SPR (Katz et al., 1995, Polonschii et al., 2010).

5.2.2 Surface chemistry

A coupling method involving activated N-hydroxysuccinimide esters is one of the most commonly used surface chemistry techniques for anchoring capture molecules to a sensor surface (Table 3, Johnsson et al., 1991, Lahiri et al, 1999). Since the target of this activated ester is any amino group that is present on the protein molecule with high probability, this coupling method is applicable to various capture agents used for SPR biosensing. To obtain highly sensitive SPR signals, the orientation of capture agents should be considered. The percentage of biochemically active capture agents that can interact with the target molecules would be higher if the orientation of the capture agents on the sensor surface can be improved. As a result of this improvement, the SPR response would be increased several times. As a typical example, the surface chemistry to immobilize proteins via hexahistidine tags (His-tag) has been used (Sigal et al., 1996). In recent years, mutated proteins, such as functional fusion proteins, have been used for achieving oriented immobilization of capture agents and simplification of the immobilization process (Terrettaz et al., 2002, Ha et al., 2007, Park et al., 2009, Le Brun et al., 2011). Some mutated proteins are already on the market as commercial layers (Athey et al., 2005).

5.2.3 Surface matrix

Polymers, polysaccharides, self-assembled monolayers, phospholipid and protein layers, among other, have all been reported as surface matrices (Table 3). One of the most important functions of the surface matrix in SPR biosensors is the suppression of non-specific adsorption of contaminants to the sensor surface. For this purpose, the introduction of oligo(ethylene glycol) molecules is highly effective (Prime & Whitesides, 1993, Sigal et al., 1998). Moreover, it is also important to increase the binding capacity of the capture agents. This factor, which determines the maximum signal variation of the SPR sensor, can control the dynamic range of the biosensing. One example of a surface matrix that has been successful in increasing the binding capacity of capture agents is the carboxymethylated dextran matrix provided by GE Healthcare (Sweden). The carboxymethylated dextran matrix provides a three-dimensional space with a thickness of 100 nm for target molecule binding (Yang et al., 2005, Johnsson et al., 1991).

5.3 Preparation of an immobilization layer on the sensor surface

To accomplish highly sensitive SPR biosensing with a nanoimprinted sensor device, the thickness of the probe layer using such as antibodies should be ~20 nm, as the sensing depth is about 40–80 nm. For this purpose, we attempted to introduce self-assembling layers of ORLA18 proteins (Orla Protein Technologies, UK) onto the sensor surface. The scaffold structure of ORLA proteins is based on the stable structure of the beta-sheet and beta-barrel mutated porin outer membrane protein (Omp) of *Escherichia coli*. It was firstly reported by the research group of J.H. Lakey in 2002 that OmpF proteins can be immobilized directly on a gold surface via thiol-gold bonds formed between the gold and the cysteine residues of the Omp protein (Terrettaz et al., 2002). Moreover, the surface loops of the monomeric porin OmpA can be replaced by anything from short peptides to larger protein domains. The advanced ORLA protein (ORLA18) is designed to present precisely oriented antibody (IgG)-binding domain structures (two Z-domains of protein A) as single layers with a thickness of ~10 nm on surfaces (Athey et al., 2005).

The surface preparation process of the ORLA18 protein layer is described below and shown in Fig. 7.

1. Treatment of the gold surface on the nanoimprinted sensor device by injecting an aqueous solution containing 1% (v/v), beta-mercaptoethanol.
2. Self assembly of the scaffold protein on the gold surface by injecting a 5 μM ORLA18 dissolved in ROG-8 buffer (Orla Protein Technologies).
3. Stabilization of the scaffold proteins and masking of the spaces between the proteins in the monolayer using 1x filler solution (Orla Protein Technologies).
4. Antibody binding on the ORLA18 protein layers by injecting a 100 μg/mL antibody dissolved in Tris-buffered saline (TBS; 10 mM Tris, pH 7.5, 150 mM NaCl) solution.

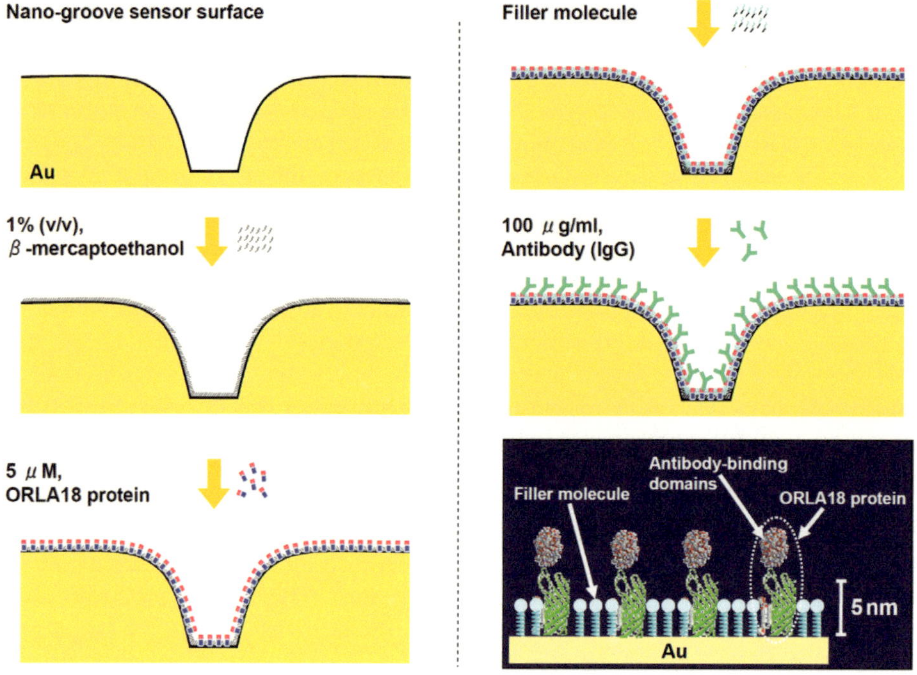

Fig. 7. Preparation process of an antibody-immobilization layer on the nanogroove sensor surface.

6. SPR biosensing using the nanoimprinted sensor device

6.1 Development of the SPR biosensor system

As a prototype of the nanoimprinted SPR biosensor system, we developed a desktop model for use in a laboratory (see Fig. 8). The dimensions of this model are W250mm × D250mm × H150mm, which is 10 times smaller than the commercialized SPR systems (Biacore-X, GE Healthcare, US).

Fig. 9 shows the optical system employed inside the prototype. The white light from the halogen lamp (LS1-LL, Ocean Optics Inc, US) is collimated and irradiated onto the sensor

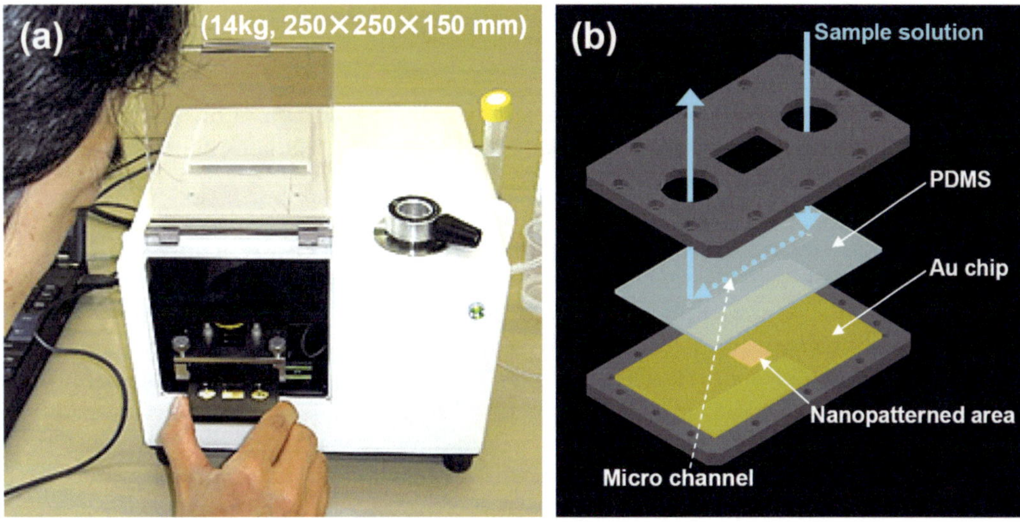

Fig. 8. Prototype of the nanoimprinted SPR biosensor system (a) and a schematic representation of the sensor chip including a microchannel (b).

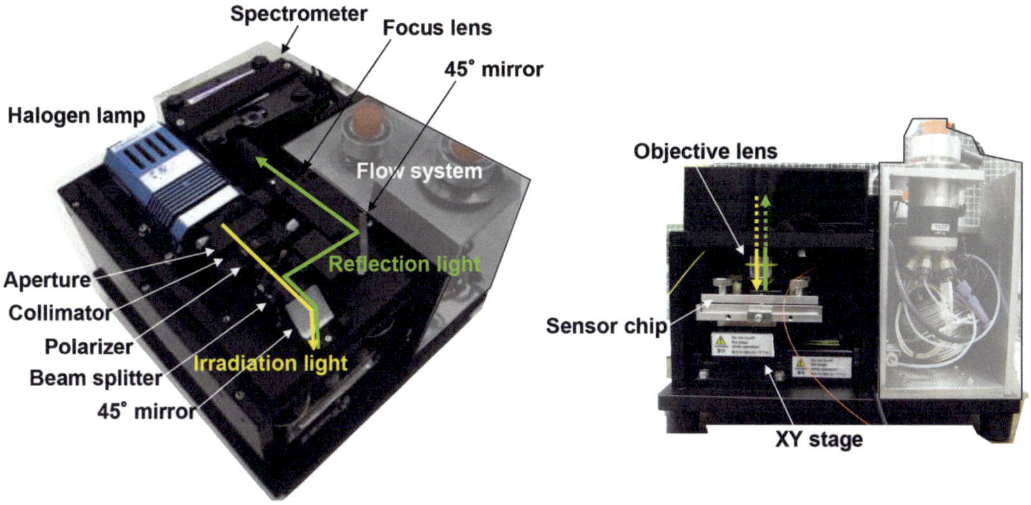

Fig. 9. Optical system inside the nanoimprinted SPR biosensor system.

surface through the objective lens (Plan N ×10, Olympus Co., Japan). The reflected light is gathered by the object lens and split by the half prism (BS CUBE NON-POL VIS 47121, Edmund Optics Inc., US) before reaching the spectrometer (USB4000, Ocean Optics Inc., USA). The resonant wavelength is analyzed by measuring the reflection spectrum data in real time. The motorized linear XY stage (SGSP15-10, Sigma Koki Co., Ltd, Japan) is located under the sensor device holder and is configured to enable multiple points on the sensor chip to be monitored by programming the detection points in advance. A correct and stable liquid flow control system is also very important. Several pumps, such as Veritas and plunger pumps, were considered for use as a flow control system in the prototype. In the

end, an electro osmotic flow (EOF) pump was selected for use. The EOF pump (RP7SP, Nano fusion Technology, Japan) is a very small-sized low-cost pump that provides a non-pulsating flow.
We attached a flow sensor (ASL1430-24, Sensirion, US) downstream of the EOF pump. The applied voltage to the EOF pump was determined under the feedback control of the flow sensor to realize a small and stable flow.

6.2 Two-dimensional monitoring of antibody-binding on the ORLA18 surface

The ORLA18 protein was immobilized on the nanogroove sensor surface according to the immobilization process shown in Fig. 7. To suppress non-specific adsorption, the remaining area was blocked using an oligo(ethylene glycol) (OEG) self-assembled monolayer composed of hydroxyl-terminated thiol ($HS(CH_2)_{11}(OCH_2CH_2)_3OH$) (Dojindo, Japan) molecules. After the docking of the ORLA18-immobilization gold substrate onto the sensor chip cassette (Fig. 8b), the SPR measurements were started. The two-dimensional variation of the SPR peak wavelength shift on the nanogroove sensor surface was monitored by the nanoimprinted SPR biosensor system of Fig. 8a. After the injection of 100 µg/ml rabbit polyclonal antibodies and IgG (Monosan, Netherlands) dissolved in TBS (pH 7.5) buffer, the specific signal corresponding to antibody-binding was confirmed in the ORLA18-immobilized area (Fig. 10, top left-hand corner of the immobilized area).

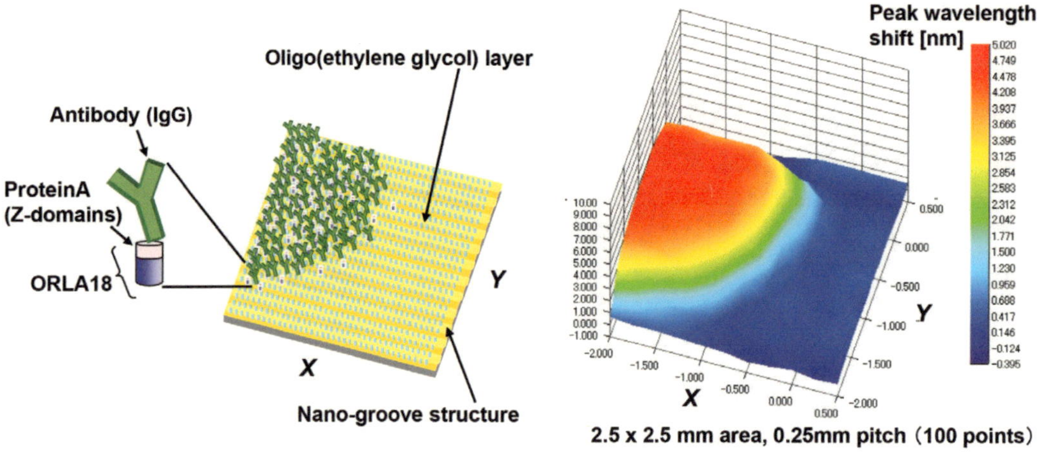

Fig. 10. 2D monitoring of the antibody-binding process on the ORLA18 surface using the nanoimprinted SPR biosensor system.

6.3 Evaluation of the sensing depth on the nanoimprinted sensor device

To demonstrate that the sensing depth is confined to a much smaller region in this sensor, we have attempted to compare the "bulk effect" between this sensor and the propagating SPR. Undiluted fetal bovine serum (FBS) purchased from Japan Bioserum (Japan) was used as a model of blood serum, which contains various proteins as background noise factors (Fig. 11).
In the propagating SPR (Biacore-X, GE Healthcare Co.), whose sensing depth is several hundred nanometers, the signal change caused by the undiluted FBS injection was about 8,000 RU, while the signal change from the binding of the antibody (IgG) dissolved in TBS

(pH 7.5) buffer was 2,100 RU. In the nanoimprinted SPR sensor, the peak shift caused by the undiluted FBS injection was 1.2 nm, while the peak shift caused by the binding of IgG dissolved in TBS (pH 7.5) buffer was 3.5 nm. The signal-to-noise ratio (IgG binding/FBS signal before washing) was 0.26 and 2.92 in the propagating SPR and the nanoimprinted SPR, respectively (Fig. 11). This shows that the nanoimprinted SPR sensor is more than 10 times less subject to bulk effects, due, for example, to the other constituents of blood and temperature fluctuations. This indicates that the sensing depth of the SPR is much smaller than that of a conventional propagating SPR sensor. This will help fabricate small-sized equipment in which temperature control is not necessary. Also, the washing protocol to separate the signal caused by the binding of the target molecules from the signal caused by the mixture of other floating biomolecules can be omitted. These advantages promise to lead to the development of protein and point-of-care chips, which are expected to become prevalent in diagnostic and healthcare applications.

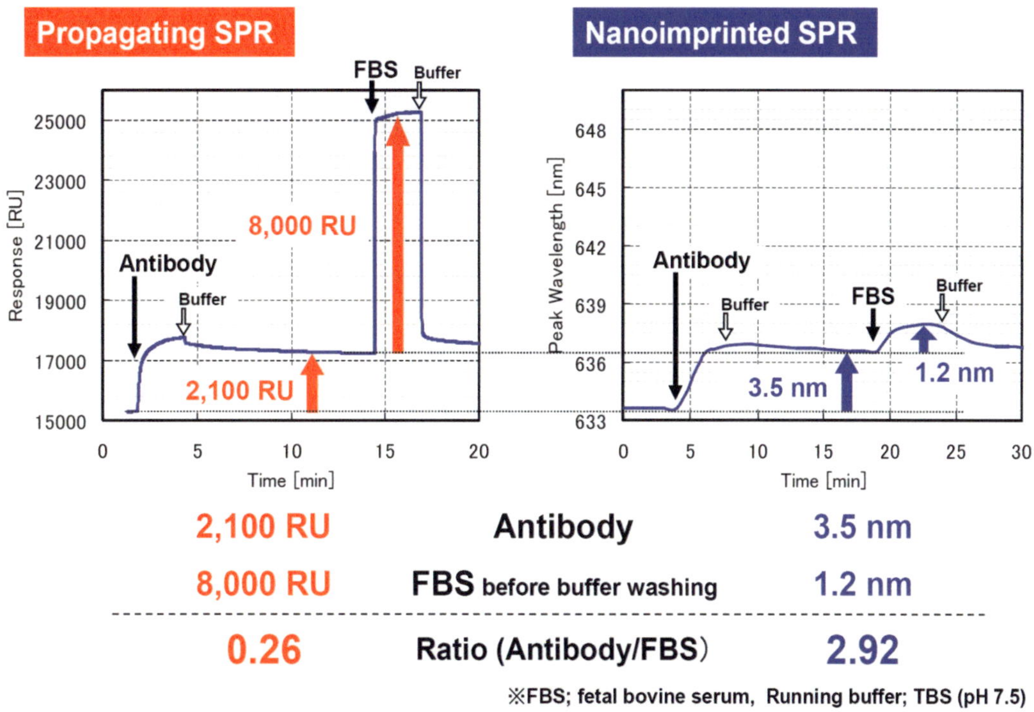

Fig. 11. Comparison of the signal-to-noise ratios of the nanoimprinted SPR and propagating SPR.

6.4 Detection of alpha-fetoprotein using the nanoimprinted SPR biosensor

Using the nanoimprinted SPR biosensor, we performed the quantitative detection of alpha-fetoprotein (AFP), a tumor marker. The AFP concentration in healthy human serum is approximately ~20 ng/ml, but its level increases markedly to over several hundred ng/ml in patients with liver cancer (Teramura & Iwata, 2007). Currently, the cut-off-value of AFP for clinical diagnosis is 200 ng/ml. Hence, the sensitive detection of the AFP using the nanoimprinted SPR system must be useful in cancer diagnosis. For the highly sensitive detection of AFP, an affinity purified rabbit polyclonal antibody (95% IgG) against human AFP was purchased from Monosan (Netherlands). Pure human AFP (a single band on SDS-PAGE) was obtained from Morinaga Institute of Biological Science (Japan). These AFP and Anti-AFP were diluted in Hepes-buffered saline (10 mM HEPES, pH 7.4, 150 mM NaCl) solution containing 0.005% (v/v) Surfactant P20 and 3 mM EDTA, which was used as a running buffer in the flow cell of the SPR system.

At first, we attempted to detect the AFP molecules on the anti-AFP-immobilized ORLA18 surface under condition 1 in Fig. 12. However, degradation of the signal was observed in low concentration. Then the detection limit of the nanoimprinted SPR biosensor was estimated to be more than several hundred ng/mL (Fig. 13). To obtain a higher variation of the SPR signal, we attempted to increase the efficiency of the antigen-antibody reaction by five times higher flow rate (100 µl/min) and two times larger than the contact time (6 min) of this reaction under condition 2. Fig. 14 shows the results of AFP detection at condition 2. The error bar indicates three standard deviations of the base line signal after the injection of a zero-concentration AFP solution. After several experiments, finally we realized that reducing the diffusion time of AFP is essential. Under condition 1 (Fig. 12), the mass-transport effect (Karlsson et al., 1991) can be larger because of the size of its flow cell. Therefore, under condition 3, we decreased the flow cell size. In this condition, the signal degradation at low concentration was observed under condition 1 to be significantly improved (Fig. 13). Then we estimated that the detection limit of AFP by the nanoimprinted SPR biosensor is ~20 ng/mL. This value already overcomes the cut-off value of 200 ng/mL in a clinical diagnosis.

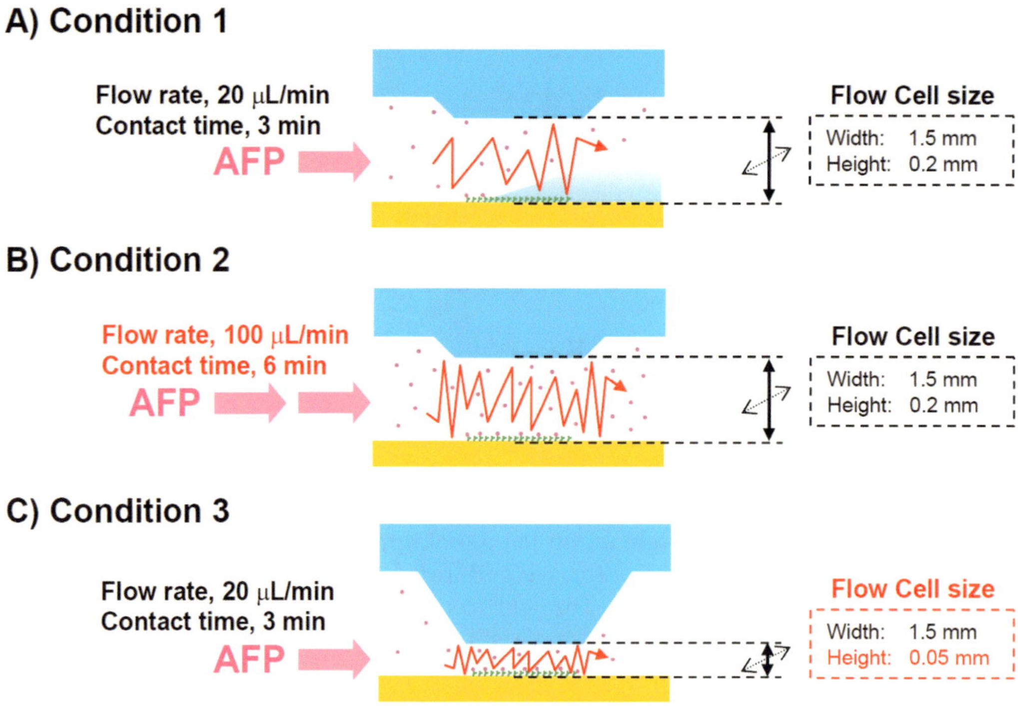

Fig. 12. Experimental conditions for AFP detection using the nanoimprinted SPR biosensor.

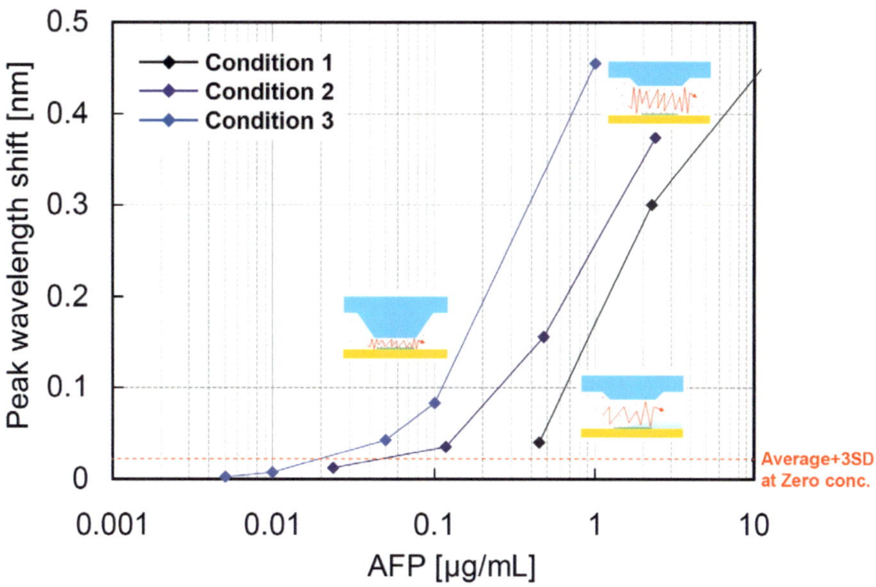

Fig. 13. Standard curves for AFP detection at different experimental conditions.

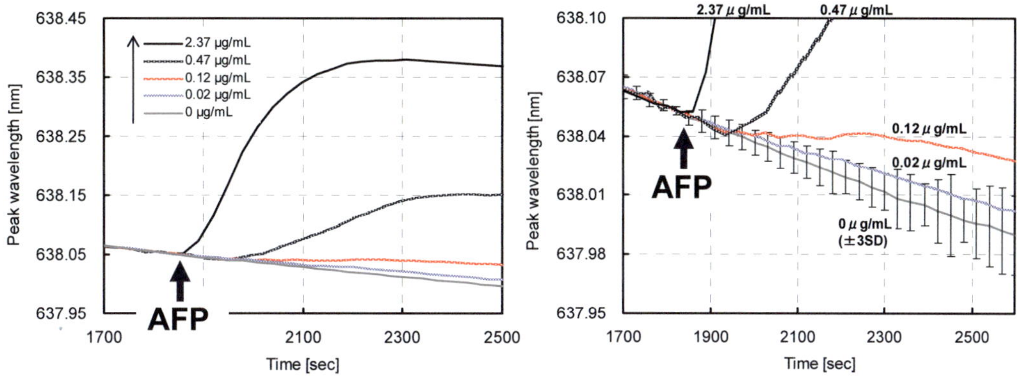

Fig. 14. Results of AFP detection using the nanoimprinted SPR biosensor. The right graphs show the expansion of the left graphs.

7. Present research - Development of palm-sized model -

Localized SPR has good potential to be used more widely as it can provide real-time, quantitative and easy operation sensing without any labeling on the target molecules. For various usages such as point-of-care testing, food analysis, and environmental tests, we have developed a palm-sized prototype based on the nanoimprinted SPR biosensor.

Fig. 15 shows a picture of the prototype. The dimensions are W77mm × D52mm × H56mm and its weight is only 240 g. The electric power used in this model is all supplied by the USB cable connected to the PC. The sensor chip is inserted from the front side into the equipment. The injection of the liquid sample through the micro channel is conducted by the

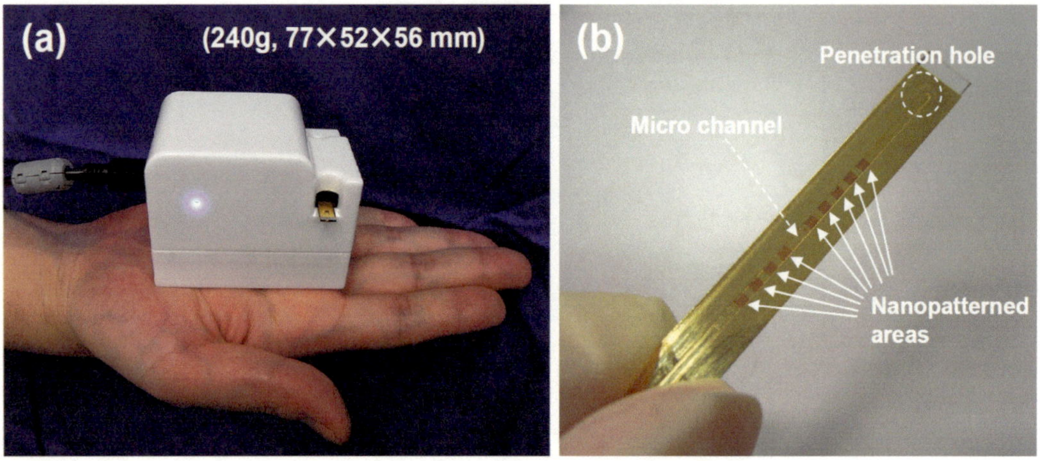

Fig. 15. Palm-sized model of the nanoimprinted SPR biosensor system (a) and the sensor chip including a micro channel (b).

syringe pressure. Fig. 16 shows the optical system of this model. A red laser (LM10-650, Kyoritsu-Electric Corporation, Japan) is used as a light source and the change of the reflection power is detected in this model. The light from the light source is split into four beams and four spot areas, which are detected at once. And the reflected light is detected by the photo-diode (S8745-01, Hamamatsu Photonics, Japan).

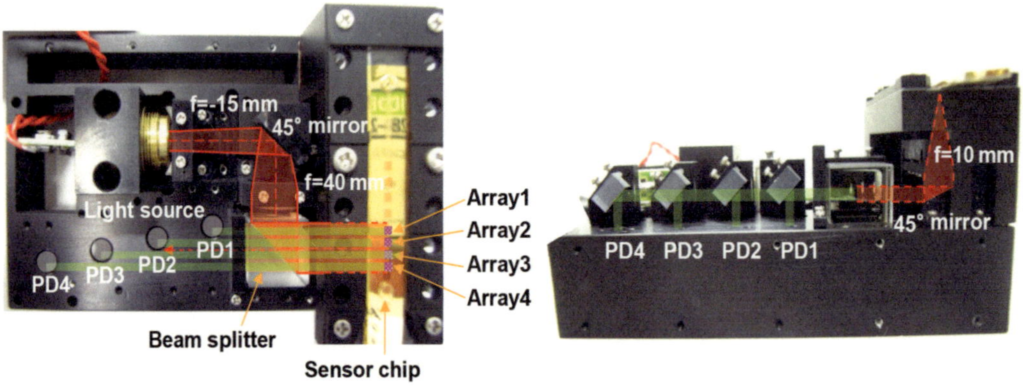

Fig. 16. Optical system inside the palm-sized nanoimprinted SPR biosensor.

To demonstrate the detection of biomolecules by using this model, we have attempted to detect avidin protein. The sensor surface is previously modified by the biotinylated alkyl thiol (BAT) layer according to the protocol below.

1. Biotin-terminated tri(ethylene glycol)hexadecanethiol (OEG-BAT) (Assemblon, USA) and 11-hydroxy-1-undecanethiol (HUT) (Dojindo, Japan) are solved in 99.5% ethanol.
2. The sensor chip was immediately immersed in the ethanol solution containing 0.95 mM OEG-BAT and 0.05 mM HUT.
3. The sensor chip is rinsed with an ethanol solution after 10 minutes of immersion.
4. The sensor chip is dried under a stream of nitrogen.

5. Inject 0.1 mg/mL NeutrAvidin (Thermo Scientific, USA) dissolved in Hepes-buffered saline (10 mM HEPES, pH 7.4, 150 mM NaCl) solution containing 0.005% (v/v) Surfactant P20 and 3 mM EDTA.

The result is shown in Fig. 17. NeutrAvidin was injected at about t=50 sec. As a result, the reflection change of 6% was observed in this system. This result indicates that the detection of biomolecules can be realized by this small and simple model.

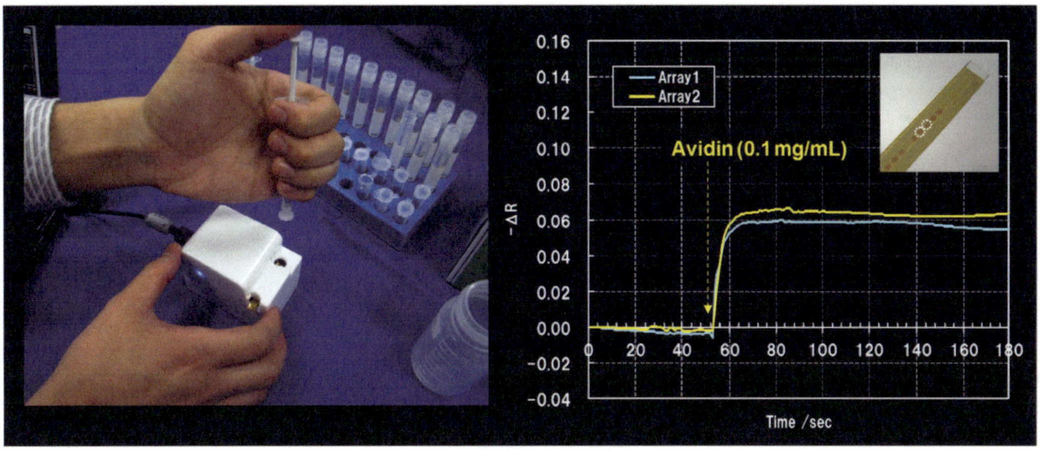

Fig. 17. Avidin protein detection using the palm-sized nanoimprinted SPR biosensor.

8. Conclusions

In this study, we accomplished a 10-times-higher signal-to-noise ratio measurement than conventional SPR using an SPR biosensor based on a gold nanogroove surface. Notably, using nanoimprinting technology, we have developed metal nanopatterns on a sensor surface with a process that has high reproducibility and throughput. Furthermore, the size of the prototype based on this detection principle was 10 times smaller than in commercialized SPR systems. Using the SPR prototype, we accomplished quantitative AFP detection as low as ~20 ng/mL. For this, 1) the smaller thickness of the probe layer and 2) the immobilization of antibodies on the sensor surface in a well-oriented manner were essential. A self-assembled fusion protein, the ORLA18 layer, was useful for accomplishing this purpose. Decreasing the size of the flow cell to reduce the diffusion time of the AFP was also very important. To the best of our knowledge, the detection limit of 20 ng/mL is the highest sensitivity achieved for direct detection of AFP using an SPR biosensor.

Recently, we were also successful in detecting AFP of about 100 pg/ml with an enhanced assay method by stepwise application of a biotinylated secondary antibody and streptavidin-bound colloidal gold. This suffices as a practical way to measure other important biomarkers such as prostate-specific antigen and carcinoembryonic antigen. Thus, the effectiveness of our SPR sensor has been demonstrated by the achievement of a high signal-to-noise ratio and highly sensitive detection of tumor marker protein. Our nanoimprinting technology-based SPR biosensor technology will have various useful applications, such as for medical diagnoses, environmental monitoring, and in the food industry.

9. Acknowledgments

We are grateful to Dr. Tetsuichi Wazawa (Graduate School of Engineering, Tohoku University) for critical reading of the abstract. This work was supported by the Core Research for Evolutional Science and Technology (CREST) project of the Japan Science and Technology Agency (JST).

10. References

Athey, D.; Shah, D.S.H.; Phillips, S.R.; Lakey, J.H. (2005). A manufacturable surface-biology platform for nano applications; cell culture, analyte detection, diagnostics sensors. *Ind. biotechnol.*, 1, 185-189

Besselink, G.A.J.; Kooyman, R.P.H.; van Os, P.J.H.J.; Engbers, G.H.M.; Schasfoort, R.B.M. (2004). Signal amplification on planar and gel-type sensor surfaces in surface plasmon resonance-based detection of prostate-specific antigen. *Anal. Biochem.*, 333, 165–173

Bonroy, K.; Frederix, F.; Reekmans, G.; Dewolf, E.; Palma, R.D.; Borghs, G.; Declerck, P.; Goddeeris, B. (2006). Comparison of random and oriented immobilisation of antibody fragments on mixed self-assembled monolayers. *J. Immunol. Methods*, 312, 167–181

Chou, S.Y.; Krauss, P.R.; Renstrom, P. J. (1995). Imprint of sub-25 nm vias and trenches in polymers. *Appl. Phys. Lett.*, 67, 3114-3116

Dostálek, J. & Homola, J. (2006). SPR biosensors for environmental monitoring. *Springer Ser. Chem. Sens. Biosens.*, Vol. 4, 191–206, ISBN 978-3-540-33918-2, Springer Berlin Heidelberg New York

Félidj, N.; Aubard, J.; Lévi, G. Krenn, J.R.; Salemo, M.; Schider, G.; Lamprecht, B.; Leitner, A.; Aussenegg, F.R.; (2002). Controlling the optical response of regular arrays of gold particles for surface-enhanced Raman scattering. *Phys. Rev. B*, 65, 075419 (1-9)

Ha, T.H.; Jung, S.O.; Lee, J.M.; Lee, K.Y.; Lee, Y.; Park, J.S.; Chung, B.H. (2007). Oriented immobilization of antibodies with GST-fused multiple Fc-specific B-domains on a gold surface. *Anal. Chem.*, 79, 546–556

Homola, J.; Yee, S. S.; Gauglitz, G. (1999). Surface plasmon resonance sensors: review. *Sens. Actuators B*, 54, 3–15

Homola, J. (2003). Present and future of surface plasmon resonance biosensors. *Anal. Bioanal. Chem.*, 377, 528–539

Huang, H.; Huang, S.; Yuan, S.; Qu, C.; Chen, Y.; Xu, Z., Liao, B.; Zeng, Y.; Paul K. Chu, P. K. (2011). High-sensitivity biosensors fabricated by tailoring the localized surface plasmon resonance property of core–shell gold nanorods. *Anal. Chimi. Acta*, 683, 242–247

Huang, L.; Reekmans, G.; Saerens, D.; Friedt, J.-M.; Frederix, F.; Francis, L.; Muyldermans, S.; Campitelli, A.; Hoof, C.V. (2005). Prostate-specific antigen immunosensing based on mixed self-assembled monolayers, camel antibodies, and colloidal gold enhanced sandwich assays. *Biosens. Bioelectron.*, 21, 483–490

Huang, N.-P.; Vörös, J.; De Paul, S.M.; Textor, M.; Spencer, N.D. (2002). Biotin-derivatized poly(L-lysine)-g-poly(ethylene glycol): a novel polymeric interface for bioaffinity sensing. *Langmuir*, 18, 220–230

Ishizuka-Katsura, Y.; Wazawa, T.; Ban, T.; K. Morigaki, K.; Aoyama, S. (2008). Biotin-containing phospholipid vesicle layer formed on self-assembled monolayer of a saccharide-terminated alkyl disulfide for surface plasmon resonance biosensing. *J. Biosci. Bioeng.*, 105, 527–535

Johnsson, B.; Löfås, S.; Lindquist, G. (1991). Immobilization of proteins to a carboxymethyldextran-modified gold surface for biospecific interaction analysis in surface plasmon resonance sensors. *Anal. Biochem.*, 198, 268–277

Karlsson, R.; Michaelsson, A.; Mattsson, L. (1991). Kinetic analysis of monoclonal antibody-antigen interactions with a new biosensor based analytical system. *J. Immunol. Methods*, 145, 229–240

Katz, B.A.; Cass, R.T.; Liu, B.; Arze, R.; Collins, N. (1995). Topochemical catalysis achieved by structure-based ligand design. *J. Biol. Chem.*, 270, 31210–31218

Kim, S.J.; Gobi, K.V.; Iwasaka, H.; Tanaka, H.; Miura, N. (2007). Novel miniature SPR immunosensor equipped with all-in-one multi-microchannel sensor chip for detecting low-molecular-weight analytes. *Biosens. Bioelectron.* 23, 701–707

Kretschmann, E. & Raether, H. (1968). Radiative decay of non-radiative surface plasmons excited by light. *Z. Naturforsch.*, 23A, 2135-2136

Kwon, Y.; Han, Z.; Karatan, E.; Mrksich, M.; Kay, B.K. (2004). Antibody arrays prepared by cutinase-mediated immobilization on self-assembled monolayers. *Anal. Chem.*, 76, 5713–5720

Ladd, J.; Taylor, A.; Jiang, S. (2006). SPR biosensors for food safety. *Springer Ser. Chem. Sens. Biosens.*, Vol. 4, 207–227, ISBN 978-3-540-33918-2, Springer Berlin Heidelberg New York

Lahiri, J.; Isaacs, L.; Tien, J.; Whitesides, G.M. (1999). A strategy for the generation of surfaces presenting ligands for studies of binding based on active aster as a common reactive intermediate: a surface plasmon resonance study. *Anal. Chem.* 71, 777–790

Le Brun, A.P.; Holt, S.A.; Shah, D.S.H.; Majkrzak, C.F.; Lakey, J.H. (2011). The structural orientation of antibody layers bound to engineered biosensor surfaces. *Biomaterials* 32, 3303–3311

Lee, J.M.; Park, H.K.; Jung, Y.; Kim, J.K.; Jung, S.O.; Chung, B.H. (2007). Direct immobilization of protein G variants with various numbers of cysteine residues on a gold surface. *Anal. Chem.*, 79, 2680–2687

Masson, J.-F.; Battaglia, T.M.; Khairallah, P.; Beaudoin, S.; Booksh, K.S. (2007). Quantitative measurement of cardiac markers in undiluted serum. *Anal. Chem.*, 79, 612-619

Nath, N. & Chilkoti, A. (2004). Label-free biosensing by surface plasmon resonance of nanoparticles on Glass: optimization of nanoparticle size. *Anal. Chem.*, 76, 5370-5378

Park, T.J.; Hyun, M.S.; Lee, H.J.; Lee, S.Y.; Ko, S. (2009). A self-assembled fusion protein-based surface plasmon resonance biosensor for rapid diagnosis of severe acute respiratory syndrome. *Talanta*, 79, 295–301

Polonschii, C.; David, S.; Tombelli, S.; Mascini, M.; Gheorghiu, M. (2010). A novel low-cost and easy to develop functionalization platform. Case study: Aptamer-based detection of thrombin by surface plasmon resonance. *Talanta*, 80, 2157–2164

Prime, K.L.; Whitesides, G.M. (1993). Adsorption of proteins onto surfaces containing end-attached oligo(ethylene oxide): a model system using self-assembled monolayers. *J. Am. Chem. Soc.*, 115, 10714–10721

Sigal, G.B.; Bamdad, C.; Barberis, A.; Strominger, J.; Whitesides, G.M. (1996). A self-assembled monolayer for the binding and study of histidine-tagged proteins by surface plasmon resonance. *Anal. Chem.*, 68, 490–497

Sigal, G.B.; Mrksich, M.; Whitesides, G.M. (1998). Effect of surface wettability on the adsorption of proteins and detergents. *J. Am. Chem. Soc.*, 120, 3464–3473

Stenberg, E.; Persson, B.; Roos, H.; Urbaniczky, C. (1991). Quantitative determination of surface concentration of protein with surface plasmon resonance using radiolabelled proteins. *J. Colloid Interface Sci.*, 143, 2, 513-526

Shah, D.S.; Thomas, M.B.; Phillips, S.; Cisneros, D.A.; Le Brun, A.P.; Holt, S.A.; Lakey, J.H. (2007). Self-assembling layers created by membrane proteins on gold. *Biochem. Soc. Trans.*, 35, 522-526

Teramura, Y. & Iwata, H. (2007). Label-free immunosensing for α-fetoprotein in human plasma using surface plasmon resonance. *Anal. Biochem.*, 365, 201–207

Terrettaz, S.; Ulrich, W.-P.; Vogel, H.; Hong, Q.; Dover, L.G.; Lakey, J.H. (2002). Stable self-assembly of a protein engineering scaffold on gold surfaces. *Protein Sci.*, 11, 1917–1925

Torrance, L.; Ziegler, A.; Pittman, H.; Paterson, M.; Toth, R.; Eggleston, I. (2006). Oriented immobilisation of engineered single-chain antibodies to develop biosensors for virus detection. *J. Vir. Methods*, 134, 164–170

Vaisocherová, H. & Homola, J. (2006). SPR biosensors for medical diagnostics. *Springer Ser. Chem. Sens. Biosens.*, Vol. 4, 229–247, ISBN 978-3-540-33918-2, Springer Berlin Heidelberg New York

Wazawa, T.; Ishizuka-Katsura, Y.; Nishikawa, S.; Iwane, A.H.; Aoyama, S. (2006). Grafting of poly(ethylene glycol) onto poly(acrylic acid)-coated glass for a protein-resistant surface. *Anal. Chem.*, 78, 2549–2556

Yang, C.-Y.; Brooks, E.; Li, Y.; Denny, P.; Ho, C.-M.; Qi, F.; Shi, W.; Wolinsky, L.; Wu, B.; Wong, D.T.; Montemagno, C.D. (2005). Detection of picomolar levels of interleukin-8 in human saliva by SPR. *Lab Chip*, 5, 1017–1023

5

Numerical Optimization of Plasmonic Biosensors

Dominique Barchiesi
GAMMA3 project (INRIA-UTT)- Charles Delaunay Institute - University of technology of Troyes 12 rue Marie Curie - BP 2060 - 10010 TROYES cedex France

1. Introduction

Since the engineering control of the deposition of nanometric gold plates on substrates the Surface Plasmon Resonance (SPR) based sensor has become one of the most successful label-free and commercially developed optical sensor, with applications to biology (Hoaa et al., 2007; Kolomenskii et al., 1997; Kretschman & Raether, 1968; Lecaruyer et al., 2006). This technique is currently employed in biomolecular engineering, drug design, monoclonal antibody characterization, virus-protein interaction, environmental pollutants detection, among other interesting problems. The basic principle of such transducer is the measurement of the sudden absorbtion of light by the thin metallic layer, under particular illumination conditions (p-polarization) and a specific angle of incidence of the illumination (Barchiesi, Kremer, Mai & Grosges, 2008; Barchiesi, Macías, Belmar-Letellier, Van Labeke, Lamy de la Chapelle, Toury, Kremer, Moreau & Grosges, 2008; Kretschman & Raether, 1968), leading to a highly sensitive device (Kolomenskii et al., 1997; Lecaruyer et al., 2006). The conditions of such absorption are linked to the plasmon resonance in metallic structure, and therefore a tiny change of the optical properties of medium above the gold plate, produces an angular shift of this absorption, due to the detuning of the resonance. The sensing principle relies therefore on the shift of the plasmonic resonance caused by the surrounding dielectric environmental change in a binding event.
The Plasmonic biosensors use the property of resonance between an illumination and the metallic part of the sensor. This resonance is used to increase the sensitivity of the biosensor and the threshold of detection. Actually, a given set of parameters of the biosensor can lead to a maximum of the absorption of the incoming light. A slight change of its immediate environment (presence/Absence of biomoecules to be detected) produces a strong change of the detected light due to the detuning of the resonance. This property is also used in cancer therapy or imaging, through metallic nanoparticles or nanoshells (Grosges, Barchiesi, Toury & Gréhan, 2008). The design of specific shapes for nanoparticles can help to tune the resonance for specific applications (Billot et al., 2006).
In the case of planar SPR (Surface Plasmon Resonance) biosensors, the reflected intensity vanishes for a specific angle of incidence. The illumination is almost totally coupled in the metal layer. A tiny change of the optical index of the upper medium, due to the presence of biomolecules, produces a measurable shift of this minimum. Therefore, to improve the efficiency of the sensor, the material and geometrical characteristics of the materials involved in the biosensor must be adjusted correctly. Surprisingly, the optimization of such structures has rarely been addressed (Ekgasit et al., 2005; Kolomenskii et al., 1997; Lecaruyer et al.,

2006) and only recently with metaheuristic methods (Barchiesi, Macías, Belmar-Letellier, Van Labeke, Lamy de la Chapelle, Toury, Kremer, Moreau & Grosges, 2008). Thus, the numerical optimization is becoming a useful tool, especially with the aim to apply to the optimization of nanostructured biosensors for which a large number of parameters has to be adjusted, making unapplicable a classical experimental design plan.
In this chapter, the requirements of such numerical optimization are put to the front, before introducing some optimization methods and discussing results. The first approach of optimization is based on deterministic methods, where a specific behavior of the bio-sensor is emphasized. For example, the influence of the thickness of the gold plate in SPR, all other parameters being fixed. More general methods of optimization are based on heuristics, and use the "random wizard," known to find what is hidden: the best parameters, much more efficiently than a systematic search, based on loops on each parameter. Among the various metaheuristic approaches, we focus on two specifics. Both are based on the bio-mymicry by numerical methods, by using life characteristics, stealing cross-over, mutation, selection, cooperation...

2. Optimization requirements: stand back and deepen the knowledge on the model

To get significant and reliable numerical results in numerical optimization, the most important requirement is having a realistic, efficient and numerically stable model. Even if this point seems to be obvious, this constraint on the model for its use for numerical optimization is not always fulfilled. Actually, numerical models entail *endogenous* (physically significant), and *exogenous* inputs. Among the exogenous parameters, some of them are linked to the mathematical model (the number of terms in series, the choice of scattering (S) or transmission (T) formulation (Li, 1994; 1996)...) and many are related to the numerical methods (the integration step size, the maximum degree of polynomials of interpolation, the stop criterion, the method of inversion, the discretization, the number of terms in series (Barchiesi et al., 2006; Barchiesi, Macías, Belmar-Letellier, Van Labeke, Lamy de la Chapelle, Toury, Kremer, Moreau & Grosges, 2008; Grosges et al., 2007; Grosges, Borouchaki & Barchiesi, 2008; Grosges et al., 2010; 2005)...)
If trends are considered as sufficient to compare experiments and numerical simulations, the exogenous inputs are often adjusted manually within the domain of physical (endogenous) parameters used for the model.
Instead, for optimization, the model is used as a black box, and the exogenous inputs must be adjusted automatically to produce stable and converged results. The model should be used blindly and remaining always reliable. This aspect of development of a stable numerical model is particularly critical in the case of resonance depiction, leading intrinsically to numerical instabilities. We encountered such a problem with FDTD (Macías et al., 2004), with evolutionary methods, the FDTD using regular Yee's cells for computation, like DDA used dipoles of the same size. This fact produced instabilities in the optimization, which prefers a continuity of the computed result with discretization. Indeed, the plasmon resonance can be described mathematically as the occurrence of a pole (in the complex plane) in the diffusion matrix, and this property has to be correctly handled. The two following sub-section illustrate two aspects of care to provide to the mathematical formulation.

2.1 The plasmon resonance and the model of biosensor

The SPR involves at least one metal layer, sometimes two, for improving the stick of the gold layer (Barchiesi, Macías, Belmar-Letellier, Van Labeke, Lamy de la Chapelle, Toury, Kremer,

Moreau & Grosges, 2008). The gold layer is the active part of the biosensor (Fig. 1). The incoming illumination is characterized by its p polarized electric field E_i (the magnetic field is parallel to the layer). The SPR biosensors use the Kretschmann configuration (Kretschmann, 1978), and therefore, the reflected (or specular) field intensity $R = |E_r|^2$ is detected. The transmitted field E_t is the probe of the biomolecules. Basically, a metal is highly reflecting. However, the launch of plasmon corresponds to the maximum of energy transfer from the illumination to the metal layer. The track of the plasmon resonance is therefore highlighted by the detection of the minimum of the reflected intensity $R(\theta)$.

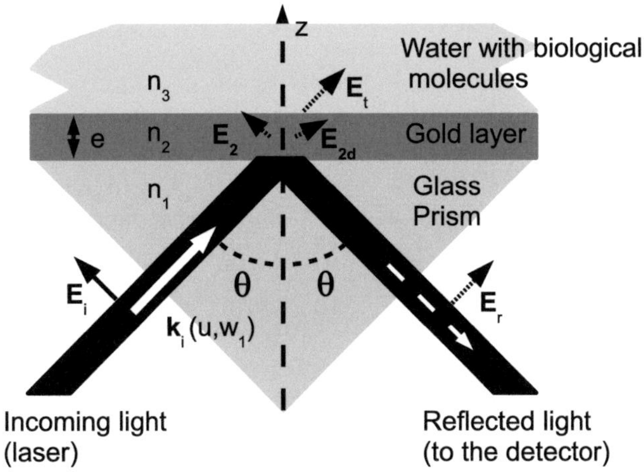

Fig. 1. Schematic of the SPR bio sensor, to be related to the Kretschmann configuration (Kretschmann, 1978).

The active part of the biosensor under consideration is the gold layer. The plasmon fingerprint corresponds to a strong decrease of R toward to 0 (Figs. 2). Therefore, the situation is slightly different from the classical electromagnetical one. In electromagnetics, the physical quantities of interest are the electromagnetic fields outside the material structures. The "input" is the incoming field and the "output" is the reflected and the transmitted fields. The (S) matrix relates the input to the output, for linear interaction of light with matter (Barchiesi, 1996; Li, 1996). On the contrary, in plasmonics, the system is the gold layer and the "output" of the system is the field inside the plate. Nevertheless, the transition between the two worlds is easy only if the property of resonance is correctly assessed. For this, the classical description of resonance by "getting something from nothing" is considered. Therefore, the field inside the gold layer must be related to the zero reflected field rather than the incoming field, through a (S') matrix. Assuming the reflected field expressed as proportional to the incoming field: $E_r = r.E_i$, the problem can be solved for plasmonics (Agarwal, 1973; Li, 1996; Raether, 1988; Simon et al., 1975). The field inside the metal film can be expressed as a sum of two fields E_2 and E_{2d} each of them associated to $\Re(w_2) > 0$ and $\Re(w_2) < 0$, w_2 being the normal to the slab components of the wave vector in gold (Fig. 1, (Born & Wolf, 1993; Simon et al., 1975)):

$$E_2 = \frac{t_{12}}{1 + r_{12} r_{23} \exp(2\imath w_2 e)} E_i \tag{1}$$

$$E_{2d} = \frac{t_{12} r_{23} \exp(2\imath w_2 e)}{1 + r_{12} r_{23} \exp(2\imath w_2 e)} E_i, \tag{2}$$

with the interface coefficients of transmission and reflection (Fresnel's coefficients):

$$r_{i,i+1} = \frac{n_{i+1}^2 w_i - n_i^2 w_{i+1}}{n_{i+1}^2 w_i + n_i^2 w_{i+1}} \text{ and } t_{i,i+1} = \frac{2n_{i+1}^2 w_i}{n_{i+1}^2 w_i + n_i^2 w_{i+1}} \quad (3)$$

To describe the resonance and to express the (S') matrix, these fields should be expressed as functions of the reflected field E_r:

$$E_2 = \frac{t_{12}}{1 + r_{12}r_{23}\exp(2\imath w_2 e)} \frac{1 + r_{12}r_{23}\exp(2\imath w_2 e)}{r_{12} + r_{23}\exp(2\imath w_2 e)} E_r \quad (4)$$

$$E_{2d} = \frac{t_{12}r_{23}\exp(2\imath w_2 e)}{1 + r_{12}r_{23}\exp(2\imath w_2 e)} \frac{1 + r_{12}r_{23}\exp(2\imath w_2 e)}{r_{12} + r_{23}\exp(2\imath w_2 e)} E_r \quad (5)$$

The resonance corresponds to a pole of the scattering coefficients:

$$s_1' = \frac{t_{12}}{r_{12} + r_{23}\exp(2\imath w_2 e)} \text{ and } s_2' = \frac{t_{12}r_{23}\exp(2\imath w_2 e)}{r_{12} + r_{23}\exp(2\imath w_2 e)} \quad (6)$$

The pole occurs if the common term of these coefficients

$$s_0' = \frac{t_{12}}{r_{12} + r_{23}\exp(2\imath w_2 e)} \quad (7)$$

$$= \frac{2n_2^2 w_1 (n_3^2 w_2 + n_2^2 w_3)}{(n_2^2 w_1 - n_1^2 w_2)(n_3^2 w_2 + n_2^2 w_3) + (n_3^2 w_2 - n_2^2 w_3)(n_2^2 w_1 + n_1^2 w_2) e^{2\imath w_2 e}} \quad (8)$$

is infinite, therefore, if the transcendent denominator vanishes. Obviously, the pole corresponds neither to the solution of $n_3^2 w_2 + n_2^2 w_3 = 0$ nor to that of $n_3^2 w_2 - n_2^2 w_3 = 0$. Consequently, the solution of this last equation $n_1 \sin(\theta) = \pm\sqrt{n_2^2 n_3^2 / (n_2^2 + n_3^2)}$, cannot be likened to the condition of plasmon excitation in a gold plate. This last expression is actually the solution for the excitation of a plasmon in a semi-infinite metal medium.

Two arguments help to better understand this result. First, it is logical to find a dependence of the plasmon in a slab, as a function of the thickness of the layer e. Then, it is necessary to find consistence between the cancelation of R and the concept of resonance.

The basic model of SPR entails a single layer of gold (thickness e, optical index n_2) deposited on a glass substrate (optical index n_1) (Fig. 1). The above medium is water of optical index n_3. The illumination is made by a p polarized plane wave, incoming on the gold layer under total internal reflection (TIR) configuration. θ is the angle between the illumination wave vector, and the normal to the layer vector. Figure 2(a) shows the computed reflected intensity $R = |r|^2$. The minimum of R depends on the thickness of the gold layer, therefore this parameter has to be optimized, to increase the efficiency of the biosensor in terms of contrast in R. The figure 2(b) shows the effect of a slight change in the optical index of the medium of detection n_3: the position of the minimum is shifted toward larger angles. Therefore, to detect a change in the optical index n_3 of the above medium, the measurement of the shift of θ, corresponding to $R \approx 0$ is achieved (Bonod et al., 2003; Lecaruyer et al., 2006).

This setup is also called Kretschmann configuration (Kretschmann, 1978) and is an object of study for undergraduates, as r and t can be easily calculated (Simon et al., 1975). The reflection coefficient r has been used in Eq. 8 and can be written as:

$$r = r_{13}(e, \theta) = \frac{n_d}{d_d} = \frac{r_{12} + r_{23}e^{2\imath w_2 e}}{1 + r_{12}r_{23}e^{2\imath w_2 e}}. \quad (9)$$

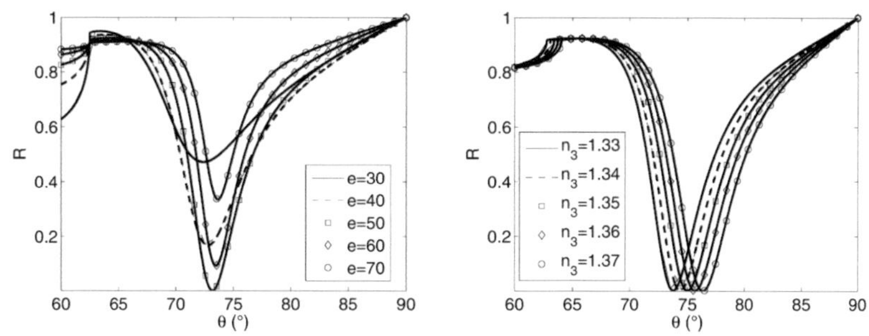

(a) $n_3 = 1.33$ (b) $e = 50$ nm

Fig. 2. Computation of the reflected field intensity $R = |r|^2$. The computation uses $n_1 = 1.5$, $n_2(\lambda_0 = 670\text{ nm}) = 0.137 + 3.797\imath$.

The vertical components of the wave vectors in each medium i can be expressed as a function of the illumination angle θ: $w_i = \frac{2\pi}{\lambda_0}\sqrt{n_i^2 - n_1^2 \sin^2(\theta)}$, where n_i is the optical index (and is a complex number for metal). This expression is not relevant for numerical study as the denominators of each $r_{i,i+1}$ can cancel. Instead, reducing to a common denominator and simplifying the fraction is necessary before numerical optimization:

$$r = \frac{n}{d} = \frac{(n_2^2 w_1 - n_1^2 w_2)(n_3^2 w_2 + n_2^2 w_3) + (n_3^2 w_2 - n_2^2 w_3)(n_2^2 w_1 + n_1^2 w_2)e^{2\imath w_2 e}}{(n_2^2 w_1 + n_1^2 w_2)(n_3^2 w_2 + n_2^2 w_3) + (n_3^2 w_2 - n_2^2 w_3)(n_2^2 w_1 - n_1^2 w_2)e^{2\imath w_2 e}}. \quad (10)$$

n is exactly the same as the denominator of s_0' (Eq. 8) which cancels at the plasmon resonance. Figure 3(a) illustrates the influence of the reduction to the same denominator of r. Obviously, both formula (Eqs. 9 and 10) give the same square modulus: $R_d = |n_d/d_d|^2$ is superimposed with $R = |n/d|^2$. Nevertheless, wrong conclusions could be drawn from the visual inspection of $|d_p|$ and $|n_p|$. For instance, the plasmon resonance could be interpreted through the increase of $|d_p|$ and the decrease of $|n_p|$ and therefore by an apparent resonance behavior. These variations, in the vicinity of the plasmon angle, seems to be produced by the Fresnel's coefficient r_{23}, but the angle for plasmon resonance differs slightly from that corresponding to the maximum of $|r_{23}|$. $|n|$ and $|d|$ have very different bearing from $|n_d|$ and $|d_d|$: $|n|$ vanishes instead of $|d|$. The first inconsistency or deficiency of the classical $r = n_d/n_p$ model is evident in Fig. 3(a): at the plasmon resonance, the numerator $|n_d|$ is close to zero and the denominator is far from zero or infinity. Nevertheless, Figs. 3(a) and 3(b), based on the $r = n/d$ model, shows clearly that the R shape is mainly related to the cancelation of the numerator n. T is also plotted: it is the transmitted intensity of light and corresponds to evanescent wave ($n_3 < n_1$ and $\sin(\theta) > n_3/n_1$) and therefore is null. Therefore, even if the field amplitude differs from zero, $T = 0$. The increase of the square modulus of the fields in the gold layer is not governed by the r_{23} maximum but on field which is reflected by the Gold/Water interface (E_{2d} in Fig. 1). This latter takes into account the thickness of gold instead of r_{23}. The vertical lines in Fig. 3(b) shows the angular position of the maximum of $|r_{23}|^2$ and of the minimum of R. This last one is located between the positions of the maximum of $|E_{2d}|$ and of the local minimum of $|E_2|$. The plasmon launch can be explained by the coupling between these two fields (rather the the reflection coefficients of each interface).

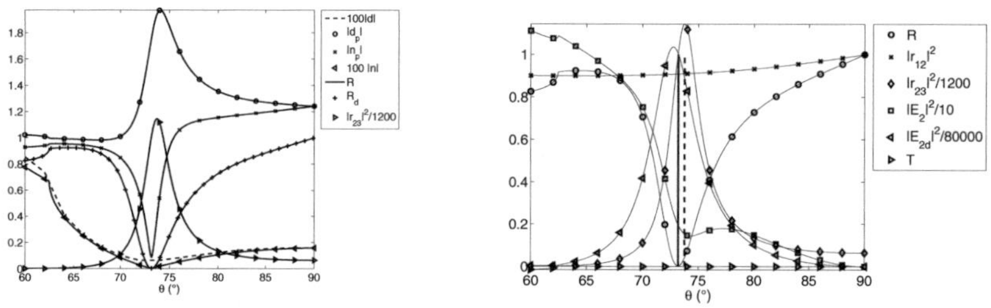

(a) (b)

Fig. 3. (a) Reflected intensity $R = |r/n|^2$, and $|n_d/d_d|^2$ (Eqs. 9,10) and numerators and denominators: $|n|$, $|d|$, $|n_p|$ and $|d_p|$. (b) Plot of the amplitude of fields inside the gold layer $|E_2|$ and $|E_{2d}|$ and of the reflection coefficient on each interface (Glass/Gold: r_{12} and Gold/Water: r_{23}. All plot are functions of the angle of incidence θ, and are computed for $n_1 = 1.5$, $n_2(\lambda_0 = 670\text{ nm}) = 0.137 + 3.797\imath$, $n_3 = 1.33$, $e = 50$ nm.

Therefore, the accurate solution of plasmon launch corresponds to $n = 0$ *ie*:

$$n = 0 = \underbrace{(n_2^2 w_1 - n_1^2 w_2)(n_3^2 w_2 + n_2^2 w_3)}_{T_1} + \underbrace{(n_3^2 w_2 - n_2^2 w_3)(n_2^2 w_1 + n_1^2 w_2)e^{2\imath w_2 e}}_{T_2}, \quad (11)$$

rather than:

$$n_3^2 w_2 - n_2^2 w_3 = 0 \Leftrightarrow \sin(\theta_{23}) = \pm\sqrt{\frac{1}{n_1^2}\frac{n_3^2 n_2^2}{n_3^2 + n_2^2}}, \quad (12)$$

which is often considered (Agarwal, 1973; Raether, 1988). Nevertheless, this solution is a complex number, the optical index n_2 of gold being complex too. Therefore, practically, the resonance cannot be exactly reached, θ being real (Barchiesi, Kremer, Mai & Grosges, 2008; Maystre & Nevière, 1977; Maystre & Nieto-Vesperinas, 1992; Neff et al., 2006). This solution cancels the second term (T_2) of the sum in Eq. 11 and reduces the value of the first one (T_1) but is clearly not the optimum (figure 3(b)).

The discussion is now made easier. The plasmon launch requires p polarisation of the illumination and $n_3/n_1 < \sin(\theta)$ (configuration which differs from that considered by Agarwal for polaritons where $n_1 = n_3$ (Agarwal, 1973)).

- The plasmon resonance is measured by the strong attenuation of $R = |r|^2$ for a specific angle of incidence, close to that cancels the real part of the numerator of r.
- The real part of d vanishes for an angle of incidence far from the angle of plasmon resonance, but its modulus is never null. Indeed, the denominator of R is not vanishing.
- The angle of incidence of the minimum of R corresponds to the value which cancel the modulus of the numerator of r. The modulus of d slightly influence the result (Fig. 3(b)).
- near the resonance, $|r_{23}|$ is drastically increased. Nevertheless, the maximum of $|r_{23}|^2$ is not localized to that of plasmon resonance. Therefore, the classical approximation based on this reflection coefficient is not relevant and cannot be used for optimization. Moreover, this approximation lies in the conclusions we could draw too rapidly from a model assuming infinite thickness of metal. Indeed, the finite thickness of gold, enables the "coupling" of the surface plasmons.

For the SPR model, let us consider both interfaces Glass/Gold and Gold/Water for the SPR: $n_1 = 1.5$, $n_3 = 1.33$. Figure 4(a) shows the dispersion curve, deduced from the canceling of R for a gold layer of thickness 50 nm. The bottom of the black well in the map is the location of the plasmon, which abscissa are the angle of incidence θ and ordinates are the wavelength. At first glance, the plasmon can be launched for each wavelength and under small variations of θ. Therefore, the influence of the optical index n_2 of gold seems to be weak. *This fact explains why the bulk values of the gold optical index can be used and gives results close the the experiments, even if it is well known that this parameters depends strongly on the mode of gold deposition.* The white continuous curve delineate the bottom of the well. The cross are the values of $\theta_{r_{23}}$ for

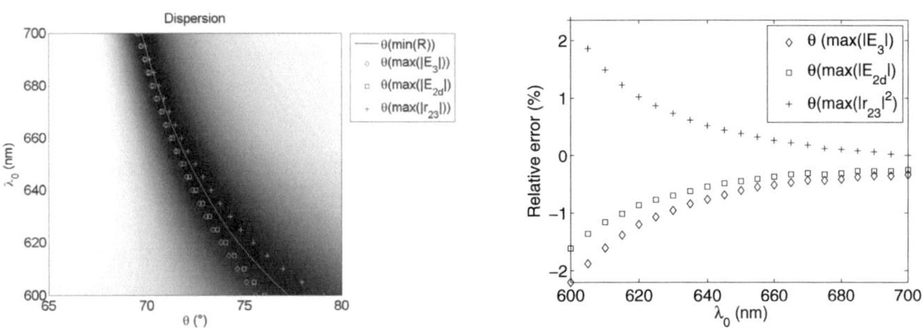

(a) (b)

Fig. 4. (a) dispersion curve $R(\theta, \lambda_0)$. The line shows the minimum of the well, the crosses indicate the positions of $r_{23}(\theta, \lambda_0) = 0$, the diamonds those of $\theta(\max(|E_3|))$. The squares correspond to the location of the maximum for the down going field in gold (E_{2d}): this field can be seen as reflected by the Gold/Water interface but takes into account the thickness of the gold layer. (b) relative error between the above mentioned angles, and the angle corresponding to the minimum of R.

the maximum of the Fresnel's coefficient of the non coupled Gold/Water interface (n_i is the optical index n_2 of gold and $n_{i+1} = 1.33$, $n_1 = 1.55$ in Eqs. 3). The diamonds are the angle θ_3 for which $T = |t|^2$ is maximum, and the square are those θ_{2d}, for the maximum of the field reflected by the Gold/Water interface in the gold layer (taking into account the "coupling"). Figure 4(b) shows the relative difference between the above mentioned angles, and $\theta(\min(R))$, in %. Some conclusions can be drawn now:

- The relative error is not negligible for optimization but if only trends are awaited, all these angles can be used. $\theta_{r_{23}}$ is greater than the plasmon angle, while θ_{2d} and θ_3 are better approximation.
- The approximations are better if λ_0 raises.
- The better approximation is always θ_{2d}. One may conclude that the plasmon resonance is mainly governed by the field reflected by the Gold/Water interface. This explains why the SPR biosensor are sensitive to any change of the optical index of the above medium (here water). Nevertheless, the thickness of gold is a critical parameter and therefore any attempt to optimize the SPR by using $|r_{23}|$ would fail.

The figure 5 illustrates the possible cancelation of R (dark zones), as a function of the real part and the imaginary part of n_2^2, the permittivity of the slab with virtual metallic optical index. For this, the thickness, the angle of incidence and the wavelength are fixed to $e = 50$ nm,

$\lambda_0 = 670$ nm and $\theta = 73^o$ (see Fig. 3(b)) to guarantee the possibility of plasmon launching. Despite all, r can be near zero for positive real part of the permittivity (n_2^2). The region of positive $\Re(n_2^2)$ define Brewster angle.

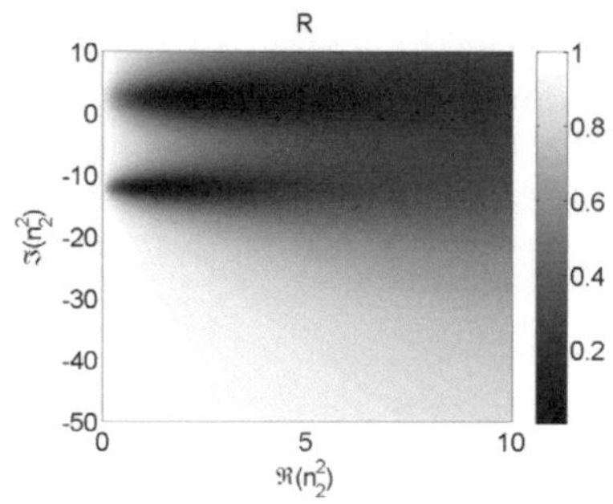

Fig. 5. R as a function of the permittivity of the layer virtual metallic material n_2^2 for $e = 50$ nm, $\lambda_0 = 670$ nm, $\theta = 73.2^o$, $n_1 = 1.5$, $n_3 = 1.33$ (Eq. 10).

The model of plasmon resonance is now well established. Nevertheless, the biosensor system is based on the detection of the angular shift of the minimum of R when n_3 varies. Therefore, the sensitivity of the biosensor must be investigated to determine if the simple minimization of R is sufficient.

2.2 The sensitivity of the SPR biosensor

The sensitivity of the SPR biosensor is related to the mode of detection. Basically, the quality of the plasmon resonance depends on the above mentioned parameters: the thickness of gold e, the wavelength λ_0 (and therefore the optical index of gold n_2) and the angle of incidence θ. But practically, a model of sensor must take into account the mode of detection of the angular shift of the plasmon resonance, under slight variations of the above optical index n_3 (Fig. 1). The detection of the angular shift is either monitored on the minimum of $R(\theta) = |r_{23}(\theta)|^2$ ($S_1 = \Delta\theta(\min(R))$), or on the maximum of slope $\max(|dR/d\theta|)$ of the same curve ($S_2 = \Delta\theta(\max(|dR/d\theta|))$). Figure 6 shows an illustration of these two modes as a function of the thickness e of the gold layer, with $n_3 = 1.330$, $\delta n_3 = 0.001$, $n_2(\lambda_0 = 670 \text{ nm}) = 0.137 + 3.797\imath$, $n_1 = 1.5$:

$$S_2 = \Delta\theta\left(\max\left(\left|\frac{dR}{d\theta}\right|\right)\right) = \theta\left(\max\left(\left|\frac{dR}{d\theta}(n_3+\delta n_3)\right|\right)\right) - \theta\left(\max\left(\left|\frac{dR}{d\theta}(n_3)\right|\right)\right) \tag{13}$$

The maximum of the visibility of the recorded signal is $V = (\max(R) - \min(R))/(\max(R) + \min(R))$. Near the plasmon resonance $\min(R) \approx 0$, but V decreases as a function of the detuning. Therefore V can be related directly to the quality of the plasmon resonance: Figs. 6(b) and 2 show that the maximum of visibility is reached when the plasmon occurs ($e \approx 52$ nm for $\lambda_0 = 670$ nm). Moreover, even if maximizing the product $V.S_2$ could be the natural target of optimization, the slight variations of the sensitivity curves can lead us to work directly on R. From here, we will try to find the best conditions of plasmon excitation *i.e.* R close to zero. Moreover, in both modes of detection, the sensitivity of the biosensor is governed by the shift of the peak and therefore exhibit the same behavior (Fig. 6(b)). Both sensitivities are increasing functions of the thickness. Therefore, the best conditions of detection are supposed to correspond to parameters closest to those of the 'best" plasmon

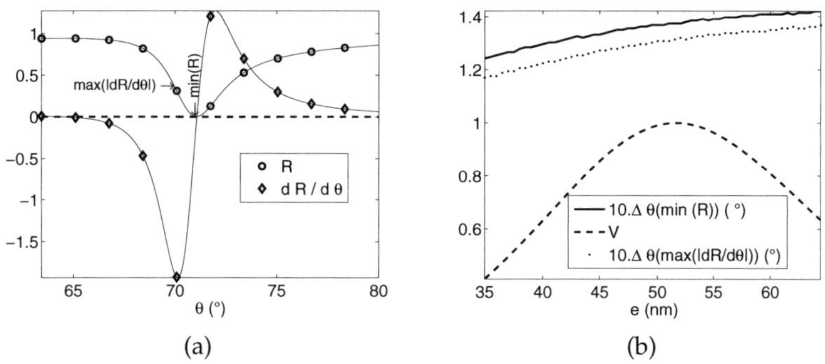

Fig. 6. (a) R and $dR/d\theta$ illustrating the two modes of detection as a function of θ. (b) Sensitivity of the biosensor as a function of the thickness of gold e, if the index of the medium of detection increases from $\delta n_3 = 0.01$. The sensitivities correspond to the angular shift of the plasmon resonance and to the shift of the maximum of the angular derivate of R. The visibility is $V = (\max(R) - \min(R))/(\max(R) + \min(R))$. The parameters are $n_3 = 1.33$, $\lambda_0 = 670$ nm, $n_2 = 0.137 + 3.797\imath$, $n_1 = 1.5$.

resonance, where sensitivity is high enough as well as visibility, *ie* when the pole is close to the real axis.
Consequently, in the following, the goal of optimization will be the minimization of R, which is directly related to the quality of the plasmon resonance.

2.3 The optimization of the gold layer thickness

We have found the conditions of plasmon launch (Eq. 11). The optimization target of the plasmon resonance is therefore the smallest value of $R = |r|^2$. Practically, to launch an efficient plasmon for the SPR biosensor, the parameters to be optimized are the angle of incidence θ, the thickness of gold e, and the incoming wavelength λ_0, the optical index of gold depending on the wavelength $n_2(\lambda_0)$. In principle, the wavelength can be imposed by the technical choice of the source of illumination and therefore, only two parameters remain free. The problem consists in finding the solutions of $|n| = 0$ (Eq 10). Even if this equation appears to be transcendent, the thickness of gold can be extracted:

$$e = -\frac{\imath}{2w_2}\log\left(-\frac{r_{12}}{r_{23}}\right) = -\frac{\imath}{2w_2}\log\left(-\frac{(n_2^2 w_1 - n_1^2 w_2)(n_3^2 w_2 + n_2^2 w_3)}{(n_3^2 w_2 - n_2^2 w_3)(n_2^2 w_1 + n_1^2 w_2)}\right) \tag{14}$$

If $n_2 = n_3$, this expression reduces to that of Eq. (2.28) in Ref. (Agarwal, 1973). Particular attention should be paid to the definition of the logarithm of complex number. It is not surprising that the mathematical solution for this thickness is a complex number. Therefore, the physical thickness e being real, the Poincaré's plot of e in the complex plane, is an obvious tool for deterministic optimization (Barchiesi, Kremer, Mai & Grosges, 2008). Both optimizations in Figs. 7 face a different methodology: Figure 7(a) consists in finding jointly the best values for e and θ, by minimizing R for each wavelength. Figure 7(b) is a Poincaré's plot (Barchiesi, Kremer, Mai & Grosges, 2008), in the phase plane of e, considering its complex value. These plots can help to choose the best set of parameters: thickness e, wavelength λ_0, and the angle θ. The best thickness is closest to the real axis (the imaginary part of e is not physical). For example, a good set of parameters is $e = 52$ nm, $\lambda_0 = 750$ nm and $\theta = 68.2^o$.

This type of plot gives also information on the sensitivity of the model to the real part of e. For instance, the shelf, close to the maximum of the $\theta = 68.2^o$ curve, near $\lambda_0 = 670$ nm, corresponds to a zone of low sensitivity of the biosensor to the imaginary part of the thickness of gold, and therefore, a zone of stability. The same curve, near $\lambda_0 = 750$ nm, exhibits an infinite derivative, and therefore much less sensitivity to the thickness e.

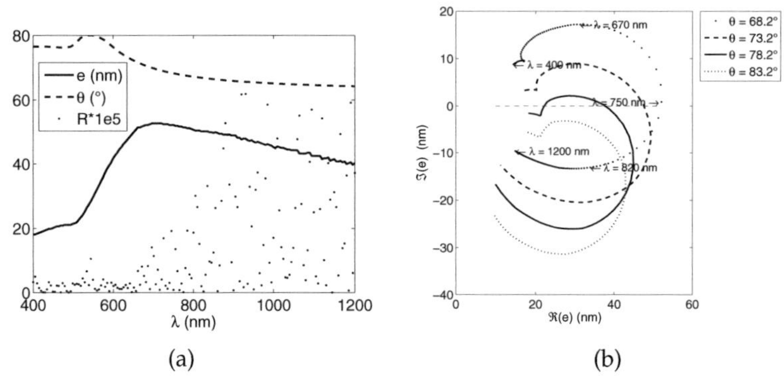

Fig. 7. Optimisation of angle θ and gold thickness e, the minimum of R is also plotted. Poincaré's plot of the best thickness e (Eq. 14), for various angles of incidence, as a function of the wavelength $\lambda_0 \in [400; 1200]$ nm.

It appears that even if the sensitivity of the SPR biosensor to the various parameters is a complex problem, it could be described by the model. The purpose of the next subsection is to evaluate the sensitivity of the model to the various parameters, through a comprehensive statistical method, where all parameters are considered simultaneously. This approach could help to evaluate the specifications for the design of biosensors.

2.4 Sensitivity of the model

The sensitivity of the model can help to evaluate what are the critical parameters in the process of fabrication of the biosensor. A Monte-Carlo method is one of the well known tools for the study of model's sensitivity. This method is based on the random generation of the endogenous parameters and on the statistical analysis of the output of the model. In the present case, a tolerance on $R \in [0, 10^{-3}]$ is fixed as well as physically acceptable interval for parameters (the input intervals in Tab. 1). To improve the efficiency of the Monte-Carlo method, an adaptation of the boundaries is proposed. A new random generation of N families $\mathbf{p}$ of random parameters is repeated at each step of a loop, until the number of families $\mathbf{p}_s$ making sure that $R(\mathbf{p_s}) \in [0, 10^{-3}]$ is greater than N. The boundaries of the space of search for each parameter are updated at each iteration, using the successful results of the previous loop. This adaptive boundary Monte-Carlo method enables to increase the number of "good" parameters $\mathbf{p}_s$, at each step, and therefore increases the convergence speed. For example, $N = 60.000$ requires less than 100 iterations in the loop. In the case of non adaptive Monte-Carlo method, the number of iterations is mostly greater than 1000. The pseudo-code of the adaptive Monte-Carlo algorithm is given (Algorithm 1).

The figure 8 shows the results that are summarized in the last column of Tab. 1 and the histograms for each parameters. The best value of the above realization of the Monte-Carlo software is also obtained: $R = 6.348^{-5}$ for $e = 52.1$ nm, $\lambda_0 = 688$ nm, $\theta = 70.5^o$ and $n_3 = 1.331$. The histograms reveals a "mode" in the $[600; 700]$ nm zone, which corresponds to

Require: α (threshold of tolerance on R), N (the number of random parameters set at each iteration). The initial boundaries of the hypercube D of acceptable parameters are set: $B_{min} = \{\min(e), \min(\lambda_0), \min(\theta), \min(n_3)\}$ and $B_{max} = \{\max(e), \max(\lambda_0), \max(\theta), \max(n_3)\}$.

[Initial random parameters set $\mathbf{p}$ generated from uniform distribution in D: $U(D)$]
$\{\mathbf{y}\} \leftarrow R(\{\mathbf{p}\})$
[Selection of the $\{p\}$ that verify $\{\mathbf{y}\} < \alpha$]
$\{\mathbf{p}_s\} \leftarrow \{\mathbf{p} \backslash \{\mathbf{y}\} < \alpha\}$
while [The sample size of $\mathbf{p}_s$ is lower than N] **do**
    $B_{min} \leftarrow \min(\mathbf{p}_s)$, $B_{max} \leftarrow \max(\mathbf{p}_s)$
    [Random generation of parameters $\{\mathbf{p}\}$ (uniform distribution in $[B_{min}, B_{max}]$: $U([B_{min}, B_{max}])$)]
    $\{\mathbf{y}\} \leftarrow R(\{\mathbf{p}\})$
    [Selection among the $\{p\}$ which verify $\{y\} < \alpha$]
    $\{\mathbf{p}_s^i\} \leftarrow \{\mathbf{p} \backslash \mathbf{y} < \alpha\}$
    $\{\mathbf{p}_s\} \leftarrow \{\mathbf{p}_s\} \bigcup \{\mathbf{p}_s^i\}$
end while
$\min(\{\mathbf{p}_s\}), \max(\{\mathbf{p}^s\})\ldots$

Algorithm 1. Pseudo-code of the adaptive Monte-Carlo algorithm. The numerical model of the SPR is denoted R and is considered stable in D.

Parameter	Input interval	Output interval	mid-height size of the peak
$e(nm)$	$[10; 80]$	$[43; 56]$	$[51.5; 52.5]$
$\theta(^o)$	$[60; 80]$	$[68; 76]$	$[70.3; 70.8]$
$\lambda_0(nm)$	$[600; 700]$	$[600; 700]$	$[680; 695]$
n_3	$[1.33; 1.34]$	$[1.330; 1.339]$	$[1.330; 1.331]$

Table 1. Parameters of the model, physically acceptable interval and tolerance revealed by the Monte-Carlo procedure. The output intervals correspond to $R < 10^{-3}$, and the statistical interval is defined by the mid-height size of the histogram of each parameter (Fig. 8).

$\lambda_0 = (682 \pm 10)$ nm, a thickness of gold $e = (52 \pm 1)$ nm, $\theta = (70.2 \pm 0.5)^o$ leading to a high sensitivity for n_3 (the peak is narrow). The sensitivity (or tolerance to variations) of parameters are obtained from the above results, and are indicated after the sign $\pm$. This study indicates that the tolerance on the thickness of gold must be better than 1 nm, that on the optical index of gold being deduced from the dispersion curve of gold in the interval $[665; 700]$ nm *i.e.* $\Re(n_2^2) \in [-16.5; -14]$ and $\Im(n_2^2) \in [1.04; 1.06]$. This last result of this sensitivity study can be considered with confidence, knowing that optical characteristics of gold are very dependent modes of deposition. Thus, the real part of permittivity is a less critical parameter for the optimization of the biosensor, than its imaginary part. This result may explain the agreement between theory and experiment, generally obtained in plasmonics, even considering the bulk optical constants, and even the more or less accurate fits of these quantities (Drude of Drude-Lorentz for example) (Kolomenskii et al., 1997; Neff et al., 2006; Raether, 1988). Despite all, these models of dispersion cannot be used if accurate optimization is awaited, the data obtained from specific measurements would be more appropriate. Another output of the sensitivity study deserves to be highlighted: the shape (less than 0.001) of the peak in Fig. 8(d) gives preliminary informations on the sensitivity of the biosensor to slight changes in the optical index of the medium of detection.

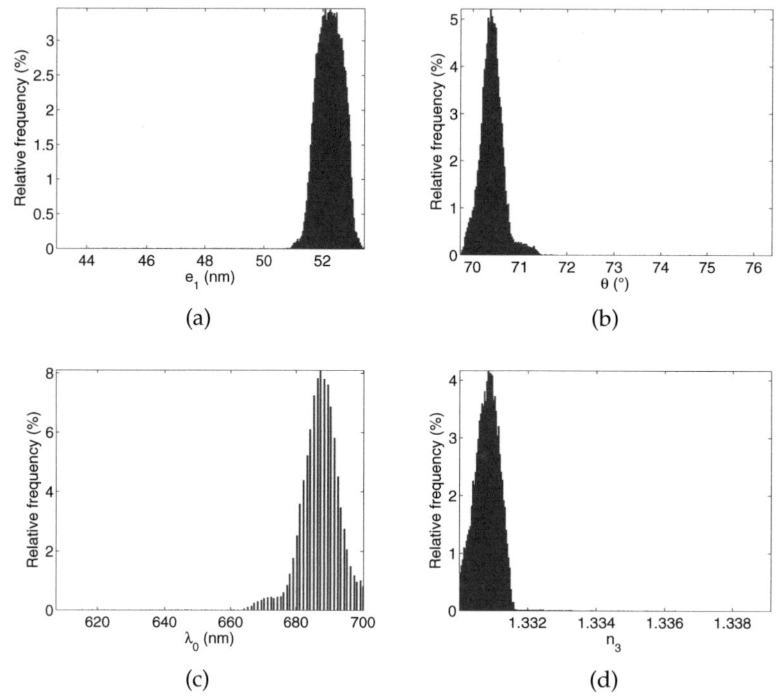

Fig. 8. Sensitivity study of the model of SPR. The involved parameters are the thickness of gold e, the angle of incidence θ, the wavelength of illumination λ_0 from which depends the optical index of gold n_2, and the optical index of the medium of detection n_3.

3. Some metaheuristic optimization methods for plasmonics

The model being established and characterized, the best values of the parameters are of interest. Models in plasmonics involve resonance and therefore the SPR is a good candidate to help to develop specific methods of optimization. Among them, two metaheuristics have been recently proposed (Barchiesi, 2009; Kessentini et al., 2011). The first one is selective and the second one is collaborative. The goal is to develop methods of optimization which could be efficient for problems in plasmonics with more degrees of freedom, especially the nanostructured biosensors. Nevertheless, to illustrate the optimization methods, we focus our study on the minimization of $R(e,\theta)$ to find the best set of parameters (e,θ) which is the most efficient to launch plasmon in the gold layer of the SPR biosensor. The wavelength of illumination is assumed to be fixed (so the index of gold), since it is imposed by choosing a laser source. In the following, we consider $\lambda_0 = 670$ nm. Of course this problem can always be solved by a systematic double loops study, but more general problems in plasmonics involve more than two parameters, and the goal is to develop a rapid method of optimization for this more general case.

The present problem being of dimension $N = 2$ (two parameters are searched: $\mathbf{p} = (\theta, e)$), a plot of R illustrates the topology of the function $R(e,\theta)$. Figure 9 exhibits the track of plasmon in the map of R, its location and shape. As expected, the best parameters for the plasmon launch, are located in a wells which shape depends on the wavelength.

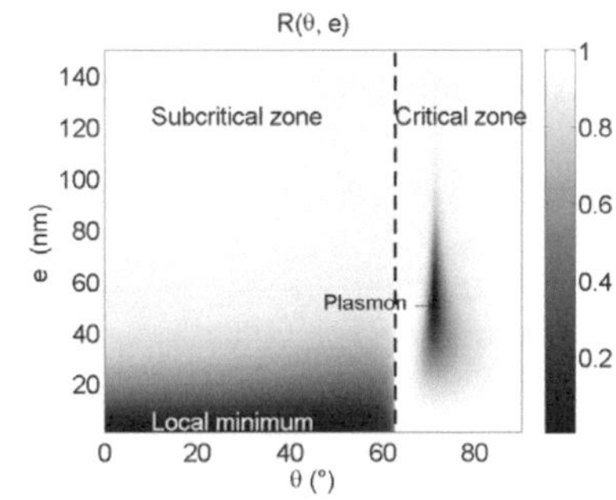

Fig. 9. Fitness function for the optimization: $R(\theta, e)$, for $n_1 = 1.5$, $n_2 = 0.1373 + 3.7975\imath$ ($\lambda_0 = 670$ nm), $n_3 = 1.33$.

In this case, the solution of the optimization can be easily determined. This problem is therefore a test for the following optimization methods.

3.1 Evolutionary method: a selective method

Among the numerous optimization schemes, the evolutionary methods are parts of the metaheuristics, based on the mimicry of nature, with the numerical mutation of the parameters considered as genes, and the selection of the bests for the breeding of the next generation (Schwefel, 1995). However, despite the apparent simplicity of the statistical method, its effectiveness depends on the addressed problem. Here, in plasmonics, the detection of sharp resonances through looking for a minimum of a complex function is under consideration. The balance between speed and diversity of research, particularly the ability to avoid local minima but to find the global optimum, must be studied carefully. In this section, we describe the classical evolutionary scheme (Schwefel, 1995) and one of its improvement (Barchiesi, 2009).

The target is the minimization of the fitness function $R(e, \theta)$ in a domain of acceptable parameters, n_3 being fixed (Fig. 1). This minimum corresponds to the best transfer of energy from the illumination to the gold layer.

The evolutionary scheme consists in four steps: initialization, recombination, mutation and selection. This process is repeated for several generations. A first population (parents) with μ parameters set (or elements) $\mathbf{p}_{m=1..\mu} = (\theta_m, e_m)$, is randomly generated. Then the parents breed to give birth to offspring (λ children): $\mathbf{p}'_{m=1..\lambda} = (\theta_i, e_i)$ (cross-over). The children mutation is used to increase the diversity of search. The selection of the μ best parameters enables to retain only the best performing in terms of fitness function. The selection is made through an elitist or non-elitist process, the first one involving also the parents in the choice of the best ones (the performance of the $\mu + \lambda$ elements is compared). A funny remark deserves to be made at this step: the elitist process is immoral because it will allow reproduction between children and parents to the next generation. The evolutionary algorithm requires strategy parameters s which enable to control the convergence of mutation (Schwefel, 1995).

The pseudo-algorithm 2 presents the steps of computation. The classical evolutionary algorithm 2 (SEM) is generic, and the crossover and mutations are unattached on the quality of the elements. Therefore, depending on the mathematical properties of the N-dimensional function R, the convergence can slow down, especially if the solution is in a narrow wells. The classical recombination uses fixed weights (Donnel & Waagen, 1995) or uniformly distributed weights for each element (Yang et al., 1997).

Classical Evolutionary Method (SEM)

Require: D domain of the N acceptable parameters $e, \theta \ldots$

Require: Fixed parameters of the model R.

Require: λ, μ, T (maximum of generations), SC stop criterion, ρ number of elements to be recombined, strategy parameters $\tau_1 \leftarrow (2.N)^{-1/2}$, $\tau_2 \leftarrow (2.\sqrt{N})^{-1/2}$
$\sigma \leftarrow 1$

[Initial population, with normal distribution of probability G or uniform law U in D]
$s_{m=1..\mu} \leftarrow \sigma.D$
$p_{m=1..\mu} \leftarrow G(D)$ or $U(D)$
$y_{m=1..\mu} \leftarrow R(p_{m=1..\mu})$

while $|y_1 - y_\mu|/|y_1 + y_\mu| > SC$ **do**

[Blind cross-over with random choice of integers n through $U(\{1, ..., \mu\})$]
$s'_{m=1..\lambda} \leftarrow \rho^{-1} \sum_\rho s_n$,
$p'_{m=1..\lambda} \leftarrow \rho^{-1} \sum_\rho p_n$

[Normal law mutation, G_i are normalized normal distribution of probability (Schwefel, 1995)]
$s''_{m=1..\lambda} \leftarrow s'_{m=1..\lambda}.\exp(\tau_1.G_2 + \tau_2.G_2)$
$p''_{m=1..\lambda} \leftarrow p'_{m=1..\lambda} + G_3.s''_{m=1..\lambda}$

[Selection (sort operator $S()$) of the μ best elements for the initial population of the next step]

if [Non Elistist] **then**
$y_{m=1..\lambda} \leftarrow R(p''_j)$
$p_{m=1..\mu} \leftarrow S(\{p''_{m=1..\lambda}\})$

else if [Ellistist] **then**
$y_{m=1..\mu+\lambda} \leftarrow R(\{p''_j, p_j\})$
$p_{m=1..\mu} \leftarrow S(\{p''_{m=1..\lambda}, p_{m=1..\mu}\})$

end if
$s_{m=1..\mu} \leftarrow s''_{m=1..\mu}$

end while

Adaptive Non Uniform Hyper Elitist Method (ANUHEM)

Require: D domain of the N acceptable parameters $e, \theta \ldots$

Require: Fixed parameters of the model R.

Require: λ, μ, T (maximum of generations), SC stop criterion, ρ number of elements to be recombined.

[Initial population with U: multidimensional uniform law in D]
$p_{m=1..\mu} \leftarrow U(D)$
$y_{m=1..\mu} \leftarrow R(p_{m=1..\mu})$

while $|y_1 - y_\mu|/|y_1 + y_\mu| > SC$ **do**

[Hyper-Elitist cross-over with random choice of integers n through $U(\{1, ..., \mu\})$]
$p'_{m=1..\lambda} \leftarrow \sum_\rho y_n^{-1} p_n / \sum_\rho y_n^{-1}$

[Adaptive Non-Uniform mutation using topology of solutions]
$b \leftarrow std(p_{m=1..\mu})/std(y_{m=1..\mu})$
$\sigma \leftarrow 1 - U([0;1])^{(1-g/T)^b}$
$p''_{m=1..\lambda} \leftarrow U_b(D,\sigma)$ {[$U_b(D,\sigma)$: multidimensional non uniform law in D with constraints $p'' \in D$]}
$y_{\mu+1..\mu+\lambda} \leftarrow R(p''_j)$

[Selection (S) of the μ best elements for the initial population of the next step]

if [Non Elistist] **then**
$p_{m=1..\mu} \leftarrow S(\{p''_{m=1..\lambda}\})$,

else if [Ellistist] **then**
$p_{m=1..\mu} \leftarrow S(\{p''_{m=1..\lambda}, p_{m=1..\mu}\})$

end if

end while

Algorithm 2. Pseudo-codes of Evolutionary Methods. R is the fitness function.

An alternative method, keeping the information on the quality of parameters during the breeding step has been proposed (Barchiesi, 2009). This Hyper-Elitist scheme (ANUHEM) is based on the balance between the variety of search (which is necessary to prevent attraction to local minima of R) through the non uniform law, and the dominance of high quality elements. The hyper elitist breeding using weighted recombination (barycentric crossover), prevents the lost of a small number of solutions near the global minimum of R. Instead, the non-uniform mutation counterbalances this strong attraction, and enables to keep the variety of search in D. The corresponding pseudo-code is on the right of Algorithm 2, to facilitate the comparison.

The ANUHEM is partially inspired by the Cooperative-Competitive scheme applied to radial basis functions networks in Ref. (Whitehead & Choate, 1996). Five cases have to be distinguished, considering $\rho = 2$ to simplify the discussion:

- If the two recombined elements are close to a global minimum of R: the weighting facilitates the convergence towards this minimum.
- If the two recombined elements are close to two separate local minimums, the offspring is near the "best" of the two ones.
- If only one recombined elements is near the global minimum, the other one may be near a local minimum of R: the recombined element is attracted by the global minimum.
- If the two recombined elements are away from the global minimum: the effect of the weighting used in recombination is lessened. The whole search space is surveyed, like with the Schwefel's recombination.
- If the two elements are close to a local minimum of R: the convergence of the algorithm to this minimum is prevented by mutation.

The mutation process in SEM uses the Gaussian distribution and the adaptation of its standard deviation, to produce offspring. Other algorithms use Cauchy or Lévy probability distributions (Lee & Yao, 2004; X. Yao & Lin, 1999). To avoid useless evaluations of R after the mutation process, which can generate offspring that are out of the domain of possible parameters, an uniform probability law is preferred. This choice is also governed by the strong local capacity escape of the uniform mutation operator (Gunter, 1997). To avoid the possible convergence toward a local minimum, the operator used in the ANUHEM is actually a "Non-Uniform" mutation proposed by Michalewicz (Michalewicz, 1992) and used for example in (Alfaro-Cid et al., 2005; Zhao et al., 2007). However, in this study, the operator has been somewhat modified as following, to deal with the detection of poles:

$$\begin{aligned}\mathbf{p}''_n = \mathbf{p}'_n + \big[(U_n - \mathbf{p}'_n).B(0.5,2) \\ -(\mathbf{p}'_n - L_n).(1 - B(0.5,2))\big] \\ .\left(1 - U^{(1-g/T)^b}\right),\end{aligned} \tag{15}$$

where U_n and L_n are the upper and lower bounds of the allowed parameters (domain D of physically acceptable values), $B(0.5,2)$ is the Bernouilli's distribution with probability $p = 0.5$ and evaluated for each parameter, U is the normalized uniform distribution (in $[0,1]$), g the generation of the evolutionary loop, T is the maximal generation number (arbitrary fixed at the beginning of the evolutionary loop) and b is a system parameter determining the degree of non uniformity (Zhao et al., 2007). In Ref. (Zhao et al., 2007), an adaptive scheme was proposed. Three possible test parameters were tested to generate offspring from the same parent, and the best one was the survivor. In this study, such a parameter cannot be fixed, due to the inhomogeneity of the fitness function. The inhomogeneity of R is given by the ratio of the standard deviation of the initial population to the standard deviation of the fitness function:

$$b = \frac{std(\mathbf{p}_i)}{std(R(\mathbf{p}_i))}. \tag{16}$$

and the non uniform distribution is given by:

$$U_b = 1 - U^{(1-g/T)^b}. \tag{17}$$

b is related to the "slope" of the solutions, in other words, to the spreading (or dispersion) of the initial population with regards to their quality, and is therefore adapted for each generation. b can differ for each of the two parameters (e, θ) and therefore takes into account the "sensitivity" of R to the variations of both parameters. At the beginning of the evolutionary loop, b is close to $(U_n - L_n)$ and the mutation is very sensitive to the variations of the fitness function and therefore to the quality of parameters. When the evolutionary algorithm converges to the global optimum, the local slope of the wells decreases like b, and the mutation operator exploration is more efficient in the wells.

Finally, in both methods (SEM and ANUHEM), the elitist selection is made among the initial and mutated elements, at each step of the evolutionary loop. Therefore, this elitist selection uses the evaluation of the quality of the parents and of the offspring (method $(\lambda + \mu) - ES$). This hyper-elitist method requires the evaluation of the fitness function with any element p_n and p''_n. Thus, these methods require time as the model used in the fitness function R must be evaluated $\mu + \lambda$ times per generation. The goal is therefore to decrease the required number of generations to reach convergence to one of the global minimums (and to detect the possible resonances).

The termination criterion is based on the convergence of the evolutionary method, the value of the global minimum being unknown in the general case. Therefore the stopping criterion is:

$$\left| \frac{R(e_\mu, \theta_\mu) - R(e_1, \theta_1)}{R(e_\mu, \theta_\mu) + R(e_1, \theta_1)} \right| < TC = 10^{-3} \tag{18}$$

When the termination criterion is reached, the evolutionary loop is stopped and a Nelder-Mead Method can be used to achieve the convergence toward the minimum of the wells of the function and to obtain the final set of parameters. Before evaluating the performances of both schemes on SPR, we introduce another method that is more collaborative than selective: the Particle Swarm Method.

3.2 Particle Swarm method: a collaborative method

The Particle Swarm Optimization (PSO) was first introduced by Kennedy and Eberhart in 1995 and imitates the swarm behaviour to search the globally best solution, which is considered as pollen for bees swarm (Kennedy & Eberhart, 1995). The swarm of parameters searches the best solution of a problem through collaboration. This metaheuristic method is based on the time dependent movement of parameters in the search space, toward the optimum. Actually, selection processes are not used in PSO, instead, reasonable displacements are chosen, based on the experience of parameters. The PSO (Kennedy & Eberhart, 1995) as well as Evolutionary Methods (Schwefel, 1995) are direct search, stochastic methods, used to find an optimal solution of a problem, described by a model, considered as a black box. So the model should be as stable as possible in the field of original research acceptable parameters. Divergences are not tolerable in the search intervals, under penalty of a failure of optimization. Contrariwise, discontinuities in the model are accepted, and test functions have been developed to check the optimization methods in that case. In plasmonics, as we noted above, one can always transform the model so that the goal becomes finding a minimum in a narrow well.

For all optimization methods, and especially metaheuristics, a universal scheme does not exist. Many improvements have been proposed, particularly to make them more effective for solving specific problems (Hu & Eberhart, 2002; Kennedy & Mendes, 2002; Liang et al., 2006; Mendes et al., 2004; Veenhuis, 2006). The main issues that have to be addressed are following:

- balancing between efficiency and rapidity: the decrease of the time of execution is critical, especially if the model requires huge computational time; but this conducts inevitably to increase the probability of attraction to any of the local optimum. The diversity of search is counterbalanced by the convergence time of the optimization;
- preventing the useless evaluations: in the evolutionary methods, the blind breeding of parameters can conduct to reduce the efficiency of method, as well as the outflow of domain for PSO.

The PSO is basically cooperative method where the set of parameters $\mathbf{p}$ at step t (corresponding to generation g in evolutionary methods) is considered as a moving particle (or bee) in the N-dimensional space of search. The particles of a swarm communicate good positions to each other and adjust their own positions $\mathbf{p}$ and velocities $\mathbf{v}$ at each step t:

$$\mathbf{v}(t+1) = \omega \mathbf{v}(t) + r_1 c_1 (\mathbf{p}_b(t) - \mathbf{p}(t)) + r_2 c_2 (\mathbf{p}_b - \mathbf{p}(t)) \quad (19)$$

$$\mathbf{p}(t+1) = \mathbf{p}(t) + \mathbf{v}(t+1) \quad (20)$$

where r_1 and r_2 are random variables between 0 and 1, $\mathbf{p}_b(t)$ is the particle best position, $\mathbf{p}_b$ is the global best, ω is the inertial weight and c_1 and c_2 are the acceleration coefficients. The parameters ω, c_1 and c_2 could be constant or time dependent (i.e. updated at each step).
After computing the new velocity, the particle moves toward a new position following Eq. 20. The particle new velocity $\mathbf{v}(t+1)$ combines its previous value and the distances between the particle current position and its own best found position i.e. its own best experience $\mathbf{p}_b(t)$ and the swarm global best $\mathbf{p}_b$. The first term of Eq. 19 is an inertia term which prevents the only local search and therefore preserves diversity in the exploration of D. Nevertheless, the inertia weight, introduced by Shi and Eberhart (Shi & Eberhart, 1998), is linearly decreasing from 0.9 to 0.4, in classical PSO. The acceleration coefficients c_1 and c_2 are generally fixed to $c_1 = 0.738$ and $c_2 = 1.51$, values that have been determined as optimal for the resolution of simple problems (Clerc, 2009) but significant efforts have been worn for improving the choice of these exogenous parameters (Zhan et al., 2009), leading to an adaptive method, by the estimation of the search state at each step. Four search states have been identified: exploration, exploitation, convergence and jumping out (Zhan et al., 2009) and adapted strategies are used to update the inertia weight and the acceleration coefficients. Finally, to avoid local optima, an elitist learning of the convergence state will permit the jump out of the likely local optima. Nevertheless, some general rules have been established to choose the cognitive parameter c_1 and the social parameter $c_2 : c_1 + c_2 < 4$ with possible priority to cognition (Carlisle & Dozier, 2001).
In the present study, we use standard PSO as reference with $c_1 = c_2 = 2$, that seems to be the most efficient choice of exogenous parameters. And we also propose an adaptive method based on the same principle as in the ANUHEM method (Barchiesi, 2009): the ANUPSO (Adaptive Non Uniform Particle Swarm Method) (Kessentini & Barchiesi, 2010a; Kessentini et al., 2011). Actually, for the plasmonic problems, a compromise between diversity search and convergence speed-up to the global optimum must be found. Consequently, the proposed adaptive PSO algorithm, will exploit topological information gathered about fitness function $R(\mathbf{p})$ at each iteration. The initialization of variables and speed for each particle is carried following the scheme proposed by Clerc (Clerc, 2009):

$$\mathbf{v}(1) = 0.5(\max(D) - \min(D)) \text{ and } \mathbf{p}(1) = U(D) \quad (21)$$

Then, the adaptation of the exogenous parameters is ensured through the non-uniform law (Eq. 17), with $b(t)$ defined in Eq. 16 :

$$\omega(t) = \max(b(t)) \text{ and } c_1 = 2U_{b-1}, c_2 = 2U_{b-1} \tag{22}$$

The domain of variation of c_i is set to include the classical values used for PSO that are mentioned above, as well as the constraint $c_1 + c_2 < 4$. All the adaptive parameters are therefore monitored by the topology of the fitness function R. Actually, $b(t)$ can be seen as the slope of the solutions, i.e. the spreading/ dispersion of the population with regards to their quality. $b(t)$ can differ for each component of $\mathbf{p}(t)$ and therefore takes into account the sensitivity of R to the variations of all parameters of $\mathbf{p}$. The only exogenous parameter is T. $b(t)$ determines the degree of non-uniformity (Zhao, 2008): the diversity of parameters increases instead the average speed of the diversity decreases, when $b(t)$ increases.
The proposed adaptive PSO (ANUPSO) can be compared to the method proposed in (Zhan et al., 2009) where the authors outlined the necessity of updating the acceleration coefficients following the three phases of optimization that are expected during the PSO loop (exploration, exploitation or convergence phase). Through the value of $b(t)$:

- ω, the inertial coefficient, is close to one in the exploration phase, then decreasing, then increasing in the exploitation state. This preserves the diversity of solutions and prevents the convergence to a local minimum. Finally it decreases toward 0 in the convergence state (when many particles are close to those for the global minimum).
- c_i, the acceleration coefficients tends toward 0 when t reaches T (Zhao, 2008)). Therefore T controls convergence and remains the only non-adaptive parameter of the method.

The values of $b(t)$, for each parameter, governs the convergence speed-up as follows:

- In the exploration state,$b(t)$ is close to one as well as $c_1(t)$ and $c_2(t)$. The value of $b(t)$ gives equal weight to the different contributions of the velocity. If the speed of the particle is too high, the particle (obtained at the generation t) leaves the search space and is therefore replaced by a random particle, through an uniform law, as in the initialization step. This contributes to the diversity at this stage.
- In the exploitation state, $b(t)$ increases and also the convergence speed-up (Zhao, 2008)
- In the final state of convergence, $b(t)$ decreases again and the wells of the objective function R are more carefully exploited.

An illustration of the performances of the the four methods is following.

3.3 Numerical study of the selective and collaborative methods

The problem under investigation is the SPR, assuming only two optimized parameters, as considered above. The best values of the thickness e of the gold layer, and of θ, the angle of illumination are searched, the goal being the minimization of $R(\theta, e)$ (Figure 9). The model is used as a black box for each method of optimization, the optimization is repeated at least 10.000 times to compute the statistics of success (converging before T generations to a solution close to the optimum) and of the number of evaluations of the model R. Let us underline again, that such method of optimization is designed to deal with much more complex models, and $dim(D) >> 2$. Therefore, the optimization must avoid useless evaluations of a time consuming model. The table 2 shows the performances of SEM, ANUHEM, PSO and ANUPSO. The domain of search is $D = [1;80]\ nm \times [\arcsin(\sqrt{\epsilon_3/\epsilon_1}); \pi/2]$. This domain is wide enough to set default behavior of the methods. The evolutionary method will give trivial solutions, out of the initial domain, corresponding to a null thickness of gold for example. The classical PSO freezes the too fast particles that would get out the domain D. Therefore, these particles are lost for the iteration of the search process. Some solutions have been proposed to overcome this problem, but are out of the scope of this study (Kessentini & Barchiesi, 2010b). Moreover, keeping in mind the objective of limiting the number of evaluations, we limit the number of generations (or iterations) to $T = 400$. This is vert constringent with regards to the classical way of bench, for which this exogenous parameter is not limited. Of course, the success rate approaches 100% for all methods, if $T > 1000$ in this case. We also fix $\mu = 5$, $\lambda = 25$ and therefore the number of particles in swarm to 30. This small number of parameters is also an encumbrance for the optimization methods. This simple test, event if only two parameters have to be optimized, pushes the methods in trenches (Tab. 2).

	SEM	ANUHEM	ANUPSO	PSO
success (%)	90%	100%	100%	100%
mean number of evaluations	6800	172	167	962

Table 2. Elitist SEM and ANUHEM, with $\lambda = 25$ and $\mu = 5$. ANUPSO and PSO, success rate and mean number of evaluations in case of success. To be considered as successful, the number of generation must be less than $T = 400$ to be considered as successful. The PSO uses $N = 30$, $c_1 = 2$, $c_2 = 2$ and ω linearly decreasing from 0.9 to 0.4. The best parameters are $e = 51$ nm and $\theta = 71^o$.

Table 2 shows that the classical methods are of course non universal and especially not convenient for plasmonics. Both improvements, using non-uniform law seem to be efficient. The best methods, under the above mentioned strong constraints are clearly the ANUPSO and the ANUHEM. Let us note that the selection scheme is elitist in this study. If not, the success rate would be worse and the number of evaluations would be increased. This illustration shows that an ideal and versatile method of optimization does not exist. Instead, some improvements have to be made to hope to reach a sufficient level of reliability. Despite all, the systematic study of double loop would require at least ten times evaluations to get the same accuracy on the optimized values.

Some of these heuristic methods have been used successfully, to optimize metal nanoparticles for the cancer therapy and imaging (Grosges, Barchiesi, Toury & Gréhan, 2008) and multilayered SPR (Barchiesi, Macías, Belmar-Letellier, Van Labeke, Lamy de la Chapelle, Toury, Kremer, Moreau & Grosges, 2008) and we hope to succeed in appliance to the more complex nanonatennas (`www.nanonatenna.eu`).

4. Conclusion

The numerical optimization of biosensors is necessary to spare time and money. In the case of plasmonics biosensors, modeling accurately the sensor is still a challenge. However, the numerical optimization requires a stable and accurate model, to be used as a black box for optimization. Even, if the model seems simple: the above model of SPR has been used for illustration, we have shown that the plasmon resonance is a tedious phenomenon, and a deep understanding of the model is necessary before optimization. On the other hand, the optimization methods themselves have to be carefully improved and tested before application to plasmonics. This still remains an open domain for physicists, biologists and theoreticians, but hopefully, solutions seem now begin to emerge.

5. References

Agarwal, G. S. (1973). New method in the theory of surface polaritons, *Phys. Rev. B* 8(10): 4768–4779.

Alfaro-Cid, E., McGookin, E. W. & Murray-Smith, D. (2005). A novel non-uniform mutation operator and its application to the problem of optimising controller parameters, *IEEE Congress on Evolutionary Computation* 2: 1555–1562.

Barchiesi, D. (1996). A 3-D multilayer model of scattering by nanostructures. application to the optimisation of thin coated Nano-Sources, *Optics Commun.* 126: 7–13.

Barchiesi, D. (2009). Adaptive non-uniform, hyper-ellitist evolutionary method for the optimization of plasmonic biosensors, *International Conference on Computers & Industrial Ingineering* pp. 542–547.

Barchiesi, D., Guizal, B. & Grosges, T. (2006). Accuracy of local field enhancement models: Toward predictive models?, *Appl. Phys. B* 84: 55–60.

Barchiesi, D., Kremer, E., Mai, V. & Grosges, T. (2008). A Poincaré's approach for plasmonics: The plasmon localization, *J. Microscopy* 229: 525–532.

Barchiesi, D., Macías, D., Belmar-Letellier, L., Van Labeke, D., Lamy de la Chapelle, M., Toury, T., Kremer, E., Moreau, L. & Grosges, T. (2008). Plasmonics: Influence of the intermediate (or stick) layer on the efficiency of sensors, *Appl. Phys. B* 93: 177–181.

Billot, L., de la Chapelle, M., Grimault, A. S., Vial, A., Barchiesi, D., Bijeon, J.-L., , Adam, P.-M. & Royer, P. (2006). Surface enhanced raman scattering on gold nanowire arrays: Evidence of strong multipolar surface plasmon resonance enhancement, *Chem. Phys. Lett.* 422(4-6): 303–307.

Bonod, N., Enoch, S., Li, L., Popov, E. & Nevière, M. (2003). Resonant optical transmission through thin metallic films with and without holes, *Opt. Express* 11(5): 482–490.

Born, M. & Wolf, E. (1993). *Principle of Optics*, Pergamon Press, Oxford.

Carlisle, C. & Dozier, G. (2001). An off-the-shelf PSO, *Proc. Particle Swarm Optimization Workshop*, pp. 1–6.

Clerc, M. (2009). A method to improve standard PSO, *Technical Report DRAFT MC2009-03-13*, France Telecom R&D.

Donnel, J. M. & Waagen, D. (1995). An empirical study of recombination in evolutionary search, *Proc. Of the Fourth Annual Conference on Evolutionary Programming*, pp. 465–478.

Ekgasit, S., Thammacharoen, C., Yu, F. & Knoll, W. (2005). Influence of the metal film thickness on the sensitivity of surface plasmon resonance biosensors, *Appl. Spectroscopy* 59: 661–667.

Grosges, T., Barchiesi, D., Toury, T. & Gréhan, G. (2008). Design of nanostructures for imaging and biomedical applications by plasmonic optimization, *Opt. Lett.* 33(23): 2812–2814.

Grosges, T., Borouchaki, H. & Barchiesi, D. (2007). Improved scheme for accurate computation of high electric near-field gradients, *Opt. Express* 15(3): 1307–1321.

Grosges, T., Borouchaki, H. & Barchiesi, D. (2008). New adaptive mesh development for accurate near-field enhancement computation, *J. Microscopy* 229(2): 293–301.

Grosges, T., Borouchaki, H. & Barchiesi, D. (2010). Three dimensional adaptive meshing scheme applied to the control of the spatial representation of complex field pattern in electromagnetics, *Appl. Phys. B* 101: 883–889.

Grosges, T., Vial, A. & Barchiesi, D. (2005). Models of near-field spectroscopic studies: Comparison between finite-element and finite-difference methods, *Opt. Express* 13: 8483–8497.

Gunter, R. (1997). Local convergence rates of simple evolutionary algorithms with Cauchy mutations, *IEEE Trans. Evol. Comput.* 4: 249–258.

Hoaa, X., Kirk, A. & Tabrizian, M. (2007). Towards integrated and sensitive surface plasmon resonance biosensors: A review of recent progress, *Biosensors and Bioelectronics* 23: 151–160.

Hu, X. & Eberhart, R. (2002). Multiobjective optimization using dynamic neighborhood particle swarm optimization, *Proc. IEEE Congress Evolutionary Computation*, IEEE, Honolulu, HI, pp. 1677–1681.

Kennedy, J. & Eberhart, R. (1995). Particle swarm optimization, *IEEE International Conference on Neural Networks*, IEEE, Path, Australia, pp. 1942–1948.

Kennedy, J. & Mendes, R. (2002). Population structure and particle swarm performance, *IEEE Congress Evolutionary Computation*, IEEE, Honolulu, HI, pp. 1671–1676.

Kessentini, S. & Barchiesi, D. (2010a). A new strategy to improve particle swarm optimization exploration ability, *Intelligent Systems (GCIS), 2010 Second WRI Global Congress on*, Vol. 1, IEEE, pp. 27 – 30.

Kessentini, S. & Barchiesi, D. (2010b). A new strategy to improve particle swarm optimization exploration ability, *2010 Seconde WRI Global Congress on Intelligent Systems*, IEEE, Wuhan, China, pp. 27–30.

Kessentini, S., Barchiesi, D., Grosges, T., Giraud-Moreau, L. & de la Chapelle, M. L. (2011). Adaptive non-uniform particle swarm application to plasmonic design, *International Journal of Applied Metaheuristic Computing (IJAMC)* 2(1): 18–28.

Kolomenskii, A., Gershon, P. & Schuessler, H. (1997). Sensitivity and detection limit of concentration and absorption measurements by laser-induced surface-plasmon resonance, *Appl. Opt.* 36: 6539–6547.

Kretschman, E. & Raether, H. (1968). Radiative decay of nonradiative surface plasmons excited by light, *Z. Naturforsch. A* 23: 2135–2136.

Kretschmann, E. (1978). The ATR method with focused light - application to guided waves on a grating, *Optics Commun.* 23(1): 41–44.

Lecaruyer, P., Maillart, E., Canva, M. & Rolland, J. (2006). Generalization of the rouard method to an absorbing thin-film stack and application to surface plasmon resonance, *Appl. Opt.* 45: 8419–8423.

Lee, C. Y. & Yao, X. (2004). Evolutionary programming using mutations based on the lévy probability distribution, *IEEE Trans. Evol. Comput.* 8: 1–13.

Li, L. (1994). Multilayer-coated diffraction gratings: Differential method of chandezon et al. revisited, *J. Opt. Soc. Am. A* 11: 2816–2828.

Li, L. (1996). Formulation and comparison of two recursive matrix algorithms for modeling layered diffraction gratings, *J. Opt. Soc. Am. A* 13(5): 1024–1035.

Liang, J. J., Qin, A., Suganthan, P. N. & S.Baskar (2006). Comprehensive learning particle swarm optimizer for global optimization of multimodal functions, *IEEE Transactions in Evolutionary Computing* 10(3): 281–295.

Macías, D., Vial, A. & Barchiesi, D. (2004). Application of evolution strategies for the solution of an inverse problem in Near-Field Optics, *J. Opt. Soc. Am. A* 21(8): 1465–1471.

Maystre, D. & Nevière, M. (1977). Sur une méthode d'étude théorique quantitative des anomalies de Wood des réseaux de diffraction, application aux anomalies de plasmons, *J. Optics (Paris)* 8: 165–174.

Maystre, D. & Nieto-Vesperinas, M. (1992). Effects of total internal reflection on the reflectivities of dielectric gratings, *J. Opt. Soc. Am. A* 9(12): 2218–2222.

Mendes, R., Kennedy, J. & Neves, J. (2004). The fully informed particle swarm: Simpler maybe better, *IEEE Transactions in Evolutionary Computing* 8: 204–210.

Michalewicz, Z. (1992). *Genetic Algorithms + Data Structure = Evolution Programs*, Springer-Verlag, New York.

Neff, H., Zong, W., Lima, A., Borre, M. & Holzhüter, G. (2006). Optical properties and instrumental performance of thin gold films near the surface plasmon resonance, *Thin Solid Films* 496: 688–697.

Raether, H. (1988). *Surface Plasmons on Smooth and Rough Surfaces and on Gratings*, Springer-Verlag, Berlin.

Schwefel, H. P. (1995). *Evolution and Optimum Seeking*, John Wiley & Sons Inc., New York.

Shi, Y. & Eberhart, R. C. (1998). A modified particle swarm optimizer, *Proc. IEEE Congress on Evolutionary Computation (CEC'98)*, Anchorage, AK, pp. 69–73.

Simon, H. J., Mitchell, D. E. & Watson, J. G. (1975). Surface plasmons in silver films - a novel undergraduate experiment, *Am. J. Phys.* 43(7): 630–636.

Veenhuis, C. (2006). Advanced meta-PSO, *Proc. IEEE Sixth International Conference on Hybrid Intelligent Systems (HIS'06)*, Rio de Janeiro, Brazil, pp. 54–59.

Whitehead, B. A. & Choate, T. D. (1996). Cooperative-competitive genetic evolution of radial basis function centers and widths for time series prediction, *IEEE Transactions on Neural Networks* 7: 869–880.

X. Yao, Y. L. & Lin, G. M. (1999). Evolutionary programming made faster, *IEEE Trans. Evol. Comput.* 3: 82–102.

Yang, J.-M., Chen, Y.-P., Horng, J.-T. & Kao, C.-Y. (1997). Applying family competition to evolution strategies for constrained optimization, *Lecture Notes in Computer Science* 1213: 201–211.

Zhan, Z.-H., Zhang, J., Li, Y. & Chung, H. S.-H. (2009). Adaptive particle swarm optimization, *IEEE Transactions on Systems, Man, and Cybernetics-Part B: Cybernetics* 39: 1362–1381.

Zhao, X. (2008). Convergent analysis on evolutionary algorithm with non-uniform mutation, *Evolutionary Computation*, IEEE, pp. 940–944.

Zhao, X., Gao, X.-S. & Hu, Z.-C. (2007). Evolutionary programming based on non-uniform mutation, *Applied Mathematics and Computation* 192: 1–11.

6

Biosensing Based on Luminescent Semiconductor Quantum Dots and Rare Earth Up-conversion Nanoparticles

Jun Zhang[1,2], Changyan Li[1,2], Wenzhi Zhao[1,2], Baocang Liu[1], Yunxia Liu[1] and Gaole Aletan[2]
[1]*College of Chemistry and Chemical Engineering,*
[2]*College of Life Science,*
Inner Mongolia University, Hohhot 010021,
P. R. China

1. Introduction

A biosensor is a device incorporating a biological sensing element either intimately connected to or integrated within a transducer, which is mainly determined by specific molecular recognition such as enzyme-substrate, antibody-antigen and so on. Currently, with the development of nanoscience and nanotechnology, more and more interest has been focused on using nanoparticles to fabricate biosensors (Alivisatos, 2004; Katz, 2004; Rosi 2005). Several kinds of biological sensors based on semiconductor quantum dots (QDs), gold nanoparticles (GNPs), carbon nanotubes (CNTs), fullerene, dendrimer nanoparticles have been presented. Semiconductor QDs are a new class of fluorescent materials for biosensor. In comparison with conventional organic dyes and fluorescent proteins, they have unique optoelectronic properties with size-tunable light emission, superior signal brightness, resistance to photobleaching and broad absorption spectra for simultaneous excitation of multiple fluorescence colors (Alivisatos, 1996). However, the use of semiconductor QDs for biosensor application still has some limitations (Jaiswal, 2004), for instance, the potential toxicity of QDs may pose risks to human health and the environment under certain conditions (Derfus, 2004). In addition, the absorption of UV and visible light by biological samples often induces autofluorescence, which interferes with fluorescent signals obtained from exogenous biomarkers. Moreover, if biological samples are prolonged exposure to UV radiation, it would cause the samples photo-damage and mutation.

The drawbacks of QDs in biosensing application have prompted the development of up-converting nanoparticles (UCNs) emerged as another class of new biosensing materials. Usually, UCNs exhibit intense visible or near-infrared light excited by near-infrared light according to the anti-stokes law. The UCNs also show a sharp emission bandwidth, long lifetime, tunable emission, high photostability, low bio-toxicity and good biocompatibility, which are less harmful to biological samples and have greater penetration depth through biological samples than conventional ultraviolet excitation. Moreover, UCNs can be easily coupled to proteins or other biological macromolecular systems and used in a variety of assay formats (Yen, 2004; Blasse, 1994). This review is composed of four sections, and is intended to summarize the recent advances in luminescent semiconductor QDs and rare earth UCNs for biosensing application. In the first section, the production mechanism, size-dependent luminescence, spectral characteristics, bioconjugation technology and potential biosensing application of semiconductor QDs are comprehensively reviewed; In the second section, the controlled synthesis, characterization, luminescence mechanism, and biosensing application of rare-earth UCNs are systemically introduced; In the third section, the comparative assessment of advantage and limitation of semiconductor QDs and rare earth UCNs in biosensing application are discussed; In the fourth section, the concluding remarks and perspective for semiconductor QDs and rare-earth UCNs in biosensing application are presented.

2. Semiconductor QDs as fluorescent labels for biosensing application

2.1 Concept of semiconductor QDs

Semiconductors have a filled band called the "valence band" and an empty band known as the "conduction band". At nanoscale dimension, the normally collective electronic properties of semiconductors become severely distorted and the electrons tend to follow the "particle in-a-box" model accounting for approximated band structure (Murray, 1993). From a quantum mechanical point of view, when a semiconductor is irradiated with light of photon energy (h_v) higher than E_g, an electron will be promoted from the valence to the conduction band, leaving a "hole" or "absence of an electron" in the valence band. Thus, this "hole" is assumed to be a "particle" with its particular effective mass and positive charge. The bound state of the electron-hole pair is called an "exciton" (Brus, 1984). The exciton can be considered a hydrogen-like system, and a Bohr approximation of the atom can be used to calculate the spatial separation of the electron–hole pair of the exciton by Eq. (1):

$$r = \frac{\varepsilon h^2}{\pi m_r e^2} \tag{1}$$

where r is the radius of the sphere, defined by the 3-D separation of the electron-hole pair, ε is the dielectric constant of the semiconductor, m_r is the reduced mass of the electron-hole pair, h is Planck's constant, and e is the charge on the electron. For many semiconductors, the masses of the electron and hole have been determined by ion cyclotron resonance and are generally in the range 0.1-3 m_e (m_e is the mass of the electron). For typical semiconductor dielectric constants, the calculation suggests that the electron-hole pair spatial separation is 1-10 nm for most semiconductors (Gaponenko, 1998).

Because the physical dimensions of a QD can be smaller than the exciton diameter, the QD is a good example of the "particle-in-a-box" calculations of undergraduate physical chemistry. In those calculations, the energies of the particle in the box depend on the size of the box. In the QD, the bandgap energy becomes size-dependent (Alivisatos, 1996; Gaponenko, 1998; Zhang, 1997; Weller, 1993; Murphy, 2002).

2.2 Optical properties of QDs

QDs are nearly spherical semiconductor particles with diameters on the order of 1-10 nm, containing roughly 200-10,000 atoms. When semiconductor QDs are smaller than their exciton Bohr radii, the quantum confinement and size-dependent effects make QDs have unique optical properties (Fig. 1): (1) single excitation, multi-emission and size-dependent; (2) large stokes shift, narrow and symmetrical fluorescence peak; (3) visible light range fluorescence and resistance to photobleaching; (4) superior signal brightness. In addition, changing QD surface functional groups, luminescent properties and stability are greatly improved and more conducive to the coupling of biological molecules. For conventional dye molecules, their narrow excitation spectrum makes the simultaneous excitation difficult in most cases, and their broad emission spectrum may cause a long tail at red wavelengths; while for semiconductor QDs, the absorbance onset and emission maximum shift to higher energy with the decrease of particle sizes (Alivisatos, 1996). The excitation tracks the absorbance, resulting in a tunable fluorescence that can be excited efficiently at any wavelength shorter than the emission peak, and therefore the characteristic narrow and symmetric spectrum can be realized regardless of the excitation wavelength (Bruchez, 1998).

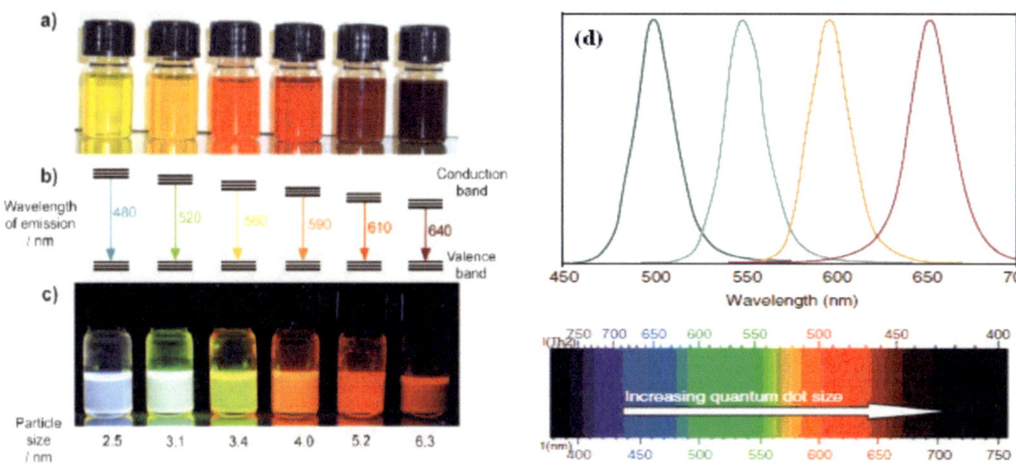

Fig. 1. Size-dependent optical properties of QDs. (a) Surface color of suspensions in toluene in visible light; (b) Schematic diagram of band gap and emission color as a function of particle size; (c) Light emission of suspensions in toluene when excited with UV light; (d) Fluorescence spectra of the QDs samples (from left to right are respectively representative 2.2, 2.9,4.1 and 7.3nm QDs). (Feldmann, 2010; Mansur, 2010; Smith, 2008).

Due to their unique optical properties, semiconductor QDs can be used as fluorescent labels for biological detection. In order to establish the utility of QDs for biological sensing application, mouse 3T3 fibroblast cells were labeled with green and red emitting CdSe/CdS nanocrystals. The green and red labels were spectrally resolved to the eye clearly under the excitation of a single light source by a laser scanning confocal microscope. Nonspecific labeling of the nuclear membrane by both the red and green probes resulted in a yellow color [Fig. 2(a)]. The intensity of the fluorescein drops quickly to autofluorescence levels, whereas the intensity of the QDs drops only slightly. Comparatively, the red QD labels are 20 times as bright, 100 times as stable against photobleaching [Fig. 2(b)] (Bruchez, 1998).
In general, QDs synthesized in nonpolar solutions using aliphatic coordinating ligands are only soluble in nonpolar organic solvents, which are not suit for biological application.

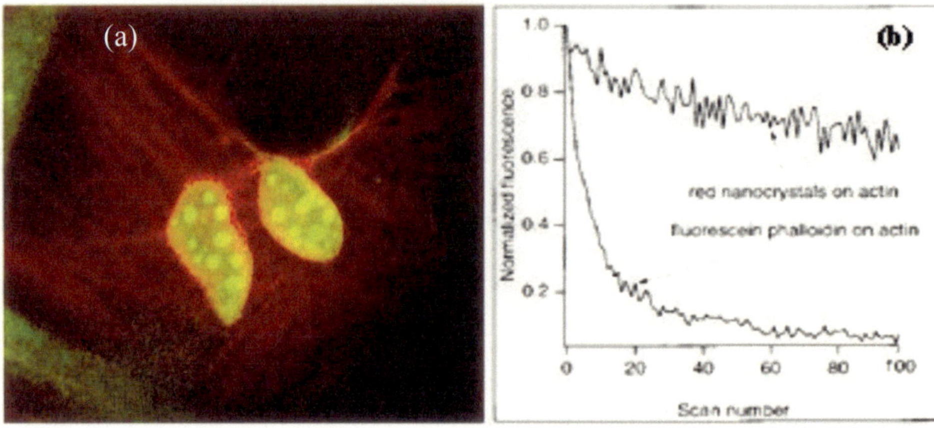

Fig. 2. Schematic diagrams of dual-color labeling and photostability. (a) The mouse 3T3 fibroblasts were labeled with dual color. (b) Sequential scan photostability comparison of fluorescein-phalloidin-labeled actin fibers compared with nanocrystal-labeled actin fibers (Bruchez, 1998).

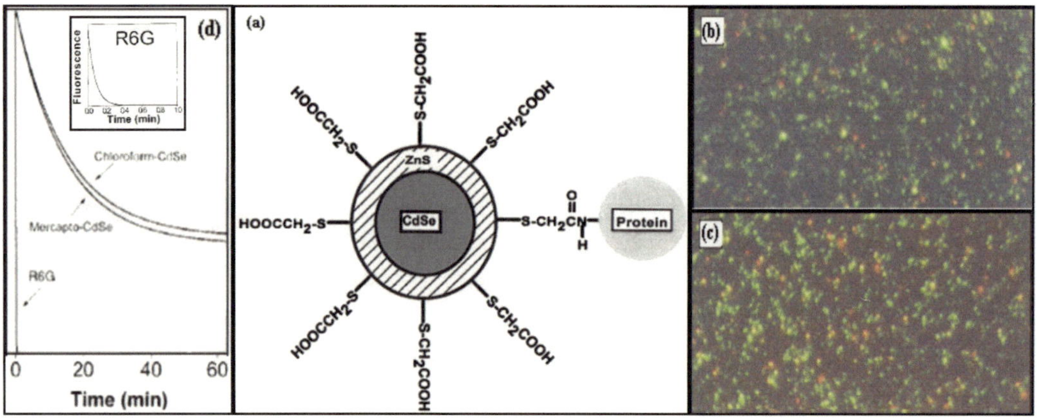

Fig. 3. (a) Scheme of a CdSe/ZnS QD covalently coupled to a protein; (b) Luminescent images obtained from the original QDs; (c) mercapto-solubilized QDs; (d) Time-resolved photobleaching curves for the original QDs, solubilized QDs and dye R6G (Chan, 1998).

Moreover, QDs have a huge surface/volume ratio, which makes them extremely unstable in solution because of the high surface energy. Hence, any route chosen to synthesize QDs should consider the stabilization of the QDs by minimizing the surface energy via "capping" and avoiding further structure growth (Weaver, 2009). Warren and coworkers presented a valuable way to solve this problem by coating CdSe QDs with higher bandgap materials such as ZnS shell in order to increase the photostability and luminescence properties of CdSe QDs (Chan, 1998). When reacting with CdSe/ZnS QDs in chloroform, the mercapto group binds to a Zn atom, and the free carboxyl group is available for covalent coupling to various biomolecules such as proteins by cross-linking to reactive amine groups [Fig. 3(a)] (Hermanson, 1996). A comparison of color luminescence images were obtained from the original QDs, water soluble QDs and protein-conjugated QDs [Figs. 3(b) and (c)], which indicated that the optical properties of QDs remain unchanged after solubilization and conjugation. The photophysical properties of QD conjugates with rhodamine 6G (R6G) was also studied. The emission of mercapto-CdSe is somehow weaker than that of single QDs, which is nearly 100 times as stable as R6G against photobleaching [Fig. 3(d)].

2.3 Synthesis of biocompatible QDs

The most common method for synthesizing water-soluble QDs is coated with a monolayer of hydrophilic thiols, typically mercaptoacetic acid (MAA), to replace the hydrophobic trioctylphosphine oxide (TOPO) coating on QDs (Chan, 1998; Hood, 2002; Duncan, 2006). But, when the MAA replace the TOPO coating on QDs, the QDs become instable accompanied by significant decreases in the quantum yield to 7% compared with TOPO-coated QDs (Kim, 2004). To overcome this problem, Alivisatos and coworkers developed an effective route to coat QDs with a cross-linked silica shell, which can be readily modified with a variety of organic functionalities such as primary amines, carboxylic acids or thiols (Gerion, 2001). The coated QDs were very stable and retained 60-80% of the quantum yield of the original QDs. Gao and coworkers developed another effective method to synthesize CdSe/ZnS QDs stabilized by a coordinating ligand (TOPO) and an amphiphilic polymer coating through hydrophobic attraction (Gao, 2004). Because of the strong hydrophobic interactions between TOPO and polymer hydrocarbon, the two layers bonds to each other and form a hydrophobic protection structure that resists hydrolysis and enzymatic degradation even under complex *in vivo* conditions. In most designs of the amphiphilic polymers, carboxylic acids provide solubility in water and can be utilized as

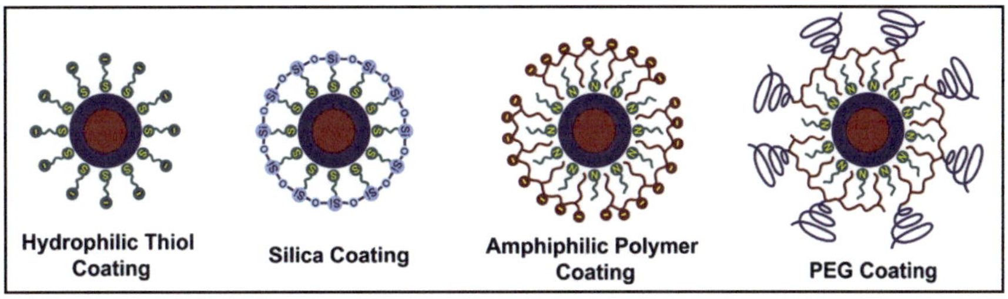

Fig. 4. Schematic diagrams of biocompatible QDs.

chemical handles for conjugation to primary amines in proteins through water soluble cross-linking reagents such as 1-ethyl-3-(3-dimethylaminopropyl) carbodiimide (EDAC). Similarly, many of these QDs also may be modified to contain polyethylene glycol (PEG) to decrease surface charge and increase colloidal stability (Fig. 4) (Dubertret, 2002 ; Smith, 2006; You, 2007; Bagwe, 2003).

2.4 Biosensing based on biocompatible QDs

On the base of the synthetic methods of biocompatible QDs, water-soluble QDs can be covalently or electrostatically bound to a biological target, which have also acted as a new class of sensor. If the QDs encapsulated in amphiphilic polymers and PEG conjugated to antibodies, it would yield specificity for a variety of antigens. In addition, QDs cross-linked to other small molecule ligands, inhibitors, peptides, or aptamers can bind with many different cellular receptors and targets (Fig. 5) (Lidke, 2004; Xing, 2007). Gao and coworkers developed multifunctional nanoparticle probes based on semiconductor QDs for prostate cancer targeting and imaging (Gao, 2004). The probes with passive and active tumor targeting behaviors were produced. This new class QDs probes contain an amphiphilic tri-block copolymer for in vivo protection, targeting-ligands for tumor antigen recognition and multiple PEG molecules for improved biocompatibility and circulation [Fig. 5(a)]. In the passive mode, antigenic tumors produce vascular endothelial growth factors, which can hyper-permeabilize the tumor-associated neovasculatures and cause the leakage of circulating macromolecules and small particles, leading to macromolecule or nanoparticle accumulation [Fig. 5(b)] (Gao, 2004; Duncan, 2003; Jain, 1999, 2001). While for active tumor targeting, antibody-conjugated QDs can track a prostate-specific membrane antigen (PSMA), which could be selected as an attractive target for imaging and therapeutic intervention of prostate cancer [Fig. 5(b)] (Gao, 2004; Schulke, 2003). This study opens new possibilities for ultrasensitive and simultaneous imaging of multiple biomarkers involved in cancer metastasis and invasion.

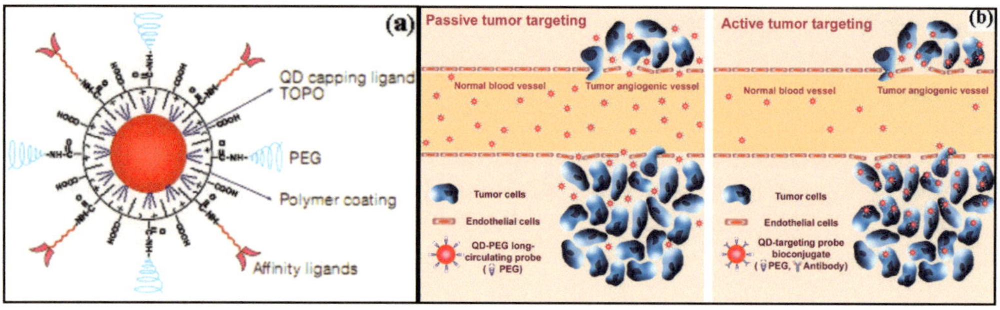

Fig. 5. Schematic illustration of bioconjugated QDs for in vivo cancer targeting and imaging. (a) Structure of a multifunctional QD probe; (b) Permeation and retention of QD probes via leaky tumor vasculatures (passive targeting) and high affinity binding of QD-antibody conjugates to tumor antigens (active targeting) (Gao, 2004).

Subsequently, Wu and coworkers demonstrated the use of 535QD-IgG and red 630QD-streptavidin to detect Her2 on the cell surface and nuclear antigens in the nucleus of SK-BR-3 cells. When the sample was observed under a fluorescence microscope, 630QD-labeled (red) nuclear antigens and 535QD-labeled (green) membrane-associated Her2 were visible simultaneously (Wu, 2003). This indicated that QDs conjugated to different secondary detection reagents can effectively detectect two cellular targets in the same cell. These results demonstrated the practicality of QDs in biological cellular real time and dynamic state imaging fields.

Fluorescence resonance energy transfer (FRET) is most commonly utilized in biosensors for detecting maltose (Medintz, 2003), aptamers (Hansen, 2006), 2,4,6-trinitrotoluene (Goldman, 2005), toxins (Goldman, 2004), and DNA (Zhang, 2005). Because of their high sensitivity, good reproducibility, and real-time monitoring capabilities, QDs are usually acted as fluorescence donors and make up of FRET with organic dyes. Medintz and coworkers designed a maltose sensor [Fig. 6(a)], in which an organic dye QSY-9 (fluorescence acceptor) was first conjugated to β-cyclodextrin (β-CD), then bonded to maltose binding protein (MBP), and at last β-CD-QSY-9/MBP complex was attached to the 560 QDs (fluorescence donors) surface through a peptide His-tag (Medintz, 2003). The optimized sensor contained 10 copies of β-CD-QSY9 bound to the QD complex, where 75% of the QD fluorescence was quenched by QSY-9. When free maltose was added, it would displace the β-CD-QSY9.

Moreover, the displacement of β-CD-QSY-9 with maltose could result in QD fluorescence increasing about 3-fold. This technique can be used to achieve the sensing of maltose. However, due to the uncertainty in the distance between the QDs and acceptors, some limitations in this sensor were arisen. In order to overcome the limitations, another maltose sensor was architected [Fig. 6(b)], in which 10 copies of Cy3 labeled MBP were first incorporated on the 530QDs surface, followed by binding of the Cy3.5 labeled β-CD, at last β-CD-Cy3.5/MBP-Cy3 complex was bound to QD through a peptide His-tag and Cy3.5 fluorescence emitted through a two-step FRET process. Sufficient fluorescence energy was initially transferred from the 530QD to MBP-Cy3, and the minimized emission energy of Cy3 was then transferred to β-CD-Cy3.5. When free maltose was added, the displacement of β-CD-Cy3.5 with maltose resulted in fluorescence increasing from Cy3 and concomitantly fluorescence decreasing from Cy3.5. The results demonstrate that the appropriately designed QD complexes with peptide immobilization tags can be used in determining small molecule concentrations in the 100 nM-10 μM range (Medintz, 2003)
Another biosensor based on combination of QDs and multi-walled carbon nanotubes (CNT) makes the detection of DNA and antigen more quickly and simply. Cui *et al* reported a highly selective, ultrasensitive, fluorescent detection method for DNA and antigen based on self-assembly of multi-walled carbon nanotubes (CNT) and CdSe QDs via oligonucleotide hybridization (Cui, 2008). This method could achieve the detection limit of 0.2 pM DNA molecules and 0.01 nM antigen molecules, and the novel detection system not only can be used for multicomponent detection and antigen-antibody immunoreaction, but also has great potential in photoelectrical biosensing application.

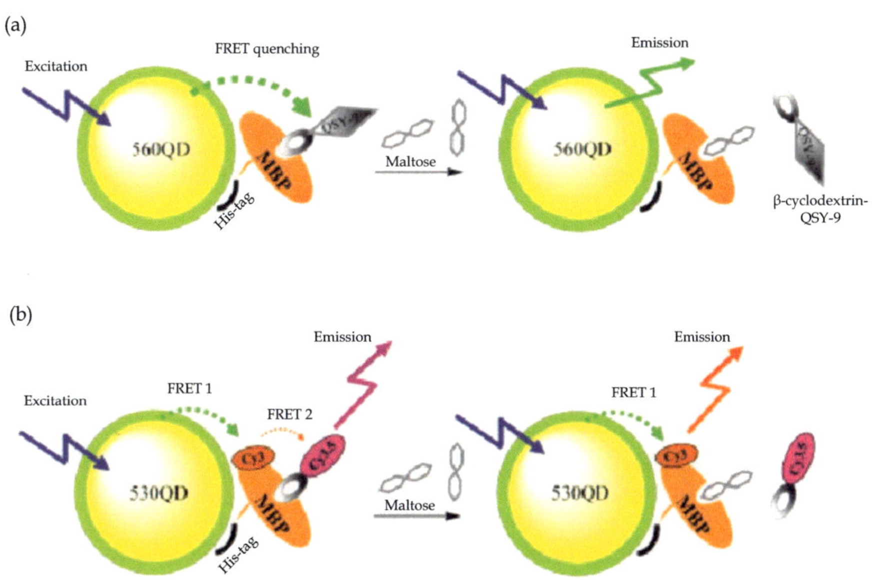

Fig. 6. QD based maltose nanosensor. (a) β-CD-QSY-9/MBP complex bound to QD through a peptide His-tag; (b) β-CD-Cy3.5/MBP-Cy3 complex bound to QD through a peptide His-tag (Zhou, 2007).

Recent advances in single-molecule detection, aptameric sensors with the surface functionalizing QDs hold exciting promise for many potential applications. Zhang *et al* developed a single-QD-based aptameric sensor through (FRET) between 605QD and Cy5 and Iowa Black RQ (Zhang, 2009). This aptamertic sensor can recognize cocaine through both signal-off and signal-on modes, indicating the higher sensitivity and more extremely low sample consumption than that of the aptameric sensors established before. With the development of aptamers for small molecules, nucleic acids, metal ions, and proteins, this single-QD-based aptameric sensor might find wide application in forensic analysis, environmental monitoring, and clinic diagnostics (Zhang, 2009).

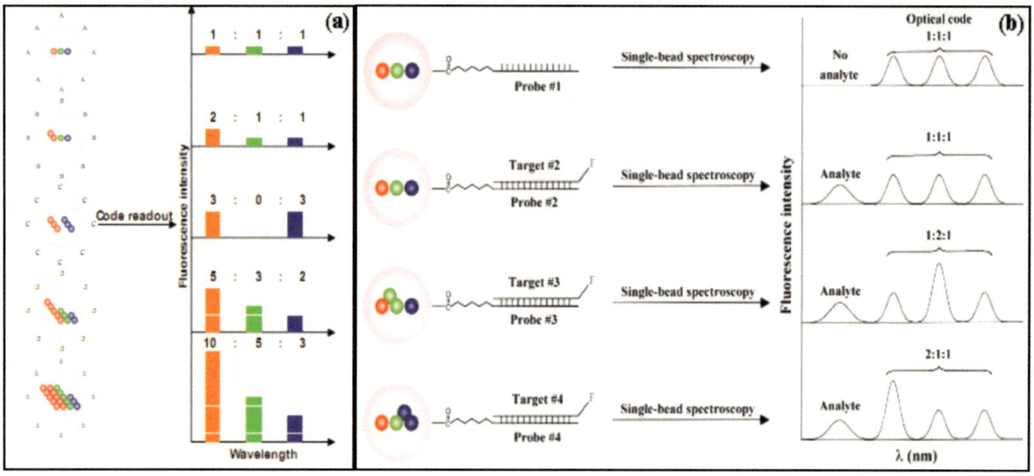

Fig. 7. Schematic illustrations of optical coding and DNA hybridization assays using QD-tagged beads (a) Optical coding based on wavelength and intensity multiplexing. Large spheres represent polymer microbeads, in which small multicolor QDs are embedded according to predetermined intensity ratios; (b) DNA hybridization assays using QD-tagged beads. Probe oligos were conjugated to the beads by crosslinking, and target DNA molecules were detected with a blue fluorescent dye such as Cascade Blue (Han, 2001).

Han and coworkers synthesized monodispersed CdSe/ZnS QDs with fluorescence emission at three primary colors (red, green and blue) (Han, 2001). Through embedding different-sized QDs into polymeric microbeads at precisely controlled intensity ratios [Fig. 7(a)], multicolor-tagged beads were prepared. Code readout is accomplished by measuring the fluorescence spectra of single beads. Their fluorescence emission wavelength can be continuously tuned by changing the particle size, and a single wavelength can be used for simultaneous excitation of different-sized QDs (Alivisatos, 1996; Han, 2001, Nirmal, 1999). On the other hand, molecular probes (A-E) may be attached to the bead surface for biological binding and recognition, such as DNA-DNA hybridization. In order to demonstrate the use of QD-tagged beads for DNA hybridization, oligonucleotide probes were conjugated to the beads by cross-linking. Target DNA molecules are directly labeled with a blue fluorescent dye such as Cascade Blue [Fig. 7(b)] (Han, 2001). Optical spectroscopy at the single-bead level yields both the coding and the target signals. Moreover, each color code corresponds to a specific DNA sequence. The coding signals can identify the DNA sequence, whereas the target signal can indicate the abundance of that sequence. A surprising finding is that the number of codes increases exponentially when multiple wavelengths and intensities are used simultaneously, for example, a

3-color/10-intensity scheme yields 999 codes, whereas a 6-color/10-intensity scheme has a theoretical coding capacity of about one million. In general, *n* intensity levels with *m* colors generate (n^m-1) unique codes (Han, 2001). If every code corresponds one type specific DNA sequence, it would be labeled every biomolecules with fluorescent code. This system made by multicolor-tagged QDs will completely change the ability of human identifying gene.

3. Rare-earth up-converting nanoparticles as fluorescent labels for biosensing application

3.1 Up-converting luminescence mechanism

Up-conversion (UC) refers to nonlinear optical processes characterized by the successive absorption of two or more pump photons via intermediate long-lived energy states followed by the emission of the output radiation at a shorter wavelength than the pump wavelength. UC processes are mainly divided into three broad classes: excited state absorption (ESA), energy transfer up-conversion (ETU), and photon avalanche (PA). All these processes involve the sequential absorption of two or more photons (Fig. 8).

In the case of ESA, the excitation takes the form of successive absorption of pump photons by a single ion. This is the basic process of up-conversion [Fig. 8(a)]. If the excitation energy is resonant with the transition from ground level G to excited metastable level E1, the phonon absorption occurs and populates E1 from G in a process known as ground state absorption (GSA). A second pump photon that promotes the ion from E1 to higher-lying state E2 results in UC emission, corresponding to the E2-G optical transition (Wang, 2009).

ETU is similar to ESA in that both processes utilize sequential absorption of two photons to populate the metastable level. The essential difference between ETU and ESA is that the excitation in ETU is realized through energy transfer between two neighboring ions. In an ETU process, each of two neighboring ions can absorb a pump phonon of the same energy, thereby populating the metastable level E1 [Fig. 8(b)]. A non-radiative energy transfer process promotes one of the ions to upper emitting state E2, while the other ion relaxes back to ground state G. The dopant concentration that determines the average distance between the neighboring dopant ions has a strong influence on the UC efficiency of an ETU process (Wang, 2009).

The phenomenon of PA was first discovered by Chivian and co-workers in Pr^{3+}-based infrared quantum counters (Chivian, 1979). PA-induced UC features an unusual pump mechanism that requires pump intensity above a certain threshold value. The PA process starts with population of level E1 by non-resonant weak GSA, followed by resonant ESA to populate upper visible-emitting level E2 [Fig. 8(c)]. After the metastable level population is established, the cross-relaxation energy transfer or ion pair relaxation occurs between the excited ion and a neighboring ground state ion, resulting in both ions occupying the intermediate level E1. The two ions readily populate level E2 to further initiate cross-relaxation and exponentially increase level E2 population by ESA, producing strong UC emission as an avalanche process (Wang, 2009).

The UC luminescent efficiency in these three processes varies considerably. ESA is the least efficient UC process. Efficient UC is possible in PA with metastable, intermediate levels that can act as a storage reservoir for pump energy. However, the PA process suffers from a number of drawbacks, including pump power dependence and slow response to excitation (up to several seconds) due to numerous looping cycles of ESA and cross-relaxation processes. In contrast, ETU is instant and pump power independent, and thus has been widely used to offer highly efficient UC (Wang, 2009; Auzel, 2004).

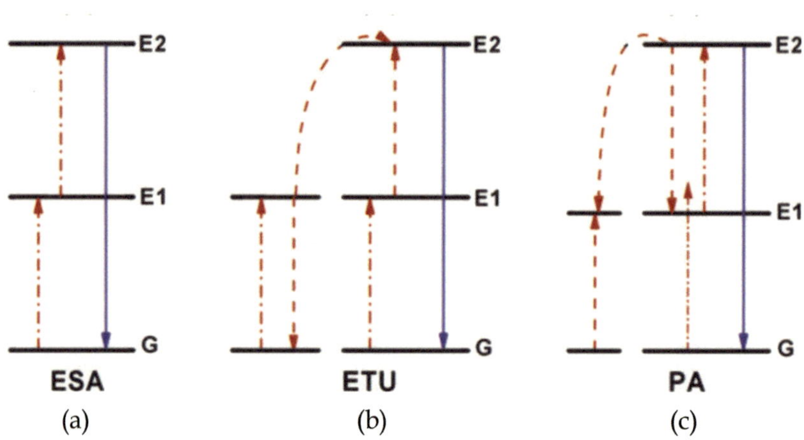

Fig. 8. Three energy transferring process diagrams of UC processes. (a) ESA; (b) ETU; (c) PA. The dashed/dotted, dashed, and full arrows represent photon excitation, energy transfer, and emission processes, respectively (Wang, 2009).

3.2 Synthesis of up-converting nanoparticles

For biological applications, UCNs should have a suitable size and surface for conjugation with biological molecules, and exhibit high intensity emission (Pires, 2006). Therefore, the synthesis of UCNs is particularly important. In general, the co-precipitation, thermal decomposition and hydro/solvo-thermal methods are most effective ways for synthesis of UCNs.

Co-precipitation is one of the most convenient techniques for synthesizing ultra-small UCNs with narrow size distribution. One of the earliest examples of this technique was demonstrated by van Veggel and co-workers, who made down-conversion LaF_3 nanocrystals doped with Ln^{3+} (Ln =Eu, Er, Nd, and Ho) (Stouwdam, 2002). The approach was expanded and refined by Chow *et al* (Yi, 2005), and UC LaF_3 nanocrystals with smaller particle size and narrower size distribution were obtained by using simple water soluble inorganic precursors. Besides, LaF_3, $NaYF_4$:Yb/Er(Tm), $LuPO_4$:Yb/Tm, and $YbPO_4$:Er nanocrystals were also synthesized via the co-precipitation approach (Heer, 2003, 2004; Yi, 2004; Zeng, 2005). The co-precipitation method is simple and quick, needing no expensive equipment and complex procedures, but requires post-heat treatment.

The thermal decomposition method is based on temporal separation of nucleation and crystal growth. It was firstly demonstrated for synthesis of highly monodispersed LaF_3 nanocrystals by Yan's group (Zhang, 2005). Later, this approach was extended as a common route to the synthesis of high quality UC $NaYF_4$ nanocrystals (Mai, 2006, Boyer, 2007). Zhao *et al* synthesized UC $NaYF_4$ nanorods, nanotubes, and flower-patterned nanodisks by an oleic acid-mediated hydrothermal method (Zhang, 2007). Recently, LaF_3:Yb/Er(Tm,Ho) nanoplates with multicolor UC luminescence were also successfully synthesized via a hybrid thermal decomposition/solvothermal method (Liu, 2007), which shows the superiorities in controlling the particle size and shape of the UCNs. However, this method needs specialized reaction vessels, expensive and air-sensitive precursors.

3.3 Optical properties of up-converting nanoparticles

Luminescent materials can absorb energy and subsequently emit the absorbed energy as radiation. According to the relative frequencies of the exciting and emitting radiations, radiant emission can be categorized into two classes of up-conversion and down-conversion. In the down-converting process, the emitting radiation obeys Stokes' law, in which the emitting radiation is of a lower energy and hence longer wavelength than the exciting light. However, for UCNs, the emitting radiation actually possesses a higher energy and smaller wavelength than the exciting wavelength, which is so-called anti-Stokes emission. As luminescent labeling materials, UCNs also show their superiority in several aspects comparing with conventional fluorescent dye or protein labels and QDs tags.

Firstly, UCNs are little analogous to QDs, even though QDs also hold a sharp emission bandwidth, long lifetime, tunable emission, high photostability and biocompatibility. The excitation and emission wavelength of UCNs are well separated from each other, which are ideal for multiplexing biological detection. Moreover, UCNs is generally made up of an inorganic host and lanthanide dopant ions embedded in the host lattice [Fig. 9(a)]. In the realization of UC processes, the crystal structure and optical property of host materials play important roles and require careful consideration. The luminescence emitted by UCNs is also dependent on the particle sizes, but it is different from quantum confinement effects as seen in QDs. The emission spectrum and color of the UCNs are associated with the host composition and particle surface properties (Lim, 2010; Mai, 2007). Generally, visible optical emissions under low pump power densities (ca. 10 W/cm^2) are only generated by using Er^{3+}, $Tm^{3+}$and Ho^{3+} as activators. In order to enhance up-converting efficiency, Yb^{3+} with a larger absorption cross-section in the NIR spectral region is frequently doped as a sensitizer in combination with the activators. In addition, UCNs can emit multicolor through the use of lanthanide-doped $NaYF_4$ nanoparticles with varied dopant ratios [Fig. 9 (d)].

Secondly, UCNs absorb NIR light and emit in the NIR or visible ranges, therefore, the penetration of NIR and the absence of autofluorescence background make the UCNs own unique ability of being imaged at a greater tissue depth. UC processes primarily rely on the ladder-like arrangement of energy levels of lanthanide dopant ions, and UC luminescence primarily originates from electron transitions between energy levels of localized dopant ions [Fig. 9(b)]. In case of the commonly used $NaYF_4$:Yb,Er nanoparticles, there are two emission peaks, one in the green region and the other in the red region [Fig. 9(c)] (Li, 2006). Recent studies show that lanthanide ions typically show a distinct set of sharp emission peaks, thus providing distinguishable spectroscopic fingerprints for accurate interpretation of the emission spectra in the event of overlapping emission spectra (Wang, 2009).

Thirdly, the UCNs are also resistant to photobleaching. A dried sample of PEI/$NaYF_4$ nanoparticles displayed no reduction in emission intensity when continually exposed to a 980 nm laser for over 7 h (Chatterjee, 2008). In addition, UCNs have lower cytotoxicity than QDs and exhibit almost no temporary and random loss of fluorescence (photo-blinking), as observed in semiconductor QDs.

3.4 Surface modification and functionalization of up-converting nanoparticles

For biological labeling applications, UCNs not only should exhibit high UC luminescence efficiency, but also need compatible with biomolecules. Most UCNs prepared by conventional strategies have no intrinsic aqueous solubility or lack functional organic moieties. Therefore, it is necessary that an additional surface treatment step should be required before bioconjugation.

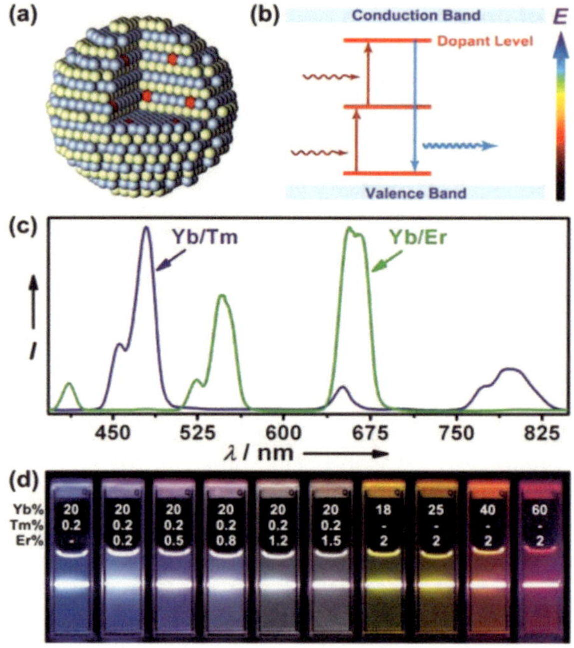

Fig. 9. (a) Structural diagram of UC nanoparticles; (b) Energy level diagram; (c) Emission spectra of cubic $NaYF_4$:Yb/Tm (20/0.2 mol%) and $NaYF_4$: Yb/Er (18/2 mol%) nanoparticles; (d) Fine tunable UC colors by adjusting the dopant ratios of lanthanide-doped $NaYF_4$ nanoparticles (Wang, 2008, 2010).

Ligand engineering, including ligand exchange, surface oxidation, ligand attraction, layer-by-layer assembly, and surface polymerization, is a common approach to generate a pendant functional group on the surface of UCNs (Fig. 10). Ligand exchange is normally realized by the reaction of UCNS with hydrophilic bifunctional molecules; while surface oxidation could be achieve by oxidizing the terminal group of native ligands to generate a pendant carboxylic functional group. Ligand attraction involves absorption of an additional amphiphilic polymer onto the nanoparticle surface through the hydrophobic van der Waals attraction between the original ligand and hydrocarbon chain of the polymer. Layer-by-layer assembly could be employed for electrostatic absorption of alternately charged polyions on the nanoparticle surface. Surface polymerization involves growing a dense cross-linked shell on the nanoparticle core by condensation of small monomers. Importance for these methods is the surface coverage with molecules consisting of additional functional groups that allow further reactions with biological entities (Cao, 2010; Boyer, 2010; Zhou, 2010; Kobayashi, 2009; Qian, 2008; Ehlert, 2008; Johnson, 2010). To some extent, the coating methods usually lead to highly stable colloidal particles in comparison with the ligand engineering method. Moreover, among various surface-coating methods, silica coating enjoys common usage by several groups, partly due to the well-established
surface chemistry of silica coating for facile bioconjugation. Distinctive feature of modified and functionalized up-converting nanoparticles is the retention of the native surface structures, thereby reducing the possibility of creating surface defects that quench the UC luminescence. However, surface modification sometimes adversely affects photophysical properties of up-converting nanoparticles.

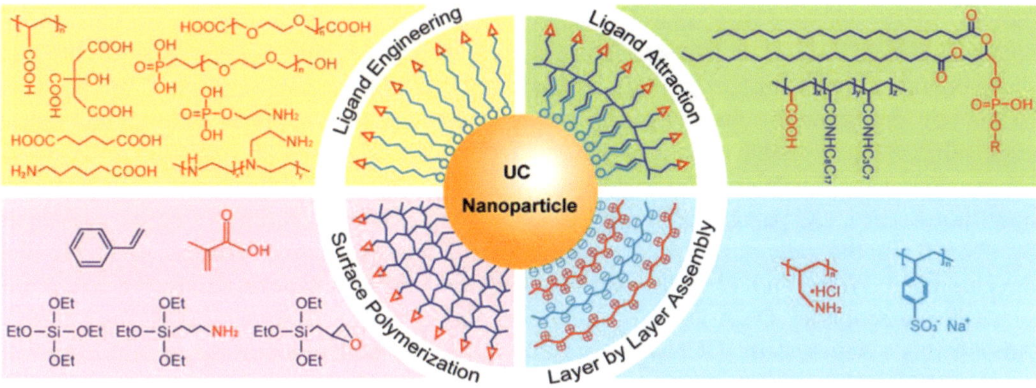

Fig. 10. Typical strategies for solubilization and functionalization of UCNs (Wang, 2010).

3.5 Application of up-converting nanoparticles for biological sensing

Application of UCNs for biological sensing can be roughly divided into two classes: one is directly observed luminescence from the UCNs, and the other is based on FRET. UCNs have been used as luminescent reporters in a variety of assays, including immune-assay, bio-affinity assay, and DNA hybridization assay as alternatives to conventional labeling agents (Zijlmans, 1999; Hampl, 2001; Corstjens, 2008; Li, 2008; Huang, 2009). A example was demonstrated by submicron-sized Y_2O_2S particles doped with Yb^{3+} and Er^{3+} ions for detection of human chorionic gonadotropin with a limit of 10 pg in a lateral flow (LF) immune-chromatographic assay format (Hampl, 2001). Another intriguing example has been demonstrated by Niedbala's group (Niedbala, 2001), in which an LF-based strip assay for the simultaneous detection of amphetamine, methamphetamine, phencyclidine, and opiates in saliva was developed by using multicolor UC particles. The architecture of the lateral flow strip is designed to accommodate up to 12 distinct test lines, in which green emitting particles were coupled to antibodies for phencyclidine and amphetamine, and blue emitting particles were coupled to antibodies for methamphetamine and morphine. In addition, each strip also contains two control lines. By analyzing the test strip for each colored phosphor, the drug molecules (amphetamine, methamphetamine, phencyclidine, and opiates) were successfully detected. The whole process was very short less than 10 min and with high sensitivity.

UCNs have also been coupled with metallic nanoparticles or organic fluorophores for FRET based biosensing. Wang *et al* developed a highly sensitive biosensor for detection of avidin by using biotinylated $NaYF_4$:Yb/Er nanoparticles as energy donors and biotinylated Au nanoparticles as energy acceptors. The 7 nm Au nanoparticles show a broad and strong absorption centered at 520 nm, which matches well with the 540 nm emission of $NaYF_4$:Yb/Er nanoparticles. Biotinylated $NaYF_4$:Yb/Er and Au nanoparticles with molecular probes can specifically interact between avidin and biotin. When the target is absent, the donor and acceptor are well separated and no FRET process is expected. In the presence of the target, the donor and acceptor will be linked in close proximity and FRET becomes significant, resulting in a decrease in emission intensity of the donor. In addition, due to UCNs with ability of reducing background autofluorescence, UCNs have also been used as luminescent reporters in genomic applications (Corstjens, 2001). As a derivative of FRET, luminescence resonance energy transfer (LRET) was firstly introduced as by Selvin

(Selvin, 1994, 2002). LRET mainly relies on the same dipole-dipole mechanism as conventional FRET, but it has its own advantage, which offers a large energy transfer distance range (>10 nm) and high reliability. Particularly, the long-lived luminescent lanthanide donors allow facile and accurate lifetime measurements to monitor biological events that are inaccessible with conventional fluorescent dyes.

UC particles have also been used in genomic biosensor. Due to the elimination of unwanted autofluorescence, UC particles can facilitate the detection and handling of target molecules by shortening the polymerase chain reaction (PCR) amplification process. In a parallel development, Wang and Li demonstrated a sandwich-hybridization assay for the ultra-sensitive detection of DNA using sub-50 nm $NaYF_4$:Yb/Er nanoparticles (Wang, 2006). Among this assay system, UCNs are modified with probe DNA strands, while magnetic nanoparticles are used and modified capture DNA strands. Upon incubation with target DNA strands, the UC and magnetic nanoparticles form binary nanoparticle aggregates. By virtue of magnetic nanoparticles, the aggregates can be easily purified and examined via UC luminescence assays (Fig. 11). Moreover the lowest detection limit of this method is ca. 10 nM and without PCR amplification.

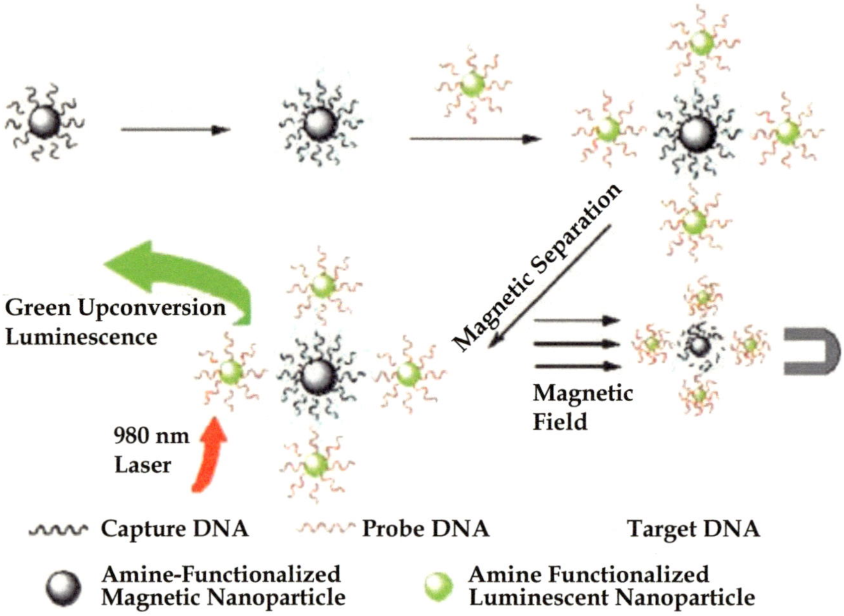

Fig. 11. Schematic illustration of the UC nanoparticle and magnetic nanoparticles-based DNA detection (Wang, 2006).

4. Comparative assessment of semiconductor QDs and rare-earth up-converting nanoparticles for biosensing application

Semiconductor QDs possess high photostability, tunable emission spectra, high quantum yields, narrow emission bandwidths, superior signal brightness, long fluorescence lifetimes, and rich surface coupling capability, so they have been widely used in a variety of biosensors (Alivisatos, 2005). QDs are down-converting materials, which emit visible fluorescence when excited by ultraviolet (UV) light or short wavelength visible light. However, when using UV light for monitoring living processes in cells and tissues, there have some potential drawbacks. In particular, if using UV light long-term irradiates living cells, it may cause DNA damage, cell death and reduce the signal-to-background ratio. Furthermore, in vivo fluorescence imaging is limited by the short penetration depth of the excitation light. In the most case, QDs have resistance to photobleaching, but sometimes they do exhibit temporary and random loss of fluorescence (photo-blinking). Currently, there are a class of NIR fluorophores such as NIR fluorescent dyes and the developed NIR quantum dots (Zhang, 2007). Though they own the abilities of deep tissue penetration and low autofluorescence as compared to visible fluorophores, they also have some disadvantages to signal detection. NIR detectors and filters are needed and the excitation and emission wavelengths are too close to each other. Furthermore, NIR dyes experienced photo-bleach and NIR QDs are cytotoxic. These factors greatly limit their application in biosensor.

Compared with QDs, UCNs absorb NIR light and emit in the NIR or visible ranges, and the excitation and emission wavelength are well separated from each other. Meanwhile, since different colored emission peaks have little overlap, sharp emission peaks, it is ideal for multiplexing bio-detection. More importantly, NIR radiation is less harmful to cells and minimizes autofluorescence from biological tissues, thereby increasing the signal-to-noise ratio significantly. UCNs exhibit almost no temporary and random loss of fluorescence (photo-blinking) as observed in QDs, which is beneficial for accurate tracking of individual UCNs (Frangioni, 2003). Of course, UCNs also own themselves shortcoming, for example, the determination of the quantum yield of UCNs becomes difficult because the standards that show up-conversion property are not available. Boyer *et al* have determined and reported the quantum yield of $NaYF_4$ UCNs with various sizes, and their quantum yields vary from 0.005% to 0.3% (Boyer, 2010). This is comparatively lower than the quantum yield of QDs, which quantum yields could attain 5-85% (Wang, 2003; Shavel, 2006). Therefore, these factors also limit, to some degree, the application of UCNs in biosensing fields.

5. Concluding remarks and perspective

This paper reviews the latest research advances in utilization of QDs and UCNs conjugates in biosensing fields based on their unique optical properties. The advantages and limitation of QDs and UCNs for biosensing applications are comparatively summarized. QDs conjugates were widely attempted in uses for imaging, targeting drug, and biosensing fields. However, the photo-blinking phenomenon, high background autofluorescence from biological tissues and toxicity to living system of QDs largely affect their potentials in biosensing application. To conquer these challenges, great efforts need to be made in control synthesis, surface modification and functionalization, luminescence modulation, and bioconjugation technology of semiconductor QDs to further improve their chemical photostability, spectra availability, surface chemistry, understand their pharmacokinetics, metabolism, degradation and safety in living system, and reduce the and toxicity. Moreover, the design and synthesis of high quality QDs with efficient NIR emission and non-toxic element composition is also desired for raising the availability of QDs in biological application. The last but not the least, with the development of QDs in biosensing application, new instrumentation and platform by integration of QDs with multifunctional nanosystem that can target, sense, image and treat diseases are also necessary to push basic research moving to clinic trial.

Partially different from semiconductor QDs, UCNs show features of chemical stability, resistance to photobleaching, large anti-Stokes shift, sharp emission peaks, and non-toxicity. Moreover, due to their unique visible emission excited by NIR light, UCNs show advantages of the deep penetration in tissue and the absence of background autofluorescence in biosensing application. However, there are still challenges for UCNs to become ideal biological labels for practical biosensing application. One of the biggest challenges that hurdles UCNs to practically used in biosensor is that the quantum yield of the UCNs is quite low, which results in the low fluorescence signals. In a relatively complicated biosensing process, the fluorescence signal may be hard to capture with normal instrumentation when using UCNs as fluorescent labels. In addition, the surface modification and functionalization of UCNs for improving their quantum yield need to be further consummated. The lack of common recognized approach and standard for determining the quantum yield of UCNs might be another challenge. The controlled synthesis and surface modification of UCNs that exhibit high colloidal stability and tailorable optical properties is always desired. Substantial efforts are also needed to focus on development of strategies for patterning UCNs on various substrates, allowing for multiplexed high-sensitivity detection in biosensor.

6. Acknowledgements

We gratefully acknowledge the financial supports from National High Technology Research and Development Program (863 program, 2010AA03A407), National Natural Science Foundation of China (20961005), Department of Science and Technology of Inner Mongolia (Public Security Foundation 208096), Inner Mongolia University Funds (10013-121008).

7. References

Alivisatos A. P. (2004). The use of nanocrystals in biological detection. *Nat. Biotechnol.*, Vol. 22, pp. 47-52.

Alivisatos A. P. (1996). Perspectives on the physical chemistry of semiconductor nanocrystals. *J. Phys. Chem.*, Vol. 100, pp. 13226-13239.

Alivisatos A. P. (1996). Semiconductor clusters, nanocrystals, and quantum dots. Science, Vol. 271, pp. 933–937.

Alivisatos A. P. Gu W. Larabell C. (2005). Quantum dots as cellular probes. *Annu. Rev. Biomed. Eng.*, Vol. 7, pp. 55–76.

Auzel F. (2004). Upconversion and anti-Stokes processes with f and d ions in solids. *Chem. Rev.*, Vol. 104, pp. 139-174.

Bagwe R. P. Zhao X. J. Tan W. H. (2003). Bioconjugated luminescent nanoparticles for biological applications. *J. Dispers. Sci. Technol.*, Vol. 24, pp. 453–464.

Blasse G. B. Grabmaier C. (1994). *Luminescent Materials*, Springer, Berlin

Boyer J. C. Cuccia L. A. Capobianco J. A. (2007). Synthesis of colloidal upconverting $NaYF_4$: Er^{3+}/Yb^{3+} and Tm^{3+}/Yb^{3+} monodisperse nanocrystals. *Nano Lett.*, Vol. 7, pp. 847-852.

Boyer J. C. Manseau M. P. Murray J. I. van Veggel F. C. J. M. (2010). Surface modification of upconverting NaYF4 nanoparticles with PEG−phosphate ligands for NIR (800 nm) biolabeling within the biological window. *Langmuir*, Vol. 26, pp. 1157–1164.

Boyer J. C. van Veggel F. C. J. M. (2010). Absolute quantum yield measurements of colloidal $NaYF_4$:Er^{3+},Yb^{3+} upconverting nanoparticles. *Nanoscale,* Vol. 2, pp. 1417–1419.

Bruchez Jr M. Moronne M. Gin P. Weiss S. Alivisatos A. P. (1998). Semiconductor Nanocrystals as Fluorescent Biological Labels. *Science*, Vol. 281, pp. 2013-2016.

Brus L. E. (1984). Electron-electron and electron-hole interactions in small metallic crystallites: The size-dependence of the lowest optically excited electronic states. *J. Chem. Phys.*, Vol. 80, pp. 4403–4409.

Cao T. Y. Yang T. S. Cao Y. Yang Y. Hu H. Li F. (2010). Water-soluble NaYF4:Yb/Er upconversion nanophosphors: Synthesis, characteristics and application in bioimaging. *Inorg. Chem. Commun.*, Vol. 13, pp. 392–394.

Chan W. C. W. Nie S. (1998). Quantum Dot Bioconjugates for Ultrasensitive Nonisotopic Detection. *Science,* Vol. 281, pp. 2016-2018.

Chatterjee D. K. Rufaihah A. J. Zhang Y. (2008.) Upconversion fluorescence imaging of cells and small animals using lanthanide doped nanocrystals. *Biomaterials*, Vol. 29, pp. 937–943.

Chivian J. S. Case W. E. Eden D. D. (1979). *Appl. Phys. Lett.*, Vol. 35, pp. 35124.

Corstjens P. van Lieshout L. Zuiderwijk M. Kornelis D. Tanke H. J. Deelder A. M. van Dam. C. J. (2008). Up-converting phosphor technology-based lateral flow assay for detection of schistosoma crculating anodic antigen in serum. *J. Clin.Microbiol.*, Vol. 46, pp. 171–176.

Corstjens P. Zuiderwijk M. Brink A. Li S. Feindt H. Niedbala R. S. Tanke H. (2001). Use of up-converting phosphor rporters in lateral-flow assays to detect specific nucleic acid sequences: A rapid, sensitive DNA test to identify human papillomavirus type 16 infection. *Clin. Chem.*, Vol. 47, pp. 1885–1893.

Cui D. X. Pan B. F. Zhang H. Gao F. Wu R. Wang J. He R. Asahi T. (2008). Self-Assembly of Quantum Dots and Carbon Nanotubes for Ultrasensitive DNA and Antigen Detection. *Anal. Chem.*, Vol. 80, pp. 7996–8001.

Derfus A. M. Chan W. C. W. Bhatia S. N. (2004). Probing the cytotoxicity of semiconductor quantum dots. *Nano Lett.*, Vol. 4, pp. 11–18.

Dubertret B. Skourides P. Norris D. J. Noireaux V. Brivanlou A. H. Libchaber A. (2002). In vivo imaging of quantum dots encapsulated in phospholipid micelles *Science*, Vol. 298, pp. 1759–1762.

Duncan R. (2006), Polymer conjugates as anticancer nanomedicines. *Nat. Rev. Cancer*, Vol. 6, pp. 688–701.

Duncan R. (2003). The dawning era of polymer therapeutics. Nat. Rev. Drug Discov., Vol. 2, pp. 347–360.

Ehlert O. Thomann R. Darbandi M. Nann. T. (2008). A four-color colloidal multiplexing nanoparticle system. *ACS Nano*, Vol. 2, pp. 120–124.

Feldmann C. Goesmann H. (2010). Nanoparticulate functional materials. *Angew. Chem. Int. Ed.*, Vol. 49, pp. 1362-95.

Frangioni J. V. (2003). In vivo near-infrared fluorescence imaging. *Curr. Opin. Chem. Biol.* Vol. 7, pp. 626–634.

Gaponenko S. V. (1998). *Optical Properties of Semiconductor Nanocrystals.* Cambridge University Press, New York

Gao X. H. Cui Y. Y. Levenson R. M. Chung W. K. L. Nie S. (2004). In vivo cancer targeting and imaging with semiconductor quantum dots. *Nat. Biotechnol.*, Vol. 22, pp. 969-976.

Gerion D. Pinaud F. Williams S. C. Parak W. J. Zanchet D. Weiss S. Alivisatos A. P. (2001). Synthesis and properties of biocompatible water-soluble silica-coated CdSe/ZnS semiconductor quantum dots, *J. Phys. Chem. B,* Vol. 105, pp. 8861–8871.

Goldman E. R. Clapp A. R. Anderson G. P. Goldman E. R. Clapp A. R. Anderson G. P. Uyeda H. T. Mauro J. M. Medintz I. L. Mattoussi H. (2004). Multiplexed toxin analysis using four colors of quantum dot fluororeagents. *Anal. Chem.,* Vol. 76, pp. 684–688.

Goldman E. R. Medintz I. L. Whitley J. L. Hayhurst A. Clapp A. R. Uyeda H. T. Deschamps J. R. Lassman M. E. Mattoussi H. (2005). A hybrid quantum dot–antibody rragment fluorescence resonance energy transfer-based TNT sensor. *J. Am. Chem. Soc.,* Vol. 127, pp. 6744–6751.

Goronkim H. et al. (1999). *In Nanostructure Science and Technology,* a worldwide study. Eds. By Siegiel R. W., Hu E. and Rocco M. C., NSTC

Hampl J. Hall M. Mufti N. A. Yao Y. M. MacQueen D. B. Wright W. H. Cooper D. E. (2001). Upconverting phosphor reporters in immunochromatographic assays. *Anal. Biochem.*, Vol. 288, pp. 176–187.

Han M. Y. Gao X. H. Su J. Z. Nie S. (2001). Quantum-dot-tagged microbeads for multiplexed optical coding of biomolecules. *Nat. Biotechnol.*, Vol. 19, pp. 631-635.

Hansen J. A. Wang J. Kawde A. N. Xiang Y. Gothelf K. V. Collins G. (2006). Quantum-dot/aptamer-based ultrasensitive multi-analyte electrochemical biosensor. *J. Am. Chem. Soc.,* Vol. 128, pp. 2228–2229.

Heer S. Kömpe K. Güdel H. U. Haase M. (2004). Highly efficient multicolour upconversion emission in transparent colloids of lanthanide-doped $NaYF_4$ nanocrystals. *Adv. Mater.*, Vol. 16, pp. 2102-2105.

Heer S. Lehmann O. Haase M. Güdel H. U. (2003), Blue, green, and red upconversion emission from lanthanide-doped $LuPO_4$ and $YbPO_4$ nanocrystals in a transparent colloidal slution. *Angew. Chem. Int. Ed.*, Vol. 42, pp. 3179-3182.

Hermanson G. T. (1996). *Bioconjugate Techniques.* Academic Press, New York

Hood J. D. Bednarski M. Frausto R. Guccione S. Reisfeld R. A. Xiang R. Cheresh D. A. (2002). Tumor regression by targeted gene delivery to the neovasculature, *Science*, Vol. 296, pp. 2404–2407.

Huang L. H. Zhou L. Zhang Y. B. Xie C. K. Qu J. F. Zeng A. J. Huang H. J. Yang R. F. Wang X. Z. (2009). Simple optical rader for upconverting phosphor particles captured on lateral flow strip. *J. IEEE Sens.*, Vol. 9, pp. 1185–1191.

Jain. R. K. (2001). Delivery of molecular medicine to solid tumors: lessons from in vivo imaging of gene expression and function. *J. Control. Release*, Vol. 74, pp. 7–25.

Jain R. K. (1999). Transport of molecules, particles, and cells in solid tumors. *Annu. Rev.Biomed. Eng.*, Vol. 1, pp. 241–263.

Jaiswal J. K. Simon S. M. (2004). Potentials and pitfalls of fluorescent quantum dots for biological imaging. *Trends. Cell Biol.*, Vol. 14, pp. 497–504.

Johnson N. J. J. Sangeetha N. M. Boyer J. C. van Veggel F. C. J. M. (2010), Facile ligand-exchange with polyvinylpyrrolidone and subsequent silica coating of hydrophobic upconverting β-$NaYF^4$:Yb^{3+}/Er^{3+} nanoparticles. *Nanoscale*, Vol. 2, pp. 771–777.

Katz E. Willner I. (2004). Integrated nanoparticle-biomolecule hybrid systems: Synthesis, properties and applications. *Angew. Chem. Int. Ed.*, Vol. 43, pp. 6042-6108.

Kim J. H. Morikis D. Ozkan M. (2004), Adaptation of inroganic quantum dots for stable molecular beacons. *Sens Actuators B*, Vol. 102, pp. 315–319.

Kobayashi H. Kosaka N. Ogawa M. Morgan N. Y. Smith P. D. Murray C. B. Ye X. Collins J. Kumar G. A. Bell H. Choyke P. L. (2009). *In vivo* multiple color lymphatic imaging using upconverting nanocrystals. *J. Mater. Chem.*, Vol. 19, pp. 6481–6484.

Li J. J. Ouellette A. L. Giovangrandi L. Coope D. E. Ricco A J. Kovacs G. T. A. (2008). Optical scanner for immunoassays with up-converting phosphorscent labels. *IEEE Trans. Biomed. Eng.*, Vol. 55, pp. 1560–1571.

Li Z. Q. Zhang Y. (2006). Monodisperse silica-coated polyvinylpyrrolidone/NaYF4 nanocrystals with multicolor upconversion fluorescence emission. *Angew. Chem. Int. Ed.*, Vol. 45, pp. 7732 -7735.

Lidke D. S. Nagy P. Heintzmann R. Arndt-Jovin D. J. Post J. N. Grecco H. E. Jares-Erijman E. A. Jovin T. M. (2004). Quantum dot ligands provide new insights into erbB/HER receptor-mediated signal transduction. *Nat. Biotechnol.*, Vol. 22, pp. 198–203.

Lim S. F. Ryu W. S. Austin R. H. (2010). Particle size dependence of the dynamic photophysical properties of NaYF4:Yb, Er nanocrystals. *Opt. Express*, Vol. 18, pp. 2309-2316.

Liu C. Chen D. (2007). Controlled synthesis of hexagon shaped lanthanide-doped LaF_3 nanoplates with multicolor upconversion fluorescence. *J. Mater. Chem.*, Vol. 17, pp. 3875-3880.

Mai H. X. Zhang Y. W. Si R. Yan Z. G. Sun L. D. You L. P. Yan C. H. (2006). High-quality sodium rare-earth fluoride nanocrystals: controlled synthesis and optical properties. *J. Am. Chem. Soc.*, Vol. 128, pp. 6426-6436.

Mai H. X. Zhang Y. W. Sun L. D. Yan C. H. (2007). Highly efficient multicolor up-conversion emissions and their mechanisms of monodisperse NaYF4:Yb,Er core and core/shell-structured nanocrystals. *J. Phys. Chem. C*, Vol. 111, pp. 13721-13729.

Mansur H. S. (2010). Quantum dots and nanocomposites. *Wiley Interdisciolinary Reviews: Nanomedicine and Nanobiotechnology*, Vol. 2, pp. 113-129.

Medintz I. L. Clapp A. R. Mattoussi H. Goldman E. R. Fisher B. Mauro J. M. (2003). Self-assembled nanoscale biosensors based on quantum dot FRET donors. *Nat. Mater.*, Vol. 2, pp. 2, 630–638.

Murray C. B. Norris D. J. Bawendi M. G. (1993). Synthesis and characterization of nearly monodisperse CdE (E = sulfur, selenium, tellurium) semiconductor nanocrystallites. *J. Am. Chem. Soc.*, Vol. 115, pp. 8706–8715.

Murphy C. J. Coffer J. L. (2002). Quantum dots: A primer. *Appl. Spectrosc.*, Vol. 56, pp. 16A-27A.

Niedbala R. S. Feindt H. Kardos K. Vail T. Burton J. Bielska B. Li S. Milunic D. Bourdelle P. Vallejo R. (2001). Detection of analytes by imunoassay using up-converting phosphor technology. *Anal. Biochem.*, Vol. 293, pp. 22–30.

Nirmal M. Brus L. E. (1999). Luminescence Photophysics in Semiconductor Nanocrystals. *Acc. Chem. Res.*, Vol. 32, pp. 407–414.

Pires M. A. Heer S. Gudel H. U. Serra O.A. (2006). Er, Yb doped yttrium based nanosized phosphors: Particle size, "host lattice" and doping ion concentration effects on upconversion efficiency. *J. Fluoresc.*, Vol. 16, pp. 461- 468.

Qian H. S. Li Z. Q. Zhang Y. (2008). Multicolor polystyrene nanospheres tagged with up-conversion fluorescent nanocrystals. *Nanotechnology*, Vol. 19, pp. 255601.

Rosi N. L. Mirkin C. A. (2005). Nanostructures in biodiagnostics. *Chem. Rev.*, Vol. 105, pp. 1547-1562.

Selvin P. R. (2002). Principles and biophysical application of lanthanide-based probes. *Annu. Rev. Biophys. Biomol. Struct.*, Vol. 31, pp. 275-302.

Selvin P. R. Rana T. M. Hearst J. E. (1994). Luminescence resonance energy transfer. *J. Am. Chem. Soc.*, Vol. 116, pp. 6029–6030.

Shavel A. Gaponik N. Eychmüller A. (2006). Factors governing the 1uality of aqueous CdTe nanocrystals:Calculations and experiment. *J. Phys. Chem. B*, Vol. 110, pp. 19280–19284.

Smith A. M. Duan H.W. Mohs A. M. Nie S. (2008). Bioconjugated quantum dots for in vivo molecular and cellular imaging. *Adv. Drug Delivery Rev.*, Vol. 60, pp. 1226-1240.

Smith A. M. Duan H.W. Rhyner M. N. Ruan G. Nie S. (2006). A systematic examination of surface coatings on the optical and chemical properties of semiconductor quantum dots. *Phys. Chem. Chem. Phys.*, Vol. 8, pp. 3895–3903.

Stouwdam J. W. van Veggel F. C. J. M. (2002). Near-infrared emission of redispersible Er^{3}+, Nd^{3+}, and Ho^{3+} doped LaF_3 nanoparticles. *Nano Lett.*, Vol. 2, pp. 733-737.

Varlamova O. A. Donovan D. P. Ma D. Gardner J. P. Morrissey D. M. Arrigale R. R. Zhan C. Chodera A. J. Surowitz K. G. Maddon P. J. Heston W. D. W. Olson W. C. (2003). The homodimer of prostate-specific membrane antigen is a functional target for cancer therapy. *Proc. Natl. Acad. Sci.*, Vol. 100, pp. 12590–12595.

Wang F. Banerjee D. Liu Y. S. Chen X. Y. Liu X. G. (2010). Upconversion nanoparticles in biological labeling, imaging, and therapy. *Analyst*, Vol. 135, pp. 1839–1854.

Wang F. Liu X. G. (2009). Recent advances in the chemistry of lanthanide-doped upconversion nanocrystals. *Chem. Soc. Rev.*, Vol. 38, pp. 976-989.

Wang F. Liu X. G. (2008). Upconversion multicolor fine-tuning: Visible to near-infrared emission from lanthanide-doped $NaYF_4$ nanoparticles. *J. Am. Chem. Soc.*, Vol. 130, pp. 5642–5643.

Wang L. Y. Li Y. D. (2006). Green upconversion nanocrystals for DNA detection. *Chem. Commun.*, Vol. 24, pp. 2557–2559.

Wang L. Yan R. Huo Z. Wang L.Zeng J. Bao J. Wang X. Peng Q. Yadong Li. (2005). Fluorescence resonant energy transfer biosensor based on upconversion-luminescent nanoparticles. *Angew. Chem. Int. Ed.*, Vol. 44, pp. 6054-6057.

Wang X. Qu L. Zhang J. Peng X. Xiao M. (2003). Surface-related emission in highly luminescent CdSe quantum dots. *Nano Lett.*, Vol. 3, pp. 1103–1106.

Weaver J. Zakeri R. Aouadi S. Kohli. P. (2009) Synthesis and characterization of quantum dot–polymer composites *J. Mater. Chem.*, Vol. 19, pp. 3198-3206.

Weller H. (1993). Colloidal semiconductor Q-particles: chemistry in the transition region between solid states and molecules. *Angew. Chem. Int. Ed.,* Vol. 32, pp. 41-53.

Wu X. Y. Liu H. J. Liu J. Q. Wu, X. Y. Liu H. J. Liu J. Q. Haley K. N. Treadway J. A. Larson J. P. Ge, N. F. Peale F. Bruchez M. P. (2003). Immunofluorescent labeling of cancer marker Her2 and other cellular targets with semiconductor quantum dots. *Nat. Biotechnol.*, Vol. 21, pp. 41–46.

Xing Y. Chaudry Q. Shen C. Kong K. Y. Zhau, H. E. W. Chung L. Petros. J. A. O'Regan R. M. Yezhelyev M .V. Simons J. W. Wang M. D. Nie S. (2007). Bioconjugated quantum dots for multiplexed and quantitative immunohistochemistry. *Nat. Protoc.*, Vol. 2, pp. 1152–1165.

Yen W. M. Weber M. J. (2004). *Inorganic phosphors: compositions, preparation and optical properties*. CRC Press, Florida

Yi G. Chow G. (2005). Colloidal LaF_3:Yb,Er, LaF_3:Yb,Ho and LaF_3:Yb,Tm nanocrystals with multicolor upconversion fluorescence. *J. Mater. Chem.*, Vol. 15, pp. 4460-4464.

Yi G. Lu H. Zhao S. Ge Y. Yang W. Chen D. Guo L. (2004). Synthesis, characterization, and biological application of size-controlled nanocrystalline NaYF4:Yb,Er infrared-to-visible up-conversion phosphors. *Nano Lett.*, Vol. 4, pp. 2191-2196.

You C. C. Chompoosor A. Rotello V. M. (2007). The biomacromolecule-nanoparticle interface, *Nano Today*, Vol. 2, pp. 34–43.

Zeng J. Su J. Li Z. Yan R. X. Li Y. D. (2005). Synthesis and upconversion luminescence of hexagonal-phase $NaYF_4$:Yb, Er^{3+} phosphors of controlled size and morphology. *Adv. Mater.*, Vol. 17, pp. 2119-2123.

Zhang C. Y. Johnson L. W. (2009). Single Quantum-Dot-Based Aptameric Nanosensor for Cocaine. Anal. *Chem.*, Vol. 81, pp. 3051–3055.

Zhang C. Y. Yeh H. C. Kuroki M. T. Wang T. H. (2005). Single-quantum-dot-based DNA nanosensor. *Nat. Mater.*, Vol. 4, pp. 826–831.

Zhang F. Wan Y. Yu T. Zhang F. Shi Y. Xie S. Li Y. Xu L. Tu B. Zhao D. (2007). Uniform nanostructured arrays of sodium rare-earth fuorides for highly efficient multicolor upconversion luminescence. *Angew. Chem. Int. Ed.*, Vol. 46, pp. 7976-7979.

Zhang J. Su J. F. Liu L. Huang Y. Mason R. P. (2007). Evaluation of red CdTe and NIR CdHgTe QDs by fluorescent imaging. *J. Nanosci. Nanotechnol.,* Vol. 8, pp. 1155-1159.

Zhang J. Z. (1997). Ultrafast studies of electron dynamics in semiconductor and metal colloidal nano-particles: effects of size and surface. *Acc. Chem. Res.*, Vol. 30, pp. 423-429.

Zhang Y. W. Sun X. Si R. You L. P. Yan C. H. (2005). Single-crystalline and monodisperse LaF_3 triangular nanoplates from a single-source precursor. *J. Am. Chem. Soc.*, Vol. 127, pp. 3260-3261.

Zhou J. Sun Y. Du X. Xiong L. Hu H. Li F. (2010). Dual-modality in vivo imaging using rare-earth nanocrystals with near-infrared to near-infrared (NIR-to-NIR) upconversion luminescence and magnetic resonance properties. *Biomaterials,* Vol. 31, pp. 3287–3295.

Zhou M. Ghosh I.(2007). Quantum dots and peptides: A bright future together. *Peptide Science,* Vol. 88, pp. 325-339.

Zijlmans H. Bonnet J. Burton J. Burton J. Kardos K. Vail T. Niedbala R. S. Tanke H. J. (1999). Detection of cell and tissue srface antigens using up-converting phosphors: A new rporter technology. *Anal. Biochem.,* Vol. 267, pp. 30–36.

7

Biosensors Based on Biological Nanostructures

Wendel A. Alves et al.*
[1]*Centro de Ciências Naturais e Humanas, Universidade Federal do ABC, Santo André, SP,*
[2]*Instituto Nacional de Ciência e Tecnologia de Bioanalítica, Campinas, SP,*
Brazil

1. Introduction

The term *biomaterials* is attributed to the materials employed to medical applications, such as ceramic implants and biopolymer scaffolds, as well as a variety of composites (Hauser e Zhang, 2010). In recent decades, researchers of distinct subjects have gathered efforts in developing new biomaterials for applications in various branches of medicine. With the advent of molecular biology and biotechnology, and knowing that many of these biomaterials are not specific for medical applications, studies have been directed to directed towards to biological and biomimetic materials preparation biological and biomimetic materials (Sanchez, Arribart *et al.*, 2005; He, Duan *et al.*, 2008; Aizenberg e Fratzl, 2009).
In this new class of materials, the peptide compounds appear as promising candidates to *building blocks* due to their easy preparation and physical and chemical stability (Cheng, Zhu *et al.*, 2007). Thus, we can propose different peptide sequences and from their self-organization to obtain structures with different geometries (spherical, cylindrical, conical) and even nanotubes and/or nanofibers (Hirata, Fujimura *et al.*, 2007) are obtained.
Peptide nanomaterials form supramolecular structures which are interconnected by intermolecular interactions such as van der Waals forces, electrostatic, hydrophobic and hydrogen bonds, among others (Cheng, Zhu *et al.*, 2007; Colombo, Soto *et al.*, 2007). Due to these characteristics, crystal engineering of supramolecular architectures has rapidly expanded in recent years, mainly due to the possibility of intermolecular interactions, structural diversity and potential applications (Sanchez, Arribart *et al.*, 2005; Cheng, Zhu *et al.*, 2007; He, Duan *et al.*, 2008; Aizenberg e Fratzl, 2009). This structural variety is possible due to the planning and construction of supramolecular architectures, as promising *building blocks* that allow the design of functional molecular materials that will display some sort of ownership of technological interest (Sanchez, Arribart *et al.*, 2005; Cheng, Zhu *et al.*, 2007; He, Duan *et al.*, 2008; Aizenberg e Fratzl, 2009).
The nanostructures obtained from biomolecules are attractive due to their biocompatibility, ability for molecular recognition and ease of chemical modification, important factors on various applications of interest. The functionalization of these materials have greatly

* Wellington Alves[1,2], Camila P. Sousa[1,2], Sergio Kogikoski. Jr.[1,2], Rondes F. da Silva[1,2], Heliane R. do Amaral[1,2], Michelle S. Liberato[1,2], Vani X. Oliveira Jr. [1], Tatiana D. Martins[3] and Pedro M. Takahashi[4]
[1]*Centro de Ciências Naturais e Humanas, Universidade Federal do ABC, Santo André, SP,* [2]*Instituto Nacional de Ciência e Tecnologia de Bioanalítica ,Campinas, SP,* [3]*Instituto de Química, Universidade Federal de Goiás, Goiânia, GO,* [4]*Departamento de Química, Universidade Federal do Espírito Santo, Vitória, ES, Brazil.*

facilitated the study of biological systems, which can be utilized in biosensor devices, catalytic activities and molecular recognition. Thus, the challenge for synthetic chemistry in the area of molecular electronics is to prepare molecules with specific and well defined functions (i.e., that can be used at a molecular level as wires, switches, diodes, etc.). The controlled assemblies of supramolecular species selected components allow the preparation of nanosize materials with quite sophisticated electronic properties (De La Rica e Matsui, 2010).

1.1 Peptide-based nanostructures

The formation of tubular peptide nanostructures has been performed using several different peptide sequences, such as heptapeptide CH_3CO-Lys-Leu-Val-Phe-Phe-Ala-Glu-NH_2, (Lu, Jacob *et al.*, 2003) and dipeptides $^+NH_3$-Phg-Phg-COO^- (Reches e Gazit, 2004) and $^+NH_3$-Phe-Trp-COO^- (Reches e Gazit, 2003). The first peptide nanotubes were obtained by M.R. Ghadiri and co-workers from cyclic compounds (Ghadiri, Granja *et al.*, 1993). The *L*-amino acids are the most used building blocks. However, *D*-amino acids can also self-assemble to form nanofibers similar to those obtained from *L*-amino acids (Poteau e Trinquier, 2005).
The properties of peptides can be modified through changes in the sequence of amino acid residues used in their preparation, providing a highly relevant factor in building these new systems (Poteau e Trinquier, 2005). Such changes were reported in a study by varying the *D*-amino acids (*D*-Alanine, *D*-Leucine and *D*-phenylanine) to obtain different peptide nanotubes (De Santis, Morosetti *et al.*, 2007). It was observed that by employing enantiomers (D, L) the possibility of obtaining different supramolecular systems arises, with possible changes in their structural and electronic properties (De Santis, Morosetti *et al.*, 2007).
One of the most commonly used peptides in synthesis of nanotubes is $^+NH_3$-Phe-Phe-COO^- .These nanotubes exhibit several unique properties such as high uniformity along the entire length of the tube, biocompatibility, stability against various solvents and thermal stability. In this sense, there are several studies that investigate the structural control of the nanotubes by changing variables such as temperature, solvent and pH (Adler-Abramovich, Reches *et al.*, 2006). The $^+NH_3$-Phe-Phe-COO^- nanotubes maintain their morphology up to 200° C, and total degradation or loss of tubular morphology occurs between 200 and 300° C (Ryu e Park, 2010). The thermal stability has been attributed to π-stacking interactions among aromatic residues that mediate the formation of structures (Reches e Gazit, 2003). The investigation of stability in different organic solvents shows that the nanotubes do not suffer morphological changes after treatment in ethanol, methanol, 2-propanol, acetone and acetonitrile (Adler-Abramovich, Reches *et al.*, 2006).
Moreover, in addition to conformational changes and the sequences of amino acids used in peptide synthesis of nanomaterials, cyclical or linear, the amount of amino acids used and the functional group of the side chains can influence the formation and possibly the desired application (Brea, Castedo *et al.*, 2007). In this case, all the proposed changes and the preparation methods are in early stages of study and require further research to better understand their formation and their influence on structural and electronic properties (Yanlian, Ulung *et al.*, 2009).

2. Preparation methods of peptide nanostructures

2.1 Obtaining nanostructures in liquid phase

The liquid phase method for obtaining nanostructures is divided in two steps. To obtain a nanostructure based on ($^+NH_3$-Phe-Phe-COO^-), for example, the first step is the dissolution

of the compound in an organic solvent (1,1,1,3,3,3-hexafluoro-2-propanol, HFP) at a concentration of 100mg mL^{-1}. In the second step, nanostructures are obtained in a spontaneous process, after the dilution in water to achieve 2mg mL^{-1} of concentration. By this protocol, $^{+}NH_3$-Phe-Phe-COO^{-} self-assemble as nanotubes of 80 to 300 nm thick.
The self-assembling mechanism in which nanotubes are produced is not yet fully understood. However, the most acceptable explanation suggests that the *π-π stacking* interactions and hydrogen bonds between aromatic rings are responsible for the material nano-organization (Reches e Gazit, 2003).
Another strategy to obtain these materials in liquid phase was proposed by Kim et al. (Kim, Han *et al.*, 2010). In this work, the authors used only pure water as solvent and submitted the system to heating and sonication to dissolve the peptide, since $^{+}NH_3$-Phe-Phe-COO^{-} present hydrophobic characteristics and do not dissolve easily in water. Nanostructures are formed after cooling pH values of the preparing media. The concentration of the dipeptide solution was susceptible to variation by the authors in order to comprehend their role in nanostructure formation. Their results showed formation of $^{+}NH_3$-Phe-Phe-COO^{-} nanowires in alkaline media, while nanotubes were formed in acidic media. Also, at high concentrations of peptide, the predominant nanostructures formed are nanowires, while at low concentrations, nanotubes are prevalent.

2.2 Nanostructure preparation in solid-vapor phase

Peptide nanostructures have been prepared by self-assembly oriented in the solid-vapor phase method, which consists of using two solvents, one to solubilize the peptide and another one to encourage the nanostructure assemble. Based on the *bottom-up* strategy, the first step consists on the formation of a peptide film onto substrate surface (usually silicon), with posterior evaporation of the solvent in the absence of humidity. In this case, the peptide film is referred to as the solid phase. The next step consists of keeping the solid film in a vapor solvent atmosphere, the commonly called vapor phase. Parameters like temperature, vapor pressure, concentration of solid film and exposure time of the film to vapor solvent govern the nanostructure formation.
Ryu et al. described this methodology as the one to obtain 1D nanostructures (Ryu e Park, 2008b; a). The authors studied the influence of temperature and water activity of a solution containing metallic salts in the nanostructures formation and they reported that nanostructures are formed at high water activity, while for activity values lower than 0.3, no nanostructures were obtained. Also, it was observed that nanostructures were only achieved at a working temperature of 100 to 150 °C. Fig. 1 shows the experimental schematic process to prepare nanowires or nanotubes in solid-vapor phase.
The role of the solvent in this process was adapted by Demirel at al. (Demirel, Malvadkar *et al.*, 2010), with a few adaptations. During this study, the concentration of the precursor solution was controlled at 2mg mL^{-1} and the solvent needed at the second step of the solid-vapor process was changed. Results show that the nanostructure morphology is related to the dielectric constant values of the solvents. For example, results showed that when formed on water, which presents a dielectric constant of 80.1, a tubular structure is obtained. Same structure are obtained when using methanol (dielectric constant of 32.6) or ethanol (24.3) as solvents, while solvents presenting dielectric constants much smaller such as toluene (2.4), chloroform (4.8) or tetrahydrofuran (7.5) do not permit the peptide self-assembling and no structure is obtained. Scanning electronic micrographs (SEM) of the nanostructure obtained at various solvents are shown in Fig. 2.

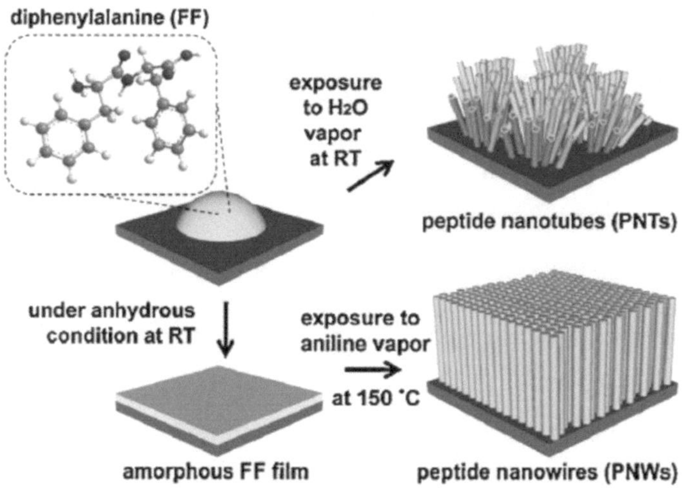

Fig. 1. Experimental scheme of obtaining peptide nanostructure using solid-vapor process. Reprinted with permission from Ryu, J. and C. B. Park (2010). "High Stability of Self-Assembled Peptide Nanowires Against Thermal, Chemical, and Proteolytic Attacks." Biotechnology and Bioengineering 105(2): 221-230 © 2010 , Wiley Ltd.

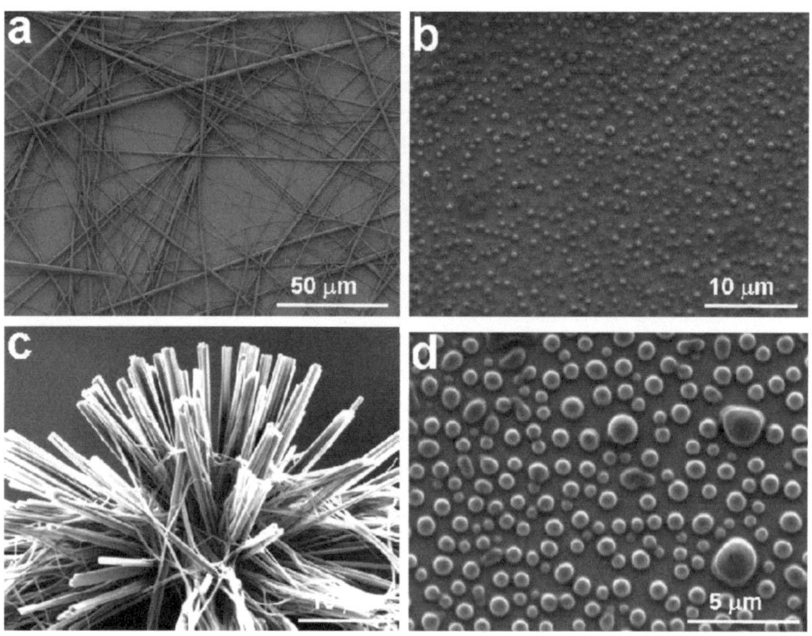

Fig. 2. SEM images of $^{+}NH_3$-Phe-Phe-COO^{-} tubes and vesicles: (a) 2mg/mL dipeptide in ethanol vaporized at 25°C, (b) 2mg/mL dipeptide in acetone vaporized at 25°C, (c) 2mg/mL dipeptide in ethanol vaporized at 80°C, and (d) 2mg/mL dipeptide in acetone vaporized at 80°C. Reprinted with permission from Demirel, G., N. Malvadkar, et al. (2010). "Control of Protein Adsorption onto Core-Shell Tubular and Vesicular Structures of Diphenylalanine/ Parylene." Langmuir 26(3): 1460-1463.© 2010 , American Chemical Society Ltd.

2.3 Obtaining nanostructures for physical vapor deposition

Recently, $^{+}NH_3$-Phe-Phe-COO^{-} nanotubes were obtained vertically oriented, employing the physical vapor deposition technique (Fig. 3) (Adler-Abramovich, Aronov *et al.*, 2009). Size and quantity of peptide nanotubes were controlled through deposition parameters adjustment such as time, solvent of preparation, temperature and distance between substrates. The peptide nanotubes formation using this technique became possible because of the low molecular weight and high volatility of precursor species. In a typical synthesis, the $^{+}NH_3$-Phe-Phe-COO^{-} is heated at 220°C in a vacuum chamber containing a clean substrate, heated at 80°C, that is located at the top of the chamber. The nanotubes formed exhibit length of hundreds of micrometers and diameters of 50 to 300nm, with morphologies similar to those from the liquid phase. This method has been employed in the fabrication of electronic devices, such as capacitors, but it can be used in the modification of electrodes for electrochemical uses.

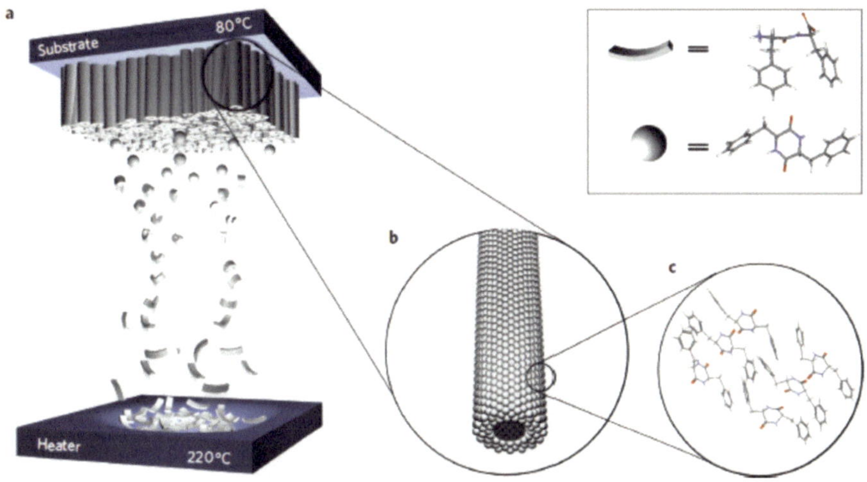

Fig. 3. Proposed assembly mechanism for the formation of vertically aligned ADNTs.
(a) Schematic of the vapor deposition technique. During evaporation, the $^{+}NH_3$-Phe-Phe-COO^{-} peptide, which is heated to 220°C, attained a cyclic structure Cyclo($^{+}NH_3$-Phe-Phe-COO^{-}) and then assembled on a substrate to form ordered vertically aligned nanotubes. (b)Illustration of a single peptide nanotube composed mainly of peptide Cyclo($^{+}NH_3$-Phe-Phe-COO^{-}).
(c) Molecular arrangement of six Cyclo($^{+}NH_3$-Phe-Phe-COO^{-}) peptides after energy minimization. A stacking interaction between aromatic moieties of the peptides is suggested to provide the energetic contribution as well as order and directionality for the initial interaction. Reprinted with permission from Shklovsky, J., P. Beker, et al. (2010). "Bioinspired peptide nanotubes: Deposition technology and physical properties." Materials Science and Engineering B-Advanced Functional Solid-State Materials 169(1-3): 62-66. © 2009 Elsevier B.V.

In a recently work, this technique was used together with photolithography to enable peptide nanotubes to assume specific positions in a silicon wafer (Shklovsky, Beker *et al.*, 2010). The authors used a photoresist wafer, with square-shaped cavities. The schematic process for the cavities preparation is in Fig. 4. According to SEM images presented in Fig. 4, dipeptide nanotubes are located over the silicon wafer, which is useful to construct integrated circuits, since the orientation and control of nanotubes material size is needed in such systems.

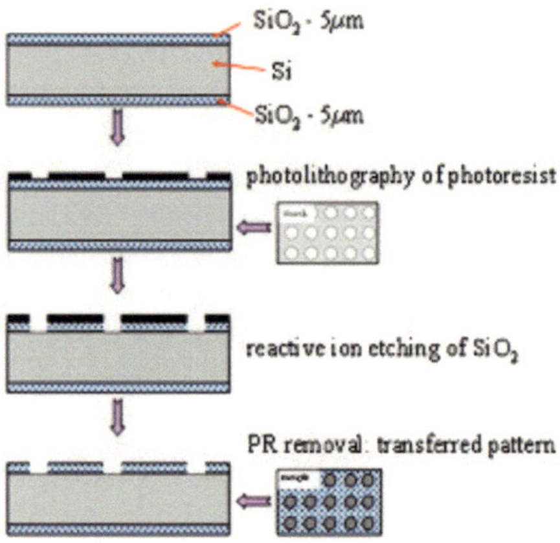

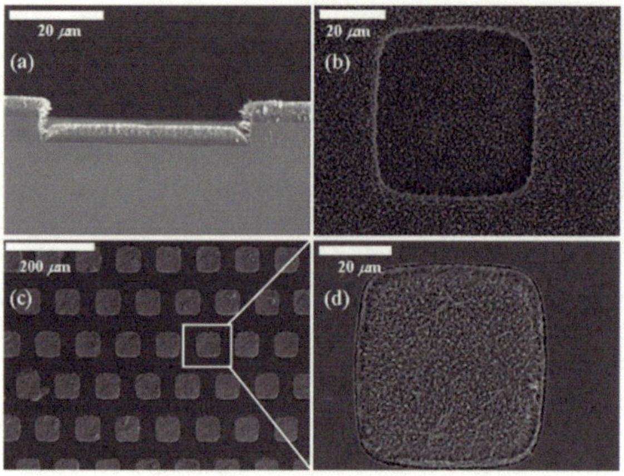

Fig. 4. Left - Schematic diagram of the peptide nanotubes bundles fabrication process. Right - SEM images of patterned arrays of peptide nanotubes fabricated by PVD. (a) Cross-section view of patterned substrate covered by peptide nanotube coating. (b) Top view of patterned substrate covered by peptide nanotube coating. (c) Top view of peptide nanotube bundles after HF release. (d) Enlargement view of image (c) Reprinted with permission from Shklovsky, J., P. Beker, et al. (2010). "Bioinspired peptide nanotubes: Deposition technology and physical properties." Materials Science and Engineering B-Advanced Functional Solid-State Materials 169(1-3): 62-66. © 2009 Elsevier B.V.

2.4 Electrospinning

The electrospinning technique is a technology that uses a high tension electric field (5-50kV) and low currents (0.5-1μA) to obtain 1D nanostructures. In this process a fluid material is accelerated and drawn trough an electric field producing structures with reduced diameters. In the work of Singh et al. (Singh, Bittner *et al.*, 2008) $^+NH_3$-Phe-Phe-COO^- nanotubes were prepared from solution in HFP. Then, this solution was diluted in water to 2.9 mmol L^{-1} of concentration and sonicated for 1 hour. Variations in the obtaining parameters of the nanostructures, like electric field, concentration, and flow injection speed on silicon wafer were investigated and their influence on the nanostructure formation was reported.

3. Functionalization of peptide nanostructures for biosensor applications

In order to obtain some new properties and increase the applicability of peptide nanomaterials, some chemical modification can be performed and materials can be functionalized to give rise to hybrid compounds. Materials that can be employed on functionalization are nanoparticles, polymers and fluorophores, among others.

Recently, Banerjee et al. reported the synthesis of peptide nanotubes containing bis(*N*-*α*-amido-glycylglycine)-1,7-heptane dicarboxylate and its modification with 2-mercaptoethylamine so as to enable its interaction with a Au substrate through a covalent bond. (Banerjee, Yu *et al.*, 2004). In this work, the nanomaterial was deposited on a Gold (Au) substrate modified with a thiol self-assembled monolayer (SAM), containing cavities that could be identified by atomic force microscopy (AFM). AFM images showed that the modification of the substrate by microfabrication techniques became viable due to the

presence of thiol groups on the outer walls of the nanotubes, which can be covalent attached to the Au substrate, allowing the modification of electrodes in specific positions.
The gold nanoparticles (GNPs) were used to ensure thermal and chemical stability and enzymatic degradation (Guha e Banerjee, 2009). In this work, β-Ala-L-Xaa (Xaa = Val / Ile / Phe, 1, 2 and 3 respectively), dipeptides were used and studies confirmed that such sequences showed thermal stability up to about 80 °C and in a wide range of pH (2–10). Guha and Banerjee have proposed the synthesis of GNPs stabilized by a peptide compound. Their analysis by X-ray diffraction indicated that the nanoparticles formed exhibit a diameter of approximately 7 nm. The influence of pH and peptide sequence used in the synthesis of the GNP coated peptide nanotubes was also studied, demonstrating that there is a relationship between pH and GNP coating that leads to a complete and uniform coverage in one specific system, while in other systems the coverage is partial and shapeless. In addition, other parameters were also varied, such as the mass ratio between the GNPs and the peptide nanotube in order to study these interactions (pH and GNP coating). Fig. 5 shows transmission electronic microscopy (TEM) images obtained for the peptide nanotubes functionalized with gold nanoparticles.

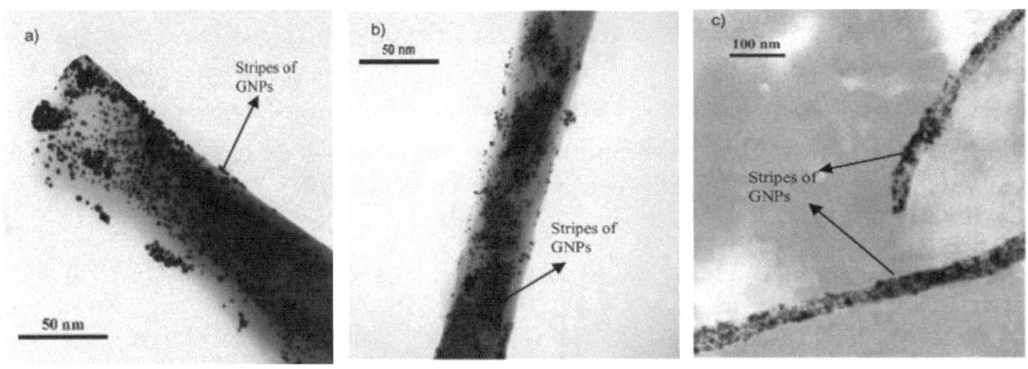

Fig. 5. (a–c) TEM images of dipeptide-capped gold nanoparticles fabricated on the outer surfaces of the dipeptide nanotube 1–3, respectively, at pH 10. It is clear from the figure that at higher pH coating of dipeptide-capped GNPs on the outer surfaces of the dipeptide nanotube is more uniform than at lower pH. Reprinted with permission from Guha, S. and A. Banerjee (2009). "Self-Assembled Robust Dipeptide Nanotubes and Fabrication of Dipeptide-Capped Gold Nanoparticles on the Surface of these Nanotubes." Advanced Functional Materials 19(12): 1949-1961.© 2009 WILEY-VCH Verlag GmbH & Co. KGaA, Weinheim

In a recent work (Martins et al., 2011 in press), the effect of controlling pH of nanotube preparation and the concentration of a doping fluorescent molecule on the final structure is carefully studied. Their results showed that structures can vary between nanotubes and nanoribbons, depending on pH of formation and their growth is influenced by the charge concentration over the nanotubes. Fig. 6 shows SEM and fluorescence microscopy images for nanostructures formed at distinct pH ranges.
Reches and Gazit studied the formation of peptide nanotubes in a solution containing Fe_3O_4 magnetite nanoparticles, , in order to verify the functionalization of peptide nanotubes with magnetic nanoparticles. (Reches e Gazit, 2006). By SEM images the presence of nanoparticles

onto a surface of peptide nanotube is easily detected. These results suggested that these hybrid systems may find application in sensors and nano(electro) mechanics devices.

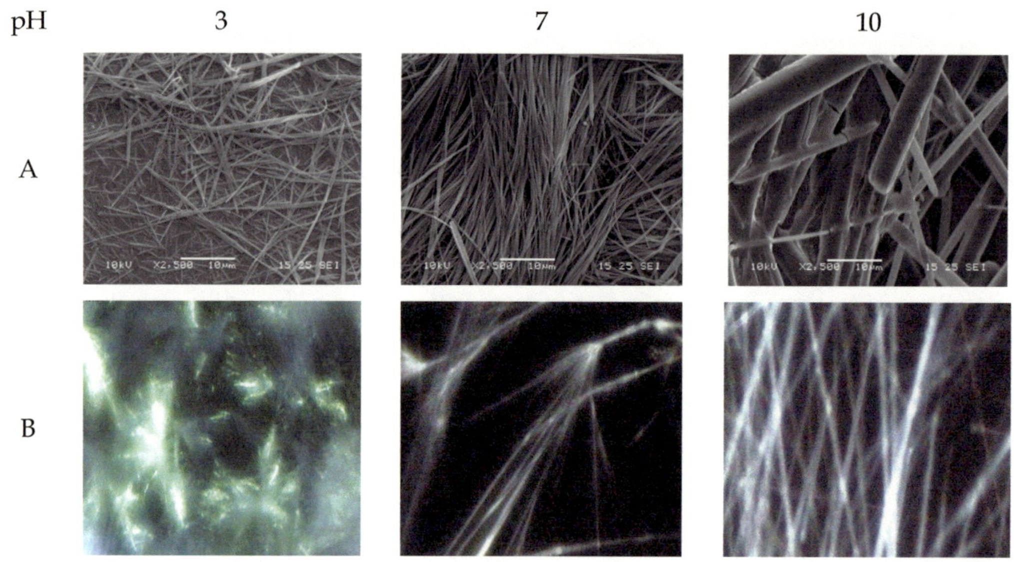

Fig. 6. (a) SEM images for nanotubes formed at the concentration of 0.002% m/m of pyrenyl moieties, (b) EPM images (200 times increased) for samples of 0.07% m/m of pyrenyl moieties. All images for samples produced at distinct pH values.

Functionalized peptide nanostructures based on platinum nanoparticles (PtNPs) were studied by Song et al. (Song, Challa *et al.*, 2004). In this work, nanotubes prepared by self-assembly of $^{+}NH_3$-D-Phe-D-Phe-COO^{-} in solution of distinct concentrations were then functionalized with PtNPs and scanning electron microscopy and Monte Carlo simulations were used to investigate them. Such analyses showed morphological changes related to concentration. At low concentrations, nanotubes were obtained, whereas at high concentrations, nanovesicles were the products. Functionalization was accomplished by adding K_2PtCl_4 and ascorbic acid to the solution of peptide nanomaterials. The formation of nanoparticles was verified by the change of solution color. Morphological characterization of nanomaterials functionalized with PtNPs was performed by TEM. These materials can find application in catalysis, among others.

Peptide nanotubes can also be used as support for the growth of semiconductor nanocrystals on the nanotubes surface. (Banerjee, Muniz *et al.*, 2007). According to the authors, it was possible to grow TiO_2, Ge and Cu_2S nanocrystals using this technique. It was also found that a simple change in pH causes significant differences in crystal size without changing their crystallographic properties.

The peptide nanomaterials can also encapsulate quantum dots (QDs), as reported by Yan and coworkers, in which a $^{+}NH_3$-Phe-Phe-COO^{-} hydrogel is treated as three-dimensional and interconnected nano-scaled fibers, that are used in the encapsulation of QDs. (Yan, Cui *et al.*, 2008). Results indicate the promising employment of such materials in nano- and biotechnology.

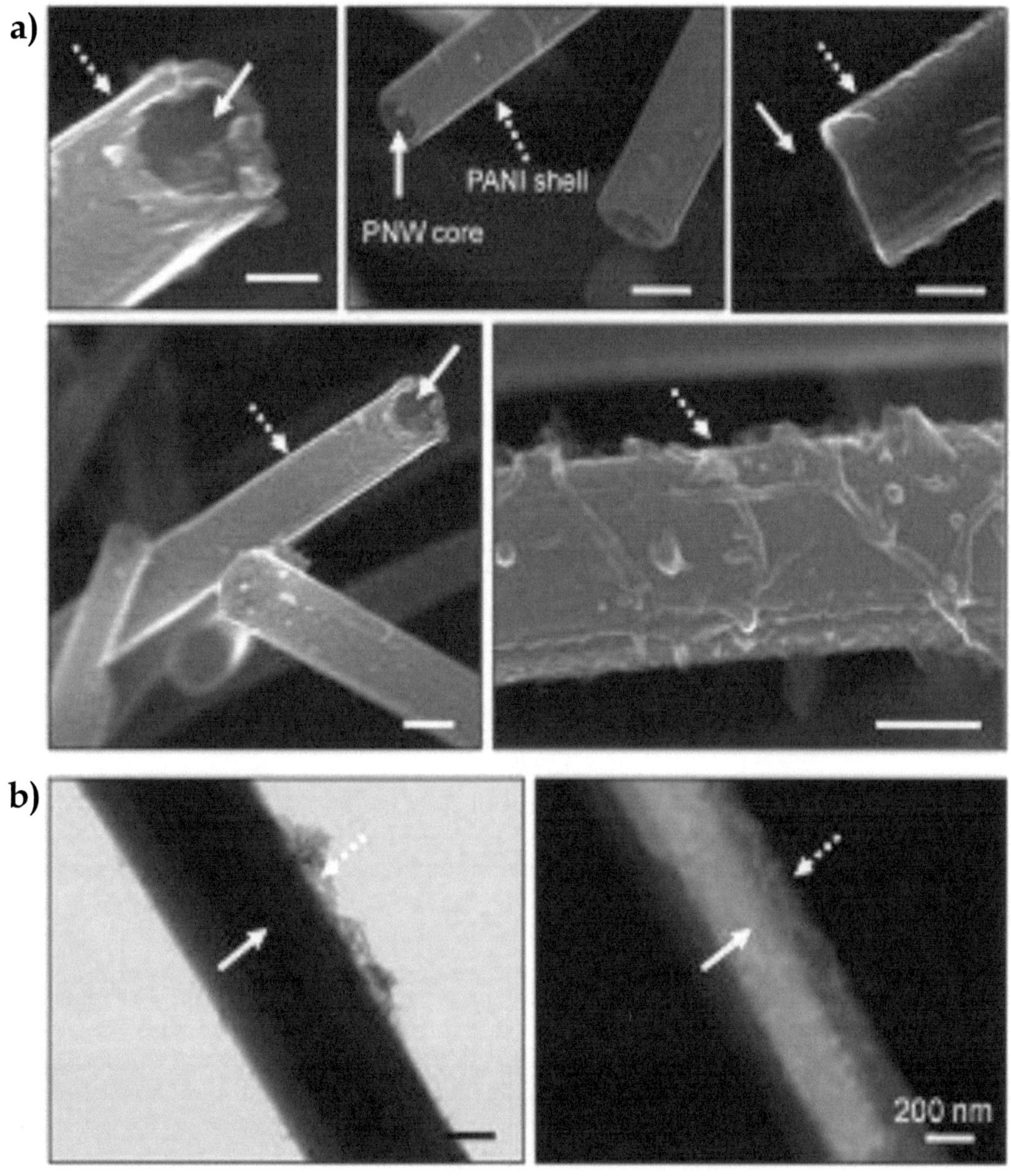

Fig. 7. (a) SEM and (b) STEM images of PNW/PANI core/shell nano- wires. Arrows indicate the PNW core (solid arrows) and PANI shell (dotted arrows). The core/shell structure of the PNW/PANI nanowires was clearly visible in STEM micrographs taken in a bright field imaging mode (left) and in a high angle angular dark field imaging mode (right). Reprinted with permission from Ryu, J. and C. B. Park (2009). "Synthesis of Diphenylalanine/Polyaniline Core/Shell Conducting Nanowires by Peptide Self-Assembly." Angewandte Chemie-International Edition 48(26): 4820-4823. © 2009 Wiley-VCH Verlag GmbH & Co. KGaA, Weinheim

The obtaining of core-shell structures between peptide nanowires (PNWs) and polyaniline (PANI) was also reported (Ryu e Park, 2009). Vertically oriented nanowires were formed by using the solid-vapor method. The nanowires were submitted to chemical modification using a polymerizing solution of ammonium persulfate (APS) containing aniline and HCl (1M) to generate the PANI shell along the sidewall of the PNWs. The SEM and scanning transmission electron microscopy (STEM) images in Fig. 7 show the presence of PANI on the nanowires. PNWs core was removed with 1,1,1,3,3,3-hexafluoride-2-propanol (HFIP). This material cam be applied as a biosensor in the detection of volatile organic compounds, glucose and hydrogen peroxide.

4. Peptide nanomaterials in biosensors

Since the Clark electrode (Clark, Wolf *et al.*, 1953), a remarkable progress has been made on the development of biosensors for clinical analyses (Yoo e Lee, 2010). A biosensor is an integrated receptor-transducer device, which is capable of providing selective quantitative or semi-quantitative analytical information using a biological recognition element (Thevenot, Toth *et al.*, 1999). This chapter will emphasize the use of peptide nanomaterials on development of electrochemical, optical and piezoelectric biosensors.

4.1 Electrochemical biosensors

Electrochemical biosensors are currently among the most popular of several types of biosensors. Particularly, carbon nanotubes (CNTs) are excellent materials for the development of biosensors (Wang e Lin, 2008), since they exhibit properties which improve the electron transfer reaction and increase the electrochemical reactivity of enzymatic products. However, CNTs are often produced using expensive techniques such as chemical vapor deposition (CVD). Such instruments usually need large-scale consumption and higher production costs. Recently, the use of peptides has attracted the attention of material science researchers. This is attributed to the biocompatibility and molecular recognition of peptides with other (bio)molecules or cells, resulting in many novel polymer-peptide hybrid molecules as surface modifiers for implants or tissue engineering applications (De La Rica e Matsui, 2010).

Electrochemical methods of analysis were first applied to peptide nanotubes by Yemini et al. In 2005. Cyclic voltammetry measurements revealed the presence of well-defined, reversible anodic and cathodic peaks indicated improved electrochemical reactivity for the potassium hexacyanoferrate with $^{+}NH_3$-Phe-Phe-COO^{-} nanotube-modified electrode. The effect of the nanotube deposition on the electrochemical process has also been investigated using chronoamperometric measurements by application of a potential of +200mV *vs.* Ag/AgCl under continuous stirring of the solution and successive additions of $K_4Fe(CN)_6$. In this case, the modified electrode has shown significant higher signal (about 2.5-fold increase) as compared to the nonmodified electrode. The increase of current can be attributed to the high electroactive surface area. The authors also explored the detection potential of peptide nanotube-modified electrodes for measuring hydrogen peroxide in phosphate buffer solution, using peroxidase and 4-acetaminophenol as mediators by applying a potential of -50 mV. The variation of the cathodic current corresponds to quinine (NAPQI) reduction, allowing indirect detection of hydrogen peroxide in solution (Sima, Cristea *et al.*, 2008). The current obtained by the modified $^{+}NH_3$-Phe-Phe-COO^{-} nanotubes electrode was four times higher than that obtained for the non-modified electrode, which is related to the increase of the functional electrode as previously suggested for CNT, which was evidenced by degradation of the nanostructures by proteinase-K on the electrode surface.

These nanotubes were further used in the construction of amperometric sensors for detection of β-nicotinamide adenine dinucleotide (NADH), hydrogen peroxide and ethanol in the absence of redox mediator (Yemini, Reches, Gazit *et al.*, 2005). In this case, the $^{+}NH_3$-Phe-Phe-COO^{-} nanotubes were used to modify a gold disk electrode surface by the self-assembly process, by using Traut's reagent (2-iminothiolane hydrochloride). The cyclic voltammetry of modified electrode in solution containing NADH has shown a significant increase in the sensitivity of the electrode (Fig. 8). The peptide nanotube-modified electrode responded significantly and rapidly to the changes in NADH concentration, as observed by amperometric measurement at +0.4 V, producing steady-state signals within less than 5 s.

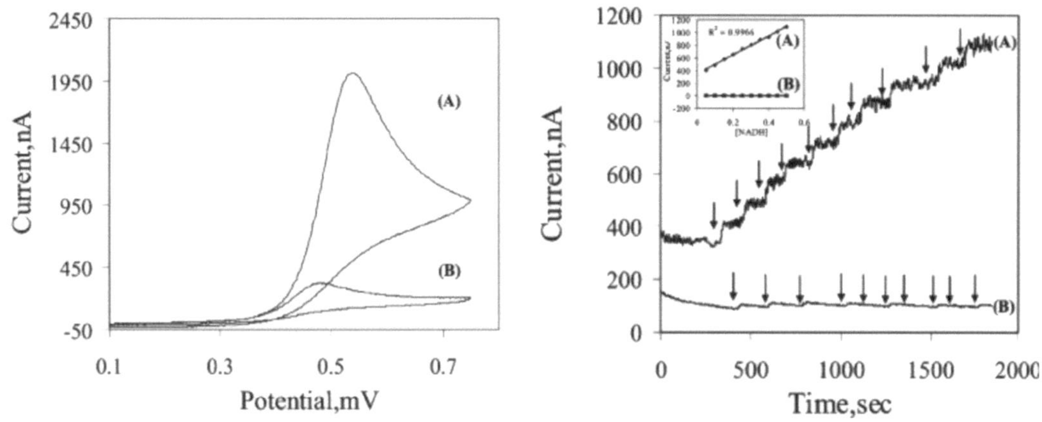

Fig. 8. Direct measurement of NADH on the peptide nanotube-based electrode. (Left) Cyclic voltammetry of (A) peptide nanotube-based electrode; (B) unmodified electrode measured in a solution containing 50 mM NADH. Scan rate, 50 mV/s. (Right) Amperometric response to successive additions of 50 µM NADH. at +0.4 V *vs.* SCE. (A) Peptide nanotube-based electrode; (B) bare electrode. Arrows indicate the addition of increasing concentrations of NADH. Reprinted with permission from Yemini, M., M. Reches, et al. (2005). "Peptide nanotube-modified electrodes for enzyme-biosensor applications." Analytical Chemistry 77(16): 5155-5159.©2005 American Chemistry Society

In developing a biosensor for glucose, Yemini and co-workers promoted the modification of the peptide nanotube-based gold electrode with glucose oxidase in presence of glutaraldehyde and PEI (polyethyleneimine). The detection mechanism is based on the determination of glucose by monitoring the hydrogen peroxide, which is produced by an enzymatic reaction between glucose oxidase, covalently linked to peptide nanotubes by glutaraldehyde on the gold electrode surface (Yemini, Reches, Gazit *et al.*, 2005). Among the applications, this biosensor can be used to detect glucose in urine and blood for the diagnosis of diabetes and also to monitor the amount of glucose during fermentation processes in food industry (Wang, 2008).

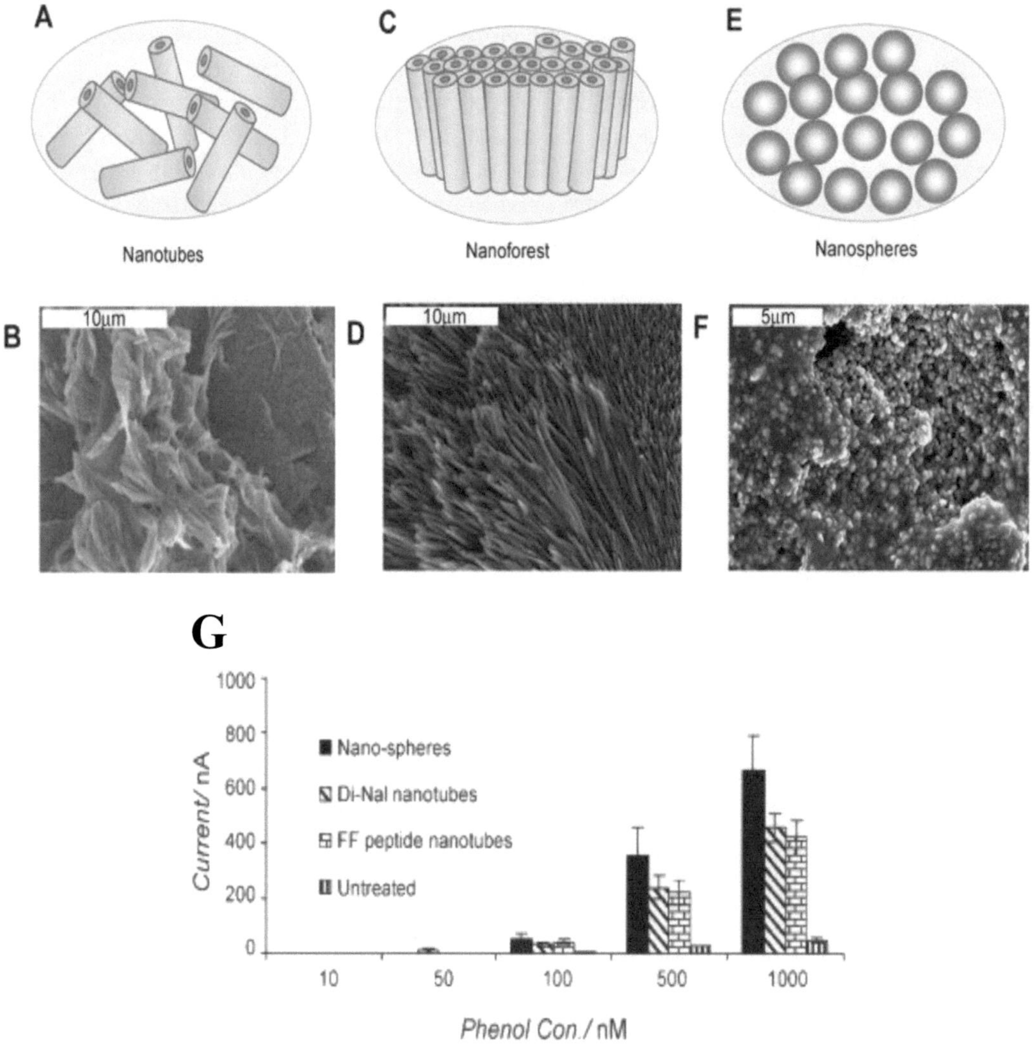

Fig. 9. Various nanoassemblies deposited on a screen-printed electrode. (a,b) $^{+}NH_3$-Nal-Nal-COO^{-} nanotubes deposited on an electrode, illustration and SEM image, respectively. (c,d) $^{+}NH_3$-Phe-Phe-COO^{-} peptide nanoforest deposited on an electrode, illustration and SEM image, respectively. (e,f) Boc-Phe-Phe-OH peptide nanospheres deposited on an electrode, illustration and SEM image, respectively. (g) Amperometric response of untreated, $^{+}NH_3$-Phe-Phe-COO^{-} nanotubes, $^{+}NH_3$-Nal-Nal-COO^{-} nanotubes, and Boc-Phe-Phe-OH peptide nanospheres on screen-printed modified electrodes to different phenol concentrations in 0.1M phosphate buffer, 0.1M KCl (pH 7.4). Measurements were performed at └ 100mV working potential versus Ag/AgC (Adler-Abramovich, Badihi-Mossberg *et al.*, 2010) Reprinted with permission from Adler-Abramovich, L., M. Badihi-Mossberg, et al. (2010). "Characterization of Peptide-Nanostructure-Modified Electrodes and Their Application for Ultrasensitive Environmental Monitoring." Small 6(7): 825-831.© 2010 Wiley-VCH Verlag GmbH & Co. KGaA, Weinheim

Recently, Adler-Abramovich and co-workers have studied the electrochemical characterization of $^{+}NH_3$-Phe-Phe-COO^- nanotubes-modified graphite electrodes and compared them to the CNT-based sensor. After that, the enzyme tyrosinase was immobilized on these nanostructure-modified electrodes for phenol detection. Various methodologies for the pattern deposition of aromatic dipeptide nanotubes and their horizontal and vertical alignment were also tested (Adler-Abramovich, Badihi-Mossberg *et al.*, 2010). For such experiment, the authors used $^{+}NH_3$-Phe-Phe-COO^- nanotubes, naphthylalanil-naphthylalanine ($^{+}NH_3$-Nal-Nal-COO^-) nanotubes, $^{+}NH_3$-Phe-Phe-COO^- nanoforests and *tert*-butoxicarbonil-Phe-Phe-OH (Boc-Phe-Phe-OH) nanospheres (Fig. 9). In this case, the tubular nanostructures have similar sensitivities, while the nanospheres show sensitivity 14 times higher compared to the untreated electrode. The electrodes modified with nanoforests showed sensitivity 17 times greater than the untreated electrode (Fig. 8). These results have been explained by the augment of the active area of the electrodes, which was confirmed by Randles-Sevcik equation. The area calculated for the bare electrode was 0.02 cm^2. After coating it with either $^{+}NH_3$-Phe-Phe-COO^- or $^{+}NH_3$-Nal-Nal-COO^- nanotubes, the surface area of the electrode was similar (0.05 cm^2). Peptide-nanosphere modification increased the surface area to 0.06 cm^2. The highest surface area, 0.07 cm2, was obtained on the electrode coated with the nanoforest. Thus, the presence of the $^{+}NH_3$-Phe-Phe-COO^- nanoforests significantly improves the sensitivity of the biosensor by increasing the surface area of the electrode and inducing electron transfer in the chemical reaction.

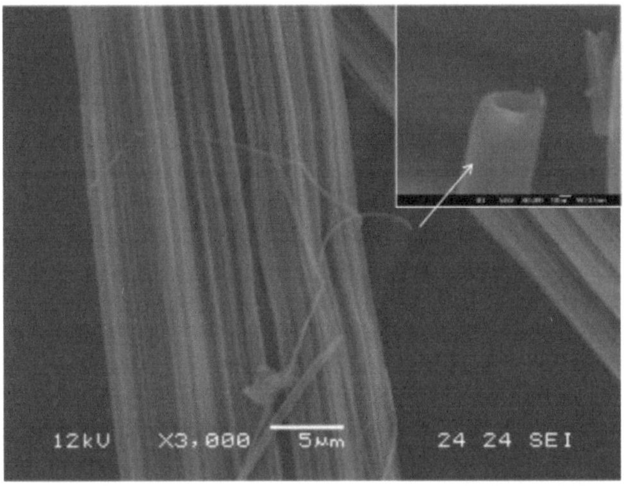

Fig. 10. SEM images showing stability of the diphenylalanine peptide nanotubes prepared in pH 7 solution containing microperoxidase-11 intercalated among the different hexagonal layers of such nanotubes. Reprinted with permission from Cipriano, T. C., P. M. Takahashi, et al. (2010). "Spatial organization of peptide nanotubes for electrochemical devices." Journal of Materials Science 45(18): 5101-5108. © Springer Science Business Media, LLC 2010

A novel biosensor for hydrogen peroxide was recently developed by combining the known properties of microperoxidase-11 (MP11) as an oxidation catalyst and the interesting properties of $^{+}NH_3$-Phe-Phe-COO^- nanotubes (PNTs) as a supporting matrix, Fig. 10, in order to allow a good bioelectrochemical interface (Cipriano, Takahashi *et al.*, 2010). In this case, the synthesized MP11/PNTs were immobilized onto the ITO electrode surface via

Layer-by-Layer (LBL) deposition, using poly(allylamine hydrochloride) (PAH) as positively charged polyelectrolyte layers. The PNTs provided a favorable microenvironment for MP11 to perform direct electron transfer to the electrode surface. The resulting electrodes showed a pair of well-defined redox peaks with formal potential at about -343 mV (*versus* SCE) in phosphate buffer solution (pH 7). The experimental results also demonstrated that the resulting biosensor exhibited good electrocatalytic activity to the reduction of H_2O_2 with a sensitivity of 9.43 μA cm^{-2} $mmol^{-1}$ L, and a detection limit of 6 μmol L^{-1} at the signal-to-noise ratio of 3. These values are expressive when compared with other procedures that involve immobilization of MP11 onto electrode surfaces that have already been reported in literature (Cipriano, Takahashi *et al.*, 2010). These values demonstrate that the PNTs can provide a bridge of electron transfer between protein and electrode. The high value obtained for the detection limit of such analyte can be related to the isolating characteristic of this material, due to wide semiconductor-like band gaps when compared to other semiconductor-like organic molecules. Moreover, we also observed that the peptides self-assembly can be influenced during the change of the pH of the solution. The study proved that the combination of PNTs with MP11 is able to open new opportunities for the design of enzymatic biosensors with potential applications in practice.

Yang and co-workers have proposed a novel approach using ionic-complementary peptides (EAK16-II) to modify a highly ordered pyrolytic graphite electrode and enhance its compatibility with enzymes for biosensor applications. The GOx was covalently immobilized on the peptide nanofiber matrix through amide bond formation between the amine groups on GOx and the carboxylate groups of glutamic acid residues on the peptide. Its catalytic activity for glucose oxidation is measured using ferrocenecarboxylic acid (FCA) as a mediator for electron transduction. The sensitivity was found to be 26 nA $mmol^{-1}L$ mm^{-2}, which is more than 6 times higher than that obtained with GOx on thiol-modified gold nanotubes and gold electrodes (~4 nA $mmol^{-1}L$ mm^{-2}) (Yang, Fung *et al.*, 2009). More recently, metalized peptide nanowires have been employed as conduits for electronic signals between a redox enzyme (NADH peroxidase) and a carbon-nanotube electrode to enhance detection sensitivity (Yeh, Lazareck *et al.*, 2007).

Another application of peptide nanotubes involves the fabrication of electrochemical immunosensors. In this case, the cyclic peptide (cyclo[(Gln-D-Leu)$_4$]) was used for the formation of nanotubes, which was later immobilized onto a substrate of carbon paste (Cho, Choi *et al.*, 2008). After that, the immobilization of antibody anti-*E. coli* O157:H7 was carried out onto the surface of the tubes. This immobilization is possible due to the bond formed between the carboxylic group present in the surface of the nanotubes and the amine groups present in the enzyme structure. This immobilization was confirmed by fluorescence microscopy images, showing the functionalization of the surface with the antibody. The antigen-antibody interaction onto the surface of the electrode modified with nanotubes was confirmed by SEM (Fig. 11) and electrochemical studies, indicating potential applications in the development of electrochemical immunosensors for detection of pathologies such as *E. coli*.

De la Rica and co-workers reported a significant improvement in the electrochemical behavior of pathogen sensors using peptide nanotubes for sensor-chip fabrication. In this work, bola-amphiphilic peptide monomers self-assembly to form peptide nanotubes and then, they were coated by antibodies in a simple incubation process (De La Rica, Mendoza *et al.*, 2008). Pathogen detection is achieved due to the difference in the dielectric properties of viral particles and water molecules. Hence, binding viruses to the peptide nanotubes decreases the permittivity of the medium surrounding the nanotube and, consequently, decreases the capacitance between electrodes. In this device configuration, the major role of the nanotubes is to concentrate targeted viruses selectively by molecular recognition at this location. At this position, impedimetric detection with the electrodes is most sensitive (De La Rica, Mendoza *et al.*, 2008).

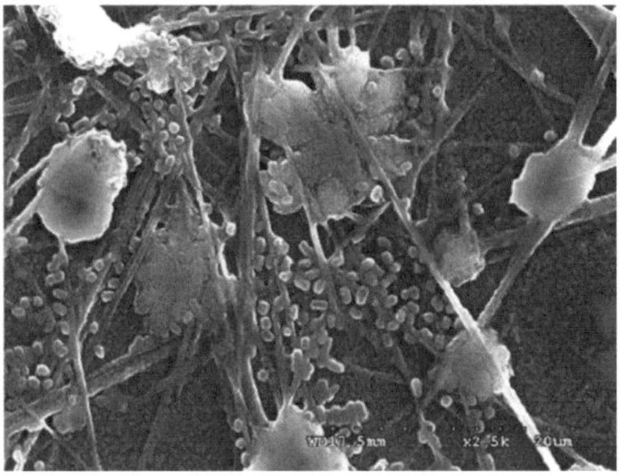

Fig. 11. SEM Image of attaching *E. coli* O157:H7 cells on the surface of peptide nanotubes by antigen–antibody interaction. Reprinted with permission from Cho, E. C., J. W. Choi, et al. (2008). "Fabrication of an electrochemical immunosensor with self-assembled peptide nanotubes." Colloids and Surfaces a-Physicochemical and Engineering Aspects 313: 95-99 © 2007 Elsevier B.V.

In another approach, membranes for dynamic sensors of ions were obtain throught the self-assembled nanotubes vertically aligned under the substrate. Motesharei et al. verified that peptide nanotubes provide channels for ion selection due to their hydrophobic character and the possibility of orientation during immobilization on the gold substrate through thiol monolayers (Motesharei Ghadiri, 1997). These channels were obtained from peptide nanotubes synthesized using D-Leu and L-Trp aminoacids (Hartgerink, Granja *et al.*, 1996). The immobilization of nanotubes onto gold substrate was oriented by thiol monolayers in two methodologies. The first methodology consisted of immersing gold substrate in an ethanolic solution containing either 1-dodecanethiol or dodecyl sulfide for 12 hours. After the formation of the monolayer, the electrode was washed with ethanol, dried in N_2 gas and immersed in an ethanolic solution (0.1 mmol L^{-1}) of cyclic peptide for 12 hours. In the second methodology the gold substrate was immersed in an ethanolic solution composed of 10 mmol L^{-1} of 1-dodecanethiol or dodecyl sulfide and cyclic peptide (0.1 mmol L^{-1}) during 12 hours. After the formation of the monolayer, the electrode was washed using ethanol, and dried in Ar.
The orientation of self-assembled cyclic peptides was verified by grazing angle FTIR spectroscopy through the band absorption of amide group compared to the band related to the N-H stretching. Such comparison is justified based on the attenuation of the stretching N-H bond caused by the presence of gold onto the horizontally-oriented nanotube.
FTIR analysis showed that both substrates modified by methodology 1, using thiol and thioether, presented greater amount of peptide tubular structures perpendicular to substrate due high intensity in peak at 1635 cm^{-1}, attributed to amine groups. The lower intense peaks

at 1686 cm^{-1} and 1549 cm^{-1} were assigned to amine groups parallel to substrate. Substrate treated by methodology 2 exhibits parallel and perpendicular alignment to substrate. Orientation mixture occurred due adsorption competition between thiol and tubular structure onto surface of gold. Therefore, the stability obtained on thiol allowed the alignment of structures. The application for ion selective channel of peptide layers was verified by cyclic voltammetry, employing three electroactive species: $[Fe(CN)_6]^{3-}$, $[Ru(NH_3)_6]^{3+}$ and $[Mo(CN)_8]^{4-}$. The electrodes prepared by methodology 2 presented good activity for less electroactive species: $[Fe(CN)_6]^{3-}$ and $[Ru(NH_3)_6]^{3+}$.

4.2 Optical sensors

Optical biosensing techniques have been widely developed because of their potential applications in a number of fields such as health care, food industry, environment monitoring and protection and in the nanotechnology field. Many are the approaches that use optical biosensor investigation techniques such as colorimetric absorbance biosensors (Song, Cheng *et al.*, 2002), which are also commercially available and conjugated polymer-based biosensors (Wang, Wang *et al.*, 2000).
Among the large variety of transducing principles that have been developed, as those mentioned in section 4.1, fluorescence-based detection has attracted the scientific community attention.

4.2.1 Fluorescence-based biosensors

Due to a number of advantages that includes high sensitivity, non-destructive characteristics of most techniques of measurements, simplicity of sensor construction and diversity of fluorescence parameters that can provide sensing properties, in this decade, fluorescence-based biosensors have been greatly exploited and developed. Their function is based on the evaluation of the optical response disturbs of a well-know fluorophore attached to or doped into the system, caused by its interaction with local constituents of the system. In the simplest sensor, the fluorophore shows binding affinity for a particular target in the system, but sometimes, more than one fluorophore incorporated at distinct locations are used in the sensor construction. (Marvin, Corcoran *et al.*, 1997) In any case, the use of fluorescent properties to sensing applications is general and versatile, but there are some requirements for the construction of the fluorescent recognition unit, such as the fluorophore structure and its photophysical mechanisms of response and the fluorescence parameters that will be determinant in detection, since in sensing applications, detection is based on a variation in fluorescence properties of a molecular recognition unit that occurs when it interacts with the target to be detected (Mcfarland e Finney, 2001).
A very interesting advantage of the use of fluorescence response on biosensor is that sensing can be achieved by using associated transduction strategies (Altschuh, Oncul *et al.*, 2006). It is well known that fluorescence properties of any dye, enclosed in an environment to which it can interact, are altered in response to those interactions (Birks, 1970; Lakowicz, 1999). Therefore, fluorescent dyes, or fluorophores, are said to be environmentally sensitive and thus, they can provide signal transduction. In the cases in which it is possible to have the fluorophore coupled to a certain region of a receptor near its binding site which can suffer a conformational change upon ligand approximation, its environment and thus its fluorescence properties change on complex formation (De Lorimier, Smith *et al.*, 2002) leading to an optical response that is related to the identity of the ligand or to the nature of

interactions and to the quantity of such ligand. These characteristics make fluorescence the most sensitive of all existing methods to detect intermolecular interaction (Lakowicz, 1999; Valeur) and, along with its characteristics of being inexpensive and easy to implement, it becomes a very attractive method to be used on sensors construction.

Therefore, materials for biosensors can be chosen based on the nature of the target, the interaction that might occur between it and a specific class of fluorophore and a photophysical process that leads to an easy-of-measure optical effect. Thus, biosensors can concentrate on evaluating the effect of interaction on steady-state fluorescence intensity, fluorescence lifetime, spectral shifts, fluorescence anisotropy and mechanisms of radioactive energy transfer such as FRET (Fluorescence Resonance Energy Transfer). (Lakowicz, 1999)

So forth, many features of fluorescent responses can be used to identify and quantitatively determine species into any environment. Even indirect optical effects are important, as in the case of the Zn(II) sensor developed by Godwin et al (Godwin e Berg, 1996), in which the FRET process informs about the quantity of Zn(II) in cells at the moment this metal binds to Zinc finger peptides. Since zinc finger peptides tightly and selectively bind zinc, with a K_d of 5.7 (+1.3) x 10^{-12} mol L^{-1} at pH 7.0 (Krizek, Merkle *et al.*, 1993), they provide an ideal proposal for a selective zinc probe. These studies showed that the activity of this fluorophore is based on changes in fluorescence energy transfer due to the metal-induced changing in conformation of this peptide.

Another approach is sensing based on fluorescence quenching. The biosensor proposed by Sharma et al. (Sharma e Gohil, 2010) is based on the evaluation of fluorescence quenching upon intermolecular interactions between a fluorescent marker and ferric ions present in the azotobactin secreted by the nitrogen-fixing bacteria Azotobacter vinelandii. The resulting fluorescence quenching is dependent on the high affinity of the fluorophore by Fe(III) ions and can be used to quantitatively determine Fe(III) in several biological media, including human serum.

Several peptides present the ability of self-assembly to form nanostructures that have found a number of interesting applications. Among them is their use as support matrix for the construction of biosensors. A common way to prepare them is to employ a fluorescent compound such as quantum dots and enzymes as receptors physically adhered to these nanostructures, as those developed by Cao et al., (Cao, Ye *et al.*, 2008) or using free enzymes and colloidal quantum dots dissolved in an aqueous solution as those developed by Costa-Fernandez et al (Costa-Fernandez, Pereiro *et al.*, 2006).

Some had aimed at the development of supports that can efficiently incorporate bioreceptors and fluorescent interacting compounds, which is the critical step for the development of biosensors and bioelectronic devices. Fabrication of enzyme-based sensors, for example, involves the incorporation of bioreceptors and quantum dots within a gel matrix. In the peptide hydrogel-based biosensor developed by Kim et al, (Kim, Lim *et al.*, 2011), which consists of a biosensing platform using encapsulation of enzyme bioreceptors and quantum dots as fluorescent markers, enzymes and quantum dots were physically immobilized within the peptide hydrogel and the resulting matrix presented some practical advantages such as simplicity of fabrication, based on the peptide property of self-assembly, very efficient diffusion of target analytes through the hydrogel and efficient encapsulation of fluorescent markers and bioreceptors. A scheme of the trapping of quantum dots into the self-assembled hydrogel as proposed by Kim et al. is shown in Fig. 12. The aim of this work was to provide an advanced sensor format and, perhaps, a protective carrier for bioreceptors. Based also on the self-assembly ability of peptides, Martins et al (Martins *et al.*,

2011 in press)showed that fluorophores such as pyrene derivatives can be sorbed onto nanostructured peptides with no effect on nanostructure formation process and depending on preparative environment, such as, preparation on distinct pH ranges, these fluorophores can be sorbed on the surface of nanostructures or intercalate to the π-stacked nanostructure, which are properties that can be exploited aiming at the delivery of components and sensor construction. This work also demonstrated that pyrene fluorescent response is dependent on the interaction with the environment in which nanostructures are found. Another approach that has been used by a number of authors (Sackmann, 1996; Kung, Kam *et al.*, 2000; Merzlyakov, Li *et al.*, 2006) is the development of supporting matrices based on bilayer lipid membranes in which the sensing property is based on monitoring changes in the electrical properties of the bilayer (Terrettaz, Ulrich *et al.*, 2001; Worsfold, Toma *et al.*, 2004). These methods present the important advantage of enabling the monitoring of single ion channel events, as shown by Cheng et al. (Cheng, Bushby *et al.*, 2001). Nevertheless, not much is known about the stability of these systems and this is a matter of concern, since earlier studies (Song e Swanson, 1999) showed that bilayers applied as matrices for optical sensors are unstable when directly attached to glass substrates for optical waveguide applications (Kelly, Grace *et al.*, 1999; Song, Shi *et al.*, 2000). A way to reduce the damaging effects of the substrate on the stability of the lipid bilayer is to use layers based on a protein linker that act as spacer layers between the substrate and the resultant bilayer, as proposed by Worsfold et al.

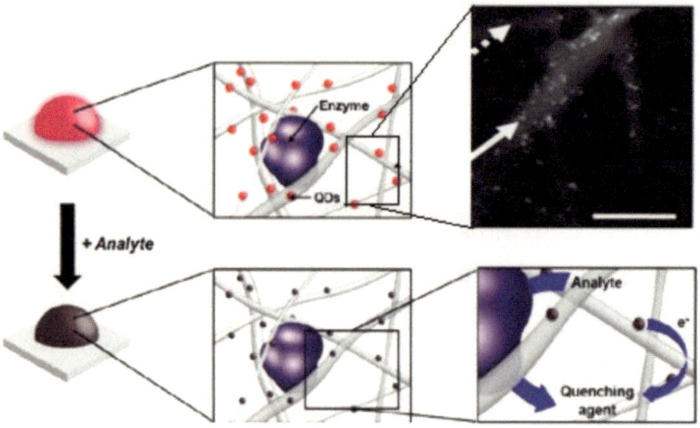

Fig. 12. Scheme of the development of a photoluminescent peptide hydrogel through the self-assembly of FmocFF building blocks and their PL quenching associated with the enzymatic detection of analytes, as shown by Kim et al. In this figure, the high photoluminescent efficiency of quantum dots on the peptide hydrogel is shown. Upon addition of analytes, a quenching agent (i.e., electron acceptor) is produced by an enzyme catalyzed reaction, which results in a decrease of luminescence of the peptide hydrogel, caused by the action of the quenching agent that absorbs the electrons of the quantum dots that were excited. The HAADF STEM image shows the nanostructure of the FmocFF hydrogel containing quantum dots. Solid and dotted arrows indicate the CdTe quantum dots and peptide nanofibers, respectively. Figure adapted from Kim et al. Reprinted with permission from Kim, J. H., S. Y. Lim, et al. (2011). "Self-assembled, photoluminescent peptide hydrogel as a versatile platform for enzyme-based optical biosensors." Biosensors and Bioelectronics 26(5): 1860-1865. © 2010 Elsevier B.V.

Fluorescence anisotropy can be used as a sensing technique due to its capability of providing a response to target binding by recording the change of rotational mobility of the fluorescent marker. Anisotropy is based on the fact that the free fluorescent sensor molecule rotates rapidly and displays a low value of anisotropy. When attached to a target, a complex of a bigger size of rotating unit is formed, leading to an anisotropy increase. This principle is employed, for example, in homogeneous fluorescence polarization immunoassay for detection of antigens or antibodies (Nielsen, Lin *et al.*, 2000), where either the antigen or the antibody can be detected in solution with the labeled fluorescent probe. The fluorescence anisotropy increases due to an increase in the size of the complex formed between the analyte and the fluorophore. Using this same principle, fluorescence polarization can also inform about the affinity of the antigen–antibody interaction (Smallshaw, Brokx *et al.*, 1998).

Fluorescence lifetime decay is also a property that can be useful in sensing activities. Based on the concept that fluorescence lifetime is representative of the interaction between a fluorophore and the environment that contains it, (Lakowicz, 1999) sensing is achieved when the difference in fluorescence lifetimes between a target-free and a target-bound forms of a sensor can be detected. The sensor constructed by Khan et al. (Khan, Saxl *et al.*, 2010) is an example. It works based on the synthesis of mutants of a glucose/galactose-binding protein (GBP), labeled with the fluorophore Badan, in order to produce a fluorescence-based glucose sensing system with an operating range compatible with continuous glucose monitoring in patients with diabetes mellitus. Results presented showed that the triple mutant H152C/A213R/L238S-Badan gave total enhance on fluorescence intensity of nearly 200% on the addition of glucose, with a binding constant, K_d =11 mM, and operating range of 1 to 100 mM, with similar responses in both buffer and serum. An enhancement on fluorescence lifetime of this mutant of 70% was also reported and the GBP mutant H152C/A213R/L238S, when labeled with Badan, showed to be suitable as a sensor of glucose monitoring in diabetes.

Another example is the sensor developed by Massey and Krull (Massey e Krull, 2010) in which the fluorescent properties of a thiazole derivative was studied for the development of a structure with application at solid-phase analyses, when immobilized. The structure, prepared by self-assembly, is capable of detection of nucleic acid hybridization. The proposal uses Neutravidin as a templating platform and combines a biotinylated probe oligonucleotide with thiazole orange as a physically immobilized intercalating dye. It works based on the assumption that intercalating fluorophores exhibits different binding affinities to single-stranded DNA (ssDNA) and double-stranded DNA (dsDNA), which provides fluorescence intensity and lifetime changes in different environments that are able to distinguish between intercalation and other binding events. In special, thiazole orange is capable of undergoing significant fluorescence enhancement upon intercalation into dsDNA. This work presented some noteworthy results. Solution-phase fluorescence lifetime data showed a biexponential behavior for sensors, suggesting intercalation as well as a significant secondary binding mode for the immobilized thiazole orange. They also found that the secondary binding mechanism for the fluorophore to DNA could be decreased, and the fluorophore could be shifted to intercalative binding modes, by simply adjusting the solution conditions, namely, by adjusting environment ionic force. This leads to a remarkable fivefold fluorescence intensity increase.

Collisional dynamic quenching produces a substantial change in lifetime. In this way, best results in lifetime sensing are obtained when determining targets that contain strong collisional quenchers of fluorescence, such as oxygen, sulfur dioxide or nitrogen oxide (Szmacinski H, 1994). Again, the disadvantage of this method is the difficulty in choosing the ideal fluorophore, since binding characteristics and optical response can vary tremendously from one molecular structure to another.

Another approach of fluorescence-based sensing is to take advantage of several fluorescence effects that occur when two dyes are put together. In this sense, the formation of a complex of two molecules, in which one of them is in its excited state, named excimer, is the property exploited in sensor construction. Its function is based on the fact that in one of the sensor states, when with bound or unbound target molecules, the two fluorophore molecules are close to each other but distant enough to form an excimer upon excitation, while in the other state they move apart and excimers are not observed. This was the idea of Yang et al. in the construction of sensors for cations (Yang, Lin *et al.*, 2001; Liao, Chen *et al.*, 2002) when constructing a sensor for anions. Furthermore, since pyrene is a fluorophore that can easily form excimers, it has been used for the construction of sensors for DNA detection, as described by Mahara et al. (Mahara, Iwase *et al.*, 2002) as it needs the formation of pyrene-conjugated oligonucleotides where excimers can occur or in sensor for protein-protein recognition, as described by Sahoo et al. (Sahoo, Narayanaswami *et al.*, 2000) Martins et al. (Martins et al., 2011 in press) showed that peptide nanostructures containing pyrene derivatives sorbed onto them can sense distinct environments, with effect on fluorescence lifetimes, even when excimer are not formed.

According to several authors, the challenge of developing these types of sensors is in the proposal of an all-serving-sensor. This has been very important because the number of systems that can be used for constructing fluorescence sensors is enormous and the focus of new research has been on enhancing fluorescence response of sensors for specific uses, in order to provide even more sensitive sensors than the search for materials to construct a single sensor that could be used in a large variety of systems.

4.3 Piezoelectric biosensors

Piezoelectricity is the crystal property to generate voltage in response to external vibration. This effect is reversible and, thus, all piezoelectric crystals vibrate in the presence of an electric field. The frequency (f) of this vibration depends on the thickness of the crystal, although it constitutes a characteristic of each crystal. This characteristic frequency changes when the crystal molecules are adsorb onto a surface. The relation between the mass transport on the surface of the piezoelectric crystal and the transduced signal is given by:

$$\Delta f = \frac{K_p f^2 \Delta m}{A}$$

where, Δf is the characteristic frequency variation, Δm is the mass change of the adsorbed material, K_p is a constant of the crystal and A is the surface area adsorbed.

As the frequency variation is proportional to the mass variation of the adsorbed material, such variation can be determined by impedance. Therefore, these biosensors contains enzymes immobilized on the piezoelectric crystals that act as transducers of the electrical signal produced at the interface. An example is a transducer to detect formaldehyde, which is formed by dehydrogenase immobilized on a quartz crystal (Kumar, 2000).

The main drawbacks of piezoelectric biosensors are the interference of atmospheric moisture on measure and the fact that they cannot be used to determine analytes in solution (Guilbault, 1991). However, piezoelectric biosensors are relatively cheap, small and produce fast responses. (Barnes, Dsilva *et al.*, 1991)
The piezoelectric materials most today are inorganic, such as $PB(Zr,Ti)O_3$. (Kobayashi, Okada *et al.*, 2010). However, these materials can only be obtained at high temperatures (~600 °C), are sensitive to defects and are not biocompatible. The evidenced piezoelectric effect in nanotubes made them useful in biological systems. Kholkin and co-workers reported that the $^{+}NH_3$-Phe-Phe-COO^{-} nanotube nanotube belongs to the $P6_1$ asymmetric group, which confer it the piezoelectricity (Kholkin, Amdursky *et al.*, 2010). AFM images were performed while a voltage V_{ac} was applied. Under these conditions, variation of the shear component of the tensor (d_{15}) was observed, suggesting a component of polarization along the axis of nanotube (Kobayashi, Okada *et al.*, 2010). These results corroborate with peptide nanotubes profiles obtained by electrostatic force microscopy (Clausen, Jensen *et al.*, 2008).
Direct quantification of the piezoelectric effect in peptide nanotubes proves tricky due to tubular geometry. However, indirect calculations showed that the coefficient d_{15} in peptide nanotubes. with ~100 nm diameter is twice lower than that observed for the bulk of $LiNbO_3$, (Smith e Welsh, 1971), ie $d_{15} \approx 35$ pm.V^{-1} (Kobayashi, Okada *et al.*, 2010). The intense piezoelectric effect observed in peptide nanotubes makes these materials promising candidates for generating "green nanopiezoelectricity", allowing the construction of biosensors that operate in direct contact with living tissues.

4.4 Implantable nanostructured biosensors

Implantable biosensors are of great impact in nanobiomedicine. However the achievement of ideal devices is not trivial and depends on factors such as biocompatibility, long-term stability, selectivity, reproducibility and miniaturization (Sadik, Aluoch *et al.*, 2009). Nanobiosensors must exhibit dimensions of elementary biomolecules (~1000 nm) such as enzymes, proteins and DNA, and are promising in the monitoring of various physical and biochemical parameters such as body temperature, oxygen and blood glucose leves (Hiller, Kranz *et al.*, 1996; Fiorito e De Torresi, 2001; Kros, Van Hovell *et al.*, 2001) (Choi, Han *et al.*, 2007). Among the applications, implantable biosensors are applied on DNA testing and pregnancy monitoring (Erdem, Karadeniz *et al.*, 2009). Implantable biosensors with continuous fluorescence for application in remote sensing of individuals (Ellis-Behnke, Liang *et al.*, 2006) have also been investigated.
Among the various materials used in the fabrication of implantable biosensors, the biocompatibility in devices based on bio-functionalized CNTs has attracted the attention of some scientists (Li, Chen *et al.*, 2006), nevertheless, the use of CNTs as implantable biosensors is questionable, since the isolated CNTs tend to cluster, increasing its cytotoxicity. (Cui, Tian *et al.*, 2005) The functionalization of carbon nanotubes with peptides has been investigated to increase its biocompatibility and solubility (Pantarotto, Partidos *et al.*, 2003; Li, Chen *et al.*, 2006). Biocompatibility of biosensors is achieved by enabling interactions between the device and the biological system.
Fabrication of implantable biosensors is subjected to several factors such as bioadaptability (biological adaptation of the physiological environment to implanted material), biostability

(absence of host immune reaction after implantation), interfacial biocompatibility (release of substance), physical analysis and morphological and mechanical properties. The biocompatibility is attributed according to the response type and the region in which the device is implanted. Thus, the biosensors are classified as bioinerts if no implant-tissue interaction; biodegradable if gradual degradation occurs on biological action, bioabsorbable, if incorporation of the implant by host tissue occurs and bioactive, if formation of new tissue at the implant-tissue interfaces occurs.
The advantages of biosensors based on peptide nanotubes are solubility in water and they can be functionalized depending on the application of interest.

5. Acknowledgment

UFABC, FAPESP, CNPq, Capes, INCT in Bioanalytics.

6. References

Adler-Abramovich, L., D. Aronov, *et al.* Self-assembled arrays of peptide nanotubes by vapour deposition. Nature Nanotechnology, v.4, n.12, Dec, p.849-854. 2009.

Adler-Abramovich, L., M. Badihi-Mossberg, *et al.* Characterization of Peptide-Nanostructure-Modified Electrodes and Their Application for Ultrasensitive Environmental Monitoring. Small, v.6, n.7, Apr 9, p.825-831. 2010.

Adler-Abramovich, L., M. Reches, *et al.* Thermal and chemical stability of diphenylalanine peptide nanotubes: Implications for nanotechnological applications. Langmuir, v.22, n.3, Jan 31, p.1313-1320. 2006.

Aizenberg, J. & P. Fratzl. Biological and Biomimetic Materials. Advanced Materials, v.21, n.4, Jan 26, p.387-388. 2009.

Altschuh, D., S. Oncul, *et al.* Fluorescence sensing of intermolecular interactions and development of direct molecular biosensors. Journal of Molecular Recognition, v.19, n.6, Nov-Dec, p.459-477. 2006.

Banerjee, I. A., G. Muniz, *et al.* Mineralization of semiconductor nanocrystals on peptide-coated bionanotubes and their pH-dependent morphology changes. Journal of Nanoscience and Nanotechnology, v.7, n.7, Jul, p.2287-2292. 2007.

Banerjee, I. A., L. T. Yu, *et al.* Thiolated peptide nanotube assembly as arrays on patterned Au substrates. Nano Letters, v.4, n.12, Dec, p.2437-2440. 2004.

Barnes, C., C. Dsilva, *et al.* A Concanavalin a-Coated Piezoelectric Crystal Biosensor. Sensors and Actuators B-Chemical, v.3, n.4, Apr, p.295-304. 1991.

Birks, J. B. Photophysics of Aromatic Molecules (Wiley monographs in chemical physics): John Wiley & Sons Ltd 1970 (Wiley Interscience)

Brea, R. J., L. Castedo, *et al.* Large-diameter self-assembled dimers of alpha,gamma-cyclic peptides, with the nanotubular solid-state structure of cyclo-[(L-Leu-D-N-Me-gamma-Acp)(4-)] 4CHCl(2)COOH. Chemical Communications, n.31, p.3267-3269. 2007.

Cao, L. H., J. Ye, *et al.* A New Route to the Considerable Enhancement of Glucose Oxidase (GOx) Activity: The Simple Assembly of a Complex from CdTe Quantum Dots and

GOx, and Its Glucose Sensing. Chemistry-a European Journal, v.14, n.31, p.9633-9640. 2008.

Cheng, J., J. C. Zhu, *et al.* Molecular modeling investigation of adsorption of self-assembled peptide nanotube of cyclo-[(1R,3S)-gamma-Acc-D-Phe](3) in CHCl3. Chemical Physics, v.333, n.2-3, Mar 30, p.105-111. 2007.

Cheng, Y. L., R. J. Bushby, *et al.* Single ion channel sensitivity in suspended bilayers on micromachined supports. Langmuir, v.17, n.4, Feb 20, p.1240-1242. 2001.

Cho, E. C., J. W. Choi, *et al.* Fabrication of an electrochemical immunosensor with self-assembled peptide nanotubes. Colloids and Surfaces a-Physicochemical and Engineering Aspects, v.313, Feb 1, p.95-99 704. 2008.

Choi, H. N., J. H. Han, *et al.* Amperometric glucose biosensor based on glucose oxidase encapsulated in carbon nanotube-titania-nafion composite film on platinized glassy carbon electrode. Electroanalysis, v.19, n.17, Sep, p.1757-1763. 2007.

Cipriano, T. C., P. M. Takahashi, *et al.* Spatial organization of peptide nanotubes for electrochemical devices. Journal of Materials Science, v.45, n.18, Sep, p.5101-5108. 2010.

Clark, L. C., R. Wolf, *et al.* Continuous Recording of Blood Oxygen Tensions by Polarography. Journal of Applied Physiology, v.6, n.3, p.189-193. 1953.

Clausen, C. H., J. Jensen, *et al.* Qualitative Mapping of Structurally Different Dipeptide Nanotubes. Nano Letters, v.8, n.11, Nov, p.4066-4069. 2008.

Colombo, G., P. Soto, *et al.* Peptide self-assembly at the nanoscale: a challenging target for computational and experimental biotechnology. Trends in Biotechnology, v.25, n.5, May, p.211-218. 2007.

Costa-Fernandez, J. M., R. Pereiro, *et al.* The use of luminescent quantum dots for optical sensing. Trac-Trends in Analytical Chemistry, v.25, n.3, Mar, p.207-218. 2006.

Cui, D. X., F. R. Tian, *et al.* Effect of single wall carbon nanotubes on human HEK293 cells. Toxicology Letters, v.155, n.1, Jan 15, p.73-85. 2005.

De La Rica, R. & H. Matsui. Applications of peptide and protein-based materials in bionanotechnology. Chemical Society Reviews, v.39, n.9, p.3499-3509. 2010.

De La Rica, R., E. Mendoza, *et al.* Label-Free Pathogen Detection with Sensor Chips Assembled from Peptide Nanotubes. Angewandte Chemie-International Edition, v.47, n.50, p.9752-9755. 2008.

De Lorimier, R. M., J. J. Smith, *et al.* Construction of a fluorescent biosensor family. Protein Science, v.11, n.11, Nov, p.2655-2675. 2002.

De Santis, P., S. Morosetti, *et al.* Peptides with regular enantiomeric sequences: A wide class of modular self-assembling architectures. Journal of Nanoscience and Nanotechnology, v.7, n.7, Jul, p.2230-2238. 2007.

Demirel, G., N. Malvadkar, *et al.* Control of Protein Adsorption onto Core-Shell Tubular and Vesicular Structures of Diphenylalanine/Parylene. Langmuir, v.26, n.3, Feb 2, p.1460-1463. 2010.

Ellis-Behnke, R. G., Y. X. Liang, *et al.* Nano neuro knitting: Peptide nanofiber scaffold for brain repair and axon regeneration with functional return of vision. Proceedings of the National Academy of Sciences of the United States of America, v.103, n.13, Mar 28, p.5054-5059. 2006.

Erdem, A., H. Karadeniz, *et al.* Single-Walled Carbon Nanotubes Modified Graphite Electrodes for Electrochemical Monitoring of Nucleic Acids and Biomolecular Interactions. Electroanalysis, v.21, n.3-5, Feb, p.464-471. 2009.

Fiorito, P. A. & S. I. C. De Torresi. Glucose amperometric biosensor based on the co-immobilization of glucose oxidase (GOx) and ferrocene in poly(pyrrole) generated from ethanol/water mixtures. Journal of the Brazilian Chemical Society, v.12, n.6, Nov-Dec, p.729-733. 2001.

Ghadiri, M. R., J. R. Granja, *et al.* Self-Assembling Organic Nanotubes Based on a Cyclic Peptide Architecture. Nature, v.366, n.6453, Nov 25, p.324-327. 1993.

Godwin, H. A. & J. M. Berg. A fluorescent zinc probe based on metal-induced peptide folding. Journal of the American Chemical Society, v.118, n.27, Jul 10, p.6514-6515. 1996.

Guha, S. & A. Banerjee. Self-Assembled Robust Dipeptide Nanotubes and Fabrication of Dipeptide-Capped Gold Nanoparticles on the Surface of these Nanotubes. Advanced Functional Materials, v.19, n.12, Jun 23, p.1949-1961. 2009.

Guilbault, G. G. Biosensors. Current Opinion in Biotechnology, v.2, n.1, Feb, p.3-8. 1991.

Hartgerink, J. D., J. R. Granja, *et al.* Self-assembling peptide nanotubes. Journal of the American Chemical Society, v.118, n.1, Jan 10, p.43-50. 1996.

Hauser, C. A. E. & S. G. Zhang. Designer self-assembling peptide nanofiber biological materials. Chemical Society Reviews, v.39, n.8, p.2780-2790. 2010.

He, Q., L. Duan, *et al.* Microcapsules containing a biomolecular motor for ATP biosynthesis. Advanced Materials, v.20, n.15, Aug 4, p.2933-2937. 2008.

Hiller, M., C. Kranz, *et al.* Amperometric biosensors produced by immobilization of redox enzymes at polythiophene-modified electrode surfaces. Advanced Materials, v.8, n.3, Mar, p.219-&. 1996.

Hirata, T., F. Fujimura, *et al.* A novel polypseudorotaxane composed of cyclic beta-peptide as bead component. Chemical Communications, n.10, p.1023-1025. 2007.

Kelly, D., K. M. Grace, *et al.* Integrated optical biosensor for detection of multivalent proteins. Optics Letters, v.24, n.23, Dec 1, p.1723-1725. 1999.

Khan, F., T. E. Saxl, *et al.* Fluorescence intensity- and lifetime-based glucose sensing using an engineered high-K-d mutant of glucose/galactose-binding protein. Analytical Biochemistry, v.399, n.1, Apr 1, p.39-43. 2010.

Kholkin, A., N. Amdursky, *et al.* Strong Piezoelectricity in Bioinspired Peptide Nanotubes. Acs Nano, v.4, n.2, Feb, p.610-614. 2010.

Kim, J., T. H. Han, *et al.* Role of Water in Directing Diphenylalanine Assembly into Nanotubes and Nanowires. Advanced Materials, v.22, n.5, Feb 2, p.583-+. 2010.

Kim, J. H., S. Y. Lim, *et al.* Self-assembled, photoluminescent peptide hydrogel as a versatile platform for enzyme-based optical biosensors. Biosensors and Bioelectronics, v.26, n.5, p.1860-1865. 2011.

Kobayashi, T., H. Okada, *et al.* A digital output piezoelectric accelerometer using a Pb(Zr, Ti)O-3 thin film array electrically connected in series. Smart Materials & Structures, v.19, n.10, Oct, p.-. 2010.

Krizek, B. A., D. L. Merkle, *et al.* Ligand Variation and Metal-Ion Binding-Specificity in Zinc Finger Peptides. Inorganic Chemistry, v.32, n.6, Mar 17, p.937-940. 1993.

Kros, A., W. F. M. Van Hovell, *et al.* Poly(3,4-ethylenedioxythiophene)-based glucose biosensors. Advanced Materials, v.13, n.20, Oct 16, p.1555-+. 2001.

Kumar, A. Biosensors Based on Piezoelectric Crystal Detectors: Theory and Application. JOM-e. 52 2000.

Kung, L. A., L. Kam, *et al.* Patterning hybrid surfaces of proteins and supported lipid bilayers. Langmuir, v.16, n.17, Aug 22, p.6773-6776. 2000.

Lakowicz, J. R. Principles of Fluorescence Spectroscopy: Springer. 1999. 725 pages p.

Li, X. J., W. Chen, *et al.* Direct measurements of interactions between polypeptides and carbon nanotubes. Journal of Physical Chemistry B, v.110, n.25, Jun 29, p.12621-12625. 2006.

Liao, J. H., C. T. Chen, *et al.* A novel phosphate chemosensor utilizing anion-induced fluorescence change. Organic Letters, v.4, n.4, Feb 21, p.561-564. 2002.

Lu, K., J. Jacob, *et al.* Exploiting amyloid fibril lamination for nanotube self-assembly. Journal of the American Chemical Society, v.125, n.21, May 28, p.6391-6393. 2003.

Mahara, A., R. Iwase, *et al.* Bispyrene-conjugated 2 '-O-methyloligonucleotide as a highly specific RNA-recognition probe. Angewandte Chemie-International Edition, v.41, n.19, p.3648-3650. 2002.

Marvin, J. S., E. E. Corcoran, *et al.* The rational design of allosteric interactions in a monomeric protein and its applications to the construction of biosensors. Proceedings of the National Academy of Sciences of the United States of America, v.94, n.9, Apr 29, p.4366-4371. 1997.

Massey, M. e U. J. Krull. Towards a fluorescent molecular switch for nucleic acid biosensing. Analytical and Bioanalytical Chemistry, v.398, n.4, Oct, p.1605-1614. 2010.

Mcfarland, S. A. & N. S. Finney. Fluorescent chemosensors based on conformational restriction of a biaryl fluorophore. Journal of the American Chemical Society, v.123, n.6, Feb 14, p.1260-1261. 2001.

Merzlyakov, M., E. Li, *et al.* Directed assembly of surface-supported bilayers with transmembrane helices. Langmuir, v.22, n.3, Jan 31, p.1247-1253. 2006.

Motesharei, K. e M. R. Ghadiri. Diffusion-limited size-selective ion sensing based on SAM-supported peptide nanotubes. Journal of the American Chemical Society, v.119, n.46, Nov 19, p.11306-11312. 1997.

Nielsen, K., M. Lin, *et al.* Fluorescence polarization immunoassay: Detection of antibody to Brucella abortus. Methods-a Companion to Methods in Enzymology, v.22, n.1, Sep, p.71-76. 2000.

Pantarotto, D., C. D. Partidos, *et al.* Synthesis, structural characterization, and immunological properties of carbon nanotubes functionalized with peptides. Journal of the American Chemical Society, v.125, n.20, May 21, p.6160-6164. 2003.

Poteau, R. & G. Trinquier. All-cis cyclic peptides. Journal of the American Chemical Society, v.127, n.40, Oct 12, p.13875-13889. 2005.

Reches, M. & E. Gazit. Casting metal nanowires within discrete self-assembled peptide nanotubes. Science, v.300, n.5619, Apr 25, p.625-627. 2003.

Formation of closed-cage nanostructures by self-assembly of aromatic dipeptides. Nano Letters, v.4, n.4, Apr, p.581-585. 2004.

Controlled patterning of aligned self-assembled peptide nanotubes. Nature Nanotechnology, v.1, n.3, Dec, p.195-200. 2006.

Ryu, J. & C. B. Park. High-Temperature Self-Assembly of Peptides into Vertically Well-Aligned Nanowires by Aniline Vapor. Advanced Materials, v.20, n.19, Oct 2, p.3754-+. 2008a.

Solid-phase growth of nanostructures from amorphous peptide thin film: Effect of water activity and temperature. Chemistry of Materials, v.20, n.13, Jul 8, p.4284-4290. 2008b.

Synthesis of Diphenylalanine/Polyaniline Core/Shell Conducting Nanowires by Peptide Self-Assembly. Angewandte Chemie-International Edition, v.48, n.26, p.4820-4823. 2009.

High Stability of Self-Assembled Peptide Nanowires Against Thermal, Chemical, and Proteolytic Attacks. Biotechnology and Bioengineering, v.105, n.2, Feb 1, p.221-230. 2010.

Sackmann, E. Supported membranes: Scientific and practical applications. Science, v.271, n.5245, Jan 5, p.43-48. 1996.

Sadik, O. A., A. O. Aluoch, *et al.* Status of biomolecular recognition using electrochemical techniques. Biosensors & Bioelectronics, v.24, n.9, May 15, p.2749-2765. 2009.

Sahoo, D., V. Narayanaswami, *et al.* Pyrene excimer fluorescence: A spatially sensitive probe to monitor lipid-induced helical rearrangement of apolipophorin III. Biochemistry, v.39, n.22, Jun 6, p.6594-6601. 2000.

Sanchez, C., H. Arribart, *et al.* Biomimetism and bioinspiration as tools for the design of innovative materials and systems. Nature Materials, v.4, n.4, Apr, p.277-288. 2005.

Sharma, M. & N. K. Gohil. Optical features of the fluorophore azotobactin: Applications for iron sensing in biological fluids. Engineering in Life Sciences, v.10, n.4, Aug, p.304-310. 2010.

Shklovsky, J., P. Beker, *et al.* Bioinspired peptide nanotubes: Deposition technology and physical properties. Materials Science and Engineering B-Advanced Functional Solid-State Materials, v.169, n.1-3, May 25, p.62-66. 2010.

Sima, V., C. Cristea, *et al.* Electroanalytical properties of a novel biosensor modified with zirconium alcoxide porous gels for the detection of acetaminophen. Journal of Pharmaceutical and Biomedical Analysis, v.48, n.4, Dec 1, p.1195-1200. 2008.

Singh, G., A. M. Bittner, *et al.* Electrospinning of diphenylalanine nanotubes. Advanced Materials, v.20, n.12, Jun 18, p.2332-+. 2008.

Smallshaw, J. E., S. Brokx, *et al.* Determination of the binding constants for three HPr-specific monoclonal antibodies and their fab fragments. Journal of Molecular Biology, v.280, n.5, Jul 31, p.765-774. 1998.

Smith, R. T. & F. S. Welsh. Temperature Dependence of Elastic, Piezoelectric, and Dielectric Constants of Lithium Tantalate and Lithium Niobate. Journal of Applied Physics, v.42, n.6, p.2219-&. 1971.

Song, J., Q. Cheng, *et al.* "Smart" materials for biosensing devices: Cell-mimicking supramolecular assemblies and colorimetric detection of pathogenic agents. Biomedical Microdevices, v.4, n.3, Jul, p.213-221. 2002.
Song, X. D., J. Shi, *et al.* Flow cytometry-based biosensor for detection of multivalent proteins. Analytical Biochemistry, v.284, n.1, Aug 15, p.35-41. 2000.
Song, X. D. & B. I. Swanson. Direct, ultrasensitive, and selective optical detection of protein toxins using multivalent interactions. Analytical Chemistry, v.71, n.11, Jun 1, p.2097-2107. 1999.
Song, Y. J., S. R. Challa, *et al.* Synthesis of peptide-nanotube platinum-nanoparticle composites. Chemical Communications, n.9, May 7, p.1044-1045. 2004.
Szmacinski H, L. J. Lifetime-based sensing. New York: Plenum Press, v.4. 1994 (InTopics in fluorescence spectroscopy (Vol. 4))
Terrettaz, S., W. P. Ulrich, *et al.* Immunosensing by a synthetic ligand-gated ion channel. Angewandte Chemie-International Edition, v.40, n.9, p.1740-1743. 2001.
Thevenot, D. R., K. Toth, *et al.* Electrochemical biosensors: Recommended definitions and classification - (Technical Report). Pure and Applied Chemistry, v.71, n.12, Dec, p.2333-2348. 1999.
Valeur, B. Molecular Fluorescence: Principles and Applications. New York: Wiley-VCH. 2001
Wang, J. Electrochemical glucose biosensors. Chemical Reviews, v.108, n.2, Feb, p.814-825. 2008.
Wang, J. & Y. H. Lin. Functionalized carbon nanotubes and nanofibers for biosensing applications. Trac-Trends in Analytical Chemistry, v.27, n.7, Jul-Aug, p.619-626. 2008.
Wang, J., D. L. Wang, *et al.* Photoluminescence of water-soluble conjugated polymers: Origin of enhanced quenching by charge transfer. Macromolecules, v.33, n.14, Jul 11, p.5153-5158. 2000.
Worsfold, O., C. Toma, *et al.* Development of a novel optical bionanosensor. Biosensors & Bioelectronics, v.19, n.11, Jun 15, p.1505-1511. 2004.
Yan, X. H., Y. Cui, *et al.* Organogels based on self-assembly of diphenylalanine peptide and their application to immobilize quantum dots. Chemistry of Materials, v.20, n.4, Feb 26, p.1522-1526. 2008.
Yang, H., S. Y. Fung, *et al.* Ionic-Complementary Peptide Matrix for Enzyme Immobilization and Biomolecular Sensing. Langmuir, v.25, n.14, Jul 21, p.7773-7777. 2009.
Yang, J. S., C. S. Lin, *et al.* Cu2+-induced blue shift of the pyrene excimer emission: A new signal transduction mode of pyrene probes. Organic Letters, v.3, n.6, Mar 22, p.889-892. 2001.
Yanlian, Y., K. Ulung, *et al.* Designer self-assembling peptide nanomaterials. Nano Today, v.4, n.2, p.193-210. 2009.
Yeh, J. I., A. Lazareck, *et al.* Peptide nanowires for coordination and signal transduction of peroxidase biosensors to carbon nanotube electrode arrays. Biosensors & Bioelectronics, v.23, n.4, Nov 30, p.568-574. 2007.
Yemini, M., M. Reches, *et al.* Peptide nanotube-modified electrodes for enzyme-biosensor applications. Analytical Chemistry, v.77, n.16, Aug 15, p.5155-5159. 2005. Novel

electrochemical biosensing platform using self-assembled peptide nanotubes. Nano Letters, v.5, n.1, Jan, p.183-186. 2005.

Yoo, E. H. e S. Y. Lee. Glucose Biosensors: An Overview of Use in Clinical Practice. Sensors, v.10, n.5, May, p.4558-4576. 2010.

8

Diamond as Functional Material for Bioelectronics and Biotechnology

Bohuslav Rezek[1], Marie Krátká[1], Egor Ukraintsev[1], Oleg Babchenko[1], Alexander Kromka[1], Antonín Brož[2] and Marie Kalbacova[2]
[1]*Institute of Physics, Academy of Sciences of the Czech Republic, Prague*
[2]*Institute of Inherited Metabolic Diseases, First Faculty of Medicine, Charles University and General Faculty Hospital in Prague*
Czech Republic

1. Introduction

Understanding the interaction between the biological environment (tissues, cells, proteins, electrolytes, etc.) and a solid surface is crucial for biomedical applications such as bio-sensors, bio-electronics, tissue engineering and the optimization of implant materials. Cells, the cornerstones of living tissue, perceive their surroundings and subsequently modify it by producing extracellular matrix (ECM), which serves as a basis to simplify their adhesion, spreading and differentiation (Shakenraad & Busscher, 1989). This process is considerably complex, flexible and strongly depends on the cell cultivation conditions including the type of the substrate. Surface roughness of the substrate plays an important role (Babchenko et al., 2009; Kalbacova et al., 2009; Kromka et al., 2009; Zhao et al., 2006), other influential factors include both the porosity (Tanaka et al., 2007) and the wettability of the substrate, the latter influencing protein conformation (Browne et al., 2004; Rezek, Ukraintsev, Michalíková, Kromka, Zemek & Kalbacova, 2009) as well as the adsorption and viability of cells (Grausova et al., 2009; Kalbacova, Kalbac, Dunsch, Kromka, Vanecek, Rezek, Hempel & Kmoch, 2007).
Materials which are commonly employed as substrates for in vitro testing are polystyrene and glass. In this context, diamond as a technological material can provide a relatively unique combination of excellent semiconducting, mechanical, chemical as well as biological properties (Nebel et al., 2007). Diamond also meets the basic requirements for large-scale industrial application, most notably, it can be prepared synthetically. Diamond can be synthesized either as a bulk material under high-pressure and high-temperature conditions, or in the form of thin films by chemical vapor deposition of methane and hydrogen on various substrates including glass and metal (Kromka et al., 2008; Potocky et al., 2007). Moreover, the application of selective nucleation makes it possible to directly grow conductive diamond microstructures, which operate e.g. as transistors or pH sensors (Kozak et al., 2010). Nowadays, it is possible to deposit diamond even on large areas (600 cm^2 or more) using linear antennas (Kromka et al., 2011; Tsugawa et al., 2010). The excellent compatibility of diamond with biological materials and environment (Bajaj et al., 2007; Grausova et al., 2009;

Kalbacova, Kalbac, Dunsch, Kromka, Vanecek, Rezek, Hempel & Kmoch, 2007; Tang et al., 1995) is of immense importance for its application in medicine. This bio-compatibility stems from the fact that diamond is a crystalline form of carbon that is mechanically, chemically and physically very stable. Despite the general chemical stability, diamond surface can be terminated by different atomic species (Rezek et al., 2003) and organic molecules (Rezek, Shin, Uetsuka & Nebel, 2007), which can alter diamond's natural properties and thus open the door for countless new applications.

For example, electrical conductance and electron affinity are both significantly influenced by surface termination of diamond by hydrogen or oxygen atoms (Chakrapani et al., 2007; Kawarada, 1996; Maier et al., 2001; Rezek et al., 2003; Ri et al., 1995). The main difference arises from the opposite dipoles of C–H and C–O bonds. Oxygen-terminated diamond is insulating, whereas the hydrogen-terminated surface causes the emergence of two-dimensional hole surface conductance on otherwise insulating diamond. These properties can be exploited for the fabrication of a planar field-effect transistor (FET), whose gate is formed solely by hydrogen surface atoms without the employment of any other insulating layers and which is sensitive to the pH of a solution (Dankerl et al., 2007; Nebel et al., 2006; Rezek, Shin, Watanabe & Nebel, 2007). The hydrogen-terminated diamond surface is also an ideal starting point for covalent bonding of other molecules such as DNA or proteins (Härtl et al., 2004; Rezek, Shin, Uetsuka & Nebel, 2007; Yang et al., 2002). On the other hand, the hydrogen-terminated diamond surface is generally less favorable for the adhesion, spreading and viability of cells than the oxidized surface (Kalbacova, Kalbac, Dunsch, Kromka, Vanecek, Rezek, Hempel & Kmoch, 2007). This difference is due to the hydrophillicity of oxygen-terminated diamond (O-diamond) in contrast to the hydrophobicity of the hydrogen-terminated diamond (H-diamond). As a result, the combination of both hydrogen- and oxygen-terminated diamond surface is very interesting for bio-electronics (Dankerl et al., 2009; Rezek, Krátká, Kromka & Kalbacova, 2010) as well as for tissue engineering (Kalbacova et al., 2008; Rezek, Michalíková, Ukraintsev, Kromka & Kalbacova, 2009).

In this chapter we present the influence of micro-structuring morphology and atomic termination of diamond surfaces on cell growth and assembly. We investigate the influence of key parameters such as the seeding concentration of cells, the type of the applied cells, the duration of cultivation, the concentration of fetal bovine serum (FBS) in the cultivation medium, the dimensions and shape of microstructures, and surface roughness. We show that the adsorption of proteins from the FBS serum is the key factor. Atomic force microscopy (AFM) both in solution and in air is applied in order to characterize the morphology of the FBS layers adsorbed on differently terminated diamond substrates. The influence of proteins and cells on the electronic properties of diamond is demonstrated by employing a field-effect transistor on hydrogen-terminated diamond, whose gate is exposed to a solution (SG-FET). These results are discussed from the point of view of fundamental physics and biology as well as the prospects in medicine.

2. Preparation of nanocrystalline diamond layers

The growth of thin-film nanocrystalline-diamond layers (NCD) was realized on silicon or glass substrates using microwave plasma enhanced chemical vapor deposition (MW-CVD) (Kromka et al., 2008; Potocky et al., 2007). The substrates were 10×10 mm^2 large and had

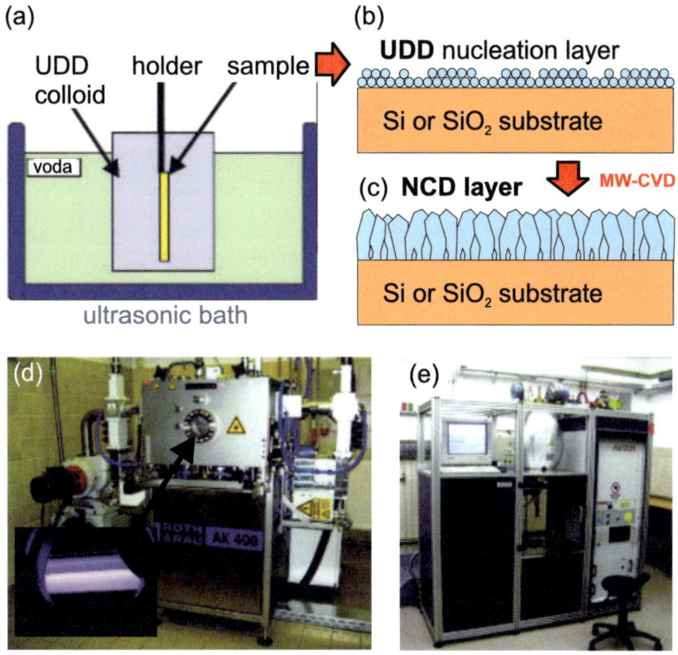

Fig. 1. Schematic depiction of the preparation procedure of thin-film diamond on glass or silicon substrates: (a) nucleation of the substrates carried out in an ultrasonic bath with ultra-dispersed diamond (UDD), (b) the resulting nucleation layer and (c) the nanocrystalline diamond layer after the microwave-plasma deposition. The deposition machines for (d) large-area growth of diamond (linear plasma) and (e) high-speed growth (focused plasma).

surface roughness < 1 nm. Before the deposition, the substrates were ultrasonically cleaned in isopropanol and deionized water and were subsequently immersed for 40 min into an ultrasonic bath with a colloidal suspension of a diamond powder (UDD – ultra-dispersed diamond; NanoAmando, New Metals and Chemicals Corp. Ltd., Kyobashi) with nominal particle size of 5 nm. This process leads to the formation of a 5- to 25-nm-thin layer of nanodiamond powder. This nucleation procedure was followed by a microwave plasma-enhanced chemical vapor deposition (MW-CVD) of diamond films. The deposition conditions were: temperature of substrates 600–800°C, 1% CH_4 in H_2, microwave power 1.4–2.5 kW, gas pressure 30–50 mbar, duration approximately 4 hours, the thickness of layers reaches 100–500 nm. The same conditions, only with methane gas switched off and process time 10 min, were used for H-termination of the diamond surface. In some cases, the nucleation and growth were repeated on the other side of the substrate, which leads to the hermetical encapsulation of the substrate by the NCD layer (Kalbacova et al., 2008; Rezek, Michalíková, Ukraintsev, Kromka & Kalbacova, 2009). The preparation procedure is schematically shown in Figure 1. This figure also depicts the photos of the set-ups for the large-area diamond growth (linear plasma) with high deposition rate (focused plasma).
NCD layer were chemically cleaned in acids (97.5% H_2SO_4 + 99% KNO_3 powder in the ratio of 4:1) at 200°C for 30 minutes. This process ensures high quality of the hydrogen-terminated surface (surface conductance in the order of 10^{-7} S/sq) (Kozak et al., 2009). The surface morphology and chemical quality of NCD layers were characterized by AFM, scanning

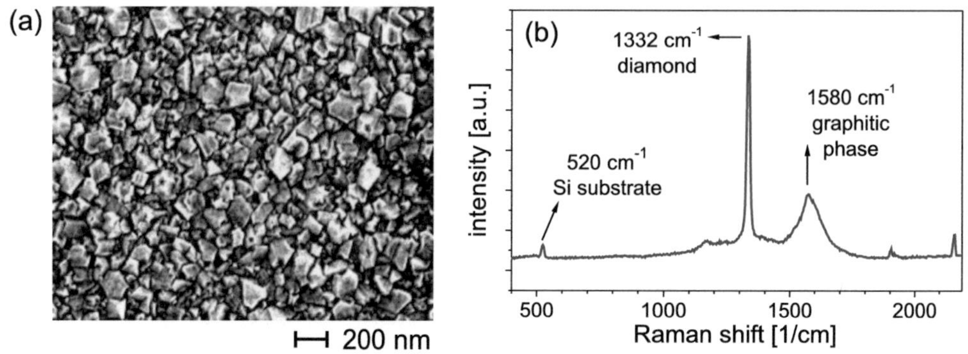

Fig. 2. Basic characteristics of a typical NCD layer on Si: (a) morphology by SEM and (b) a typical Raman-scattering spectrum.

electron microscopy (SEM) and Raman spectroscopy. Roughness evaluated in the tapping AFM regime is 15 – 30 nm rms (1×1 μm^2 area), grain size as measured by SEM is 50 – 150 nm (see Figure 2(a)). The grains exhibit clear facets that evidences their crystalline diamond form. Raman spectroscopy (excitation wavelength 325 nm) confirmed the diamond character of the layers (see Figure 2(b)). With a small alteration of the deposition conditions, grain sizes of even several hundreds of nanometers can be reached.

3. Cell growth on diamond with surface nanostructures

To produce nanostructured diamond surfaces the NCD films were first masked with: i) 5 nm diamond nanoparticles using the ultrasonic treatment in UDD colloidal suspension, ii) 30 nm nickel particles prepared by deposition of 3 nm nickel layer on diamond and its treatment in hydrogen plasma for 5 min (Babchenko et al., 2009). Subsequent etching of diamond nanostructures was performed by reactive ion etching (RIE) system (Phantom LT RIE System, Trion Technology) at about 100°C for 300 s using 2 sccm of CF_4 and 50 sscm of O_2. Remaining nickel masks were then removed by a wet etching process. Finally, the diamond surfaces were treated in r.f. oxygen plasma to obtain hydrophilic character of the surface that is suitable for cellular adhesion (Kalbacova, Kalbac, Dunsch, Kromka, Vanecek, Rezek, Hempel & Kmoch, 2007).

Scanning electron microscopy (SEM) images of the NCD films with nanoparticle masks and after the RIE process are shown in Figure 3a-b and 3e-f. Diamond nanoparticle mask resulted in a formation of isolated cone-like structures (height 5–100 nm, diameter up to 80 nm) randomly spread on the remaining NCD film. Mask made of the nickel nanoparticles resulted in a formation of upright, densely packed diamond nanorods with the height of 120–200 nm and diameter 20–40 nm. Diamond nanoparticles are obviously (and expectably) not enough resistant to the plasma etching process. Therefore, the surface exhibit lower density of cone-like structures. Nickel nanoparticles were able to withstand the whole etching period, hence the nanorods were formed.

These nanostructured diamond surfaces were used as artificial substrates for growth of human osteoblast-like cells. Human osteoblast-like cells (SAOS-2; DSMZ, Germany) were plated on the samples in 25,000 cells/cm^2 concentration and grown in the McCoy's 5A medium without phenol red (BioConcept) supplemented with 15% heat-inactivated fetal

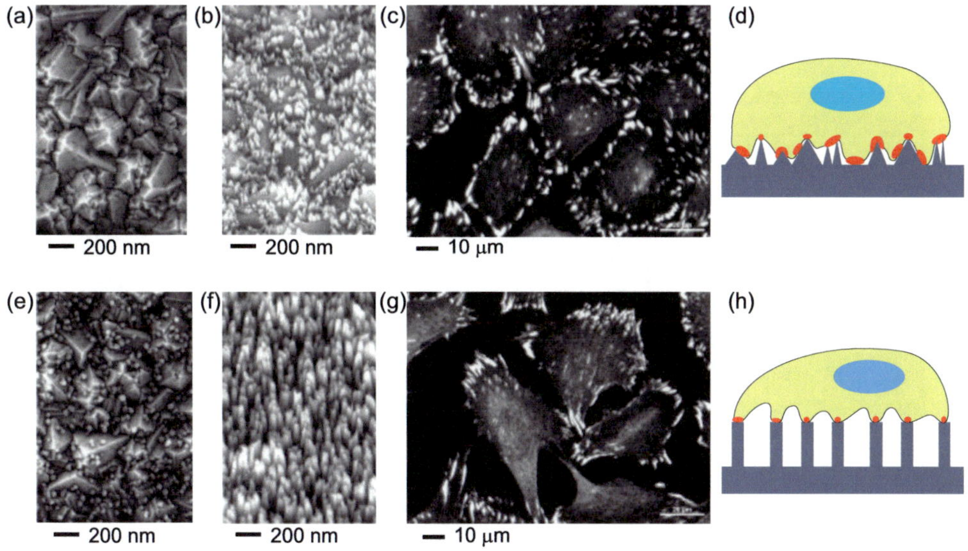

Fig. 3. Scanning electron microscopy (SEM) image of the NCD layer (a) with diamond nanoparticle mask and (b) resulting nanostructured surface (nano-cones) after plasma etching. (c) Fluorescence microscopy image of stained focal adhesions (vinculin) of osteoblast-like cells on the surface with nano-cones. (d) Schematic drawing of cellular adhesion on the nano-cones (focal adhesions – red, nucleus – blue, cytoskeleton – green). Same measurements for the case on nickel nanoparticle mask and diamond nanorods are shown in (e-h).

bovine serum (PAA), 20 U penicillin and 20 μg/ml streptomycin in a humidified 5% CO_2 atmosphere at 37°C. Resulting morphology of focal adhesions of SAOS-2 cells was characterized by immunofluorescent staining of vinculin (1:150, Sigma, anti-mouse Alexa 568) and imaging in the epi-fluorescence microscope (Nikon E-400).
The fluorescence images are shown in Figure 3c and 3g, next to the SEM images. Based on the fluorescence images, osteoblasts exhibit generally well spread fibroblast-like morphology on both substrates. During the 48h incubation the cells went through one cell cycle. This also indicates general substrate suitability. However, the size and shape of highlighted focal adhesions differ on each type of the nanostructures. Osteoblasts cultivated on relatively short and broad nano-cones form well pronounced large focal adhesions with intensive vinculin staining indicating bigger surface available for adhesion and thus stronger adhesion contacts between cell and diamond. On the other hand, cells cultivated on relatively high and thin nanorods form very thin and fine focal adhesions indicating weaker adhesion. This is schematically shown in Figure 3d and 3h. Another crucial role in cell-diamond interaction play atoms terminating the diamond surface.

4. Cell growth on diamond with atomic micro-patterns

To characterize influence of diamond surface atoms on the arrangement of cells, NCD layers with hydrogen and oxygen surface atoms forming microscopic patterns of widths from 30 to 200 µm were fabricated as follows. Positive photoresist ma-P1215 (micro resist technology GmbH, Germany) was spin-coated on the NCD surface an micro-patterned by

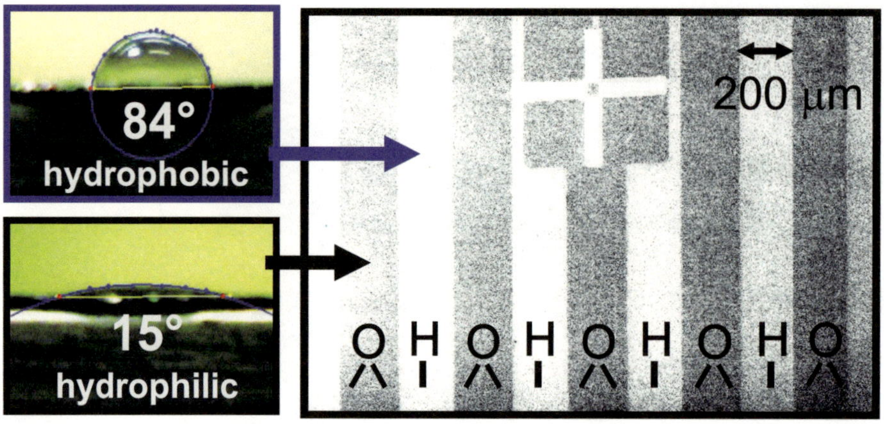

Fig. 4. SEM image of a nanocrystalline-diamond layer with 200-μm-wide stripes with alternating hydrogen and oxygen termination. Light stripes correspond to the hydrogen surface due to its low electron affinity. The cross in the upper part of the image is made up of a thin layer of gold and serves as a mark for the differentiation of particular stripes. Typical measurements of wetting angle on the two types of diamond surfaces (uniformly terminated) are shown along the left side of the SEM image.

optical lithography. Afterwards, the NCD layers were exposed with a photolithographic mask in high-frequency oxygen plasma (power 300 W, duration 3 minutes), which gives rise to the oxidation of the surface, and, consequently, to the formation of hydrophilic patterns. The wetting angle of water on oxygen-terminated diamond was $< 20^\circ$, in contrast to about 80° on the hydrogen-terminated diamond. The morphology of the surface remains unchanged during this procedure. Figure 4 shows how the microscopic stripe patterns look look like in an electron microscope (hydrogen and oxygen stripes have different SEM contrast due to different electron affinity).

Before cell plating, the NCD layers were sterilized using either UV irradiation or 70% ethanol treatment for 10 minutes. In most experiments, the cell line of human bone cells (osteoblasts – SAOS-2 cells; DSMZ GmbH) were used. The cells were plated on diamond in the concentrations ranging from 2,500 (sub-confluent coverage) to 10,000 cells/cm^2 (confluent coverage, when the cells are in direct contact with each other) and immersed in the McCoy's 5A (BioConcept) medium, which contains penicillin (20 U/ml) and streptomycin (20 μg/ml) and different concentrations of FBS (0–15%). Then, the cells were cultivated in an incubator at 37°C in 5% CO_2 for 48h. We used osteoblasts because SAOS-2 is a standard cell line, whose properties are stable even for long timespans. This is why we are able to compare the results of different experiments, as well as our results with the literature. Other cell types were also applied for comparison: human periodontal ligament fibroblasts (HPdLF; Lonza) and human cervical carcinoma cells (HeLaG; DSMZ GmbH).

Adhesion and morphology of cells were characterized by fluorescent staining of actin stress fibers (in green) and cell nuclei (in blue) using the protocol described in (Kalbacova, Roessler, Hempel, Tsaryk, Peters, Scharnweber, Kirkpatrick & Dieter, 2007). The staining was visualized using the E-400 epifluorescence microscope (Nikon); digital images were acquired with a DS-5M-U1 Color Digital Camera (Nikon).

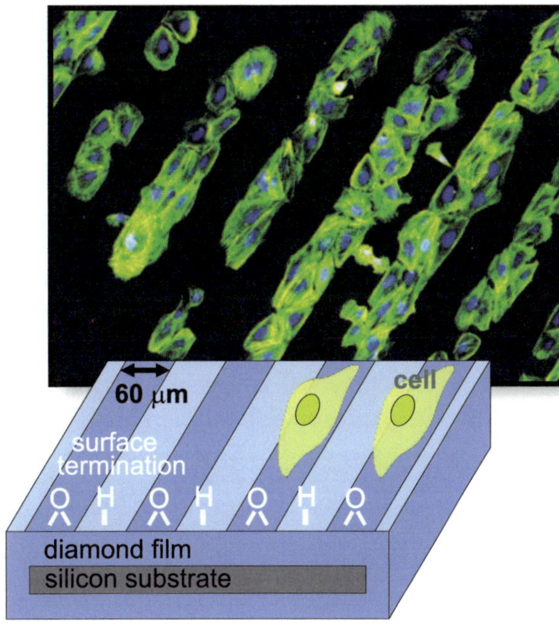

Fig. 5. Microscopic fluorescence image illustrates how osteoblastic cells (SAOS-2) preferentially self-assemble on oxygen-terminated diamond after a 48h cultivation in McCoy's 5A medium with 15% FBS on H-/O-diamond stripes of 60 µm width. Starting cell concentration was 2,500 cells/cm^2. Fluorescence microscopy shows actin filaments in green and cell nuclei in blue. The scheme under the image further clarifies the situation.

When the osteoblastic cells were plated and grown on the H-/O-terminated microstructures, they self-assembled preferably on the oxygen-terminated diamond surface. A scheme and fluorescence image shown in Figure 5 give an example of such behavior for the case of 60-µm-wide stripes. The cells' preference is independent of the width of the stripes between 30 and 200 µm (Rezek, Michalíková, Ukraintsev, Kromka & Kalbacova, 2009) and of the surface roughness between 20 and 500 nm rms (Michalíková et al., 2009). However, the shape of cells was found to be influenced by surface roughness (Kalbacova et al., 2009; Kromka et al., 2009) and the width of microstructures (Kalbacova et al., 2008; Rezek, Michalíková, Ukraintsev, Kromka & Kalbacova, 2009). Cells grown on narrow O-stripes (30 µm i.e. comparable with the size of the cell) are elongated and form chain-like structures. On the other hand, cells growing on wider stripes (60, 100 a 200 µm – larger than the typical cell size) spread over the whole width of the stripe. The H-/O-diamond boundary forms a sharp interface for cell adhesion.

Figure 6 confirms that other types of cells are also able of controlled self-assembly on H-/O-diamond stripes. Human fibroblasts (HPdLF) and cervical carcinoma cells (HeLaG) were plated on NCD samples with 30-µm-wide stripes and were cultivated for 48h. Cells exhibit a different morphology, however, their preference for O-diamond remains unchanged. Selective growth of cells on H-/O-diamond is also influenced by the seeding concentration, which is illustrated in Figure 7. At low concentrations (2,500 cells/cm^2), the cells grow predominantly on the oxygen-terminated surface, where the cells have enough room to

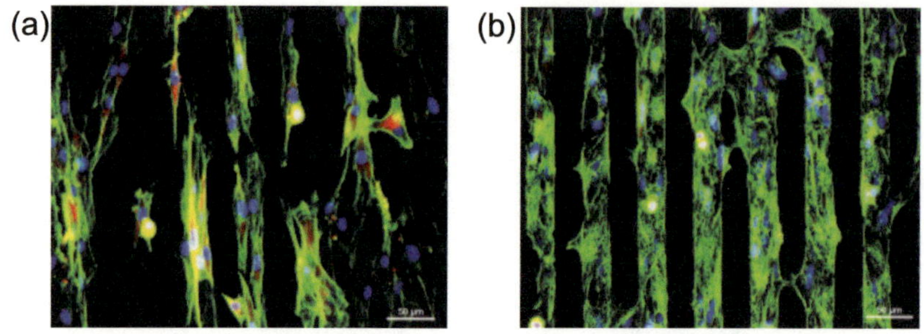

Fig. 6. Fluorescence image of (a) fibroblasts (HPdLF) and (b) cervical-carcinoma cells (HeLaG), which were cultivated for 48h on 30-µm-wide H-/O-diamond stripes. Starting cell concentration was 2,500 cells/cm^2, medium was supplemented with 15% FBS. Fluorescence microscopy shows actin filaments in green and cell nuclei in blue.

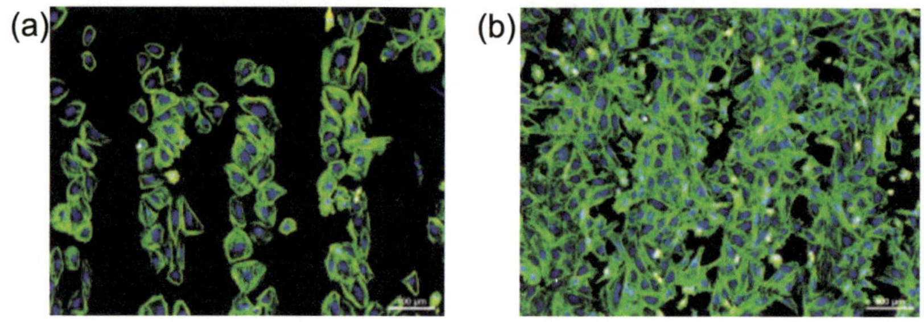

Fig. 7. Fluorescence images of osteoblasts, which were cultivated for 48h on 100-µm-wide H-/O-diamond stripes with starting cell concentrations: (a) 2,500 cells/cm^2, (a) 10,500 cells/cm^2. Fluorescence microscopy shows actin filaments in green and cell nuclei in blue.

spread on a hydrophilic area (Figure 7(a)). On the other hand, cells plated at high seeding concentrations (10,000 cells/cm^2) colonize also the hydrogen-terminated surface (Figure 7(b)). The FBS serum is another factor which has impact on the selective growth of cells. Figure 8 depicts the influence of FBS in the cultivation medium on the arrangement of cells on the H-/O-diamond terminated stripes. The range of concentrations between 5% and 15% does not significantly influence the cell adhesion (image for 15% FBS concentration is shown). Nevertheless, cells plated in a medium without FBS assemble of the surface independently of the surface termination. The cells' preference for a particular type of surface is thus presumably determined by the FBS proteins and not by a direct interaction between diamond surface dipoles and the cells. This is why the properties of FBS layers adsorbed on different types of diamond surfaces were investigated.

5. Morphology of protein layers on H-/O-diamond

Adsorption, adhesion and conformation of FBS layers on diamond were studied using AFM (Ntegra, NTMDT). The AFM measurements were carried out in air and in solution both in contact and tapping regimes. Doped silicon cantilevers (Multi75Al, BudgetSensors) with typical spring constant of 3 N/m, resonant frequency 75 kHz in air and 30 kHz in solution and nominal tip radius $<$ 10 nm were used. Polished monocrystalline diamond was used as a substrate to minimize the influence of its surface

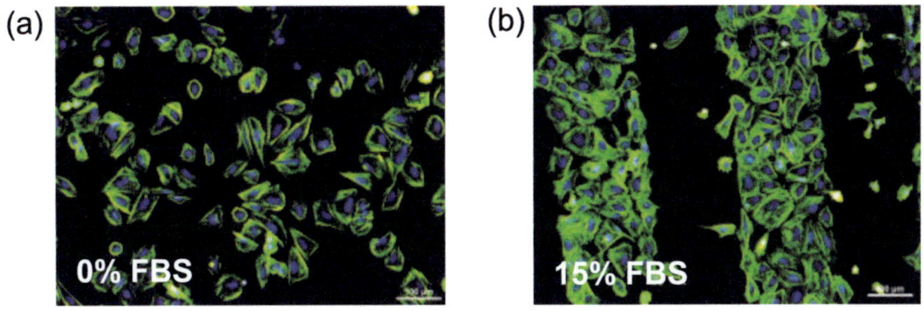

Fig. 8. Fluorescence images of osteoblasts, which were cultivated for 48h on 100-µm-wide H-/O-diamond stripes with different starting concentrations of fetal bovine serum: (a) 0%, (a) 15%. Fluorescence microscopy shows actin filaments in green and cell nuclei in blue. In the 0% case, the cells were plated without the serum, however, the serum was added after 2 hours to allow cells to grow for next 48 h.

morphology on the layers. Surface terminations were prepared in the same way as in the case of NCD films. The thickness of the protein layer was determined using the nanoshaving method, in which a part of the protein layer is removed by means of the AFM tip in contact mode and subsequently the profile of the resulting step in height is measured in oscillating (tapping) mode (Rezek et al., 2006; Rezek, Shin, Uetsuka & Nebel, 2007; Rezek, Ukraintsev, Michalíková, Kromka, Zemek & Kalbacova, 2009). Polished monocrystalline diamond is an ideal substrate for this method, because it is flat and hard.

Proteins were adsorbed on the surface of diamond from 15% FBS solution (Biowest) in McCoy's 5A medium (BioConcept). Two adsorption methods were applied: (i) either a drop of the solution was deposited on the substrate by a pipette, the substrate was then kept in a humid chamber for 10 minutes and was subsequently rinsed with water, or (ii) the adsorption was carried out directly in a fluid cell of AFM microscope with a subsequent *in-situ* measurement. Both methods yielded comparable results. The protein monolayer formed on the diamond surface within several seconds after the application (Rezek, Ukraintsev, Michalíková, Kromka, Zemek & Kalbacova, 2009).

AFM nanoshaving experiments showed that the thickness of the protein layer adsorbed from the solution is (4 ± 2) nm on O-diamond and (1.5 ± 2) nm on H-diamond (Rezek, Ukraintsev, Michalíková, Kromka, Zemek & Kalbacova, 2009). Thus, FBS layers formed on both types of diamond surfaces. Figure 9 presents a detailed topography and a phase map of the protein layers measured in AFM. Standard deviation values (i.e. RMS – root-mean-square) of the height and phase signals together with the characteristic lateral size of the features (L_x) determined by means of the autocorrelation function are shown below the images. In the case of the topography, RMS value corresponds to surface roughness. Roughness of the FBS layer on H-diamond (0.6 nm) is approximately $3\times$ smaller when compared to the O-diamond layer (1.7 nm). Besides, the features on the surface are of different shapes and sizes (12 and 18 nm, respectively). The phase signal exhibits an even more pronounced difference. Whereas in the H-diamond case the phase image of the FBS layer consists of dark dots correlating with the protrusion in topography, the O-diamond phase image is characterized by much larger light areas, which correlates with round structures in topography. In air AFM experiments in air, such differences in topography and phase channel were not observed (Rezek, Ukraintsev, Michalíková, Kromka, Zemek & Kalbacova,

2009). This discrepancy results from the fact that FBS layers are not in their natural environment (solution).

Atomic force spectroscopy then showed that a characteristic sawtooth profile in tip-surface interaction of 500 ± 100 pN force in the adhesion part of the curve (negative force) can be detected (Rezek, Michalíková, Ukraintsev, Kromka & Kalbacova, 2009). Typical curves are shown in Figure 9(e). Similar values of forces and interactions were detected in force curves on glass-adsorbed proteins where they were attributed to the stretching of the proteins by the AFM tip (Popov et al., 2007). The character of the force curves is thus a proof that the FBS proteins are adsorbed on both types of diamond surfaces.

Based on these AFM measurements, we propose a model of the conformation of proteins adsorbed on diamond surfaces (Rezek, Ukraintsev, Michalíková, Kromka, Zemek & Kalbacova, 2009). This model is schematically depicted in Figure 9(f). On hydrophobic surfaces, the denaturation of proteins (i.e. negative conformational change) occurs because their hydrophobic core sticks to the hydrogen-terminated surface. On hydrophilic surfaces, on the other hand, the proteins remain in their natural globular shape. This is why AFM detects a different shape, height and energy dissipation (phase) on the protrusions on the surface. Similar behavior of proteins was observed also on other materials (Browne et al., 2004).

6. Electronic effects on the diamond-protein-cell interface

Hydrogen-terminated stripes surrounded by oxygen-terminated areas were further utilized as conductive channels of *p*-type SG-FET transistors (Rezek, Shin, Watanabe & Nebel, 2007), which serves as a tool for the characterization of the influence of adsorbed proteins and cells grown on them on the electronic properties of diamond (Rezek, Krátká, Kromka & Kalbacova, 2010). The top-view and cross-section diagrams of the SG-FET transistor are shown in Figures 10(a) and 10(b), respectively. Electrical contacts were prepared by the sputtering of thin metal layers (10 nm Ti and 50 nm Au) over a photolithographic mask and the subsequent application of the lift-off technique. The transistor was insulated from the electrolyte using a layer of photoresist (1.5-µm-thick ma-P1315 or 5-µm-thick SU8-3050). Within the active area of the transistor, openings of about 60×60 µm^2 were introduced to this insulating layer. These openings exposed the surface of the 20-µm-wide conductive channel and partly also the surrounding oxidized surface (about 20 µm from each side) (Rezek, Krátká, Kromka & Kalbacova, 2010). The transistor gate was generated by the immersion of this active area in the solution (electrolyte), which is in contact with an Ag/AgCl reference electrode. The gate is insulated solely by hydrogen surface atoms without the employment of any other insulating layers.

Output and transfer SG-FET transistor characteristics were measured using two Keithley K327 source-measure units connected according to Figure 10(a). Characteristics were acquired in the following solutions: (a) McCoy's 5A medium, (b) McCoy's 5A medium with 15% FBS and (c) McCoy's 5A medium with Britton-Robinson buffer at pH = 7. In order to ensure that the acquired characteristics represent stable data, all the measurements were repeated three times. Output characteristics in Figure 10(c) confirms that nanocrystalline-based transistors are fully functional in solution and its behavior under gate voltage is in accord with what is expected for a *p*-type channel. This functionality was reached even in NCD layers as thin as 100 nm with the average grain size of (80 ± 50) nm. The influence of the adsorption of proteins and

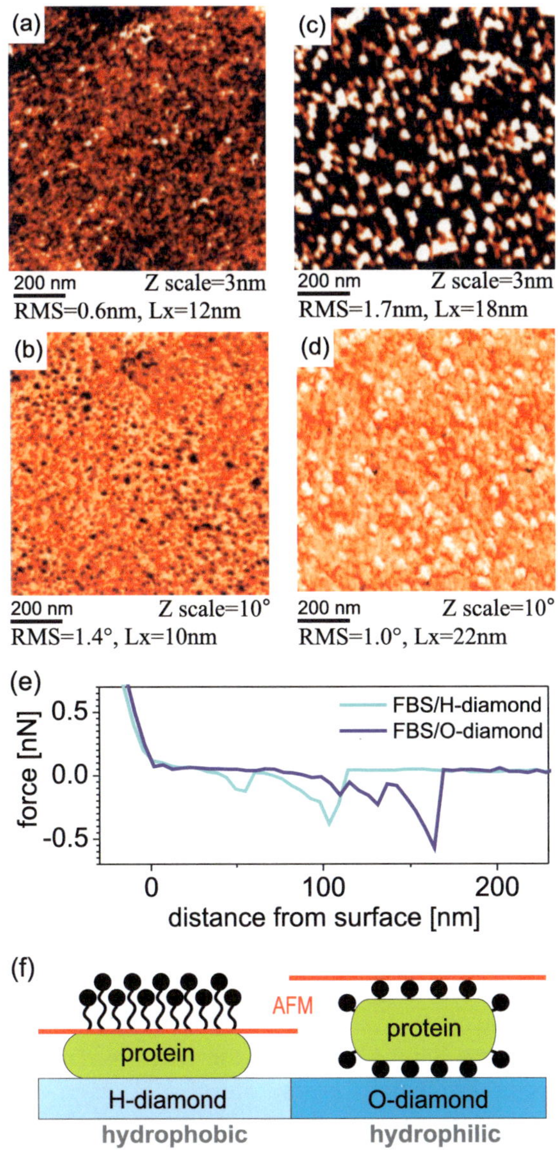

Fig. 9. Atomic force microscopy (AFM) on hydrogen- and oxygen-terminated diamond surfaces with an adsorbed FBS layer in FBS/McCoy's medium: topography and phase (a-b) of FBS/H-diamond, (c-d) FBS/O-diamond. Values of standard deviation (RMS) of the height and phase channel and characteristic lateral size of the features (L_x) below the images were determined using the autocorrelation function. (e) Typical atomic force spectroscopy curves for an FBS layer on hydrogen- and oxygen-terminated diamond surface. (f) Model of the conformation of proteins on hydrogen- and oxygen-terminated diamond surface. Hydrophobic core in green, the black spheres represent polar groups surrounding the core in aqueous environment. The red line denotes the height of the protein as detected by AFM in solution.

subsequent growth of cells on the electronic properties of diamond is easily discernible in Figure 10(c), which represents transfer characteristics of a pristine diamond transistor (blue), the same transistor after the adsorption of FBS (red) and after SAOS-2 cell cultivation (green). All characteristics were acquired in the McCoy's 5A medium, source-drain voltage was kept constant during all the measurements (−0.6 V; this setting corresponds to the amplification regime of the transistor). A slight hysteresis effect was observed in all transfer characteristics. Current flowing through the SG-FET transistor decreased after the application of FBS and the transfer characteristics shifted approximately by −45 mV for $I_{ds} = -0.6$ nA. Another shift roughly by −78 mV was observed after the cultivation of cells, giving rise to an overall shift of about −123 mV. Apart from the shift, the steepness of the slope (transconductance) defined as $g_m = \delta I_{ds}/\delta Ug$ decreased from 9.5 to 8.3 nS at $I_{ds} = -0.6$ nA. Rinsing the sample with the McCoy's medium (Rezek, Krátká, Kromka & Kalbacova, 2010) had only little impact on the characteristics. Transistor gate (leakage) currents were in the order of 10 pA. Typically, FBS adsorption on the surface reduced the gate currents as FBS forms additional layer on the diamond surface. Yet in some cases the currents slightly increased (to about 40 pA) as a result of the adsorption of proteins (Rezek, Krátká, Kromka & Kalbacova, 2010).

7. Discussion

Interaction of cells with as-grown and nanostructured diamond surfaces indicates that the diamond surface morphology can be tailored in a controlled way with respect to bio-technological and bio-medical requirements. It also demonstrates that quite wide range of diamond surface morphologies is acceptable for the cell growth. This is in agreement with other experiments on diamond films where hierarchically modified substrate roughness was employed (Kalbacova et al., 2009).

In the case of nanostructured diamond surfaces, amount of vinculin detected by fluorescence microscopy can be used an indication of the cell motility on the substrate because vinculin generally serves as a stabilizing protein in the focal adhesion (Fernandez et al., 1992). Increased expression of vinculin on the nano-cones promotes the cell adhesion and reduces the cell motility. On the nano-rods, solitary cells have more chance to move and search the entire space, whereas cells in confluent layer could be easily peeled off.

In the case of hydrogen- and oxygen-terminated microstructures, cells preferably self-assemble on the oxygen-terminated surface. The growth of cells over the hydrogen-terminated areas, mostly at high cell concentrations, is presumably enabled by their linkage to the O-diamond layers because individual cells exhibit poor adhesion to H-diamond and reduced metabolic activity (Kalbacova, Kalbac, Dunsch, Kromka, Vanecek, Rezek, Hempel & Kmoch, 2007; Kalbacova et al., 2008). Very probably, cells communicate, exchange growth factors and various stimuli and gradually form the extracellular matrix (ECM). In this way, they modify the surface with proteins and proteoglycans underneath them to overcome the unfavorable properties of the substrate. This process then makes it possible for the cells to grow also over the electrically conductive H-diamond areas, if these are surrounded by O-diamond areas. This effect was exploited during the incubation of cells in field transistors.

Figure 8 clearly demonstrates that the FBS proteins are the factor whose influence determines the cell adhesion on the diamond layer. As the protein adsorption proceeds much more rapidly than the transport of cells to the surface, the interaction of the cell with the diamond

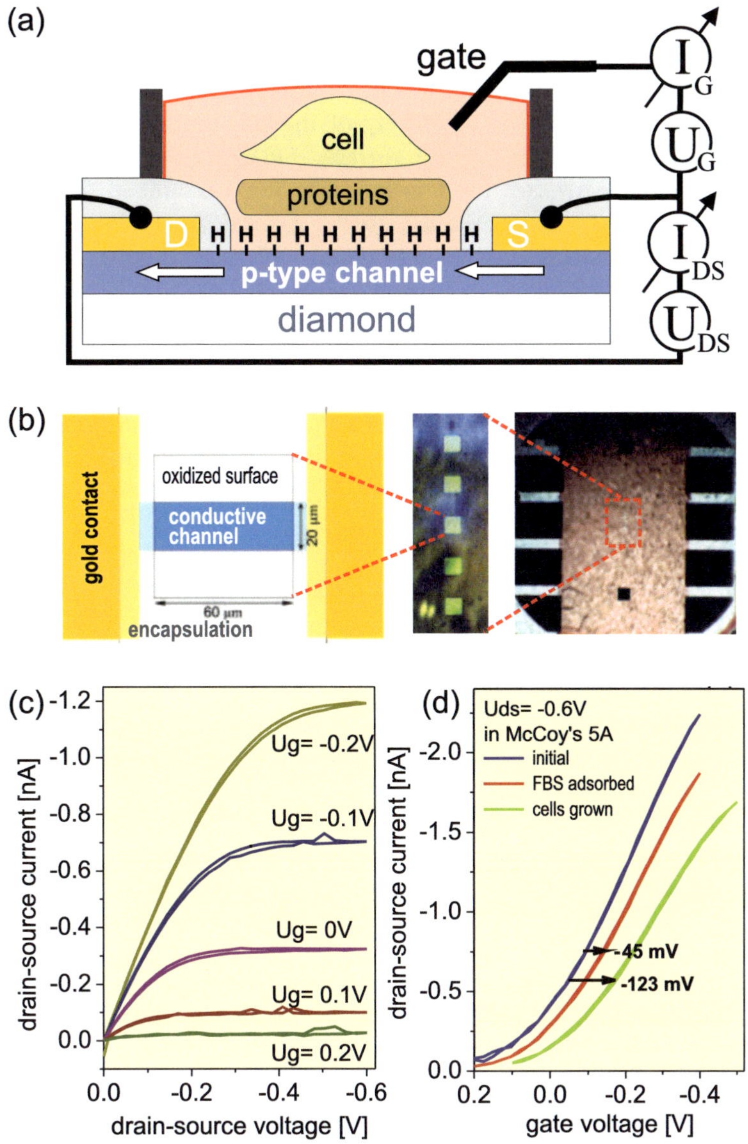

Fig. 10. (a) Diagram of a solution-gate field-effect transistor (SG-FET) based on the surface conductivity of hydrogen-terminated diamond. The insulation of the SG-FET gate is ensured merely by the hydrogen termination of the diamond channel surface. Thus, proteins and cells react directly with the surface of diamond. (b) Top-view: hydrogen-terminated conductive microscopic channel is surrounded by insulating oxygen-terminated areas and the active area is determined by the hole in the insulating layer. A chip contains several such areas, as is demonstrated in the optical image of the whole chip (10×10 mm^2 with 5 transistors) on the right. (c) Output characteristics of SG-FET transistor from nanocrystalline diamond in McCoy's 5A solution with gate potential between −0.2 and 0.2 V. (d) Transfer characteristics of a transistor in McCoy's 5A solution at the beginning of the experiment (blue), after the adsorption of proteins from FBS (red) and after 48h cell cultivation (green)

substrate very likely results from the nature of this adsorbed layer. AFM measurements show that proteins adsorb on both types of surfaces, which agrees well with experiments carried out on other materials, where albumin adsorbs both on hydrophilic and on hydrophobic surfaces (Browne et al., 2004). The selectivity of the cell growth is thus not determined by FBS adsorbing solely on a one type of surface. Other factors, such as denaturation of proteins on hydrophobic surfaces, need to be taken into account in order to successfully explain the selective adsorption. Detailed study of surface morphology using the AFM method clearly confirms that differences in surface roughness, morphology as well as phase contrast between the protein layers on H- and O-diamond exist. When on H-diamond, the FBS proteins probably adopt the conformation when their epitopes (e.g. adhesion mediated RGD sequences of peptides) are hidden, thus not providing optimal conditions for cell adhesion. A similar difference in protein morphology was observed on polystyrene substrates (Browne et al., 2004). This is why the wetting properties of a surface seem to be the most influential factor for the growth of cells, whereas other specific properties of diamond layers do not play such an important role. As we have shown, this phenomenon is general and valid also for other types of cells.

The above described preference of the cells for oxygen-terminated surface on H/O-patterned diamond is detectable as early as during the first two hours of adsorption in the 15% FBS supplemented medium (Rezek, Michalíková, Ukraintsev, Kromka & Kalbacova, 2009). However, the pattern is not yet as sharp as after 48h because the cells did not have enough time to spread on the surface. On the other hand, in a control experiment without FBS the patterned self-assembly was not observed. This implies that even the initial stage of the assembly is strongly influenced by the FBS proteins. In this stage, cells move and actively explore their surrounding environment.

Other factors that can influence the selective cell growth include a different adhesion of cells and proteins to hydrogen- and oxygen-terminated surface. Also a differences in composition of the protein layer on each type of surface can play role. Adhesion of cells to the hydrogen-terminated diamond lowered by as much as 40% was observed in the presence of FBS in comparison to oxygen-terminated diamond (Rezek, Ukraintsev, Kromka, Ledinský, Brož, Nosková, Hartmannová & Kalbacova, 2010). Furthermore, fibronectin, one of the FBS components, was found to have the crucial influence on the selective growth of cells (Rezek, Ukraintsev, Kromka, Ledinský, Brož, Nosková, Hartmannová & Kalbacova, 2010). Detailed composition of the FBS layer on diamond, however, has not yet been successfully identified.

In the medium without FBS, the cells cannot detect any protein layer and thus they are in direct contact with the NCD substrate. After a short time (2 hours), the cells are not yet fully spread, but their contacts (focal complexes) with the substrate are already detectable (Rezek, Michalíková, Ukraintsev, Kromka & Kalbacova, 2009). In general, the adhesion mechanism is not yet understood. After further cultivation time (48 hours) in the medium where FBS was added, the cells assume normal shapes and growth takes place properly at the spots where the cells initially attached (see Figure 8(a)) because they had enough time to produce their own extracellular matrix and adapt the surface underneath them. The hydrogen- or oxygen-termination of diamond (without the initial activity of the FBS proteins) is, therefore, not the sole factor determining the cells selectivity by itself.

From the point of view of electronic properties of the diamond-protein-cell system, SG-FET diamond transistor exhibits a shift in transfer characteristics towards negative gate voltages after the FBS proteins adsorbed on the surface and subsequently the cells were cultivated on top of them. This is a clear sign of a lowered transistor's conductivity. This effect cannot be fully explained solely by the electrostatic field effect. The most important discrepancy here consists in the fact that the major FBS proteins (albumin, fibronectin, vitronectin) as well as cell membranes are negatively charged under physiologic pH. Thus, their presence near the gate of a p type transistor should increase the I_{ds} current flowing through the transistor, which is not the case. As was already mentioned, proteins become denatured on a hydrophobic surface and their hydrophobic core sticks to the surface. Consequently, they can modify the initial equilibrium of the conductive layer, which is a result of the equilibrium of chemical potentials of the diamond and the solution (Chakrapani et al., 2007; Maier et al., 2000). A negative shift occurs as a result of the change of the material properties of diamond (i.e. its conductivity), which is in accord with the lowered steepness of the slope of the transfer curve (transconductance). Sometimes observed increase in the SG-FET gate currents indicates that proteins can lower the electronic barrier of the diamond-electrolyte system resulting from the surface C–H dipoles (Rezek, Krátká, Kromka & Kalbacova, 2010) and can therefore simplify the charge transfer across the interface with the solution. The primary FBS monolayer persists on the surface (Rezek, Ukraintsev, Michalíková, Kromka, Zemek & Kalbacova, 2009; Ukraintsev et al., 2009) and cannot be easily removed by common rinsing methods, even when detergents and enzymes are employed. This explains the stability of the shift in the SG-FET transistor's transfer characteristics.

A further negative shift in transfer characteristics was observed after the cultivation of cells on the device. This shift cannot be ascribed to the cells themselves, because it persists even after the cells are removed. Possible reasons for this shift include the fact that osteoblastic cells attach to the surface only in a limited number of spots (the so-called focal adhesion), which cannot cover the whole gate area, and the remaining cells are not in direct contact with the substrate surface (Kalbacova et al., 2009). Moreover, cells on H-diamond do not tend to spread and adhere but they rather form bridges to O-diamond if it is in close proximity (Kalbacova et al., 2008). The adhesion of osteoblasts is then mediated by proteins, i.e. another FBS protein layer exists between the cell and the diamond surface. This is why the most part of a cell membrane is presumably further than the Debye length in the medium, which amounts to < 10 nm due to the presence of salts and other ionic compounds in the cultivation medium. As a result, we deduce that the shift after the cultivation of cells is a result of a change in the adsorbed layer of proteins, which remains on the diamond surface even after rinsing (Rezek, Ukraintsev, Michalíková, Kromka, Zemek & Kalbacova, 2009; Ukraintsev et al., 2009). Cells can actively participate at such changes because osteoblasts continually modify their surrounding environment and subsequently produce their own ECM. Based on the above reasoning, a model of the interface between the channel of the diamond SG-FET and the cell medium containing proteins and cells can be constructed (Rezek, Krátká, Kromka & Kalbacova, 2010). Figure 11 depicts a schematic concept of this model. The model presumes common cell-plating conditions when the cultivation medium contains FBS proteins.

Further research should answer the question concerning the composition of the layers adsorbed on diamond and the possibility of direct electrical detection of the function of cells

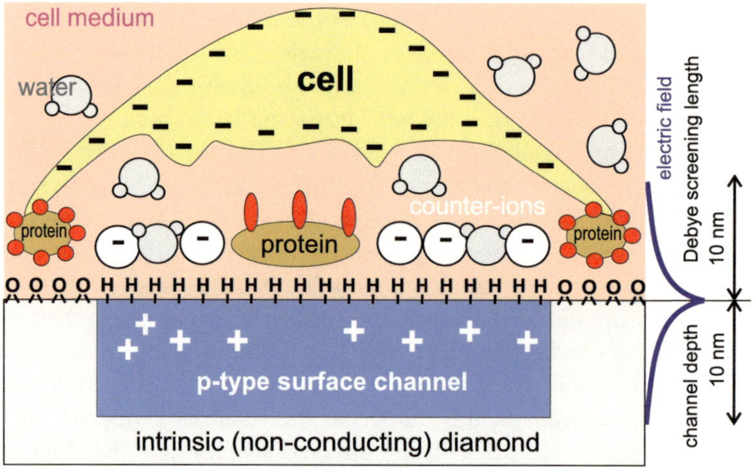

Fig. 11. Schematic sketch of the interface between the surface-condutive SG-FET channel and cell medium containing proteins and cells. The electric field and its reach over the interface is depicted on the right. It demonstrates that the interaction is limited to distances of several tens of nm.

using the interface with diamond, as has already been suggested for neurons (Dankerl et al., 2009).

8. Conclusions

We have demonstrated some of the crucial properties and discussed prospective application of diamond for biomedicine. We showed that nanostructuring of diamond surfaces can be used to tailor adhesion and growth of the cells. We also demonstrated that the combination of oxygen- and hydrogen-terminated surfaces allows for the controlled self-assembly of cells into microstructures. Cells preferably adhere to oxygen-terminated areas, this effect is general and occurs for various types of cells. The best selectivity is achieved for low seeding cell concentrations (2,500 cells cm^2) regardless of the geometry of the surface and usual range of FBS concentrations (5 to 15%). Higher seeding concentrations make it possible for the cells to colonize even the less suitable hydrogen-terminated surface, which is electrically conductive and thus can be utilized in electronic components. Cells plated in the medium without FBS colonize the surface independently of the microstructures. Consequently, the cells' preference stems from the properties of the proteins on H- and O-diamond and it is not a direct consequence of the cells' interaction with diamond surface dipoles. Atomic force microscopy revealed the existence of a thin film (2–4 nm) of proteins on both types of surfaces, however, adopting different conformations on different terminations. Based on these measurements, we propose a model of how the proteins arrange on diamond as a result of the wettability of the surfaces, similarly to other materials. Apart from the protein conformation, other factors, such as the composition and different adhesion of the FBS layer on H- and O-diamond, can contribute the preferential growth of cells.

Electronic effects on the diamond-protein-cell interface were characterized by the SG-FET transistors based on the surface conductivity of nanocrystalline diamond and having the gate insulated solely by hydrogen surface atoms. We show that these transistors are fully operational and can serve as a transducer (and partly also as an amplifier) of the characteristics of biological material and environment to electrical impulses. Adsorption of proteins from the FBS-enriched cultivation medium and subsequent cultivation of cells on it led to a shift in transfer characteristics of the transistor in the range of as much as a hundred mV. This shift is the result of the adsorption of a thin film of proteins onto the diamond surface as was confirmed by AFM. The key finding here is that these shifts cannot be solely due to electrostatic field effect because the field effect acts in the opposite direction. We propose a model in which the proteins replace the ions close to the diamond surface. The negative shift in the transfer characteristics then results from a change in the material property of diamond (its conductivity), which is in accord with a lowered steepness of the slope (i.e. transconductance) of the measured curves. Related changes in SG-FET gate currents suggest that the FBS layer can block and under certain conditions also promote the transfer of charge across the interface between diamond and the solution. The above findings and conclusions are significant for prospective application of the unique properties of diamond in biosensors and biotechnologies that can be exploited in medicine as well as other fields.

This research was carried out through the financial support of the projects KAN400100701 (AVČR), IAAX00100902 (GAAV), LC510 (MŠMT), LC06040 (MŠMT), MSM0021620806 (MŠMT), 202/09/H041 (GAČR), institutional Research Plan AV0Z10100521, scholarship of J.E. Purkyně Fellowship (BR, AK) and Fellowship 2010 L´Oreal-UNESCO for Women in Science (MK). Zdenka Poláčková, Vlastimil Jurka, Karel Jurek, and Lenka Michalíková are acknowledged for technical support. Software libraries TAFLAB for the measurement software were developed and kindly provided by Dr. Antonín Fejfar.

9. References

Babchenko, O., Kromka, A., Hruska, K., Kalbacova, M., Broz, A. & Vanecek, M. (2009). Fabrication of nano-structured diamond films for saos-2 cell cultivation, *phys. stat. sol. (b)* 206: 2033.

Bajaj, P., Akin, D., Gupta, A., Sherman, D., Shi, B., Auciello, O. & Bashir, R. (2007). Ultrananocrystalline diamond film as an optimal cell interface for biomedical applications, *Biomed. Devices* 9: 787–794.

Browne, M. M., Lubarsky, G. V., Davidson, M. R. & Bradley, R. H. (2004). Protein adsorption onto polystyrene surfaces studied by xps and afm, *Surf. Sci.* 553: 155.

Chakrapani, V., Angus, J. C., Anderson, A. B., Wolter, S. D., Stoner, B. R. & Sumanasekera, G. U. (2007). Charge transfer equilibria between diamond and an aqueous oxygen electrochemical redox couple, *Science* 318: 1424.

Dankerl, M., Eick, S., Hofmann, B., Hauf, M., Ingebrandt, S., Offenhäusser, A., Stutzmann, M. & Garrido, J. A. (2009). Diamond transistor array for extracellular recording from electrogenic cells, *Adv. Funct. Mater.* 19: 2915.

Dankerl, M., Reitinger, A., Stutzmann, M. & Garrido, J. A. (2007). Resolving the controversy on the ph sensitivity of diamond surfaces, *phys. stat. sol. RRL* 2: 31.

Fernandez, J. L. R., Geiger, B., Salomon, D. & Ben-Ze'v, A. (1992). Overexpression of vinculin suppresses cell motility in balb/c 3t3 cells, *Cell. Motil. Cytoskeleton* 22: 127.

Grausova, L., Bacakova, L., Kromka, A., Vanecek, M., Rezek, B. & Lisa, V. (2009). Molecular markers of adhesion, maturation and immune activation of human osteoblast-like MG63 cells on nanocrystalline diamond films, *Diam. Relat. Mater.* 18: 258.

Härtl, A., Schmich, E., Garrido, J. A., Hernando, J., Catharino, S. C. R., Walter, S., Feulner, P., Kromka, A., Steinmüller, D. & Stutzmann, M. (2004). Protein-modified nanocrystalline diamond thin films for biosensor applications, *Nature Mat.* 3: 736.

Kalbacova, M., Kalbac, M., Dunsch, L., Kromka, A., Vanecek, M., Rezek, B., Hempel, U. & Kmoch, S. (2007). The effect of SWCNT and nano-diamond films on human osteoblast cells, *phys. stat. sol. (b)* 244(11): 4356.

Kalbacova, M., Michalíková, L., Barešová, V., Kromka, A., Rezek, B. & Kmoch, S. (2008). Adhesion of osteoblasts on chemically patterned nanocrystalline diamonds, *phys. stat. sol. (b)* 245: 2124.

Kalbacova, M., Rezek, B., Baresova, V., Wolf-Brandstetter, C. & Kromka, A. (2009). Nano-scale topography of nanocrystalline diamonds promotes differentiation of osteoblasts, *Acta Biomaterialia* 5: 3076.

Kalbacova, M., Roessler, S., Hempel, U., Tsaryk, R., Peters, K., Scharnweber, D., Kirkpatrick, C. & Dieter, P. (2007). The effect of electrochemically simulated titanium cathodic corrosion products on ros production and metabolic activity of osteoblasts and monocytes/macrophages, *Biomaterials* 28: 3263–3272.

Kawarada, H. (1996). Hydrogen-terminated diamond surfaces and interfaces, *Surf. Sci. Rep.* 26(7): 205.

Kozak, H., Kromka, A., Babchenko, O. & Rezek, B. (2010). Directly grown nanocrystalline diamond field-effect transistor microstructures, *Sensor Lett.* 8: 482.

Kozak, H., Kromka, A., Ledinský, M. & Rezek, B. (2009). Enhancing nanocrystalline diamond surface conductivity by deposition temperature and chemical post-processing, *phys. stat. sol. (a)* 206: 276.

Kromka, A., Babchenko, O., Izak, T., Hruska, K. & Rezek, B. (2011). Linear antenna microwave plasma cvd deposition of diamond films over large areas, *Vacuum* p. in press.

Kromka, A., Rezek, B., Kalbacova, M., Baresova, V., Zemek, J., Konak, C. & Vanecek, M. (2009). Diamond seeding and growth of hierarchically structured films for tissue engineering, *Adv. Eng. Mater.* 11: B71.

Kromka, A., Rezek, B., Remeš, Z., Michalka, M., Ledinský, M., Zemek, J., Potměšil, J. & Vaněček, M. (2008). Formation of continuous nanocrystalline diamond layer on glass and silicon at low temperatures, *Chem. Vap. Deposition* 14: 181.

Maier, F., Riedel, M., Mantel, B., Ristein, J. & Ley, L. (2000). Origin of surface conductivity in diamond, *Phys. Rev. Lett.* 85: 3472.

Maier, F., Ristein, J. & Ley, L. (2001). Electron affinity of plasma-hydrogenated and chemically oxidized diamond (100) surfaces, *Phys. Rev. B* 64: 65411.

Michalíková, L., Rezek, B., Kromka, A. & Kalbacova, M. (2009). CVD diamond films with hydrophilic micro-patterns for self-organisation of human osteoblasts, *Vacuum* 84: 61.

Nebel, C. E., Rezek, B., Shin, D., Watanabe, H. & Yamamoto, T. (2006). Electronic properties of h-terminated diamond in electrolyte solutions, *J. Appl. Phys.* 99: 033711.

Nebel, C. E., Shin, D., Rezek, B., Tokuda, N., Uetsuka, H. & Watanabe, H. (2007). Diamond and biology, *J. R. Soc. Interface* 4: 439.

Popov, C., Kulisch, W., Reithmaier, J., Dostalova, T., Jelinek, M., Anspach, N. & Hammann, C. (2007). Bioproperties of nanocrystalline diamond/amorphous carbon composite films, *Diamond Relat. Mater.* 16: 735.

Potocky, S., Kromka, A., Potmesil, J., Vorlicek, Z., Vanecek, M. & Michalka, M. (2007). Investigation of nanocrystalline diamond films grown on silicon and glass at substrate temperature below 400° c, *Diamond Relat. Mater.* 16: 744–747.

Rezek, B., Krátká, M., Kromka, A. & Kalbacova, M. (2010). Effects of protein inter-layers on cell-diamond fet characteristics, *Biosens. Bioelectron.* 26: 1307.

Rezek, B., Michalíková, L., Ukraintsev, E., Kromka, A. & Kalbacova, M. (2009). Micro-pattern guided adhesion of osteoblasts on diamond surfaces, *Sensors* 9: 3549.

Rezek, B., Sauerer, C., Nebel, C. E., Stutzmann, M., Ristein, J., Ley, L., Snidero, E. & Bergonzo, P. (2003). Fermi level on hydrogen terminated diamond surfaces, *Appl. Phys. Lett.* 82: 2266.

Rezek, B., Shin, D., Nakamura, T. & Nebel, C. E. (2006). Geometric properties of covalently bonded DNA on single-crystalline diamond, *J. Am. Chem. Soc.* 128: 3884.

Rezek, B., Shin, D., Uetsuka, H. & Nebel, C. E. (2007). Microscopic diagnostics of DNA molecules on mono-crystalline diamond, *phys. stat. sol. (a)* 204: 2888.

Rezek, B., Shin, D., Watanabe, H. & Nebel, C. E. (2007). Intrinsic hydrogen-terminated diamond as ion-sensitive field effect transistor, *Sens. Actuators B* 122: 596.

Rezek, B., Ukraintsev, E., Kromka, A., Ledinský, M., Brož, A., Nosková, L., Hartmannová, H. & Kalbacova, M. (2010). Assembly of osteoblastic cell micro-arrays on diamond guided by protein pre-adsorption, *Diam. Relat. Mater.* 19: 153.

Rezek, B., Ukraintsev, E., Michalíková, L., Kromka, A., Zemek, J. & Kalbacova, M. (2009). Adsorption of fetal bovine serum on H/O-terminated diamond studied by atomic force microscopy, *Diam. Relat. Mater.* 18: 918.

Ri, S. G., Mizumasa, T., Akiba, Y., Hirose, Y., Kurosu, T. & Iida, M. (1995). Formation mechanism of p-type surface conductive layer on deposited diamond films, *Jpn. J. Appl. Phys.* 34: 5550.

Shakenraad, J. & Busscher, H. (1989). Cell-polymer interactions:the influence of protein adsorption, *Colloid Surf.* 42: 331–343.

Tanaka, M., Takayama, A., Ito, E., Sunami, H., Yamamoto, S. & Shimomura, M. (2007). Effect of pore size of self-organized honeycomb-patterned polymer films on spreading, focal adhesion, proliferation, and function of endothelial cells, *J. Nanosci. Nanotechnol.* 7: 763–772.

Tang, L., Tsai, C., Gerberich, W., Kruckeberg, L. & Kania, D. (1995). Biocompatibility of chemical-vapour-deposited diamond, *Biomaterials* 16(6): 483–488.

Tsugawa, K., Ishihara, M., Kim, J., Koga, Y. & Hasegawa, M. (2010). Nanocrystalline diamond film growth on plastic substrates at temperatures below 100°c from low-temperature plasma, *Phys. Rev. B* 82: 125460.

Ukraintsev, E., Rezek, B., Kromka, A., Broz, A. & Kalbacova, M. (2009). Long-term adsorption of fetal bovine serum on H/O-terminated diamond studied in-situ by atomic force microscopy, *phys. stat. sol. (b)* 246: 2832.

Yang, W., Auciello, O., Butler, J. E., Cai, W., Carlisle, J. A., Gerbi, J. E., Gruen, D. M., Knickerbocker, T., Lasseter, T. L., J. N. Russel, J., Smith, L. M. & Hamers, R. J. (2002). DNA-modified nanocrystalline diamond thin films as stable, biologically active substrates, *Nature Mat.* 1: 253.

Zhao, G., Zinger, O., Schwartz, Z., Wieland, M., Landolt, D. & Boyan, B. D. (2006). Osteoblast-like cells are sensitive to submicron-scale surface structure, *Clin. Oral. Implant. Res.* 17: 258.

9

New Generation Biosensors Based on Ellipsometry

Bora Garipcan[1,*], M. Oğuzhan Çağlayan[2] and Gökhan Demirel[3]
[1]*Institute of Biomedical Engineering, Boğaziçi University, Istanbul*
[2]*Chemical Engineering Department, Cumhuriyet University, Sivas*
[3]*Bio-inspired Materials Research Lab., Department of Chemistry, Gazi University, Ankara*
Turkey

1. Introduction

1.1 What is a biosensor?

There is a big demand for the fast, reliable and low-cost systems for the detection, monitoring and diagnosis of biological molecules and diseases in medicine (Sharma, 1994; D`Orazio, 2003; Mohanty and Kougianos, 2006). Of course, this demand is not restricted only in the field of medicine; for environmental pollutant monitoring, detection of food borne pathogens and potential danger of bioterrorism. Therefore, researchers from various fields such as; physics, chemistry, biology, engineering and medicine interested in the developing, constructing and manufacturing of new sensing devices to get more efficient and reliable information (Figure 1.); (Mohanty and Kougianos, 2006).

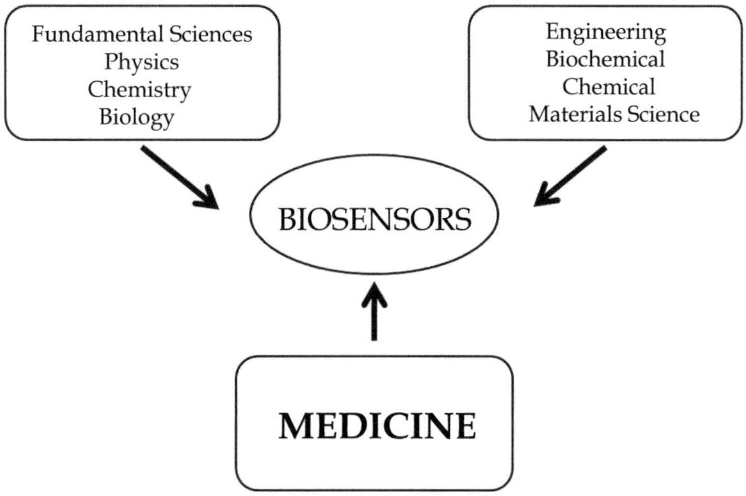

Fig. 1. Biosensors; an excellent example of multi and interdisciplinary research area.

* Dr. Bora Garipcan is currently working at Institute of Biomedical Engineering as a Part time instructor.

Biosensors are the most impressive and useful devices which correspond to these purposes. In the literature about biosensors, there are two common articles which describe the term biosensor as "a biosensor is a chemical sensing device in which a biologically derived recognition entity is coupled to a transducer, to allow the quantitative development of some complex biochemical parameter," and "a biosensor is an analytical device incorporating a deliberate and intimate combination of a specific biological element (that creates a recognition event) and a physical element (that transduces the recognition event)" by S.P.J. Higson and D.M. Fraser, respectively (Fraser, 1994; Higson, 1994; Mohanty and Kougianos 2006). In another words, a biosensor is commonly defined as an analytical device which is used mostly for the recognition of target biological molecules, macromolecules, and atoms which can also be named as analytes. Typically, a biosensor consists of three main components: first one; a biological recognition part that is responsible for the specific interaction with analyte second one; a transducer which transduces the biological interaction to an electrical signal and third one; an output system (Vo-Dinh and Cullum, 2000). In figure 2, main parts of a typical biosensor are schematized.

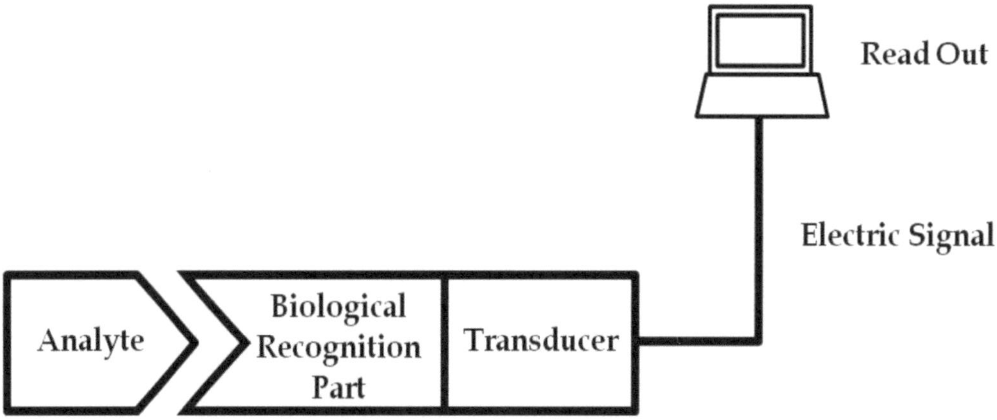

Fig. 2. Shematic representation of main parts of a typical biosensor.

1.2 History of biosensors

Most probably the first biosensors were canaries which have been used in coal mines since 1911 to monitor gas leakage. Up to early 1960`s the developments in this field were mostly in chemical sensing devices as glass electrodes for sensing hydrogen ion concentration and oxygen electrodes. In 1962, Clark made the first study on biosensors which was an amperometric enzyme biosensor for the detection of glucose (Table 1 summarizes the historical development of biosensors) (Clark, 1962). In this historical study, Clark used platinum (Pt) electrodes to detect oxygen. The enzyme glucose oxidase (GOD) was entrapped by using a piece of dialysis membrane. The change at the enzyme activity depending on the surrounding oxygen concentration was monitored by this amperometric enzyme electrode biosensor (Clark, 1962). After this milestone study, there are numerous studies have been done to monitor the interaction of target biomolecules (enzymes, Deoxyribonucleic acid (DNA), antibodies, cells, viruses etc.) and molecules (amino acids, metal ions, etc) with their complementary molecules (Justino, 2010). Today, in the nanotechnology era, quantum dots, nanowires, nanotubes and nanoparticles are being used as new biosensing devices to get more efficient and reliable information from diagnosis and monitoring of biomolecules (Figure 3) (Yogeswaran and Chen, 2008; Ghoshal, 2010, Palma, 2010).

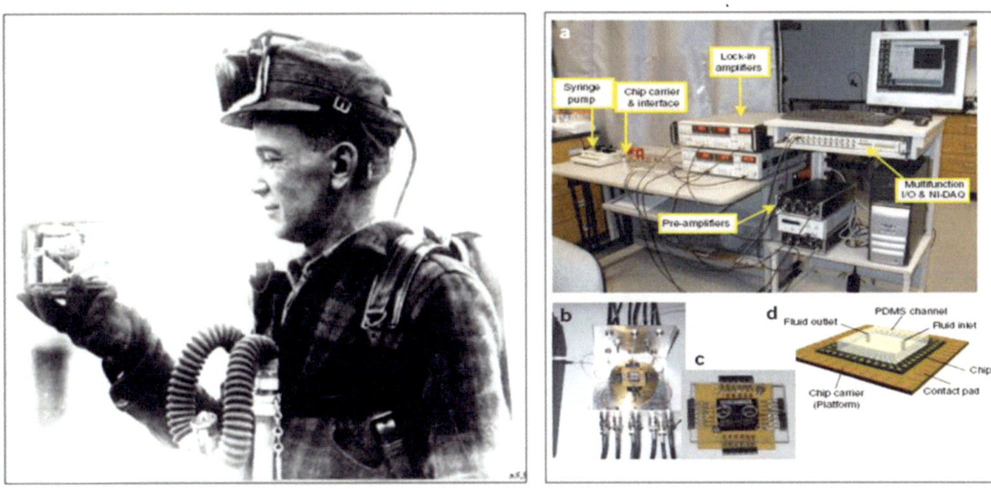

(a) (b)

Fig. 3. A survey of progress in biosensing devices at 100 years (a) The first biosensors were canaries which have been used in coal mines (Copyrighted Google), (b) Silicon nanowire biosensors are the latest biosensing devices (Copyrighted Nature Publishing Group).

1.3 Recognition parts and immobilization

The recognition part probably is the most crucial part of a biosensor, because the selectivity relies on the interaction between the target biomolecules (analytes) and the molecules immobilized on the surface of a biosensor. Analytes mostly in biosensors are such as; enzymes, antibodies, DNA, oligonucleotides, oligopeptides, carbohydrates, cells, bacteria, microorganisms, viruses and tissues (Vo-Dinh and Cullum, 2000). However, sometimes analytes can be macromolecules, chemicals and even if atoms, especially in biosensors that monitor the environmental pollutants. The complementary of biomolecules are immobilized on the surface of biosensors and sometimes biomimetic structures, polymers (molecular imprinted), synthetic molecules (especially in drug research using computational chemistry), oligonucleotides (ODNs) and atoms can be used to interact with the target biomolecules (analytes). Table 2, shows the specific interactions of biomolecules which are commonly used in biosensing devices to increase specificity and discriminate between different substances exist in the same environment (Vo-Dinh and Cullum, 2000).

There are several factors which affect the performance of a biosensor such as sensitivity, calibration, background signal, hysteresis, long-term stability, dynamic response and biocompatibility (Justino, 2010). Immobilization of biomolecules (molecules those are responsible for the specific interactions with the analytes) is one of the important steps of constructing a biosensing device that directly or indirectly influence the performance of a biosensor. Immobilization is a technique used for the fixation of biomolecules such as enzymes, antibodies or other proteins, oligopeptides, oligonucleotides, DNA, cells, microorganisms, organelles, physically or chemically onto (or into) a solid support for increasing the stability, repeated and long term usability of biosensors (Tang, 2002; Chou, 2002; Manelli, 2003).

Year	Type of Sensor	References
1911	Canaries have been used as biosensors	Hernandez, 2008
1922	First glass pH electrode	Hughes,1922
1956	First oxygen electrode	Clark, 1957
1962	First biosensor: an amperometric enzyme electrode for glucose	Clark, 1962
1969	First potentiometric biosensor: urease immobilized on an ammonia electrode to detect urea	Guilbault and Montalvo, 1967
1970	First ion selective Field Effect Transistor (ISFET)	Bergveld, 1970
1975	First fiber-optic sensor : an indicator immobilized to measure carbon dioxide or oxygen	Opitz and Lübbers, 1975
1975	First commercial biosensor (Yellow springs instruments glucose biosensor)	Magner, 1998
1980	First fiber optic pH sensor for in vivo blood gases	Peterson, 1980
1982	First fiber optic-based biosensor for glucose	Schultz, 1982
1983	First surface plasmon resonance (SPR) immunosensor	Liedberg, 1983
1990	SPR based biosensor by Pharmacia BIACore	Jonsson, 1991
2000	Ellipsometric Biosensors	Arwin, 2001
Current	Quantum dots, nanoparticles, nanowires, nanotubes, etc	Ghoshal, 2010

Table 1. Historical development of biosensors.

Analyte	Complemantary
Antibody	Antigen
Enzyme	Substrate
Carbohydrates	Receptors
Cells	Receptors
Drug	Receptors
ssDNA	Complementary DNA
Metal ions	Aminoacids

Table 2. The specific interactions of biomolecules which are commonly used in biosensing devices.

Biomolecules can be immobilized physically through; hydrophobic, ionic or Van der Wall's interactions to a solid matrix or by covalently immobilized to chemically activated surfaces. Physical attachment of molecules can be very effective in many cases; however, in some applications it fails due to weakness of the interaction of biomolecules with the biosensor surface. Covalent immobilization is often used for the molecules those do not adsorb, weakly adsorb or improperly adsorbed by using physical immobilization. In covalent immobilization, bioactivity of molecules (enzymes, protein 3D structure) can be sustained, shows less non specific adsorption and greater stability of the immobilized biomolecules (Tang, 2002; Chou, 2002; Su and Li, 2004). Proteins are much more sensitive to their physiological environments and can be easily denaturized by physical and chemical effects. Protein`s 3D conformation must not change during immobilization procedure. However, on the other side, DNA molecules are much more stable and durable to harsh physical and chemical conditions (Sharma and Rogers, 1994; Pişkin and Garipcan 2004; Pişkin 2009,).

As stated above the text, immobilization procedure is very important step for manufacturing biosensing devices so that, immobilization reaction should have several characteristics for effective, sensitive, selective and long-term usable biosensors. These are;

- The coupling reaction of biomolecules and activated groups on the biosensor surface should occur rapidly, to use low amounts of reagents for feasible and economical immobilization,
- The chemistry which will be used for immobilization should require little, if any, no post-synthetic modification of biosensor surface before immobilization,
- Immobilized molecules must be in an oriented and homogeneous manner, because orientation of biomolecules during the immobilization procedure is very important for proper interaction of target biomolecules and probe molecules (molecules responsible to interact with the target biomolecules) on the surface of the biosensor. As an example, antibody-antigen interaction occurs from the antigen binding regions of antibodies. If, the antigen binding regions of an antibody interact with the biosensor surface, proper interaction will not occur between antibody and antigen molecules.
- Surface density of the probe molecules should be optimized.

  Low density surface coverage of probe molecules will decrease the interaction of probe molecules with target biomolecules and resulted in low detection signal value,

  High surface densities may result steric hindrance between the covalently immobilized probe molecules and the target biomolecules,
- If necessary, to avoid steric hindrance and for correct orientation of the probe molecules on the surface and using a spacer arm can be critical and make the probe molecules available to interact with the target biomolecules,
- During immobilization procedure, it should be avoided for any deformation on the 3D-structures of the probe molecules (especially in the case of protein-based probes),
- None or minimum nonspecific interactions of the probe molecules with the biosensor surface will be desired, immobilization reaction should be only occur via specific functional groups (amino, carboxylic acid, aldehyde, epoxy, etc.) on the biosensor surface and probe molecules (Pişkin and Garipcan, 2004; Pişkin 2009).

1.4 Transducers

When a target biomolecule interacts with the immobilized probe molecules on a biosensor surface, depending on the application; a physical, chemical or biological change is observed. This change is converted to a measurable signal by a detecting device which is called, a transducer. These physical, chemical and biological changes can be pH, electro-active substance formation and/or consumption, heat, light, mass and viscosity. The magnitude of the measurable electrical signal is proportional with the concentration of the target biomolecules. Transducers are the key components of the biosensors. Transducers can be categorized according to the fundamentals of the physical or chemical changes as optical, electrochemical, acoustic (mass based) and thermal transducers (Vo-Dinh and Cullum, 2000).

Optical transducers are one of the most common types of transducers used in biosensors which are based on the measuring of the changes in light. After the interaction of the target molecules and probe molecules, a change in light intensity, polarization, phase, peak position, and angular wavelength will be observed and this change can be measured and converted to an electrical signal by optical transducers (Borisov and Wolfbeis, 2008). As mentioned above, optical transducers are widely used in biosensors; however electrochemical transducers are also very common due to simplicity of construction and low cost. A change at electrical potential, current, conductance and impedance can be measured and converted to an electrical signal by electrochemical transducers (Ronkainen, 2008). Also, Field Effect Transistors (FETs) based biosensors which use one type of electrochemical transducer become very promising when integrated with semi-conductor nanowires (Patolsky, 2007; He, 2010) and Carbon Nanotubes (Yang, 2007; Hu, 2010) due to their high selectivity and low detection levels. Acoustic transducers are a relatively new concept in biosensing applications that their principle is based on responding to mass accumulation on the biosensors surface. Piezoelectric crystals (Quartz Crystal Microbalance Biosensors) are the most common acoustic transducers which involve the generation of electric currents from a vibrating crystal. The frequency of vibration is affected by the mass of material adsorbed on its surface, which could be related to changes in a reaction (Cooper and Singleton, 2007; Karamollaoğlu, 2009). There are also thermal and micro cantilever based transducers are being used as detection devices which are based on a processes measuring the production or absorption of heat and the change in the resonant frequency of the cantilevers (Micrometer-sized cantilevers, started to be used for sensing purposes shortly after the invention of the atomic force microscope (AFM) in 1986), respectively (Ricciardi, 2010; Muhlen 2010).

1.5 Classification of biosensors

Biosensors can be classified according to their recognition part [enzyme, antibody (immunosensors), nucleic acid, tissue, microbial, polysaccharide, etc] or transducers (optical, electrochemical, acoustic, thermal, etc.) (Justino, 2010). Classification according to transducers seems much more logical then recognition part, because using only the biological component does not give much information about the biosensing device. Hence using both recognition part and transducer (even if using the sub type of the transducer) together is the best way to describe the type of biosensors, as an example Ellipsometry based DNA biosensors (Figure 4) (Demirel, 2008).

Table 3 gives an overview of biosensors which are classified according to transducer and recognition parts. A brief summary of the transducer fundamentals and literature will be discussed in this section. As mentioned, electrochemical transducers are also very common due to simplicity of construction and low cost (Ronkainen, 2008). Ion et al, have chosen organophosphate pesticides as target molecules and acetylcholinesterase as probe molecules and constructed voltammetric enzyme biosensors (Ion, 2010) where voltammetry refers to the measurement of current resulting from the application of a potential (Kissenger and Heineman, 1996; Ronkainen, 2008). In amperometry, changes in current generated by the electrochemical oxidation or reduction are monitored directly with time while a constant potential is maintained at the working electrode with respect to a reference electrode. It is the absence of a scanning potential that distinguishes amperometry from voltammetry (Barlett, 2008; Ronkainen, 2008).

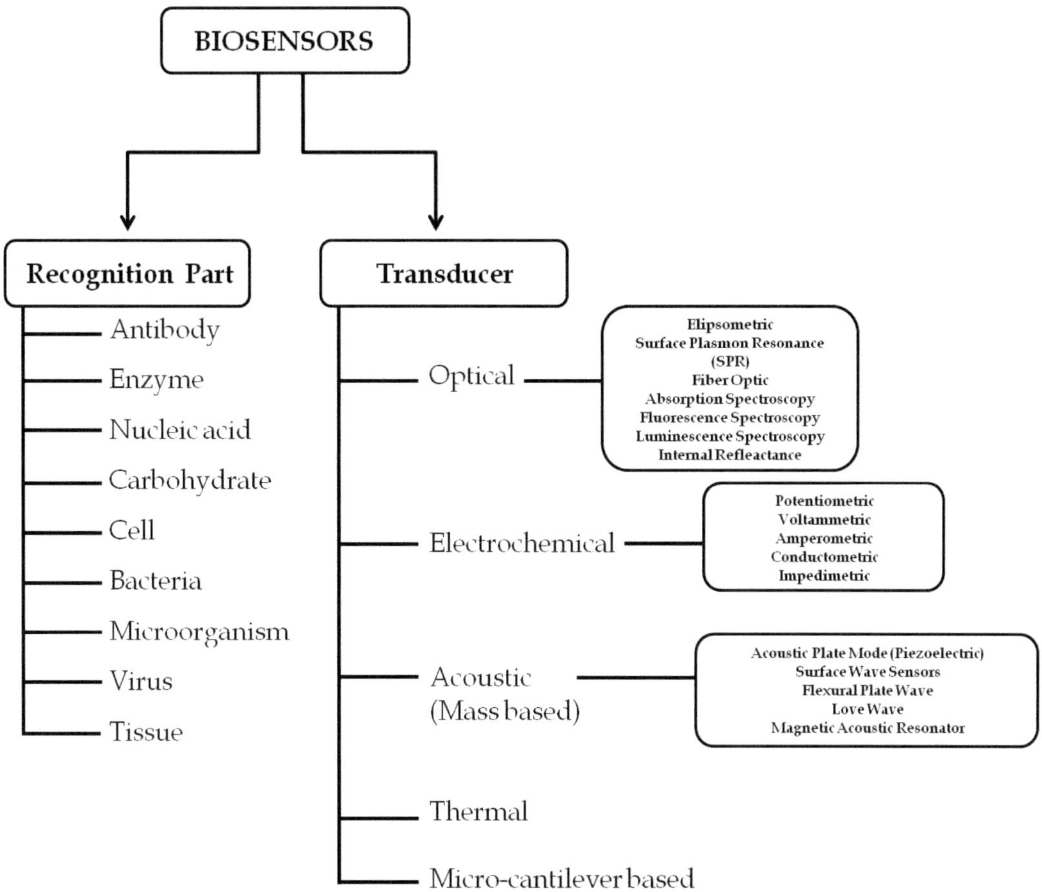

Fig. 4. The classification of biosensor according to recognition parts and transducers.

Salazar et al., have designed an amperometric enzyme biosensor for the detection of H_2O_2 in brain fluid by immobilizing Prussian blue on the biosensor surface (Salazar, 2010). Potentiometry is the branch of electroanalytical chemistry in which potential is measured under the conditions of no current flow (Eggins, 2002; Ronkainen, 2008). A DNA biosensor was developed by Wu et al (Wu, 2009) and a cell electrochemical biosensor for monitoring hydroquinone cytotoxicity on conductive polymer modified electrode surface by Wang et al (Wang, 2010) were two examples of potentiometric electrochemical biosensors. Impedimetry is an ac method that describes the response of an electrochemical cell to small amplitude sinusoidal voltage signal as a function of frequency (Prodmidis, 2010). An impedimeric electrochemical DNA biosensor was designed by Bonani et al., for detection of Single Nucleotide Polymorphism (Bonanni, 2010). Conductometric detection relys on the changes in the electrical conductivity of the the solution (Anh, 2004; Ronkainen, 2008). Korpan et al, used an conductometric enzyme biosensor for the detection of formaldeyhde by using formaldeyde dehydrogenase as probe molecule (Korpan, 2010). The quartz crystal microbalance, QCM, and is undoubtedly the oldest and the most recognized acoustic sensor. QCM technique involves the generation of electric currents from a vibrating crystal. The frequency of vibration is affected by the mass of material adsorbed on its surface, which could be related to changes in a reaction (Cooper and Singleton, 2007; Karamollaoğlu, 2009). In a study by Wang et al, a QCM immunosensor was developed for the detection of γ-Aminobutyric acid (Wang and Muthuswamy, 2008), in an another study QCM immunosensor for monitoring Aflatoxin B1 was developed by Wang et al (Wang and Gan, 2009a). Karamollaoğlu et al was constructed an interesting DNA QCM biosensor for the detection of Genetically Modified Organisms (GMOs) (Karamollaoğlu, 2009). Love wave sensors are acoustic devices that employ Love waves, propagating shear-horizontal acoustic waves that are confined to the surface region of a substrate by applying a thin overlayer that acts as a waveguide. In common with many other acoustic sensors, the principle of measurement is that the propagation of the acoustic wave through the solid medium of the sensor is affected by changes in the adjacent medium that contains the analyte of interest (Dinh, 2010). An acoustic Love wave immunosensor was developed by Saitakis at al, for the detection of major histocompatibility complex class I HLA-A2 proteins (Saitakis, 2008). Micrometer-sized cantilevers, started to be used for sensing purposes shortly after the invention of the atomic force microscope (AFM) in 1986. A change in the resonant frequency of the cantilevers is caused by a change in mass and/or stiffness of the cantilever, and this change can be measured (Ricciardi, 2010; Muhlen 2010). An microcantilever based immunosensor was designed by Muhlen at al, for the detection of Activated Leukocyte Adhesion Molecule (ALCAM) (Muhlen, 2010). In an another study by Ricciardi et al, immunosensor and receptor based microcantilever biosensors were developed for angiopoietin using angiopoitein antiboy and protein A probe molecules, respectively. (Ricciardi, 2010). Wang et al, have used imaging ellipsometry as an immunosensor in a model study to monitor the interaction of bovine serum albumin (BSA), fibrinogen and immunoglobulin- G with their antibodies (Wang and Jin, 2003). In another, study by Demirel et al, have shown that ellipsometry could also be used to monitor DNA hybridization (Demirel, 2008). Surface plasmon resonance (SPR) biosensors are also very well known optical biosensors which have been found many applications in this field. Milkani et al have constructed a SPR based DNA biosensor for oligonucleotide mismatch detection (Milkani, 2010) and Frasconi have shown that SPR based biosensors can also be used as a drug sensor (Frasconi, 2010). Fiber-optic biosensors (FOBS) use optical fibers as the transduction element, and rely exclusively on optical transduction mechanisms for detecting target biomolecules where as Kapoor et al, have detected trophic factor by immobilizing the Anti- signal transducer and activators of transcription 3 (STAT-3) antibody on an optical fiber (Kapoor, 2004). Not only biomolecules can be detected, but chemicals like 1-2 dichloroethane was sensed with enzyme immobilized fiber optic biosensors (Derek and Müller, 2006). A more detailed description on ellipsometry and SPR biosensors will be given in next section.

Transducer	Recognition Part	Target Molecules	Probe Molecules	Ref.
Optical/ Ellipsometry	Immunosensor	Bovine Serum Albumin (BSA) Fibrinogen Immunoglobulin-G	Anti-BSA Antibody Anti-Fibrinogen AntibodyAnti-Immunoglobulin-G Antibody	Wang, 2003
Optical/ Ellipsometry	DNA	Oligonucleotide	Complementary Oligonucleotide	Demirel, 2008
Optical/SPR	DNA	Oligonucleotide mis match detection	Complementary and non-complementary Oligonucleotide	Milkani, 2010
Optical/SPR	Drug	Neomycin, Kanamycin, Streptomycin Antibiotics	Imprinted Boronic acid functionalized Au nanoparticles	Frasconi, 2010
Optical/ Fiber Optic	Immunosensor	Trophic factor	Anti- signal transducer and activators of transcription 3 (STAT-3) antibody	Kapoor, 2004
Optical/ Fiber Optic	Enzyme	1,2 Dichloroethane	Haloalkane dehalogenase	Derek, 2006
Electrochemical/ Voltammetric	Enzyme	Organophosphate pesticides	Acetylcholinesterase	Ion, 2010
Electrochemical/ Amperometric	Enzyme	H_20_2 in brain fluids	Prussian Blue	Salazar, 2010
Electrochemical/ Potentiometric	DNA	DNA hybridization	Complementary DNA	Wu, 2009
Electrochemical/ Potentiometric	Cell	Hydroquinone cytotoxicity	Conductive polymers	Wang, 2010
Electrochemical/ Impedimetric	DNA	Single Nucleotide Polymorphism	Complementary Oligonucleotide	Boranni, 2010
Electrochemical/ Conductometric	Enzyme	Formaldehyde	Formaldehyde dehydrogenase	Korpan, 2010
Acoustic/ QCM Quartz Crystal Microbalance	Immunosensor	γ-Aminobutyric acid (GABA)	Anti-GABA Antibody	Wang, 2008

Transducer	Recognition Part	Target Molecules	Probe Molecules	Ref.
Acoustic/ QCM Quartz Crystal Microbalance	Immunosensor	Aflatoxin-B1	Anti- Aflatoxin-B1 Antibody	Wang, 2009a
Acoustic/QCM Quartz Crystal Microbalance	DNA	Genetically ModifiedMicroorganis ms (GDOs)	Complementary Oligonucleotide	Kara- mollaoğlu 2009
Acoustic/ Love Wave	Immunosensor	Major histocompatibility complex classI HLA-A2 proteins	Anti- HLA-A2 protein Antibody	Saitakis, 2008
Acoustic/LSAW Leaky Surface Acoustic Wave	Peptide-DNA	Human papilla virus	Complementary Oligonucleotide	Wang, 2009b
Microcantilever based	Immunosensor	Activated Leukocyte Cell Adhesion Molecule (ALCAM)	Anti-ALCAM Antibody	Muhlen, 2010
Microcantilever based	Immunosensor and Receptor	Angiopoietin-1	Anti-Angiopoeitin-1 Antibody Protein A	Ricciardi , 2010

Table 3. Overview of biosensors and transducers.

2. Ellipsometry based biosensors

In this chapter, we will specifically focus on the new generation biosensor systems based on ellipsometry for the detection of biological molecules (i.e. DNA and protein). Before discussing the sensor applications, it is useful to give some basic principles of ellipsometry for further understanding. Traditionally, ellipsometry is an optical and reflection-based technique which is mostly used for determining optical properties of materials and micro-structural parameters such as layer thicknesses, porosity and crystal orientation through ellipsometric data (Azzam and Bashara, 1972; Azzam and Bashara, 1977). In an ellipsometric measurement, fundamentally, the change in polarization, or more precisely, the polarization states after and before reflection which depend on surface properties are measured (Figure 5).
The incident light is not only reflected on the thin film surface but also penetrates into the outermost substrate material under the film surface. As a result, it reflects and refracts further at each interface and obtained ellipsometric data include information for investigated material within the penetration depth of the light (Poksinski and Arwin, 2006). In an ellipsometry, two experimental parameters (also called ellipsometric angles), ψ and Δ, defined as the relative amplitude and phase difference for p- and s-polarized light, before and after reflecting on sample surface are usually measured. They are defined by the ratio ρ

of the complex reflection coefficients R_p for light polarized parallel and R_s for perpendicular to the plane of incidence as,

$$\rho = \frac{Rp}{Rs} = \tan\psi \exp(i\Delta) \quad (1)$$

Ellipsometry does not provide the relevant informations about the structure and the investigated materials directly. In most cases, an appropriate optical model has to be established and nonlinear regression has to be applied to obtain reliable data for investigated materials. In the presence of biological molecules, further ellipsometric modeling is also needed because of their low refractive indexes and nanometer range thicknesses. More detailed informations for ellipsometry and data analysis can be found elsewhere (Poksinski and Arwin, 2006; Arwin, 2001; Arwin, 2000; Aspnes and Palik, 1985).
There are various types of ellipsometer for measuring two ellipsometric parameters, such as fixed polarizer, rotating polarizer, nulling and phase modulating. Ellipsometers can also utilize fixed wavelength or multiple wavelength light source. In monochromatic ellipsometers, typically a diode laser is used. Some versions utilize two or more diodes in order to expand measurement capability. More sophisticated ellipsometers utilize polychromatic light source and a monochromator for spectrophotometric measurements, which is more versatile than single wavelength ellipsometers. Additionally, angle modulation is necessary for an ellipsometric measurement. Angle modulation is performed either by automatic motorized controller or by manual adjustment. For angle modulation this two arm, light source and detector parts, are assembled on a goniometer, of which complexity also determine the type/price of the ellipsometer. Finally, if a monochromatic light source is used in the ellipsometer system, one may use an optical setup and preferably a CCD camera for monitoring and mapping of the surface, which system called as "imaging ellipsometer".

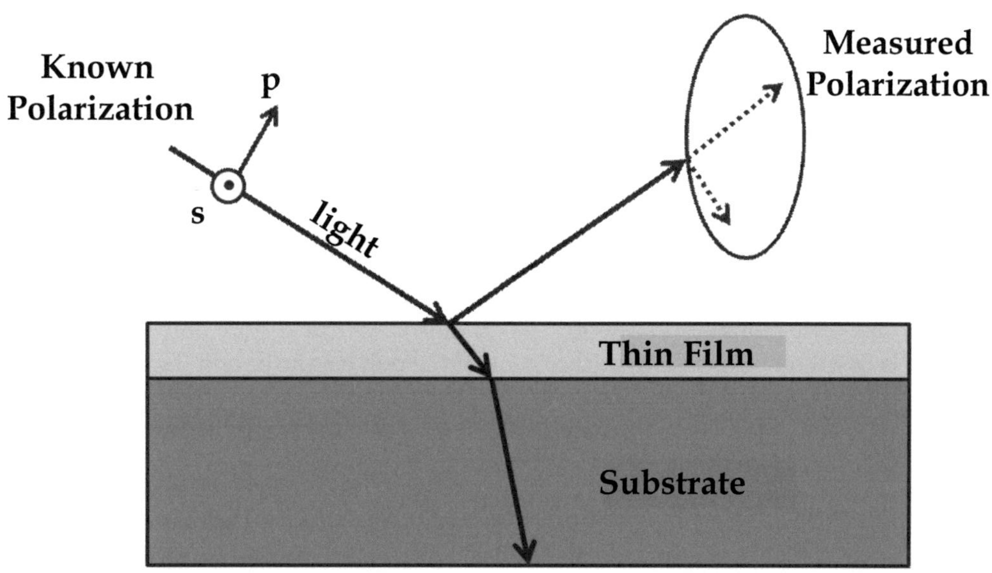

Fig. 5. The fundamental of ellipsometry.

Some of the advantages and disadvantages of ellipsometry are tabulated in Table 4. Ellipsometry has remarkable features such as high precision of the measurement, very high thickness sensitivity, fast measurement, wide application area, real-time observations, feedback control of processing and no contact with the investigated materials. Beyond these superiorities, it has also some drawbacks. The most important drawback of ellipsometry is the necessity of an optical model in data analysis. Another problem is the spot size of a light beam used for ellipsometry. Typically, they are several millimeters and caused to the low spatial resolution of the measurement. Characterization of small absorption coefficients is also rather difficult (Arwin, 2001).

Advantages	**Disadvantages**
- Non-destructive measurement	- Indirect analysis
- Large measurement range (nm to μm)	- optical model for data analysis
- Real Time monitoring	- low spatial resolution
- Fast Measurements	- Difficulty in the characterization of low absorption coefficients
- High Thickness sensitivity	
- No reference necessity	

Table 4. Some important advantages and disadvantages of Ellipsometry

Since the first application of ellipsometry to monitor antigen and antibody interactions (Rothen, 1945), ellipsometry based sensor systems have been attracted more interest for variety of applications due to the superior features, recently. The main reason of the using ellipsometry in sensor application is about reflection based technique and therefore, highly sensitive to changes taking place on the surface because of it only measures polarization change of light beam and blind to light scattering or absorption in the beam path (Arwin, 2001). As a result, any reference material is not needed like in many other techniques. Ellipsometry can also be used in explosive, corrosive or high temperature environments due to the non-electric technique. With well-collimated lasers it is possible to develop systems for remote sensing. Ellipsometry is a label-free technique and no markers are needed. In sensor applications, multi-sensing is also possible due to the each ellipsometric measurements provide two data which gives additional information (Arwin, 2001).

Basically, different sensing principles can be used in ellipsometry based biosensor systems. The simplest one is the based on affinity mechanism. In this case, a sensing layer, mostly antigen, aptamer or single stranded DNA, is formed on a substrate via chemical or physical modification methods. The changes in the Ψ and Δ depending on the interaction with target molecules are then monitored. Another possibility is to use a thin polymer layer. This princibles is based on the swelling or shrinking of the polymer layer and thereby to changes in the film optical properties and thickness. In porous materials, pore filling by adsorption on the inner walls of pores or capillary condensation are also useful sensing mechanisms (Arwin, 2001).

Beyond the conventional applications of ellipsometry, recently, total internal reflection ellipsometry (TIRE) is used for monitoring the ultrathin films in aqueous environments which is essential for biosensor and other *in situ* applications. A known technique, Surface Plasmon Resonance (SPR) is an evanescent wave technique which consists of a coupler to interact evanescent wave with surface-dielectric interface (Sutherland and Dahne, 1987). The detection system of a SPR sensor essentially consists of a monochromatic and p-polarized (i.e. electrical vector of light is parallel with the plane of incidence) light source, a glass prism (used as coupler), a thin metal film in contact with the base of the prism (plasmon source) and a photodetector. In order to couple an evanescent wave, a total internal reflection mechanism is used. A useful and widely used coupler configuration is Kretschmann configuration (Kretchmann and Raether, 1968). Obliquely incident light on the base of the prism exhibits total internal reflection for angles larger than the critical angle. This causes an evanescent field to extend from the prism into the metal film (Figure 6.). Intensity of this evanescent field logarithmically decays from the coupler surface into the next media. Generally, effective intensity of evanescent waves in Kretschmann configuration is maintained up to half of the wavelength of incident light (i.e. 250 nm for 500 nm - green - incident light).

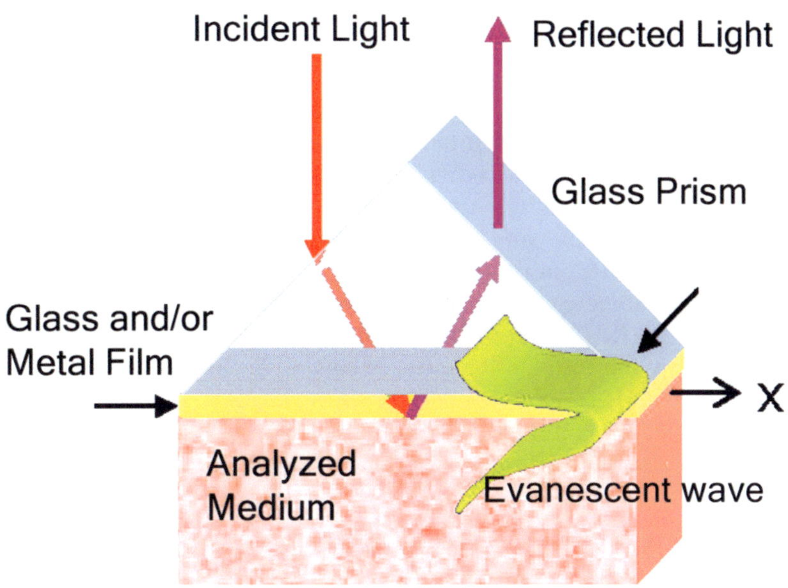

Fig. 6. The Principles of SPREE.

In conventional SPR systems, this evanescent field can couple to an electromagnetic surface wave, a surface plasmon at the metal/liquid interface. Coupling is achieved at a specific angle of incidence, or specific wavelength. In particular, reflected light intensity goes through a minimum at resonance angle for angle modulation. It should be noted that evanescent field is used for various applications such as intensity enhancement by nanoparticles. Plasmon resonance is highly sensitive to change in refractive index, or dielectric constant of the analyzed medium adjacent to the metal surface. Any change in the local refractive index and therefore the permittivity (ε) either by way of bulk index change or, as for instance in the case of biosensor, by the binding of an analyte to the surface plasmon polaritions active interface thus changes the SPR excitation conditions. If the ellipsometric parameters are measured with attenuated total reflection coupling of surface plasmon waves, this technique called as surface plasmon resonance ellipsometry (or surface plasmon resonance enhanced ellipsometry, SPREE) (Arwin, 2004). SPREE shows several

similarities to SPR techniques. A major and advantageous difference is that in SPR only the intensity information for reflection of p-polarized light is measured. However, in ellipsometry, properties of both p-polarized and s-polarized light are measured. The polarization state change at the probed interface (analyzed medium) is primarily due to the reflectance associated with total internal reflection (TIR) at a dielectric interface with composition change at interface. Particularly for biosensing, the binding of analytes to the surface cause thickness changes (t) and changes in complex refractive index ($N=n-i\kappa$) which are likely be determined by Δ and ψ parameters measured by ellipsometry (Venketosubbaro, 2006). Ellipsometry is more complex technique than SPR but has some advantages over SPR techniques. The s-polarization provides a reference for the overall intensity transmittance and with Δ parameters, phase information is also utilized, in addition to amplitude (intensity) information.
Another exciting application of evanescent waves with ellipsometry is Localized Surface Plasmon Resonance (LSPR) enhanced ellipsometry (Caglayan, 2009). In the first group of plasmonic ellipsometry sensors, the system based on propagating surface plasmons in thin metallic layers, so called Surface Plasmon Polaritions (SPPs). The second group utilizes metal nanostructures. Similarly to flat metal films, metal nanoparticles exhibit charge density oscillations giving rise to very intense and confined electromagnetic fields so called LSPRs. In this method, TIRE measurements are likely enhanced by immobilizing metal nanoparticles on sensor surface within useful depth of evanescent field. However, the basis of SPR-TIRE and LSPR-TIRE are generally confused with total internal reflection ellipsometry (TIRE). The TIRE, in principle, is based on spectroscopic (or more primitively single wavelength) ellipsometry performed under condition of total internal reflection. It should be noted that, in TIRE method which is proposed by Poksinski, there is no ultrathin metal film coated below the coupler, the latter is needed for SPR conditions (Poksinski and Arwin, 2006). Thus, for TIRE measurements there is no need a plasmon coupling at the coupler-analyzed medium interface. TIRE configuration is similar to Kretschmann configuration and utilizes TIR. This configuration is suitable for monitoring and analysis of thin semitransparent films, even they are in aqueous media, which is common for biosensor applications.

3. Conclusion

Ellipsometry techniques have several unique advantages for biosensor applications not only it does not require labeling of molecules as do fluorescence measurements, but also it can provide high precision of the measurement, very high thickness sensitivity, fast measurement, wide application area, real-time observations, feedback control of processing and no contact with the investigated materials etc. Beyond the current applications of ellipsometry in immunoassays and DNA sequencing, we believe that if multiplexing reading, in-field using, affordable price and scale up protocols could be solved for ellipsometric detections, these systems would be useful for next generation sensor systems. Moreover, integrated ellipsometry techniques, such as optical fibers, AFM and waveguide systems, will be appeared the future researching priorities. The integration with MEMS (or NENS) system to enable the multiplexing and miniaturizing will be another trend for ellipsometry based biosensors. Multifunctional biosensor which not only sense refractive index variation or phase shift but also other critical parameters, such as molecule structure and orientation change, will also attracting more and more interests.

4. Acknowledgment

We would like to gratefully acknowledge the Gazi University for the financial support (Project No. 05/2010-83 and 05/2010-17).

5. References

Anh, T. M., Dzyadevych, S. V., Van, M. C., Renault, N. J., Duc, C. N. & Chovelon, J. M. (2004). Conductometric tyrosinase biosensor for the detection of diuron, atrazine and its main metabolites. *Talanta*, 63, 365-370.

Arwin, H. (2000). Ellipsometry on thin organic layers of biological interest: characterization and applications. *Thin Solid Films*, 377-378, 48-56.

Arwin, H. (2001). Is ellipsometry suitable for sensor applications? *Sensors and Actuators A*, 92, 43-51.

Arwin, H., Poksinski, M. & Johansen, K. (2004). Enhancement in ellipsometric thin film sensitivity near surface plasmon resonance conditions. *Physica Status Solidi A*, 205, 817-820.

Aspnes, D. E. & Palik, E. D. (1985). Handbook of optical constants of solids. p.89. Academic Press, Orlando, ISBN: 0125444206 9780125444200.

Azzam, R. M. A. & Bashara, N. M. (1972). Generalized ellipsometry for surfaces with directional preference: application to diffraction gratings. *Journal of The Optical Society of America*, 62, 1521-1523.

Azzam, R. M. A. & Bashara, N. M. (1977). Ellipsometry and polarized light. p. 153-267. North-Holland, Netherland, ISBN: 0444870164.

Bartlett, P.N. (2008). Bioelectrochemistry fundamentals, experimental techniques and applications, p. 39-86. John Wiley & Sons, West Sussex, England, ISBN: 978-0-470-84364-2.

Bergveld, P. (1970). Development of an ion sensitive solid-state for neurophysiological measurements. *IEEE Trans.*, BME–17, 70.

Bonanni, Alessandra., Pumera, Martin. & Miyahara, Yuji. (2010). Rapid, sensitive, and label-free impedimetric detection of a single-nucleotide polymorphism correlated to kidney disease. *Analytical Chemistry*, 82, 3772–3779.

Caglayan, M. O., Demirel, G., Sayar, F., Otman, B., Celen, B. & Piskin, E. (2006). Stepwise formation approach to improve ellipsometric biosensor response. *Nanomedicine*, 5, 152-161.

Clark, L. C. & Lyons, C. (1962). Electrode systems for continuous monitoring in cardiovascular surgery. *Annals of the New York Academy of Sciences*, 102, 1, 29-45.

Demirel, G., Çağlayan, O. M., Garipcan, B., Pişkin, E. (2008). A novel DNA biosensor based on ellipsometry. *Surface Science*, 602, 952–959.

Derek, C. W., Cord, M. & Kenneth, R. F. (2006). Development of a fiber optic enzymatic biosensor for 1,2-dichloroethane. *Biotechnology Letter*, 28, 883–887.

Dinh, D. H., Pascal, E., Vellutini, L., Bennetau, B., Rebière, D., Dejous, C., Moynet, D., Belin, C. & Pillot, J. P. (2010). Novel optimized biofunctional surfaces for Love mode surface acoustic wave based immunosensors, *Sensors and Actuators B*, 146, 289–296.

D'Orazio, P. (2003). Biosensors in clinical chemistry. *Clinica Chimica Acta*, 334, 41–69.

Eggins, B. R. (2002). *Chemical sensors and biosensors*. 12-26. John Wiley & Sons, West Sussex, England, ISBN: 0471899143.

Frasconi, M., Tel-Vered, R., Riskin, M., & Willlner, I. (2010). Surface plasmon resonance analysis of antibiotics using imprinted boronic acid-functionalized Au nanoparticle composites. *Analytical Chemistry*, 82, 2512–2519.

Fraser, D. M. (1994). Glucose biosensors—The sweet smell of success. *Medical Device Technology*, 5, 9, 44–47.

Ghoshal, S., Mitra, D., Roy, S., & Majumder, D. D. (2010). Biosensors and biochips for nanomedical applications: A review. *Sensors & Transducers Journal,* 113, 2, 1-17.

Guilbault, G. G. & Montalvo, J. (1969). A urea specific enzyme electrode. *Journal of American Chemical Society,* 91, 2164.

He, Y., Fan, C. & Lee, S. T. (2010). Silicon nanostructures for bioapplications. *Nano Today,* 5, 282—295.

Hernandez, F. J. (2008). Design of biosensors exploiting conformational changes in biomolecules. *PhD Thesis,* Universitat Rovira I Virgili, 18.

Higson, S. P. J., Reddy, S. M, & Vadgama P. M.. (1994). Glucose enzyme and other biosensors: Evolution of a technology. *Engineering Science and Education Journal*, 3, 1, 41–48.

Hu, P., Zhang, J., Li, L., Wang, Z., O'Neill, W. & Estrela, P. (2010). Carbon nanostructure-based field-effect transistors for label-free chemical/biological sensors, *Sensors,* 10, 5133-5159.

Hughes, W. S., (1922). The potential difference between glass and electrolytes in contact with water. *Journal of American Chemical Society,* 44, 2860-2866.

Ion, C. A., Ion, I., Celetu, A., Gherase, D., Moldavan, A. C., Iosub, R. & Dinescu, A. (2010). Acetylcholinesterase voltammetric biosensors based on carbon nanostructurechitosan composite material for organophosphate pesticides. *Materials Science and Engineering C,* 30, 817–821.

Justino, I. L. C., Rocha-Santos, A. T. & Duarte, C. A. (2010). Review of analytical figures of merit of sensors and biosensors in clinical applications. *Trends in Analytical Chemistry*, 29, 10, 1172—1183.

Kapoor, R., Kaur, N., Nishanth, T. E., Halvorsen, W. S., Bergey, J. E. & Prasad, N. P. (2004). Detection of trophic factor activated signaling molecules in cells by a compact fiber-optic sensor. *Biosensors and Bioelectronics*, 20, 345–349.

Karamollaoğlu, I., Öktem, A. H. & Mutlu, M. (2009) QCM-based DNA biosensor for detection of genetically modified organisms (GMOs), *Biochemical Engineering Journal*, 44, 142–150.

Kissinger, P. T. & Heineman, W. R. (1996). Laboratory techniques in electroanalytical chemistry, p. 51-125. Marcel Dekker Inc, New York, NY, USA. ISBN: 0824794451.

Korpan, I. Y., Soldatkin, O. O., Sosoyska, F. O., Klepach, M. H., Csöregi, E., Vocanson, F., Jaffrezic-Renault, N. & Gonchar, V. M. (2010). Formaldehyde-sensitive conductometric sensors based on commercial and recombinant formaldehyde dehydrogenase. *Microchim Acta*, 170, 337–344.

Kretschmann, E. & Raether, H. (1968). Radiative decay of non-radiative surface plasmons excited by light. *Naturforsch*, 23, 2135-2136.

Liedberg, B., Nylander, C. & Lundstrom, I. (1983). Surface plasmon resonance for gas detection and biosensing. *Sensors Actuators A*, 4, 299-304.

Mannelli, I., Minunni, M., Tombelli, S. & Mascini, M. (2003). Quartz crystal microbalance (QCM) affinity biosensor for genetically modified organisms (GMOs) detection. *Biosensors and Bioelectronics*, 18, 129-140.

Martín-Palma, J. R., Manso, M. & Torres-Costa, V. (2009). Optical biosensors based on semiconductor nanostructures. *Sensors*, 9, 5149-5172.

Milkani, E., Morai, S., Lambert, R. C. & McGimpsey, W. G. (2010). Detection of oligonucleotide systematic mismatches with a surface plasmon resonance sensor. *Biosensors and Bioelectronics*, 25, 1217–1220.

Mohanty, P. S. & Kougianos, E. (2006). Biosensors: A tutorial review, IEEE Potentials, March-April, 35-40.

Opitz, N. & Lübbers, D. W. (1975). A new fast responding optical method to measure PCO_2 in gases and solutions. *European Journal of Physiology*, 355, R210.

Patolsky, F., Timko, P. B., Zheng, G. & Lieber, M. C. (2007). Nanowire–based nanoelectronic devices in the life sciences. *MRS Bulletin*, 32, 142-149.

Peterson, J. I., Goldstein, S. R. & Fitzgerald, R. V. (1980). Fiber optic pH probe for physiological use. *Analytical Chemistry*, 52, 864-869.

Piskin, E., Garipcan, B., & Duman, M., Probe Immobilization Techniques in Array Technologies, Detection of Highly Dangerous Pathogens, Kostic, Tanja., Butaye, Patrick., & Schrenzel Jacques. 83-102. Wiley-VCH, ISBN: 978-3-527-32275-6.

Piskin, E. & Garipcan, B. (2004). Biochips: focusing on surfaces and surface modification. *Advances in Experimental Medicine and Biology*, 553, 149-166.

Poksinski, M. & Arwin, H. (2006). Proteins at solid-liquid interfaces. p. 105-120. Springer-Verlag, Berlin, ISBN: 13978354032657.

Prodromidis, I. M. (2010). Impedimetric immunosensors-A review. *Electrochimica Acta*, 55, 4227–4233.

Ricciardi, C., Fiorilli, S., Bianco, S., Canavese, G., Ferrante, I., Digregorio, G., Marasso, L. S., Napione, L. & Bussolino, F. (2010). Development of microcantilever-based biosensor array to detect Angiopoietin-1, a marker of tumor angiogenesis. *Biosensors and Bioelectronics*, 25, 1193–1198.

Ronkainen, J. N., Halsall, H. B. & Heineman, R. W. (2010). Electrochemical biosensors. *Chemical Society Reviews*, 39, 1747–1763.

Rothen, A. (1945). The ellipsometer: an apparatus to measure thickness of thin surface films. *Review of Scientific Instruments*, 16, 26-30.

Saitakis, M., Tsortos, A., Gizeli, E. (2010). Probing the interaction of a membrane receptor with a surface-attached ligand using whole cells on acoustic biosensors. *Biosensors and Bioelectronics*, 25, 1688–1693.

Salazar, P., Martin, M., Roche, R., O'Neill, R. D. & González-Mora, J. L. (2010). Prussian blue-modified microelectrodes for selective transduction in enzyme-based amperometric microbiosensors for in vivo neurochemical monitoring. *Electrochimica Acta*, 55, 6476–6484.

Schultz, J. S., Mansouri., S. & Goldstein, I. J. (1982). Affinity sensor: a new technique for developing implantable sensors for glucose and other metabolites. *Diabetes Care*, 5, 3, 245-253.

Sergiy, B. M. & Otto, W. S. (2008). Optical biosensors. *Chemical Review*, 108, 423-461.

Sharmat, A. & Rogers, R. K. (1994). Biosensors. *Measurement Science and Technology*, 5 461-472.

Shu-Fen, C., Win-Lin, H., Jing-Min, H. & Chien-Yuan, C. (2002). Development of an immunosensor for human ferritin, a nonspecific tumor marker, based on a quartz crystal microbalance. *Analytica Chimica Acta*, 453, 181–189.

Su, X. L. & Li, Y. (2004). A self-assembled monolayer-based piezoelectric immunosensor for rapid detection of Escherichia coli O157:H7. *Biosensors and Bioelectronics*, 19, 563–574.

Turner, A. B. F., Karube, I. & Wilson, G. S. (1987). Biosensors: fundamentals and applications. p. 655, Oxford University Press, New York, ISBN:0198547242.

Tang, A. X. J., Pravda, M., Guilbault, G. G., Piletsky, S. & Turner, A. P. F. (2002). Immunosensor for okadaic acid using quartz crystal microbalance. *Analytica Chimica Acta*, 471, 33- 40.

Vo-Dinh, T. & Cullum, B. (2000). Biosensors and biochips: advances in biological and medical diagnostics. *Fresenius Journal of Analytical Chemistry*, 366, 540–551.

Venketosubbaro, S. N., Beaudry, Y., Zhao, R. & Chipman, R. (2006). Evanescent-imaging ellipsometry based microarray reader. *Journal of Biomedical Optics*, 11, 1-9.

Von Muhlen, G. M., Brault, D. N., Knudsen, M. S., Jiang, S. & Manalis, R. S. (2010). Label-free biomarker sensing in undiluted serum with suspended microchannel resonators. *Analytical Chemistry*, 82, 1905-1910.

Wang, H. Zhan., & Jin, G. (2003). A label-free multisensing immunosensor based on imaging ellipsometry. *Analytical Chemistry*, 75, 6119-6123.

Wang, T. & Muthuswamy, J. (2008). Immunosensor for detection of inhibitory neurotransmitter γ-aminobutyric acid using quartz crystal microbalance. *Analytical Chemistry*, 80, 8576–8582.

Wang, L. & Gan, X. X. (2009a). Biomolecule-functionalized magnetic nanoparticles for flow-through quartz crystal microbalance immunoassay of aflatoxin B1. *Bioprocess Biosystem Engineering*, 32, 109–116.

Wang, Y., Chen, M., Zhang, L., Ding, Y., Luo, Y., Xu, Q., Shi, J., Cao, L. & Fu, W. (2009b). Rapid detection of human papilloma virus using a novel leaky surface acoustic wave peptide nucleic acid biosensor. *Biosensors and Bioelectronics*, 24, 3455–3460

Wang, Y., Chen, Q. & Zeng, X. (2010). Potentiometric biosensor for studying hydroquinone cytotoxicity in vitro. *Biosensors and Bioelectronics*, 25, 1356–1362.

Wu, J., Chumbimuni-Torres, Y. K., Galik, M., Thammakhet, C., Haake, A. D. & Wang, J. (2009). Potentiometric detection of DNA hybridization using enzyme-induced metallization and a silver ion selective electrode. *Analytical Chemistry*, 81, 10007–10012.

Yogeswaran, U. & Chen, S. M. (2008). A review on the electrochemical sensors and biosensors composed of nanowires as sensing material. *Sensors*, 8, 290-313.

10

Mathematical Modeling of Biosensors: Enzyme-substrate Interaction and Biomolecular Interaction

A. Meena, A. Eswari and L. Rajendran
Department of Mathematics, The Madura College, Madurai- 625011, Tamilnadu, India

1. Introduction

The vast majority of chemical transformations inside cells are carried out by proteins called enzymes. Enzymes accelerate the rate of chemical reactions (both forward and backward) without being consumed in the process and tend to be very selective, with a particular enzyme accelerating only a specific reaction. Enzymes are important in regulating biological processes, for example, as activators or inhibitors in a reaction. To understand the role of enzyme kinetics, the researcher has to study the rates of reactions, the temporal behaviours of the various reactants and the conditions which influence the enzyme kinetics. Introduction with a mathematical bent is given in the books by (Rubinow, 1975), (Murray, 1989), (Segel, 1980) and (Roberts, 1977). Biosensors are analytical devices made up of a combination of a specific biological element, usually an enzyme that recognizes a specific analyte (substrate) and the transducer that translates the biorecognition event into an electrical signal (Tuner et al., 1987; Scheller et al., 1992). Amperometric biosensors may utilize one, two, three or multi enzymes (Kulys, 1981). The classical example of mono enzyme biosensor might be the biosensor that contains membrane with immobilized glucose oxidase. The glucose oxidase specifically oxidizes glucose to hydrogen peroxide that is determined ampero-metrically on platinum electrode (Kulys, 1981). The amperometric biosensors measure the current that arises on a working electrode by direct electrochemical oxidation or reduction of the biochemical reaction product. The current is proportionate to the concentration of the target analyte. The biosensors are widely used in clinical diagnostics, environment monitoring, food analysis and drug detection because they are reliable, highly sensitive and relatively cheap. However, amperometric biosensors possess a number of serious drawbacks.

One of the main reasons that restrict the wider use of the biosensors is the relatively short linear range of the calibration curve (Nakamura et al., 2003). Another serious drawback is the instability of bio-molecules. These problems can be partially solved by the application of an additional outer perforated membrane (Tuner et al., 1987; Scheller et al., 1992; Wollenberger et al., 1997). To improve the productivity and efficiency of a biosensor design as well as to optimize the biosensor configuration a model of the real biosensor should be built (Amatore et al., 2006; Stamatin et al., 2006). Modeling of a biosensor with a perforated membrane has been already performed by Schulmeister and Pfeiffer (Schulmeister et al., 1993). The proposed one-dimensional-in-space (1-D) mathematical model does not take into consideration the geometry of the membrane perforation and it also includes effective diffusion coefficients. The quantitative value of diffusion coefficients is limited, for one dimensional model (Schulmeister et al., 1993). Recently, a two-dimensional-in-space (2-D) mathematical model has been proposed taking into consideration the perforation geometry (Baronas et al., 2006; Baronas, 2007). However, a simulation of the biosensor action based on the 2-D model is much more time-consuming than a simulation based on the corresponding 1-D model. This is especially important when investigating numerically peculiarities of the biosensor response in wide ranges of catalytically and geometrical parameters. The multifold numerical simulation of the biosensor response based on the 1-D model is much more efficient than the simulation based on the corresponding 2-D model.

1.1 Biomolecule model and Enzyme substrate interaction

A Biomolecular interaction is a central element in understanding disease mechanisms and is essential for devising safe and effective drugs. Optical biosensors usually involves biomolecular interaction, they are very often used for affinity relation test.

The catalytic event that converts substrate to product involves the formation of a transition state. The complex, when substrate S and enzyme E combine, is called the enzyme substrate complex C, etc. Enzyme interfaced biosensors involve enzyme-substrate interaction, two significant applications are: monitoring of human glucose and monitoring biochemical reaction at a single cell level. Normally, we have two ways to set up experiments for biosensors: free enzyme model and immobilized enzyme model. The mathematical and computational model for these two models are very similar, at here we are going to investigate the free enzyme model. Recently (Yupeng Liu et al., 2008) investigate the problem of optimizing biosensor design using an interdisciplinary approach which combines mathematical and computational modeling with electrochemistry and biochemistry techniques. Yupeng Liu and Qi Wang developed a model for enzyme-substrate interaction and a model for biomolecular interaction and derived the free enzyme model for the non-steady state using simulation result. To my knowledge no rigorous analytical solutions of free enzyme model under steady-state conditions for all values of reaction/diffusion parameters γ_E, γ_S and γ_P have been reported. The purpose of this communication is to derive asymptotic approximate expressions for the substrate, product, enzyme and enzyme-substrate concentrations using variational iteration method for all values of dimensionless reaction diffusion parameters γ_S,γ_E and γ_P .

2. Mathematical formulation and solution of the problem

The enzyme kinetics in biochemical systems have traditionally been modelled by ordinary differential equations which are based solely on reactions without spatial dependence of the various concentrations. The model for an enzyme action, first elucidated by Michaelis and Menten suggested the binding of free enzyme to the reactant forming an enzyme-reactant complex. This complex undergoes a transformation, releasing the product and free enzyme. The free enzyme is then available for another round of binding to a new reactant. Traditionally, the reactant molecule that binds to the enzyme is termed the substrate S, and the mechanism is often written as:

$$E + S \underset{k-1}{\overset{k_1}{\leftrightarrow}} C \xrightarrow{kcat} E + P \tag{1}$$

This mechanism illustrates the binding of substrate S and release of product P. E is the free enzyme and C is the enzyme-substrate complex. k_1, k_{-1} and k_{cat} denote the rates of reaction of these three processes. Note that substrate binding is reversible but product release is not. The concentration of the reactants in the equation (1) is denoted by lower case letters

$$s = [S]\,,\ e = [E],\quad c = [C],\quad p = [P] \tag{2}$$

The law of mass action leads to the system of following non-linear reaction equations [15]

$$D_S \frac{d^2 s}{dx^2} - k_1 es + k_{-1} c \ = 0 \tag{3}$$

$$D_e \frac{d^2 e}{dx^2} - k_1 es + (k_{-1} + k_{cat})c \ = 0 \tag{4}$$

$$D_c \frac{d^2 c}{dx^2} + k_1 es - (k_{-1} + k_{cat})c \ = 0 \tag{5}$$

$$D_p \frac{d^2 p}{dx^2} + k_{cat} c = 0 \tag{6}$$

where k_1 is the forward rate of complex formation and k_{-1} is the backward rate constant. All species are considered to have an equal diffusion coefficient ($D_s = D_p = D_e = D_c = D$). The boundary conditions are

$$\frac{ds}{dx} = 0,\ \frac{dp}{dx} = 0,\ \frac{de}{dx} = 0,\ \frac{dc}{dx} = 0, \text{ when } t > 0 \text{ and } x = 0 \tag{7}$$

$$s = s_0,\ \frac{dp}{dx} = 0,\ \frac{de}{dx} = 0,\ \frac{dc}{dx} = 0, \text{ when } t > 0 \text{ and } x = L \tag{8}$$

Adding Eqs. (4) and (5), we get,

$$d^2 e / dx^2 \ + d^2 c / dx^2 = 0 \tag{9}$$

Using the boundary conditions and from the law of mass conservation, we obtain

$$e = e_0 - c \tag{10}$$

With this, the system of ordinary differential equations reduce to only two, for s and c, namely

$$D \frac{d^2 s}{dx^2} - k_1 e_0 s + (k_1 s + k_{-1})c = 0 \tag{11}$$

$$D\frac{d^2c}{dx^2}+k_1e_0s-(k_1s+k_{-1}+k_{cat})c=0 \tag{12}$$

By introducing the following parameters

$$u=\frac{s}{s_0},\ v=\frac{c}{e_0},\ w=\frac{p}{e_0},\ X=\frac{x}{L},\ \gamma_S=\frac{k_{-1}L^2}{D},\ \gamma_E=\frac{k_1s_0L^2}{D},\ \gamma_P=\frac{k_{cat}L^2}{D} \tag{13}$$

Now the given two differential equations reduce to the following dimensionless form (Yupeng Liu et al., 2008):

$$\frac{d^2u}{dX^2}-\gamma_Eu+(\gamma_S+\gamma_Eu)v=0 \tag{14}$$

$$\frac{d^2v}{dX^2}+\gamma_Eu-(\gamma_S+\gamma_Eu+\gamma_P)v=0 \tag{15}$$

$$\frac{d^2w}{dX^2}+\gamma_Pv=0 \tag{16}$$

where γ_E, γ_S and γ_P are the dimensionless reaction diffusion parameters. These equations must obey the following boundary conditions:

$$\frac{du}{dX}=0,\ \frac{dv}{dX}=0,\ \frac{dw}{dX}=0 \text{ when } X=0 \tag{17}$$

$$u=1,\ \frac{dv}{dX}=0,\ \frac{dw}{dX}=0 \text{ when } X=1 \tag{18}$$

3. Variational iteration method

The variational iteration method (He, 2007, 1999; Momani et al., 2000; Abdou et al., 2005) has been extensively worked out over a number of years by numerous authors. variational iteration method has been favourably applied to various kinds of nonlinear problems (Abdou et al., 2005; He et al., 2006). The main property of the method is in its flexibility and ability to solve nonlinear equations (Abdou et al., 2005). Recently (Rahamathunissa and Rajendran, 2008) and (Senthamarai and Rajendran, 2010) implemented variational iteration method to give approximate and analytical solutions of nonlinear reaction diffusion equations containing a nonlinear term related to Michaelis-Menten kinetic of the enzymatic reaction. More recently (Manimozhi et al., 2010) solved the non-linear partial differential equations in the action of biosensor at mixed enzyme kinetics using variational iteration method. (Loghambal and Rajendran, 2010) applied the method for an enzyme electrode where electron transfer is accomplished by a mediator reacting in a homogeneous solution. (Eswari and Rajendran, 2010) solved the coupled non linear diffusion equations analytically for the transport and kinetics of electrodes and reactant in the layer of modified electrode. Besides its mathematical importance and its links to other branches of mathematics, it is widely used in all ramifications of modern sciences. In this method the solution procedure is very simple by means of Variational theory and only few iterations lead to high accurate solution which are valid for the whole solution domain. The basic concept of Variational iteration method is given in Appendix A.

4. Analytical solution of the concentration and current using Variational iteration method

Using variational iteration method (He, 2007, 1999) (refer Appendix A), the concentration of the substrate and the enzyme-substrate are

$$\begin{aligned} u(X) = 1 - a + 0.5\gamma_E\left[1 + ab - b - (\gamma_S/\gamma_E)b - a\right]X^2 + 0.083\gamma_E\left[2a - 1 - ab - (\gamma_S/\gamma_E)\right]X^4 \\ + 0.1\gamma_E\left[1 - a + (\gamma_S/\gamma_E)\right]X^5 - 0.03\gamma_E\left[1 + (\gamma_S/\gamma_E)\right]X^6 + 0.05a\gamma_E X^7 - 0.02a\gamma_E X^8 \end{aligned} \quad (14)$$

$$\begin{aligned} v(X) = b + 0.5\gamma_E\left[b - ab + ((\gamma_S/\gamma_E) + (\gamma_P/\gamma_E))b - 1 + a\right]X^2 + \\ +0.083\gamma_E\begin{bmatrix}((\gamma_S/\gamma_E) + (\gamma_P/\gamma_E)) \\ -2a + 1 + ab\end{bmatrix}X^4 \\ +0.1\gamma_E\left[a - 1 - ((\gamma_S/\gamma_E) + (\gamma_P/\gamma_E))\right]X^5 + \\ +0.03\gamma_E\left[1 + ((\gamma_S/\gamma_E) + (\gamma_P/\gamma_E))\right]X^6 \\ -0.05a\gamma_E X^7 + 0.02a\gamma_E X^8 \end{aligned} \quad (15)$$

where

$$a = \frac{7}{5}\left[\frac{\gamma_S + \gamma_P - 29\gamma_E + 30b(\gamma_S + \gamma_P + \gamma_E)}{\gamma_E(28b - 27)}\right] \quad (16)$$

$$\begin{aligned} b = \frac{1}{2}\left[(2100(\gamma_S + \gamma_E) + 10500\gamma_P)\gamma_E\right]^{-1} \\ \text{x}\begin{bmatrix} 9820\gamma_E\gamma_P - 25200\gamma_S + 2000\gamma_S\gamma_E + 4100\gamma_E^2 + 25200\gamma_P - 20(1595160\gamma_E\gamma_S\gamma_P + \\ 3175200\ (\gamma_E\gamma_S + \gamma_E\gamma_P + \gamma_P\gamma_S) + 1587600(\gamma_E^2 + \gamma_P^2 + \gamma_S^2). + 3175200\gamma_P\gamma_S \\ +112564\gamma_E^2\gamma_P\gamma_S - 786240\gamma_E^2\gamma_P + 1325520\gamma_E\gamma_P^2 + 276676\gamma_E^2\gamma_P^2 - 1676\gamma_E^3\gamma_P \\ +269640\gamma_E\gamma_S^2 + 274680\gamma_S\gamma_E^2 + 11449\gamma_E^2\gamma_S^2 + 428\gamma_E^3\gamma_S + 5040\gamma_E^3 + 4\gamma_E^4)^{1/2} \end{bmatrix} \end{aligned} \quad (17)$$

Equations (14), (15), (16) and (17) represent the analytical expressions of the substrate $u(X)$ and enzyme-substrate $v(X)$ concentration. From the equation (15), we can also obtain the dimensionless concentration of enzyme

$$\begin{aligned} e(X) &= e(t)/e_0 = 1 - v(\tau) \\ &= 1 - b + 0.5\gamma_E\left[b - ab + ((\gamma_S/\gamma_E) + (\gamma_P/\gamma_E))b - 1 + a\right]X^2 + 0.083\gamma_E\begin{bmatrix}((\gamma_S/\gamma_E) + (\gamma_P/\gamma_E)) \\ -2a + 1 + ab\end{bmatrix}X^4 \\ &+ 0.1\gamma_E\left[a - 1 - ((\gamma_S/\gamma_E) + (\gamma_P/\gamma_E))\right]X^5 + 0.03\gamma_E\left[1 + ((\gamma_S/\gamma_E) + (\gamma_P/\gamma_E))\right]X^6 \\ &- 0.05a\gamma_E X^7 + 0.02a\gamma_E X^8 \end{aligned} \quad (18)$$

The dimensionless concentration of the product is given by

$$w(X) = 0.0335X^2 + 0.0167\gamma_P X^2 - 0.0333X^2(X-1)^2 - 0.0667X^3 - 0.0833\gamma_P X^4 + 0.0333X^4 + 0.1000\gamma_P X^5 - 0.00033\gamma_P X^6 \tag{19}$$

5. Numerical simulation

The non-linear differential equations (14-16) are solved by numerical methods. The function pdex4 in SCILAB software which is a function of solving the boundary value problems for differential equation is used to solve this equation. Its numerical solution is compared with variational iteration method in Figure 1*a*-c, 2*a*-c, 3 and it gives a satisfactory result for various values of γ_E, γ_S and γ_P. The SCILAB program is also given in Appendix C.

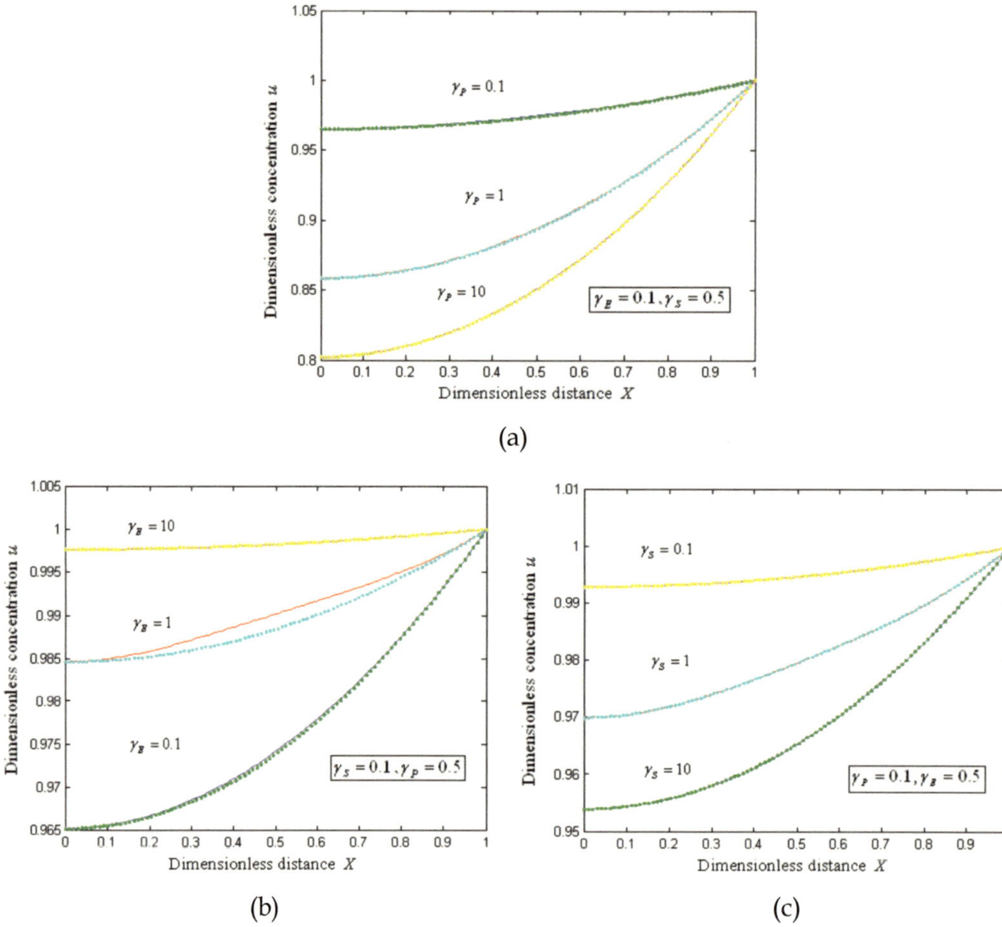

Fig. 1. Profile of the normalized concentrations of the substrate *u*, were computed using equation (14) for various values of γ_S, γ_E and γ_P when the reaction/diffusion parameters (a) $\gamma_E = 0.1,\ \gamma_S = 0.5$ (b) $\gamma_S = 0.1,\ \gamma_P = 0.5$ (c) $\gamma_P = 0.1,\ \gamma_E = 0.5$. The key to the graph: (__) represents the Eq. (14) and (.) represents the numerical results.

6. Results and discussion

Equations (14) and (15) are the new and simple analytical expressions of normalized concentration profiles for the substrate $u(X)$ and enzyme-substrate $v(X)$. The approximate solutions of second order differential equations describing the transport and kinetics of the enzyme and the substrate in the diffusion layer of the electrode are derived.
Fig. 1a-c, we present the series of normalized concentration profile for a substrate $u(X)$ as a function of the reaction/diffusion parameters γ_E, γ_S and γ_P. From this figure1a, it is inferred that, the value of $u \approx 1$ for all small values of γ_P, γ_E. Also the value of u increases when γ_P decreases when γ_E and γ_S small. Similarly, in fig1b, it is evident that the value of concentration increases when γ_E increases for small values of γ_S and γ_P. Also value of concentration of substrate increases when γ_S decreases (Refer fig1c).

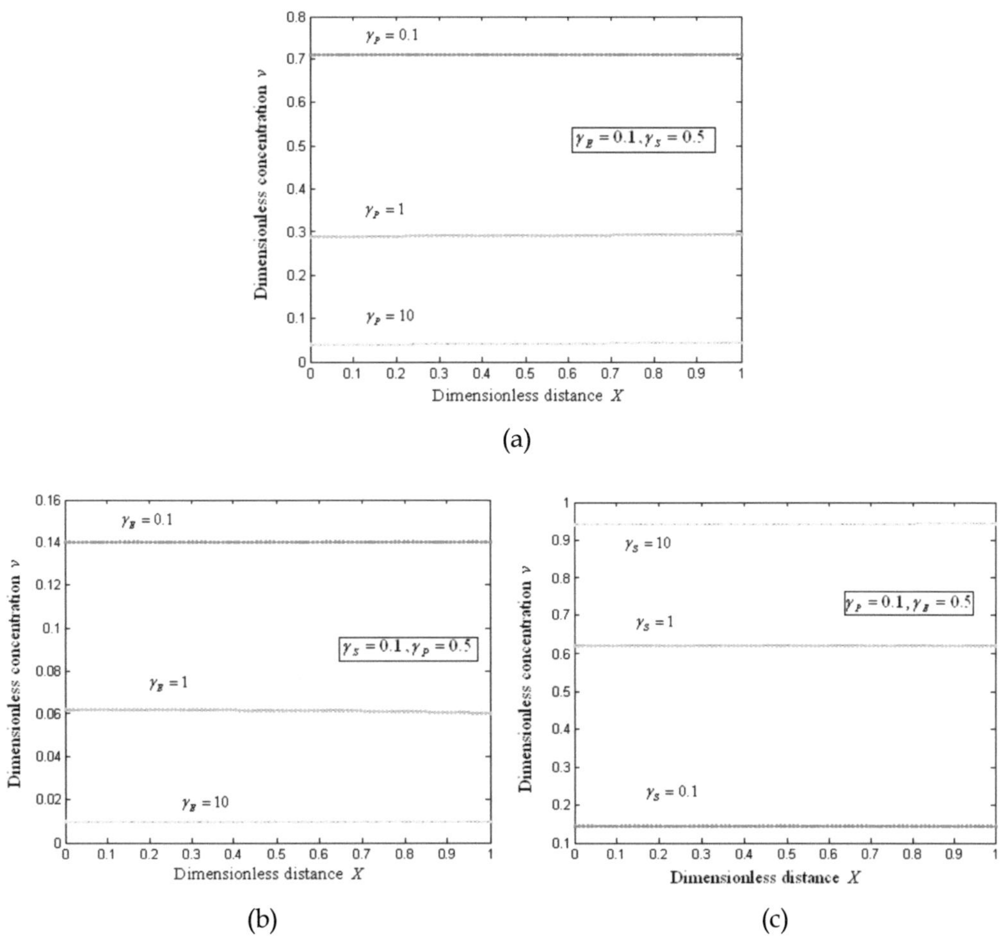

Fig. 2. Profile of the normalized enzyme-substrate complex v, were computed using equation (15) for various values of γ_S, γ_E and γ_P when the reaction/diffusion parameters (a) $\gamma_E = 0.1,\ \gamma_S = 0.5$ (b) $\gamma_S = 0.1,\ \gamma_P = 0.5$ (c) $\gamma_P = 0.1,\ \gamma_E = 0.5$. The key to the graph: (__) represents the Eq. (14) and (…) represents the numerical results.

Fig. 2*a-c* shows the normalized steady-state concentration of enzyme-substrate $v(X)$ versus the dimensionless distance X for various values of dimensionless parameters γ_E, γ_S and γ_P. From these figure, it is obvious that the values of the concentration $v(X)$ reaches the constant value for various values of γ_E, γ_S and γ_P. In figure 2*a-b*, the value of enzyme-substrate $v(X)$ decreases when the value of γ_P and γ_E are increases for $\gamma_E = 0.1, \gamma_S = 0.5$ and $\gamma_S = 0.1, \gamma_P = 0.5$. In Fig. 2*c*, the concentration $v(X)$ increases when γ_S increases.

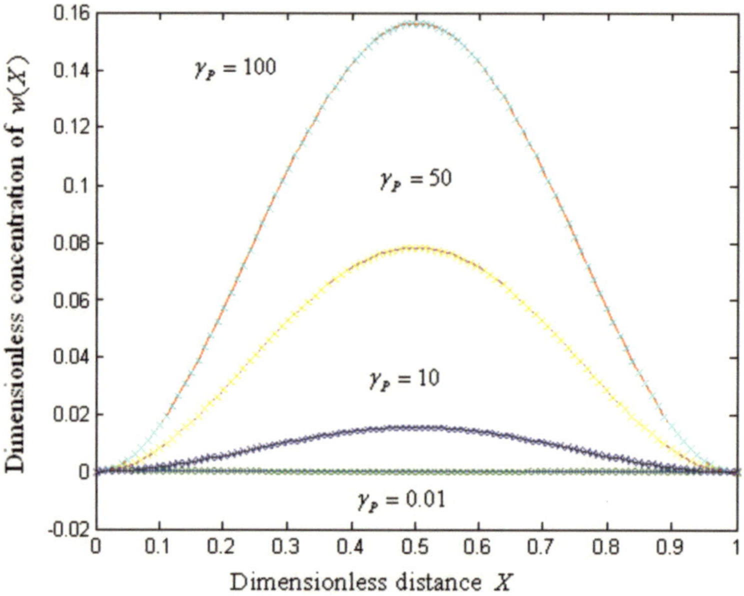

Fig. 3. Profile of the normalized concentration of product w for various values of γ_P. The curves are plotted using equation (19). The key to the graph: (__) represents the Eq. (19) and (++) represents the numerical results.

Fig. 3 shows the dimensionless concentration profile of product $w(X)$ using Eq. (20) for all various values of γ_P. Thus it is concluded that there is a simultaneous increase in the values of the concentration of $w(X)$ as well as in γ_P. Also the value of concentration is equal to zero when $X = 0$ and 1. From the Fig. 3, it is also inferred that, the concentration $w(X)$ increases slowly and then reaches the maximum value at $X = 0.5$ and then decreases slowly. In the Figs. 1*a-c*, 2*a-c* and 3 our steady-state analytical results (Eqs. (14, 15, 19)) are compared with simulation program for various values of γ_E, γ_S and γ_P.

In Fig. 4*a-b*, we present the dimensionless concentration profile for an enzyme as a function of dimensionless parameters for various values of γ_E, γ_S and γ_P. From this figure, it is confirmed that the value of the concentration increases when the value of γ_P increases for various values of γ_E and γ_S.

7. Conclusion

In this paper, the coupled time-independent nonlinear reaction/diffusion equations have been formulated and solved analytically using variational iteration method. A simple, straight forward and a new method of estimating the concentrations of substrate, product, enzyme-substrate complex and enzyme are derived. we have presented analytical expressions corresponding to the concentration of the substrate and concentration of the enzyme-substrate complex and enzyme interms of the parameters, γ_E, γ_S and γ_P. Moreover, we have also reported a simple and closed form of an analytical expression for the steady state concentration of the product for different values of the parameter γ_P. This solution procedure can be easily extended to all kinds of system of coupled non-linear equations with various complex boundary conditions in enzyme-substrate reaction diffusion processes (Baronas et al., 2008).

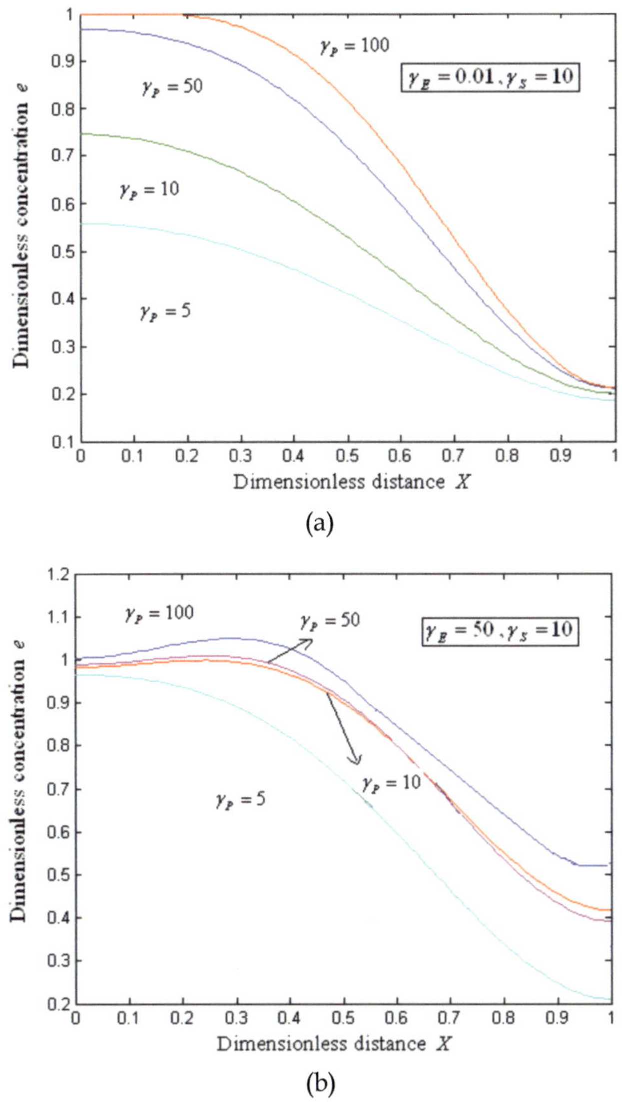

Fig. 4. Profile of the normalized concentration enzyme e for various values of γ_S, γ_E and γ_P when the reaction/diffusion parameters (a) $\gamma_E = 0.01$, $\gamma_S = 10$ (b) $\gamma_E = 50$, $\gamma_S = 10$. The curves are plotted using equations (18).

Appendix A

In this appendix, we derive the general solution of non-linear reaction eqns. (14) to (16) using He's variational iteration method. To illustrate the basic concepts of variational iteration method (VIM), we consider the following non-linear partial differential equation (Scheller et al., 1992; Wollenberger et al., 1997; Nakamura et al., 2003; Amatore et al., 2006)

$$L[u(x)] + N[u(x)] = g(x) \tag{A1}$$

where L is a linear operator, N is a nonlinear operator, and $g(x)$ is a given continuous function. According to the variational iteration method, we can construct a correct functional as follows [10]

$$u_{n+1}(X) = u_n(X) + \int_0^x \lambda \left[L[u_n(\xi)] + N[\tilde{u}_n(\xi)] - g(\xi) \right] d\xi \tag{A2}$$

where λ is a general Lagrange multiplier which can be identified optimally via variational theory, u_n is the nth approximate solution, and $\tilde{u}_n$ denotes a restricted variation, i.e., $\delta\tilde{u}_n = 0$. In this method, a trail function (an initial solution) is chosen which satisfies given boundary conditions. Using above variation iteration method we can write the correction functional of eqn. (10) as follows

$$u_{n+1}(X) = u_n(X) + \int_0^x \lambda_1 \left[u''_n(\xi) - \gamma_E \widetilde{u_n(\xi)} + \gamma_S \widetilde{v_n(\xi)} + \widetilde{\gamma_E u_n(\xi) v_n(\xi)} \right] d\xi \tag{A3}$$

$$v_{n+1}(X) = v_n(X) + \int_0^x \lambda_2 \left[v''_n(\xi) + \gamma_E \widetilde{u_n(\xi)} - \gamma_S \widetilde{v_n(\xi)} + \widetilde{\gamma_E u_n(\xi) v_n(\xi)} \right] d\xi \tag{A4}$$

$$w_{n+1}(X) = w_n(X) + \int_0^x \lambda_3 \left[w''_n(\xi) + \gamma_P \widetilde{v_n(\xi)} \right] d\xi \tag{A5}$$

Taking variation with respect to the independent variable u_n and v_n, we get

$$\delta u_{n+1}(X) = \delta u_n(X) + \delta \int_0^x \lambda_1 \left[u''_n(\xi) - \gamma_E \widetilde{u_n(\xi)} + \gamma_S \widetilde{v_n(\xi)} + \widetilde{\gamma_E u_n(\xi) v_n(\xi)} \right] d\xi \tag{A6}$$

$$\delta v_{n+1}(X) = \delta v_n(X) + \delta \int_0^x \lambda_2 \left[v''_n(\xi) + \gamma_E \widetilde{u_n(\xi)} - \gamma_S \widetilde{v_n(\xi)} + \widetilde{\gamma_E u_n(\xi) v_n(\xi)} \right] d\xi \tag{A7}$$

$$\delta w_{n+1}(X) = \delta w_n(X) + \delta \int_0^x \lambda_3 \left[w''_n(\xi) + \gamma_P \widetilde{v_n(\xi)} \right] d\xi \tag{A8}$$

where λ_1 and λ_2 are general Lagrangian multipliers, u_0 and v_0 are initial approximations or trial functions, $\overbrace{\tilde{u}_n(\xi)}$, $\overbrace{\tilde{v}_n(\xi)}$ and $\overbrace{u_n(\xi)v_n(\xi)}^{\sim}$ are considered as restricted variations i.e $\delta\tilde{u}_n = 0$, $\delta\tilde{v}_n = 0$ and $\delta\tilde{u}_n\tilde{v}_n = 0$. Making the above correction functional (A5) and (A6) stationary, noticing that $\delta u_n(0) = 0$, $\delta v_n(0) = 0$ and $\delta u_n(0)v_n(0) = 0$.

$$\delta u_n:\ 1 + \lambda_1(\xi)\big|_{\xi=\tau} = 0\,,\ \delta v_n{:}1 + \lambda_2(\xi)\big|_{\xi=\tau} = 0 \tag{A9}$$

$$\delta u_n: -\lambda_1'(\xi) + \varepsilon\lambda(\xi)\ \big|_{\xi=\tau},\ \delta v_n: -\lambda_2'(\xi) + k\lambda(\xi)\big|_{\xi=\xi} = 0 \tag{A10}$$

The above equations are called Lagrange-Euler equations. The Lagrange multipliers, can be identified as

$$\lambda_1(\xi) = \lambda_2(\xi) = \lambda_3(\xi) = \xi - X \tag{A11}$$

Substituting the Lagrangian multipliers and $n = 0$ in the iteration formula (eqns. (A3) and (A4)) we obtain,

$$u_1(X) = u_0(X) + \int_0^x (\xi - X)\left[u''_0(\xi) - \gamma_E u_0(\xi) + \gamma_S v_0(\xi) + \gamma_E u_0(\xi)v_0(\xi)\right] d\xi \tag{A12}$$

$$v_1(X) = v_0(X) + \int_0^x (\xi - X)\left[v''_0(\xi) + \gamma_E u_0(\xi) - (\gamma_S + \gamma_P)v_0(\xi) + \gamma_E u_0(\xi)v_0(\xi)\right] d\xi \tag{A13}$$

$$w_1(X) = w_0(X) + \int_0^x (\xi - X)\left[w''_0(\xi) + \gamma_P v_0(\xi)\right] d\xi \tag{A14}$$

Assuming that its initial approximate solution which satisfies the boundary condition (11) have the form

$$\begin{aligned} u_0(x) &= 1 - a + aX^2 \\ v_0(x) &= b + X^2(X-1)^2 \\ w_0(x) &= b_1X^2(X-1)^2 \end{aligned} \tag{A15}$$

By the iteration formula (A10) and (A11) we obtain the equations (14) and (15) in the text.

Appendix B

function pdex4

```
m = 0;
x = linspace(0,1);
t = linspace(0,1000);
sol = pdepe(m,@pdex4pde,@pdex4ic,@pdex4bc,x,t);
u1 = sol(:,:,1);
```

```
u2 = sol(:,:,2);
u3 = sol(:,:,3);
figure
plot(x,u1(end,:))
title('Solution at t = 2')
xlabel('Distance x')
ylabel('u1(x,2)')
figure
plot(x,u2(end,:))
title('Solution at t = 2')
xlabel('Distance x')
ylabel('u2(x,2)')
figure
plot(x,u3(end,:))
title('Solution at t = 2')
xlabel('Distance x')
ylabel('u3(x,2)')
% --------------------------------------------------------------
function [c,f,s] = pdex4pde(x,t,u,DuDx)
c = [1; 1; 1];
f = [1; 1; 1] .* DuDx;
l=1;
m=1;
n=10;
F=-m*u(1)+(l+m*u(1))*u(2);
F1=m*u(1)-(l+m*u(1)+n)*u(2);
F2=n*u(2);
s=[F; F1; F2];
% --------------------------------------------------------------
function u0 = pdex4ic(x);
u0 = [1; 0; 1];
% --------------------------------------------------------------
function [pl,ql,pr,qr] = pdex4bc(xl,ul,xr,ur,t)
pl = [0; 0; 0];
ql = [1; 1; 1];
pr = [ur(1)-1; 0; 0];
qr = [0; 1; 1];
```

Appendix C

Nomenclature and units

Symbol	Meaning	Usual dimension
s	Concentration of the substrate	mole cm $^{-3}$
c	Concentration of the enzyme-substrate complex	mole cm $^{-3}$

e	Concentration of the enzyme	mole cm $^{-3}$
p	Concentration of the product	mole cm $^{-3}$
s_0	Bulk concentration of the substrate	mole cm $^{-3}$
e_0	Bulk concentration of the enzyme	mole cm $^{-3}$
D_S	Diffusion coefficient of the substrate	cm ^{2} sec $^{-1}$
D_C	Diffusion coefficient of the enzyme-substrate complex	cm ^{2} sec $^{-1}$
D_e	Diffusion coefficient of the enzyme	cm ^{2} sec $^{-1}$
D_P	Diffusion coefficient of the product	cm ^{2} sec $^{-1}$
D	Diffusion coefficient	cm ^{2} sec $^{-1}$
x	Distance	cm
L	Length	cm
k_1	The forward rate of complex formation.	sec $^{-1}$
k_{-1}	The backward rate constant	sec $^{-1}$
k_{cat}	The rate of catalytic reaction	sec $^{-1}$
u	Dimensionless concentration of substrate	None
v	Dimensionless concentration of enzyme-substrate complex	None
w	Dimensionless concentration of product	None
γ_E ,γ_S,γ_P	Dimensionless reaction/diffusion parameter	None

8. References

[1] Amatore C.; Oleinick A.; Svir I.; da Mota N; Thouin L. (2006). Theoretical Modeling and Optimization of the Detection Performance: a New Concept for Electrochemical Detection of Proteins in Microfluidic Channels, Nonlinear Analysis modeling and control. Vol.11, pp. 345-365

[2] Abdou MA.; Soliman AA.(2005). New applications of variational iteration method, Physica D: Nonlinear Phenomena, Vol. 211, No. 1-2, pp.1-8

[3] Baronas R.; Kulys J.; Ivanauskas F. (2006). Computational Modelling of Biosensors with Perforated and Selective Membranes, Journal of Mathematical Chemistry. Vol. 39, No. 2, pp. 345–362.

[4] Baronas R. (2007). Numerical simulation of biochemical behaviour of biosensors with perforated membrane, I. Zelinka, Z. Oplatkova, A. Orsoni (Eds.), 214–217.

[5] Baronas R.; kulys J. (2008). Modelling Amperometric Biosensors Based on Chemically Modified Electrodes. Sensors, Vol. 8, pp. 4800.

[6] Eswari A.; Rajendran L. (2010). Application of variational iteration method and electron transfer mediator/catalyst composites in modified electrodes, Natural Science, Vol.2, No.6, pp. 612-625.

[7] He JH. (2007). Variational iteration method-some recent results and new Interpretations. Journal of Computational Applied Mathematics, Vol. 207, pp. 3.

[8] He JH. (1999). Variational iteration method- a kind of non-linear analytical Technique: some examples, International Journal of Nonlinear Mechanisms. Vol. 34, No. 4, pp. 699.

[9] He J H.; Wu XH. (2006). Construction of solitary solution and compacton-like solution by variational iteration method. Chaos Solitons Fractals, Vol. 29, No. 1, pp. 108.

[10] Loghambal S.; L. Rajendran. (2010). Analysis of Amperometric Enzyme electrodes in the homogeneous mediated mechanism using Variational iteration method. International Journal of Electrochemical Science, Vol. 5, pp. 327-343.

[11] Kulys J. (1981). Analytical systems based on immobilized enzymes, Mokslas, Vilnius, p. 200, Russia.

[12] Murray JD. (1989). Mathematical Biology, 109, Springer Verlag.

[13] Momani S.; Abuasad S. (2000). Application of He's variational iteration method to Helmholtz equation. Chaos Solitons fractals, Vol. 27, No. 5, pp. 1119.

[14] Manimozhi P.; Subbiah A.; L. Rajendran. (2010). Solution of steady-state substrate concentration in the action of biosensor response at mixed enzyme kinetics. Sensors and Actuators B. Vol. 147, pp. 290-297

[15] Nakamura H.; Karube I. (2003). Current research activity in biosensors Anal. Bioanal. Chem. Vol. 377, pp. 446–468.

[16] Rubinow, SI. (1975). Introduction to Mathematical Biology, Newyork, Wiley.

[17] Roberts, DV. (1977). Enzyme kinetics. Cambridge, Cambridge University press.

[18] Rajendran L.; Rahamathunissa G. (2008). The Application of He's variational iteration method to nonlinear boundary value problems in enzyme-substrate reaction diffusion processes: Part 1.The steady-state amperometric response, Journal of Mathematical Chemistry, Vol. 44, pp. 849-861.

[19] Segel LA. (1980). Mathematical models in molecular and cellular Biology, Cambridge University press.

[20] Scheller F.; Schubert F. (1992). Biosensors, vol. 7, Elsevier, Amsterdam.

[21] Stamatin I.; Berlic C.; Vaseashta A. (2006). On the computer-aided modelling of analyte–receptor interactions for an efficient ensor design. Thin Solid Films, Vol. 495, pp. 312-315.

[22] Schulmeister T.;Pfeiffer D. (1993). Mathematical modelling of amperometric enzyme electrodes with perforated membranes, Biosensors and Bioelectronics,Vol. 8, pp. 75–79.

[23] Senthamarai R.; Rajendran L. (2010). System of coupled non-linear reaction diffusion processes at conducting polymer ultramicroelectrodes, Electrochimica Acta, Vol. 55, pp. 3223-3235.

[24] Turner APF.; Karube I.; Wilson GS. (1987). Biosensors: Fundamentals and Applications, Oxford University Press, Oxford.

[25] Wollenberger U.; Lisdat F.; Scheller FW. (1997). Frontiers in Biosensorics 2, Practical Applications, Birkhauser Verlag, Basel.

[26] Yupeng Liu; Qi Wang. (2008). Proceedings of the 4th WSEAS International Conference on Cellular and MOLECULAR BIOLOGY, BIOPHYSICS and BIOENGINEERING (BIO '08'), Proceedings of the 2nd WSEAS International Conference on COMPUTATIONAL CHEMISTRY (COMPUCHEM '08') eds. Stamatios kartalopoulos, Andris Buikis, Nikos Mastorakis, Luigi Viadareanu, p. 38.

11

Numerical Analysis and Simulation of Fluidics in Nanogap-Embedded Separated Double-Gate Field Effect Transistor for Biosensor

Maesoon Im[1,*] and Yang-Kyu Choi[2]
[1]*University of Michigan, Ann Arbor*
[2]*Korea Advanced Institute of Science and Technology (KAIST)*
[1]*United States of America*
[2]*Republic of Korea*

1. Introduction

For detection of diverse biomolecules, researchers have developed a wide variety of biosensors, using, for example, fluorescent imaging (Oh et al., 2005), piezoelectric properties (Yang et al., 2006), nano-mechanical properties (Fritz et al., 2000), electrochemical properties (Drummond et al., 2003), conducting properties (Reed et al., 1997; Cui et al., 2001; Patolsky et al., 2007), and so on. Although some of these techniques show ultra-high sensitivity, they require labelling processes for analytes or bulky and expensive equipment for measurement. Label-free detection without necessity of an external apparatus is important in point-of-care testing (POCT) devices (Kost et al., 1999; St-Louis 2000; Tierney et al., 2000), which enable fast and easy on-site detection of biomolecules for health monitoring.

In terms of integration with peripheral CMOS circuitry for realizing a more affordable POCT system, biosensors based on a field-effect transistor (FET) scheme have notable advantages (Schöning & Poghossian, 2002). Hence, FET-based biosensors have been actively studied (Begveld, 2003; Schöning & Poghossian, 2002) since the first report of an ion-sensitive solid-state device (Begveld, 1970). In most FET-based biosensor devices (Schöning & Poghossian, 2002; Kim et al., 2006; Sakata et al., 2007), variation of threshold voltage on a scale of tens of mV was obtained in the detection of biomolecules, and the fabrication process was not fully compatible with conventional CMOS technology. Recently, our group reported a new concept for a FET-based biosensor utilizing dielectric constant change inside nanogaps embedded in a FET device (Im, H. et al., 2007).

In our previous work (Im et al., 2011), we successfully detected the antigen and antibody of avian influenza (AI), which can cause human fatality. Avian influenza antigen (AIa) and antibody (anti-AI) showed a large degree of signal change (*i.e.* a high signal-to-noise ratio) with a fabricated nanogap-embedded separated double-gate field effect transistor (hereafter referred to as "nanogap-DGFET"), shown in Fig. 1 (Im et al., 2011). Fig. 2 shows scanning

* M. Im was with the Department of Electrical Engineering, KAIST, Daejeon 305-701, Republic of Korea. He is now with the Department of Electrical Engineering and Computer Science, University of Michigan, Ann Arbor, MI 48109 USA.

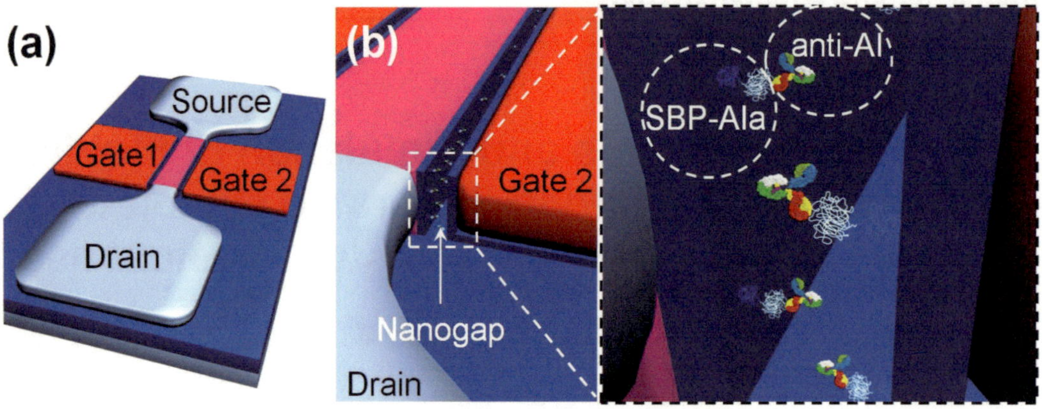

Fig. 1. (a) Schematic diagram of a nanogap-embedded separated double-gate field effect transistor (nanogap-DGFET). (b) Magnified view of the nanogap near the drain and gate 2. Dotted box conceptually shows immobilized avian influenza antigen conjugated with silica binding protein (SBP-AIa) (Gu et al., 2009) and avian influenza antibody (anti-AI) inside the nanogap. Reprinted with permission from (Im et al., 2011) © Copyright 2011 IEEE.

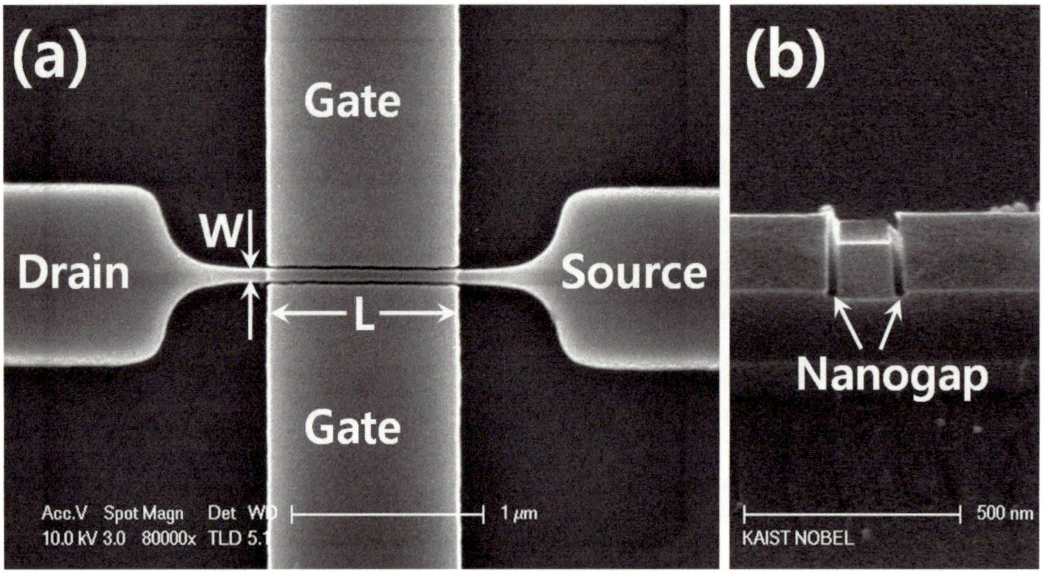

Fig. 2. Scanning electron microscopy images of the fabricated device. (a) Top view of nanogap-embedded seperated double-gate filed effect transistor. The width (W) and the length (L) of this transistor are 150 nm and 1μm, respectively. (b) Cross-sectional view of a nanogap in test pattern. The width of nanogap is 30 nm.

electron microscopy (SEM) images of the fabricated nanogap-DGFET device. Large signal change is a desirable feature in a handheld size apparatus for POCT application (Tierney et al., 2000). Moreover, the electrical signal of the nanogap-DGFET biosensor does not depend on the Debye length (Siu & Cobbold, 1979), which is a function of the ionic strength of the sample solution (Schöning & Poghossian, 2002). This is because the nanogap-DGFET devices are measured in a quasi-dry state, and the detection principle is based on the permittivity change rather than charge effect of biomolecules. On the other hand, the electrical signal of FET biosensors changes significantly with the ionic concentration of the sample solution (Stern et al., 2007). For general POCT application, it is not easy to control the ionic concentration precisely with any real human sample, such as blood serum, urine, or saliva. Therefore, this feature of Debye-screening-free sensing is another advantage of the nanogap-DGFET, together with moderate sensitivity and large signal change (Im, H. et al., 2007; Gu et al., 2009).

In studies of nanogap-based biosensors (Haguet et al., 2004; Yi et al., 2005), it is very important to understand the fluidics in the nanogap (Brinkmann et al., 2006) because most biomolecules are immobilized and coupled inside a nanogap immersed in a water-based solution. In order to examine the fluidic characteristics in the nanogap of nanogap-DGFET devices, theoretical calculations and numerical simulations are performed in this study. Three-dimensional simulation results dynamically visualize the process of liquid filling the nanogap.

2. Fluidics in the nanogap of the nanogap-DGFET

The mechanism by which the nanogap is filled with the sample solution is an important aspect of the nanogap-DGFET. In the wet etching process of the nanogap, the liquid fills the nanogap by chemically-assisted injection of liquid, *i.e.* the nanogap is filled with a diluted fluoric acid solution while being etched (Im et al., 2011). The SEM image in Fig. 2(b) clearly shows the resultant nanogap structure from wet etching. However, in real experiments for the detection of biomolecules, the sample solution containing analytes should enter the nanogap for immobilization of biomolecules such as DNAs, antibodies, antigens, and so on. If the nanogap cannot be wetted by the sample solution, the nanogap-DGFET cannot be used as a biosensor. Filling the nanogap with the solution presents challenges, as the gap is initially filled with air before applying the sample solution and is in a nanometre dimension, and thus the surface tension of the liquid has significant effects.

As performed in a previous work (Brinkmann et al., 2006), it is worthwhile to estimate the fluidic properties inside the nanogap of the nanogap-DGFET with a simplified model and theoretical calculations before three-dimensional simulation results are discussed.

2.1 Capillary pressure in the nanogap

The liquid is expected to be injected by capillary force rather than by gravity into the nanogap of the nanogap-DGFET owing to the nanometre scale of the gap. Therefore, capillary pressure inside the nanogap is an essential aspect of the fluidic behaviour of the sample solution that will be loaded in the nanogap. This section discusses modelling and computation of the capillary pressure inside the nanogap.

Fig. 3 is a schematic illustration showing notations of symbols used in the modelling and calculation. The sample solution in the nanogap can be modelled as shown in Fig. 4. It is apparent that the entire region except for the nanogap will become wet immediately after introduction of the sample liquid on top of the device, because the exposed surface of the nanogap-DGFET is a native oxide, which is hydrophilic. If the nanogap is initially filled with air, we can assume that two sidewalls (*i.e.* gate side and channel side) in the nanogap are native oxide and the other two sidewalls are water applied to the system. Therefore, the capillary pressure (ΔP) inside the nanogap (shown in Fig. 4) with the sample solution of water can be expressed as the following equation (Im, M. et al., 2007):

$$\Delta P = \frac{2}{G}\gamma \cos\theta_{SiO_2} + \frac{2}{L}\gamma \cos\theta_{water} \quad (1)$$

where γ is the liquid surface tension of the sample solution, θ_{SiO2} is the contact angle of silicon dioxide, θ_{water} is the contact angle of water (full wetting), G is the width of the nanogap, and L is the length of the nanogap, as shown in Fig. 3 and Fig. 4. For the sample solution of water, capillary pressures estimated with Equation (1) are plotted in Fig. 5. In the case of nanogap length of 1μm, the capillary pressure (ΔP) is about 3.38MPa.

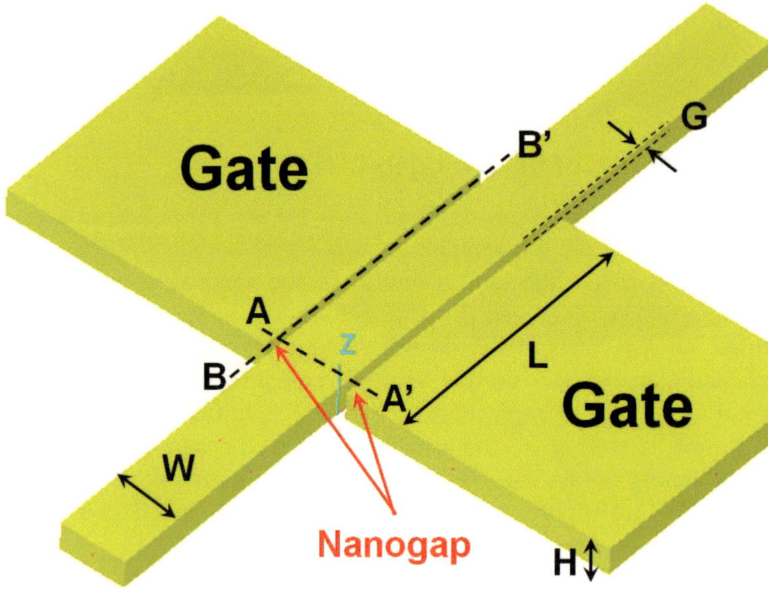

Fig. 3. Schematic diagram showing notation of symbols used in calculations and simulations.

2.2 Theoretical calculation of the nanogap filling depth

The sample solution continues to enter the nanogap if the capillary force is larger than the pressure difference between the pressure inside the nanogap (P_x) and the atmospheric pressure (P_0=0.1MPa). In the worst case where air cannot be evacuated from the nanogap, the pressure inside the nanogap will be increased by compressed air and will have a relationship delineated as follows:

$$P_x = P_0 \times \frac{H}{H - x} \quad (2)$$

where H is the height of the nanogap. Since the water meniscus will stop at the condition of $\Delta P=P_x-P_0$, we can calculate that the water meniscus can move to x=97nm of a 100-nm-deep nanogap (H=100nm) even in the worst case, *i.e.* the nanogap is filled with compressed air.

This calculation result means that capillary pressure is sufficient to deliver the water to the bottom surface of the nanogap. We will confirm this result with three-dimensional simulations in the following section.

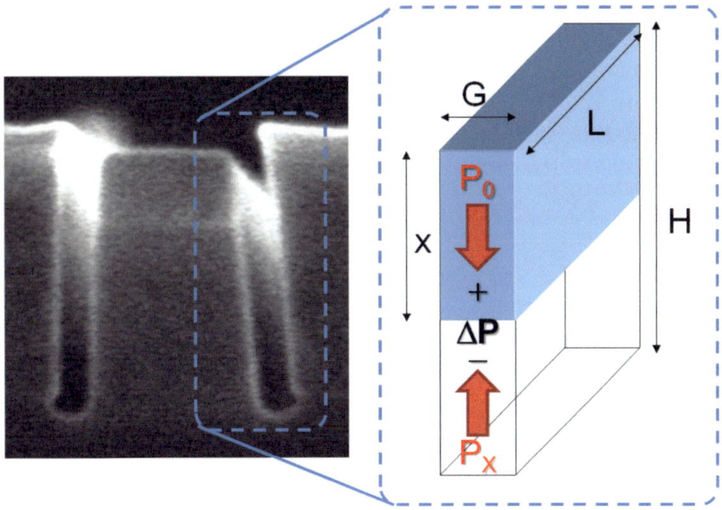

Fig. 4. A capillary force modeling of the nanogap highlighted by the dotted box in the SEM image displaying AA′ direction as shown in Fig. 3. *G* is the nanogap width, *L* is the nanogap length, *H* is the nanogap height, *x* is the water penetration depth, P_0 is the atmospheric pressure, P_x is the pressure inside the nanogap, and ΔP is the pressure difference between P_x and P_0.

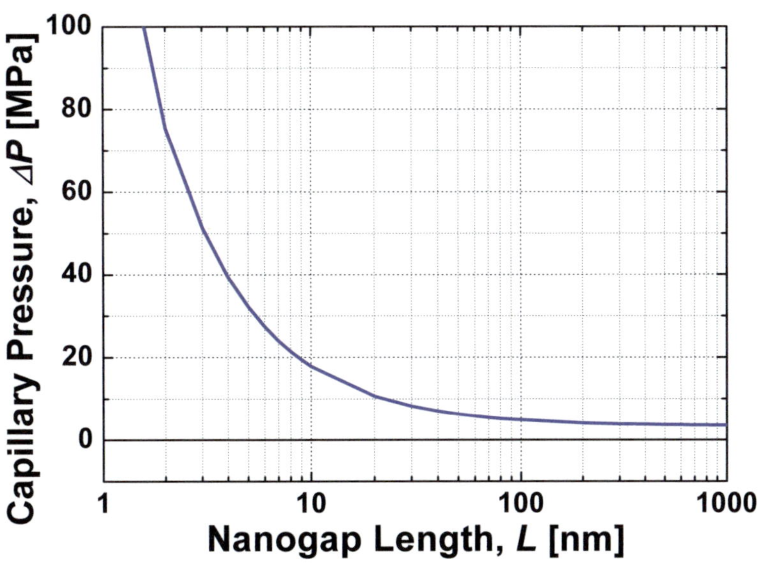

Fig. 5. A plot of capillary pressures as a function of the nanogap length, where *G*=30nm, θ_{SiO2}=45°, θ_{water}=0°, and γ=72.5mN/m for the sample solution of water.

3. Numerical simulations of the nanogap filling process

Although a study on the fluidics on a nanogap was previously carried out (Brinkmann et al., 2006) to support earlier results with a nanogap biosensor (Haguet et al., 2004), only theoretical calculations were presented. In order to visualize the nanogap filling and support the calculation results provided in previous section, three-dimensional simulations were also performed using CFD-ACE+™ (CFD Research Corporation, Huntsville, Alabama, USA) with the structure shown in the inset of Fig. 3. CFD-ACE+™ is a commercial software for multiphysics simulation, and has been used in previous microfluidic studies (Jen et al., 2003; Kobayashi et al., 2004; Rawool et al., 2006; Rawool & Mitra, 2006; Yang et al., 2007; Im et al., 2009).

3.1 Simulation setup

The finite element method is applied with structured grids, as shown in Fig. 6. In order to observe the fluidic behaviour in nanogaps, fine meshes are used in the nanogaps, as highlighted by the red dotted box in Fig. 6. On top of the nanogap-DGFET structure shown in Fig. 3, 1.5-μm-high regions are additionally assigned for an initial water position mimicking introduction of a water droplet on the nanogap-DGFET. The total number of cells is 205,760 in 28 structured zones. Flow and Free Surfaces (VOF) modules are used in this simulation. In the VOF module, the surface reconstruction method is chosen to be 2nd Order (PLIC), and surface tension is considered. The wetting angle of the sidewall in the nanogaps is assumed to be 45 deg due to the presence of native oxide. In addition to surface tension, gravitational force is also considered along the Z-direction, as shown in Fig. 3. The reference pressure of 100,000 N/m^2 (0.1 MPa) is set as the atmospheric pressure. Table 1 summarizes the physical properties of water used in this simulation study.

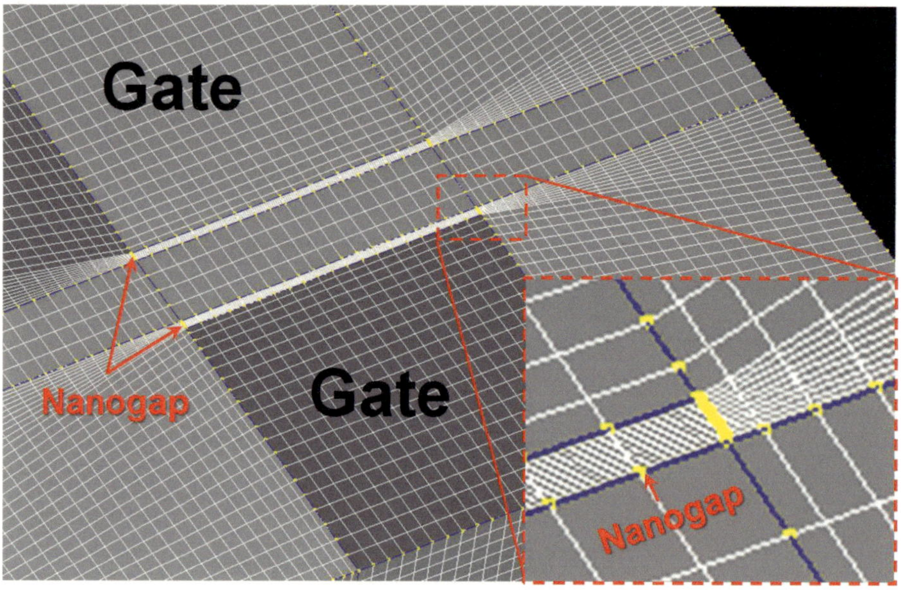

Fig. 6. Grid shapes for structured meshes for simulation. The dotted red box shows fine meshes in the nanogap region.

Physical property	Value	Comment
Density (kg/m^3)	1000	Constant
Viscosity (m^2/s)	1×10^{-6}	Constant (Kinematic)
Surface tension (N/m)	0.0725	Constant

Table 1. Properties of water in the numerical simulation

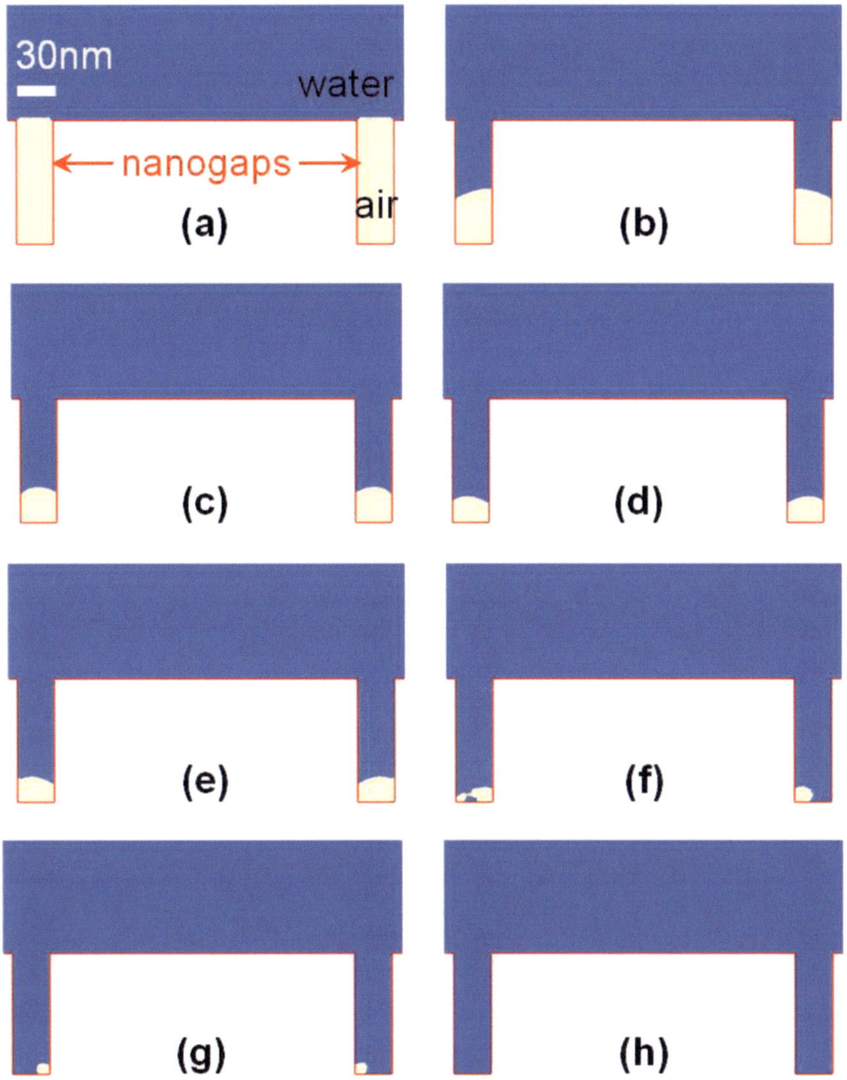

Fig. 7. Nanogap filling of the sample solution of water at the nanogap edge indicated as AA′ in Fig. 5. At various instants of (a) 0 nsec (Initially, air is in the nanogap) (b) 95 nsec (c) 163 nsec (d) 315 nsec (e) 573 nsec (f) 643 nsec (g) 650 nsec (h) 681 nsec (Finally, the nanogap is filled with the sample solution)

3.2 Simulation results: nanogap filling

Fig. 7 shows the water meniscus positions at various instants from the nanogap edge which is denoted as AA′ in Fig. 3. Air inside the nanogap is continuously squeezed and compressed by marching water along the sidewalls of the nanogap. Finally, the entire region of the nanogap becomes filled with water, as confirmed in Fig. 7(h).

It is noteworthy that the wetting speeds are different at the centre and at the edge of the nanogap in the simulation results. Positions of the water meniscus are plotted in Fig. 8; the nanogap is completely filled with water within 700 nsec at the edge of the nanogap; however, it takes longer than that at the centre of the nanogap.

From the calculation results in the previous section and the simulation results in this section, we can find an interesting aspect of the fluidics in the nanogap. The length of the nanogap is effectively reduced after some portion of the nanogap is wetted, because wetting occurs from the edge of the nanogap. With a shorter nanogap, it is straightforward that the capillary pressure becomes greater, as shown in Fig. 5. As a consequence, we can conclude that the nanogap can be fully wetted with the sample solution by this sort of positive feedback.

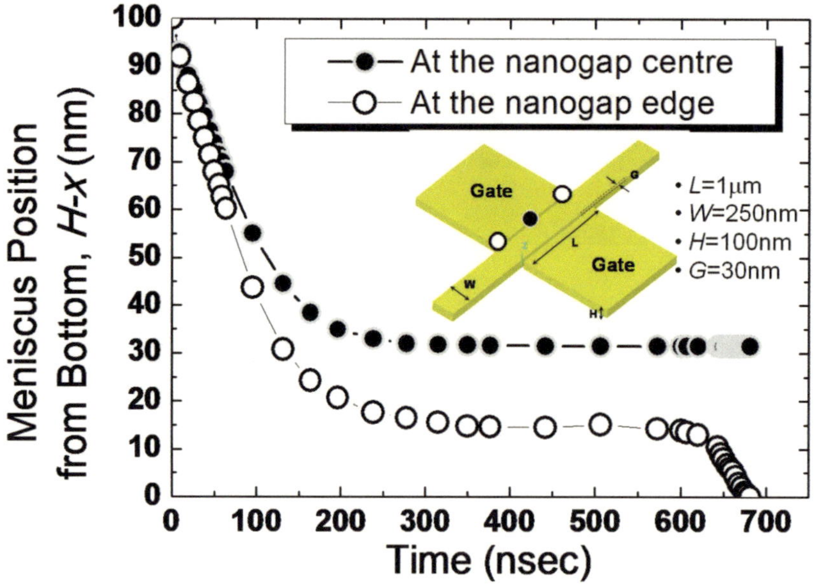

Fig. 8. Water meniscus positions as a function of time in the simulation structure shown in the inset (L=1μm, W=250nm, H=100nm, and G=30nm). Hollow circles mean meniscus positions at the nanogap edge and solid circles mean meniscus positions at the nanogap centre.

The plateau in the graph of Fig. 8 is attributed to the pressure of the compressed air being too high for the capillary pressure to overcome for further advancement. This phenomenon is confirmed by monitoring pressure changes inside the nanogap together with corresponding water meniscus positions. As shown by the dotted boxes in Fig. 9, the pressure inside the nanogap increases gradually as the meniscus advances to the bottom of the nanogap. In the process of nanogap filling, there is a period where only pressure increment is observed without meaningful progress of the water meniscus locations.

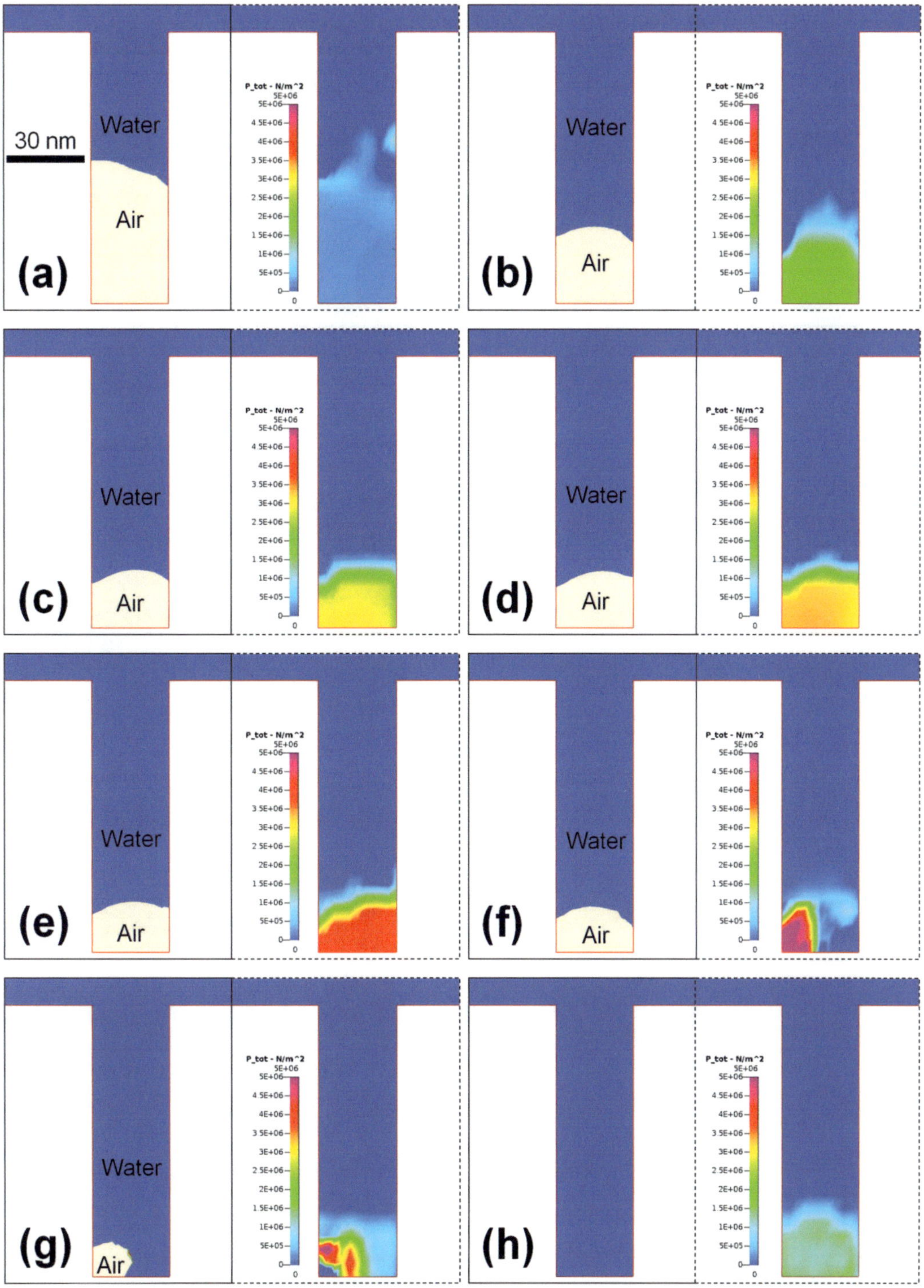

Fig. 9. Water meniscus positions (shown in solid boxes) in the nanogap with corresponding pressure changes (shown in dotted boxes).

3.3 Simulation results: expelling air bubbles from the nanogap

As shown in Fig. 9, air trapped inside the nanogap is pressurized by the capillary pressure of water above the air. Then, where does the air finally go? By careful observation of the simulation results, we can see air bubbles appear and disappear repeatedly inside the nanogap, as shown in Fig. 10.

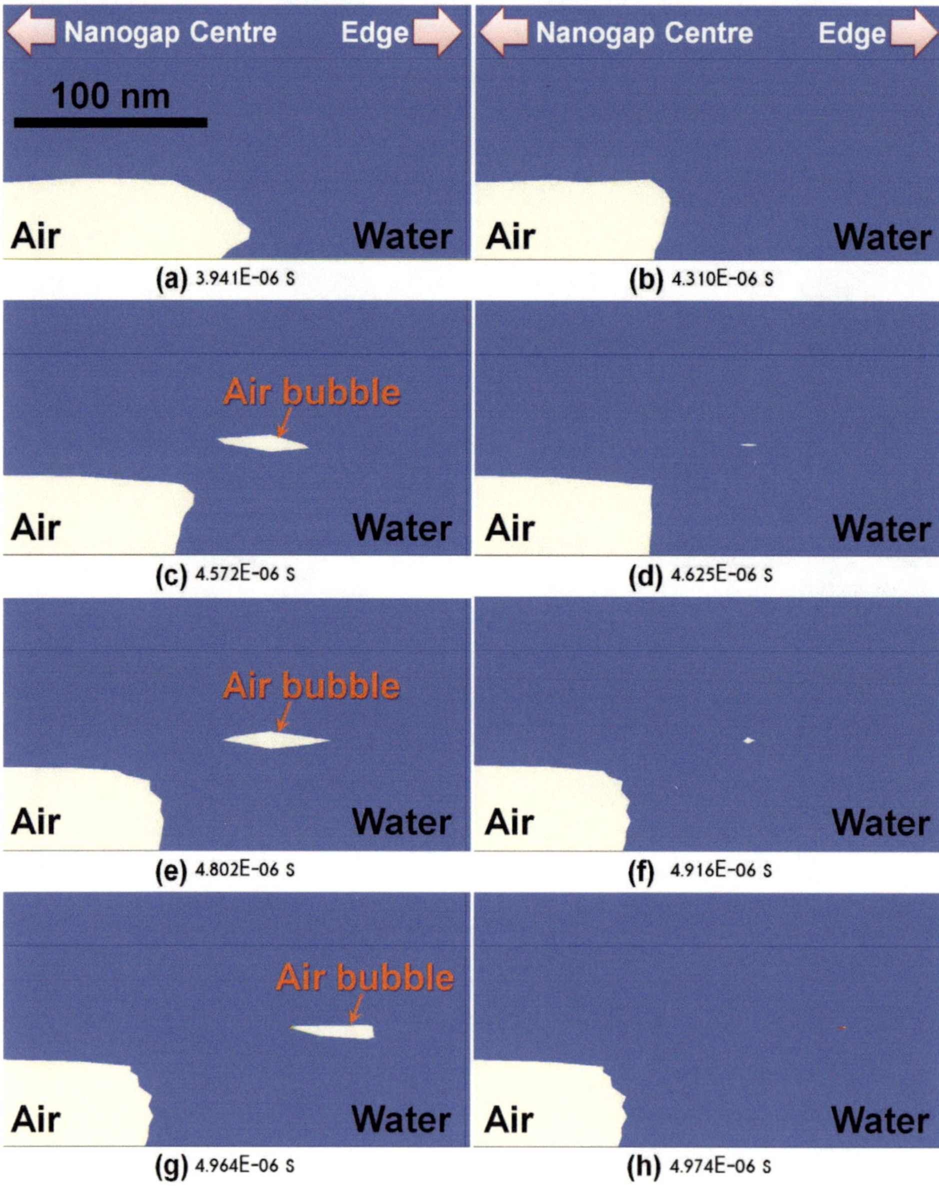

Fig. 10. Movement of water meniscus in the direction of BB′ shown in Fig. 5. (Closed-up views near the B′ side) (a) 3.941 μsec (b) 4.310 μsec (c) 4.572 μsec (d) 4.625 μsec (e) 4.802 μsec (f) 4.916 μsec (g) 4.964 μsec (h) 4.974 μsec. Air bubbles appears and disappears repeatedly to lower the pressure of the air trapped inside the nanogap.

Because water continuously compresses the air in the nanogap with capillary pressure, it is analyzed that a certain threshold pressure is necessary for the trapped air to evacuate an air bubble against the capillary pressure. After the appearance of air bubbles, which occurs with reduced pressure of the trapped air, the water meniscus proceeds further toward the nanogap centre by additional compression of trapped air. Generated air bubbles from the trapped air last for a period of a few tens of nanoseconds to three hundreds nanoseconds. By repetition of this process (*i.e.* pressure reduction by air bubbles and further compression), the nanogap is gradually filled with water.

From the simulation, the threshold pressure for generation of air bubbles is estimated to be around 5MPa, which is 50 times the atmospheric pressure (0.1MPa). As shown in Figs. 9(f) through 9(h), trapped air is eliminated after the pressure reaches roughly 5MPa. Air bubbles cannot be seen in Fig. 9, because they will appear in different places, as shown in Fig. 10.

3.4 Simulation results: velocity vectors

The blue arrows in Fig. 11 represent velocity vectors of water and air in designated meshes. These velocity vectors are obtained from the plane 5 nm away from the nanogap edge, as shown in the figure. In the initial stage of nanogap filling, as shown in Fig. 11(a), air exits quickly from the nanogap by advancing water. After velocity reduction of air, as seen in Fig. 11(b), the velocity direction of air changes toward the nanogap centre in the stage of compressing air, as shown in Fig. 11(c). Finally, if some plane is filled with water, water will fill the trapped air region at the nanogap centre, and consequently the velocity vectors are oriented toward the centre of the nanogap, as shown in Fig. 11(d).

Fig. 12 shows velocity vectors when water cannot advance because compressed air resists against the water. It is shown that the velocity vectors are oriented upward at the water/air interface due to high pressure, represented by green colour in Fig. 12(b), which indicates pressure of around 2MPa.

4. Conclusions

In this chapter, nanogap-DGFET's fluidic characteristics are discussed with theoretical calculations as well as numerical simulations. Theoretical computation based on appropriate modelling predicts that almost complete filling of the nanogap with water is possible. Three-dimensional simulations using CFD-ACE+TM support the theoretical calculations. Various characteristics such as water meniscus position, pressure distribution, and velocity vectors in the simulation results have been analyzed in detail for comprehensive understanding of the process of nanogap filling in the nanogap-embedded biosensor. The sample solution of water is expected to completely fill the nanogap by capillary pressure. These results indicate that biomolecules in a water-based sample solution can be successfully delivered to sensing regions (*i.e.* nanogaps) in nanogap-DGFET devices.

5. Acknowledgment

This work was supported in part by a National Research Foundation of Korea (NRF) grant funded by the Korean Ministry of Education, Science and Technology (MEST) (No. 2010-0018931), in part by the National Research and Development Program (NRDP, 2010-0002108) for the development of biomedical function monitoring biosensors, which is also

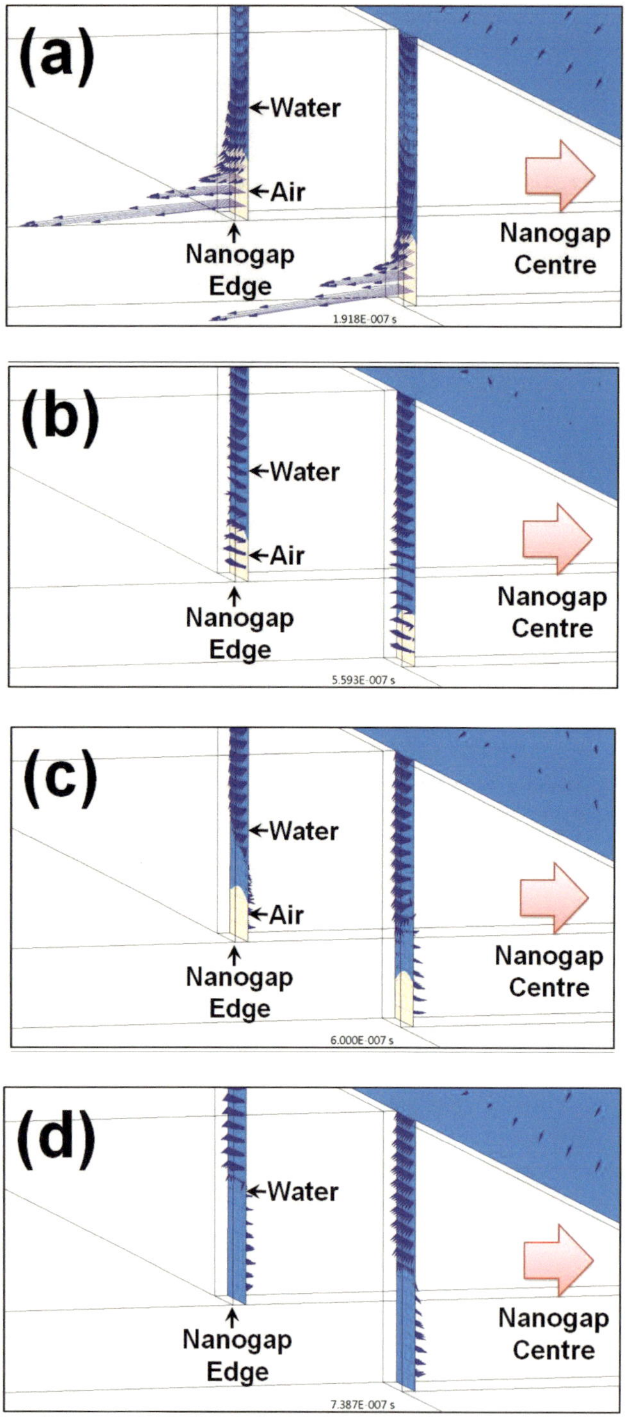

(a) 191.8 nsec after beginning of water penetration, air exits with fast velocity from the nanogap by capillary force of water from the top. Velocity vectors of water are toward the bottom of the nanogap.

(b) 559.3 nsec after beginning of water penetration, air still exits with reduced velocity from the nanogap. Water is being supplied from the top of the nanogap.

(c) 600.0 nsec after beginning of water penetration, the direction of air velocity vectors is changed toward the nanogap centre due to additional capillary force from the nanogap edge which is completely filled with water. As shown in Fig. 8, the nanogap edges become wet before the nanogap centre does.

(d) 738.7 nsec after beginning of water penetration, water at the lower part of nanogap moves to the nanogap centre to fill the remainder of the nanogap at this region, as described in Fig. 10.

Fig. 11. Distribution of velocity vectors (shown as blue arrows) of air and water at 5 nm away from a nanogap edge.

funded by the Korean Ministry of Education, Science and Technology. The work of M. Im was supported in part by the Brain Korea 21 Project, the School of Information Technology, KAIST, 2009. The authors would like to thank Mr. Jae-Hyuk Ahn, Dr. Jin-Woo Han, Dr. Tae Jung Park, and Prof. Sang Yup Lee for their help in the fabrication and analysis of real nanogap-DGFET devices in a previous study that motivated this work.

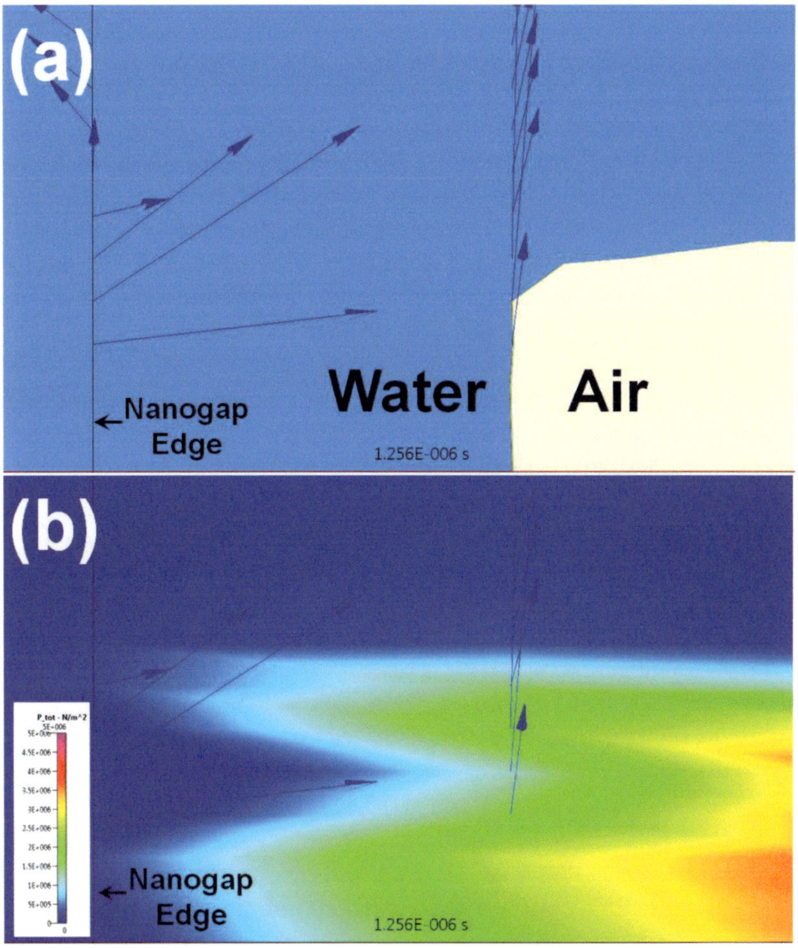

Fig. 12. Velocity vectors in the direction of BB' shown in Fig. 5 with (a) water/air boundary and (b) pressure distribution.

6. References

Bergveld, P. Development of an ion-sensitive solid-state device for neurophysiological measurements. *IEEE Transactions on Biomedical Engineering*, Vol. BME-17, No. 1, (January 1970), pp. 70-71, ISSN 0018-9294.

Bergveld, P. Thirty years of Isfetology what happend in the past 30 years and what may happen in the next 30 years. *Sensors and Actuators B : Chemical*, Vol. 88, No. 1, (January 2003), pp. 1-20, ISSN 0925-4005.

Brinkmann, M. ; Blossey, R. ; Marcon, L. ; Stiévenard, D. ; Dufrêne, Y. F. & Melnyk, O. Fluidics of a Nanogap. *Langmuir*, Vol. 22, No. 23, (October 2006), pp. 9784–9788, ISSN 0743-7463.

Cui, X. D. ; Primak, A. ; Zarate, X. ; Tomfohr, J. ; Sankey, O. F. ; Moor, A. L. ; Moore, T. A. ; Gust, D. ; Harris, G. & Lindsay, S. M. Reproducible measurement of single-molecule conductivity. *Science*, Vol. 294, No. 5542, (October 2001), pp. 571-574, ISSN 0036-8075.

Drummond, T. G. ; Hill, M. G. & Barton, J. K. Electrochemical DNA sensors. *Nature Biotechnology*, Vol. 21, No. 10, (October 2003), pp. 1192-1199, ISSN 1087-0156.

Fritz, J. ; Baller, M. K. ; Lang, H. P. ; Rothuizen, H. ; Vettiger, P. ; Meyer, E. ; Güntherodt, H.-J. ; Gerber, Ch. & Gimzewski, J. K. Translating biomolecular recognition into nanomechanics. *Science*, Vol. 288, No. 5464, (April 2000), pp. 316-318, ISSN 0036-8075.

Gu, B. ; Park, T. J. ; Ahn, J.-H. ; Huang, X.-J. ; Lee, S. Y. & Choi, Y.-K. Nanogap field-effect transistor biosensors for electrical detection of avian influenza. *Small*, Vol. 5, No. 21, (November 2009), pp. 2407-2412, ISSN 1613-6810.

Haguet, V. ; Martin, D. ; Marcon, L. ; Heim, T. ; Stiévenard, D. ; Olivier, C. ; El-Mahdi, O. & Melnyk, O. Combined nanogap nanoparticles nanosensor for electrical detection of biomolecular interactions between polypeptides. *Applied Physics Letters*, Vol. 84, No. 7, (February 2004), pp. 1213-1215, ISSN 0003-6951.

Im, H. ; Huang, X.-J. ; Gu, B. & Choi, Y.-K. A dielectric modulated field-effect transistor for biosensing. *Nature Nanotechnology*, Vol. 2, (June 2007), pp. 430-434, ISSN 1748-3387.

Im, M. ; Cho, I.-J. ; Yun, K.-S. & Yoon, E. Electromagnetic actuation and microchannel engineering of a polymer micropen array integrated with microchannels and sample reservoirs for biological assay patterning. *Applied Physics Letters*, Vol. 91, No. 12, (September 2007), 124101(3pp), ISSN 0003-6951.

Im, M. ; Im, H. ; Kim, D.-H. ; Lee, J.-H. ; Yoon, J.-B. & Choi, Y.-K. (2009). Analysis of a superhydrophobic microlens array surface : as a microchannel wall for pressure drop reduction, *Proceedings of Thirtheenth Internation Conference on Miniaturized Systems for Chemistry and Life Sciences (μTAS2009)*, pp. 162-164, ISSN 1556-5904, Jeju, South Korea, November 1-5, 2009.

Im, M. ; Ahn, J.-H. ; Han, J.-W. ; Park, T. J. ; Lee, S. Y. & Choi, Y.-K. Development of a point-of-care testing platform with a nanogap-embedded separated double-gate field effect transistor array and its readout system for detection of avian influenza. *IEEE Sensors Journal*, Vol. 11, No. 2, (February 2011), pp. 351-360, ISSN 1530-437X.

Jen, C.-P. ; Wu, C.-Y. ; Lin, Y.-C. & Wu, C.-Y. Design and simulation of the micromixer with chaotic advection in twisted microchannels. *Lab on a chip*, Vol. 3, (April 2003), pp. 77-81, ISSN 1473-0197.

Kim, D.-S. ; Park, J.-E. ; Shin, J.-K. ; Kim, P.K. ; Lim, G. & Shoji, S. An extended gate FET-based biosensor integrated with a Si microfluidic channel for detection of protein complexes. *Sensors and Actuators B: Chemical*, Vol. 117, No. 2, (October 2006), pp. 488–494, ISSN 0925-4005.

Kobayashi, I. ; Mukataka, S. & Nakajima, M. CFD simulation and analysis of emulsion droplet formation from straight-through microchannels. *Langmuir*, Vol. 20, No. 22, (September 2004), pp. 9868-9877, ISSN 0743-7463.

Kost, G. J. ; Ehrmeyer, S. S. ; Chernow, B. ; Winkelman, J. W. ; Zaloga, G. P. ; Dellinger, R. P. & Shirey, T. The laboratory-clinical interface : point-of-care testing. *Chest*, Vol. 115, No. 4, (April 1999), pp. 1140-1154, ISSN 0012-3692.

Oh, S. W. ; Moon, J. D. ; Lim, H. J. ; Park, S. Y. ; Kim, T. ; Park, J. B. ; Han, M. H. ; Snyder, M. & Choi, E. Y. Calixarene derivative as a tool for highly sensitive detection and oriented immobilization of proteins in a microarray format through noncovalent molecular interaction. *The FASEB Journal*, Vol. 19, No. 10, (August 2005), pp. 1335-1337, ISSN 0892-6638.

Patolsky, F. ; Timko, B. P. ; Zheng, G. & Lieber, C. M. Nanowire-based nanoelectronic devices in the life sciences. *MRS Bulletin*, Vol. 32, No. 2, (February 2007), pp. 142-149, ISSN 0883-7694.

Rawool, A. S. ; Mitra, S. K. & Kandlikar, S. G. Numerical simulation of flow through microchannels with designed roughness. *Microfluidics and Nanofluidics*, Vol. 2, No. 3, (February 2006), pp. 215-221, ISSN 1613-4982.

Rawool, A. S. & Mitra, S. K. Numerical simulation of electroosmotic effect in serpentine channels. *Microfluidics and Nanofluidics*, Vol. 2, No. 3, (February 2006), pp. 261-269, ISSN 1613-4982.

Reed, M. A. ; Zhou, C. ; Muller, C. J. ; Burgin, T. P. & Tour, J. M. Conductance of a molecular junction. *Science*, Vol. 278, No. 5336, (October 1997), pp. 252-254, ISSN 0036-8075.

Sakata, T. & Miyahara, Y. Direct transduction of allele-specific primer extension into electrical signal using genetic field effect transistor. *Biosensors and Bioelectronics*, Vol. 22, No. 7, (February 2007), pp. 1311–1316, ISSN 0956-5663.

Schöning, M. J. & Poghossian, A. Recent advances in biologically sensitive field-effect transistors (BioFETs). *Analyst*, Vol. 127, No. 9, (August 2002), pp. 1137–1151, ISSN 0003-2654.

Siu, W. M. & Cobbold, R. S. C. Basic properties of the Electrolyte-SiO2-Si system: physical and theoretical aspects. *IEEE Transactions on Electron Devices*, Vol. ED-26, No. 11, (November 1979), pp. 1805–1815, ISSN 0018-9383.

Stern, E. ; Wagner, R. ; Sigworth, F. J. ; Breaker, R. ; Fahmy, T. M. & Reed, M. A. Importance of the debye screening length on nanowire field effect transistor sensors. *Nano Letters*, Vol. 7, No. 11, (October 2007), pp. 3405–3409, ISSN 1530-6984.

St-Louis, P. Status of point-of-care testing : promise, realities, and possibilities. *Clinical Biochemistry*, Vol. 33, No. 6, (August 2000), pp. 427-440, ISSN 0009-9120.

Tierney, M. J. ; Tamada, J. A. ; Potts, R. O. ; Eastman, R. C. ; Pitzer, K. ; Ackerman, N. R. & Fermi, S. J. The GlucoWatch biographer : a frequent automatic and noninvasive glucose monitor. *Annals of Medicine*, Vol. 32, No. 9, (December 2000), pp. 632-641, ISSN 0785-3890.

Yang, C.-K. ; Chang, J.-S. ; Chao, S. D. & Wu, K.-C. Two dimensional simulation on immunoassay for a biosensor with applying electrothermal effect. *Applied Physics Letters*, Vol. 91, No. 11, (September 2007), 113904 (3pp), ISSN 0003-6951.

Yang, Y. T. ; Callegari, C. ; Feng, X. L. ; Ekinci, K. L. & Roukes, M. L. Zeptogram-scale nanomechanical mass sensing. *Nano Letters*, Vol. 6, No. 4, (April 2006), pp. 583-586, ISSN 1530-6984.

Yi, M. ; Jeong, K.-H. & Lee, L. P. Theoretical and experimental study towards a nanogap dielectric biosensor. *Biosensors and Bioelectronics*, Vol. 20, No. 7, (January 2005), pp. 1320-1326, ISSN 0956-5663.

12

Fabrication of Biosensors Using Vinyl Polymer-grafted Carbon Nanotubes

Seong-Ho Choi, Da-Jung Chung and Hai-Doo Kwen
Department of Chemistry, Hannam University, Daejeon 305-811, Republic of Korea

1. Introduction

A biosensor is commonly defined as a device incorporating a bioreceptor connected to a transducer, which converts an observed response into a measurable signal proportional to analyte concentration which then is conveyed to a detector (Eggins, 1996). As demonstrated in Fig. 1, a biosensor consists of a bio-element and a sensor-element. A specific bio-element, including enzyme, antibody, microorganism, cell, and DNA, recognizes a specific analyte, and a sensor element transduces the change in the biomolecules into an electrical signal. Biosensors can be classified either by their bioreceptor or their transducer. Biosensors are known as enzymatic biosensors (enzymes), genosensors (DNAs), immunosensors (antibodies), etc. depending on the bioreceptors used. Biosensors can also be divided into several categories based on the transduction process, such as electrochemical, optical, piezoelectric, and thermal/calorimetric. Among these, electrochemical biosensors are the most widespread, numerous and successfully commercialized devices of biomolecular electronics (Dzyadevych et al., 2008).

Much literature on carbon nanotube (CNT)-based biosensors has been published over the past several years because CNTs have the following advantages: (1) small size with large surface area, (2) high sensitivity, (3) fast response time, (4) enhanced electron transfer and (5) easy protein immobilization on CNT-modified electrodes, coupled with the fact that several methods have been developed (J. Wang & Musameh, 2003a; J. Wang et al., 2003b; Y. Saito et al., 1993). These properties make CNTs ideal for use in electrochemical biosensors and nanoscale electronic devices. Such potential applications would greatly benefit from CNTs in promoting the electron-transfer reaction of biomolecules, including catecholamine neurotransmitters (J. Wang et al., 2002a), cytochrome *c* (J. Wang et al., 2002b), ascorbic acid (Z. H. Wang et al., 2002), NADH (Musameh et al., 2002), and hydrazine compounds (Zhao et al., 2002). The insolubility of CNTs in most solvents is a major barrier for developing such CNT-based biosensing devices. Therefore, surface modification is necessary for CNT materials to be biocompatible and to improve solubility in common solvents and selective binding capability to biotargets.

There are two main approaches for surface modification of CNTs: a non-covalent wrapping or adsorption and covalent chemical tethering. The non-covalent approach includes surfactant modification, polymer wrapping, and polymer absorption via various adsorption forces, such as van der Waals and π-stacking interactions. The advantage of non-covalent modification is that the structures and mechanical properties of CNTs remain intact.

However, the force between the CNTs and the wrapping molecules is very weak, which means that the load may not be transferred efficiently from the polymer matrix to the CNT filler (Islam et al., 2003). The covalent functionalization of CNT surfaces can improve the efficiency of load transfer from matrix to nanotubes. However, it must be noted that the process to obtain functional groups may introduce defects on the walls of nanotubes. These defects will lower the strength of the reinforcing component. Therefore, there will be a trade-off between the strength of the interface and the strength of the CNT filler (Eitan et al., 2003). The covalent functionalization of CNTs is most frequently initiated by introducing carboxylic acid groups using nitric acid oxidation (Men et al., 2008; J. Shen et al., 2007; Kitano et al., 2007). Thereafter, small molecules (Kooi et al., 2002; Liu, 2005; Tasis et al., 2003) or polymer chains (Kang & Taton., 2003; O. K. Kim et al., 2003) can be chemically attached to the CNTs by esterification and amidation reactions via the carboxylic acid moieties. The chemical modification is an especially attractive target, as it can improve solubility (Bahr et al., 2001) and processing ability and allows the unique properties of CNTs to be coupled to other types of materials.

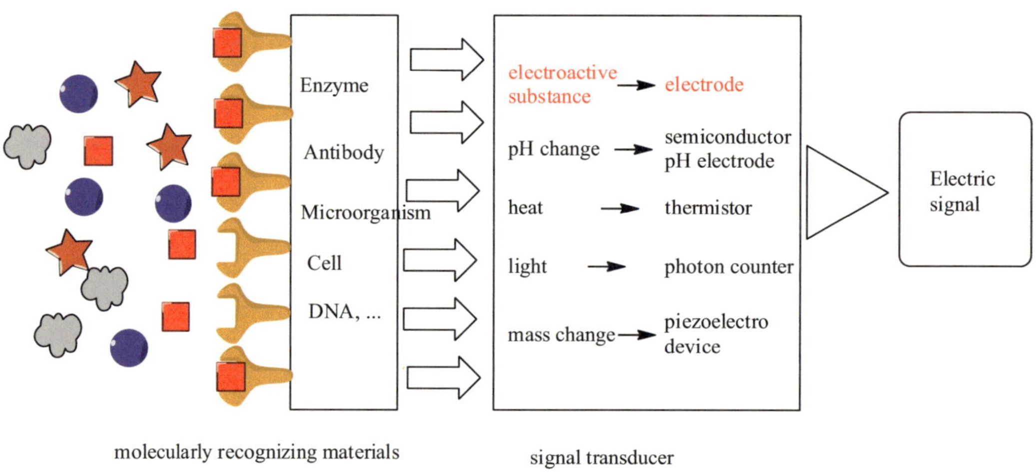

Fig. 1. Schematic diagram for the principal of the biosensors.

Radiation-induced graft polymerization (RIGP) is a useful method for the introduction of functional groups into polymer *matrices* using specially selected vinyl monomers. There have been several reports on RIGP of polar monomers onto the surface of polymer substrates with hydrophobic properties to obtain hydrophilic properties for versatile applications (Choi & Nho, 1999a, 1999b; Choi et al., 1999, 2000a 2000b, 2001; S. K. Kim et al., 2010). RIGP can be easily modified for the surface of CNTs to induce free radicals on the surface of nanotubes in aqueous solution and organic solvents at room temperature. Figure 2 shows the introduction of functional groups, such as hydroxyl, carboxyl, and sulfonic acid onto the CNT surface (Oh et al., 2006a) and fullerene (Chung et al., 2011) using free radicals generated during γ-ray irradiation.
In this chapter, we describe the fabrication of biosensors using vinyl polymer-grafted carbon nanotubes prepared by RIGP. Various vinyl monomers used for functionalization of CNTs will be introduced. The obtained vinyl polymer-grafted CNTs are used as biosensor supporting materials to increase sensitivity and affinity for biomolecules. The characterization and application of the four biosensor types are: (1) Enzyme-free biosensors

based on chemical reaction, (2) Enzymatic biosensors based on functional group-MWNTs, (3) Bacterial biosensors based on polymer grafted MWNTs, and (4) E-DNA biosensors based on polymer grafted MWNTs, as summarized in Fig. 3.

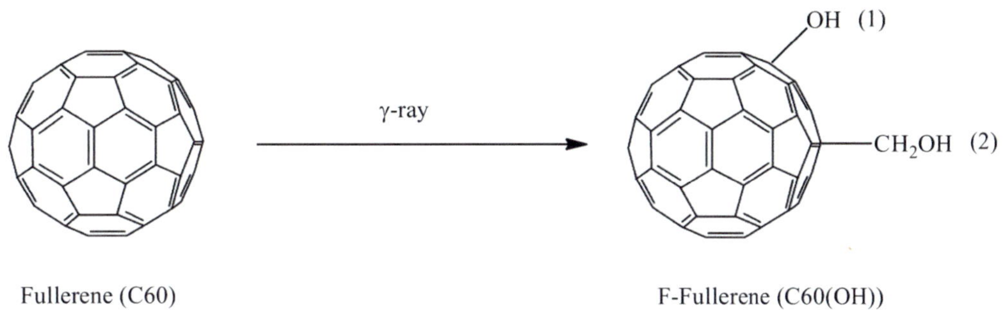

$$(1)\ H_2O \xrightarrow{\gamma\text{-ray}} E_{aq}^{-}, H^{+}, H^{\cdot}, OH^{\cdot}, H_2O_2, H_2$$

$$(2)\ CH_3OH + OH^{\cdot} \longrightarrow H_2O + CH_2OH^{\cdot}$$

Fig. 2. Radiolytic functionalization possible mechanism of Fullerene (C60) in H_2O/MeOH mixture solution.

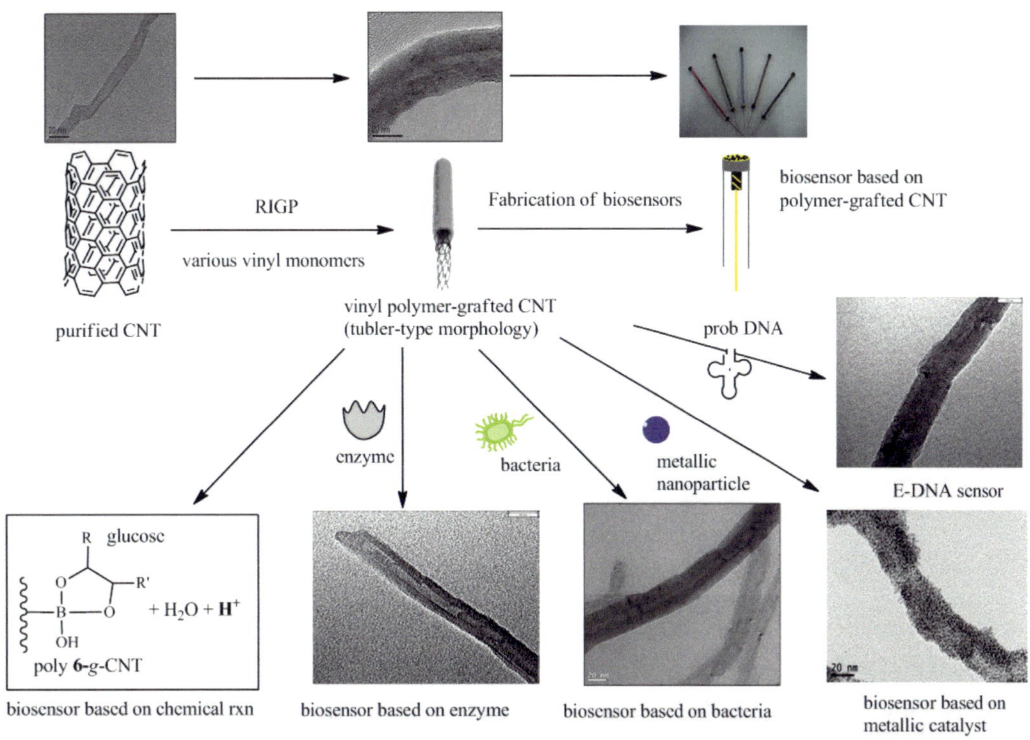

Fig. 3. Schemetic fabrication of biosensor based on vinyl polymer-grafted MWNT.

2. Enzyme-free biosensor based on chemical reaction

Numerous methods based on enzyme immobilization for human cholesterol assays have been developed, including colorimetric, spectrometric and electrochemical methods (Crumbliss et al., 1993; Shumyantseva et al., 2004). The use of enzymes in the fabrication of sensors has advantages due to their rapid, selective, and sensitive nature. However, there exist some practical problems related to the use of enzymes in analytical devices due to their short lifetime and low reusability since they are easily affected by temperature, humidity, and pH (Gavalas & Chaniotakis, 2000, 2001). To address these issues, non-enzymatic sensors based on the direct electrocatalytic oxidation of glucose are being investigated for their stability, simple fabrication, reproducibility, low cost, and freedom from oxygen limitation, unlike enzyme-based sensors (Lee et al., 2009). In this section, we discuss the preparation and characterization of enzyme-free biosensors based on boronic acid-modified and metallic nanoparticles-immobilized CNTs.

2.1 Chemical reaction between boronic acid containing group modified carbon surface and target molecules

Boronic acids (-$B(OH)_2$) can interact with cyanides (Badugu et al., 2004a) and fluorides (Cesare & Lakowicz, 2002a), which have been explored for sensor development. Boronic acids binding with diols (J. Wang et al., 2005) have been mostly studied in developing fluorescent carbohydrate sensors. Boronic acids act as an electron withdrawing group in its neutral form, -$B(OH)_2$, and as an electron donation group in its anionic form, -$B(OH)_3^-$.

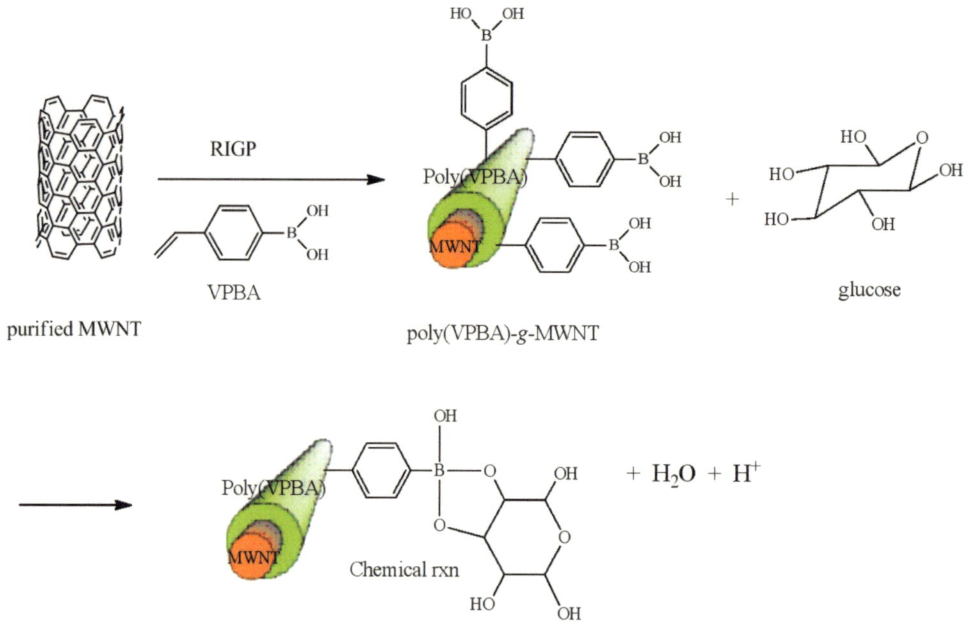

Fig. 4. Preparation of non-enzymatic biosensor based on chemical reaction by RIGP.

The feasibility of tear glucose sensing was tested using a daily disposable contact lens embedded with boronic acid-containing fluorophores which act as a potential alternative to current invasive glucose monitoring techniques (Badugu et al., 2004b). The boronic acid probes in the contact lens could continuously monitor the tear glucose levels in the range of 50-500 μM. The boronic acid group showed higher affinity for D-fructose and smaller affinity for D-glucose (Cesare & Lakowicz, 2002a). This means that the use of the boronic acid group for sensing sugars is strongly dependent on the molecular geometry and the aromatic species where boronic acid is present.

Poly(VBAc)-grafted MWNTs are of great interest for the preparation of enzyme-free sensors because of the boronic acid group they contain. 4-Vinylphenyl boronic acid (VPBA) was used to functionalize the surface of multi-walled carbon nanotubes (MWNTs) since it possesses both hydrophobic and hydrophilic properties (D. S. Yang et al., 2010). The vinyl group of the monomer attaches to the surface of MWNTs because of a hydrophobic-hydrophobic interaction, while the functional group of the monomer comes to the surface in an aqueous solution because of a hydrophilic-hydrophilic interaction. When irradiated, the radical polymerization of the monomer on the surface of MWNTs occurs to form grafted vinyl polymer PVBAc-g-MWNTs. Boronic acid in PVBAc-g-MWNTs couples with diols of glucose to form a boronic acid diester group, as shown in Figure 4 (D. S. Yang et al., 2010). The boronic acid content of PVBAc-g-MWNTs was 296 mg/g, as determined by titration. The diols are linked covalently and the reaction is fast and completely reversible (Cesare & Lakowicz, 2002b). The cyclic voltammograms of PVBAc-g-MWNTs in 0.1 M phosphoric buffer solution displayed an excellent linear response to glucose concentration in the range 1.0–10 mM.

2.2 Catalytic reaction of the target molecules on the surface of metallic nanoparticle-modified MWNT

Recently, an enzyme-free hydrogen peroxide (H_2O_2) biosensor was developed based on nano-conducting polymer composites (MWNT–PEDOT nanoparticles) (K. C. Lin et al., 2010). The use of enzyme-free H_2O_2 biosensors is important in chemical, food and environmental applications. More enzyme-free H_2O_2 biosensors have been developed based on modified carbon fiber microelectrodes (Y. Wang et al., 1998), vanadium-doped zirconias (Domenecha & Alarcon, 2002) and Fe_3O_4 (M. S. Lin & Leu, 2005).

Nanoscale materials of metal (Ag, Au, Pd, Pt, etc.), alloy (Pt-Ru), carbon and polymers are very attractive for a variety of applications including optical and electronic nanodevices, and chemical and biological nanosensors. Nanoparticles offer higher catalytic efficiency than bulk materials due to their large surface-to-volume ratio (Yu et al., 1999; S. J. Kim et al., 2008).

Initial research developing non-enzymatic sensors focused on the use of nanocrystalline metals, such as Pt and Au, especially Pt-based amperometric electrodes (S. J. Park et al., 2003; Song et al., 2005). However, such Pt-based glucose sensors lacked sufficient selectivity and sensitivity due to chemisorbed intermediates and electroactive species. The desire for better and cheaper electrocatalysts has resulted in bimetallic systems being developed. Pt-Au (Habrioux et al., 2007; H. Liu et al., 1992), Pt-Pb (Cui et al., 2007; Bai et al., 2008; J. Wang et al., 2008; Sun et al., 2001), and Pt-Ru (Xiao et al., 2009) have all displayed high electrocatalytic activity for glucose oxidation.

Effective fabrication of electrocatalysts also depends on the support material (Hsu et al., 2008). Catalyst dispersion and utilization have been shown to improve supporting Pt-Ru nanoparticles on high-surface area carbon materials, such as CNTs, carbon nanofibers, carbon nanocoils and carbon nanohorns (Steigerwalt et al., 2002; Hyeon et al., 2003; K. Park et al., 2004; R. Yang et al., 2005). A systematic study has shown that MWNTs are the best of the carbon based electrocatalyst supports (Reddy & Ramaprabhu, 2007). In principle, MWNTs are seamless cylinders. However, they often have defects where the attachment of Pt-based alloy nanoparticles most likely occurs.

In a preliminary report, Pt-Ru nanoparticles were deposited on the surfaces of various carbon supports, including Vulcan XC-71, Ketjen-300, Ketjen-600, single-walled carbon nanotubes (SWNTs), and MWNTs for use as fuel cell catalysts using γ-ray irradiation without anchoring agents (Choi et al., 2003a, 2003b; Oh et al., 2006; Hwang et al., 2008). The metal (Ag or Pd) and alloy (Pt-Ru) nanoparticles were also deposited on the surfaces of SWNTs (Oh et al., 2005, 2006a, 2006b, 2008) and porous carbon supports using γ-irradiation without anchoring agents (Seo et al., 2008). However, metallic alloy nanoparticles aggregated on the surfaces of the carbon supports due to their hydrophobic nature. This aggregation was overcome by modifying the surface of the carbon support to give it hydrophilic properties. This was done by *in-situ* polymerization of β-caprolactone, methacrylate and pyrrole using oxidizing agents as initiators (Bae et al., 2010). The polymer-stabilized bimetallic (Pd-Ag) nanoparticles were prepared by γ-irradiation in organic solvents and used as catalysts for hydrogenation of *cis,cis*-1,3-cyclooctadiene (Choi et al., 2005). Pt- Ru nanoparticles were then deposited on the polymer-wrapped MWNT supports to produce a direct methanol fuel cell (DMFC) anode catalyst (Choi et al., 2010).

Pt-Ru nanoparticles have also been deposited on functional polymer (FP)-grafted MWNTs by RIGP, to produce an anode catalyst for DMFCs (D. S. Yang et al., 2011). This method involved two steps: grafting the functional polymer onto the MWNTs by RIGP; and then depositing the Pt-Ru nanoparticles onto the MWNTs by radiation-induced reduction. Pt-M nanoparticles on FP-MWNT supports have also been prepared via a one-step process initiated by free radicals and hydrated electrons generated during γ-irradiation in an aqueous solution.

The catalytic efficiencies of the Pd/C and Pd-M/C particles in various Suzuki-type and Heck-type reactions were examined (S. J. Kim et al., 2008; M. R. Kim & Choi, 2009). In the Suzuki-type reactions, the catalytic efficiency (measured by the yield of the product) decreases in the order of Pd-Cu/C > Pd/C > Pd-Ag/C > Pd-Ni/C. The reaction yield with Pd-Ni/C was much lower than those with other particles. Generally the carbon-supported Pd and Pd-M nanoparticles showed excellent capabilities as a catalyst for carbon–carbon coupling reaction such as Suzuki- and Heck-type reactions.

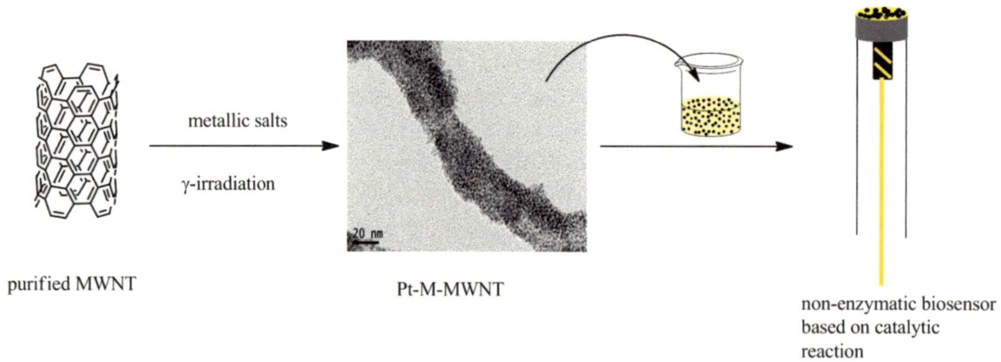

Fig. 5. Radiotic preparation of non-enzymatic biosensor based on catalytic oxidation.

Non-enzymatic glucose sensors employing polyvinylpyrrolidone (PVP) modified-MWNTs with highly dispersed Pt-M (M = Ru and Sn) nanoparticles (Pt-M/PVP@MWNTs) were fabricated by radiolytic deposition (Kwon et al., 2011). The Pt-M nanoparticles were found to be well-dispersed and exhibit alloy properties on the MWNT supports. Electrochemical testing showed that these non-enzymatic sensors had larger currents (mA) than that of a bare glassy carbon (GC) electrode and PVP modified-MWNTs. The prepared biosensor with Pt-Ru nanoparticles for glucose has good sensitivity, linear range, and a lower detection limit in NaOH electrolyte. These non-enzymatic sensors can effectively avoid interference from ascorbic acid and uric acid in NaOH electrolyte.

3. Enzymatic biosensors based on vinyl polymer grafted-MWNTs prepared by RIGP

3.1 Enzymatic biosensors

The first enzyme electrode was an amperometric type of biosensor developed by Clark and Lyons (Clark & Lyons, 1962). A soluble biomaterial glucose oxidase was held between membranes and the oxygen uptake was measured with an oxygen electrode. Since then, enzyme-based electrochemical biosensors have been widely used in medical and pharmaceutical applications, food safety and environmental monitoring, defense and security. Health care is the main area using biosensor applications today for monitoring blood glucose levels and diabetes. Also, potential applications exist for the reliable detection of urea in renal disease patients either at home or in the hospital. Industrial applications are used to improve manufacturing processes leading to better yield and product quality, such as monitoring the production of alcohol during the fermentation process. Furthermore, biosensors help to meet environmental legislation through monitoring of phenolic compounds contained in industrial waste water, much of which is toxic to the environment.

Electrochemical biosensors incorporating enzymes with nanomaterials, which combine the recognition and catalytic properties of enzymes and the electronic properties of various nanomaterials, are the desired materials with synergistic properties originating from the components of the hybrid composites. Many enzymes have been employed to prepare various kinds of biosensors using carbon nanotubes (CNTs) (Chakraborty & Raj, 2007; Male et al., 2007; Arvinte et al., 2008). Usually, enzymes are immobilized onto CNTs by physical adsorption (Guan et al., 2005) and covalent bonding (Patolsky et al., 2004; Y. J. Zhang et al., 2005). Various vinyl monomers, such as acrylic acid (AAc), methacrylic acid (MAc), glycidyl methacrylate (GMA), maleic anhydride (MAn), and 4-vinylphenylboronic acid (VPBAc), are used to functionalize CNTs prior to immobilizing enzymes onto CNTs. Figure 6 shows the vinyl monomers which possess both hydrophobic and hydrophilic properties. Polymer-CNT nanocomposites have been obtained by γ-irradiation polymerization of various vinyl monomers. The obtained vinyl polymer-grafted CNTs are used as biosensor support materials to increase sensitivity and affinity for biomolecules.

Tyrosinase-immobilized biosensors were fabricated based on Poly(AAc)-g-MWNT and Poly(Man)-g-MWNT by RIGP of AAc and MAn on the surface of MWNTs, (#1 and 4 in Fig. 6). The biosensor was then prepared on an indium tin oxide (ITO) glass electrode via a hand-casting of chitosan solution with tyrosinase-immobilized Poly(AAc)-g-MWNT (#1 in Fig. 6) and Poly(Man)-g-MWNT (#4 in Fig. 6) respectively. The sensing ranges of biosensors were 0.2–0.9 mM and 0.1–0.5 mM concentrations for phenol in phosphate buffer solution. Various parameters influencing biosensor performance have been optimized for pH,

temperature, and the response to various phenolic compounds. The biosensor was then tested on phenolic compounds contained in commercial red wines (K. I. Kim et al., 2010).
A tyrosinase-immobilized biosensor with hydroxyl group-functionalized MWNTs was also developed for phenol detection (J. H. Yang et al., 2009). The hydroxyl group-modified MWNTs include poly(GVPB)-g-MWNT and poly(HEMA) prepared by RIGP (#5 and 6 in Fig. 6). The biosensor response was in the range of 0.6–7.0 mM and 0.05–0.35 mM for phenol in a phosphate buffer solution, respectively. The biosensor was then optimized for pH, temperature, and other phenolic compounds in commercial red wines. As a result, the amount of phenolic compounds in commercial red wines are in the range of 68.5~655.0 mg/L, which was calculated from a calibration curve of phenol on a biosensor based on poly(GVPB)-g-MWNTs.

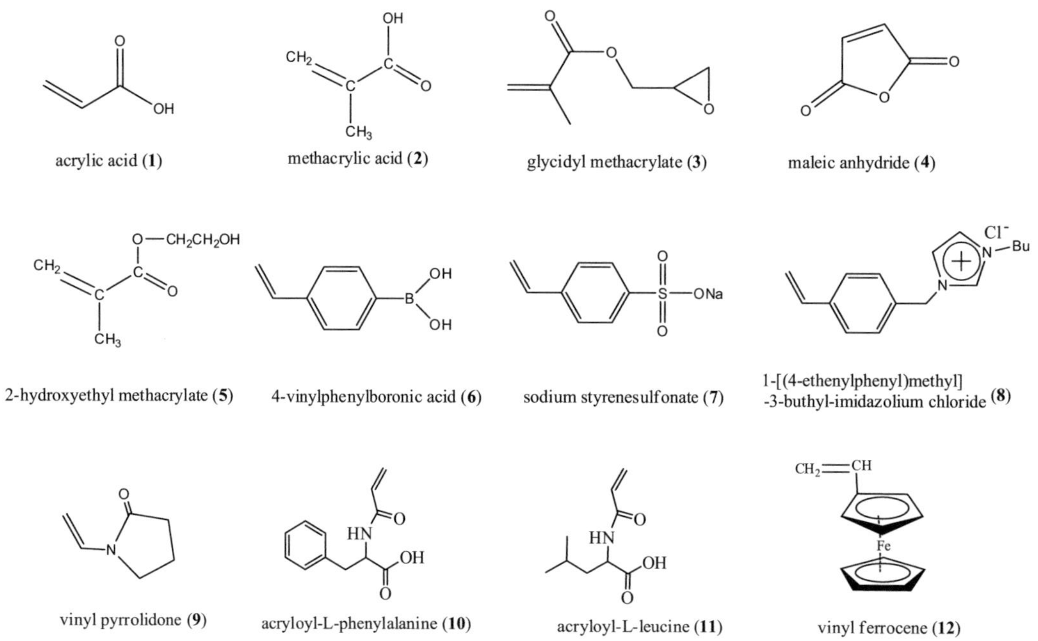

Fig. 6. The used vinyl monomers in Choi lab. for radiation-induced grafting onto carbon nanotubes.

Direct electrochemistry of biological enzymes has been studied with ion liquids (ILs) in both theoretical and practical applications since ILs are considered to be suitable media for supporting a biocatalytic process with high polarity, non-coordination power, high selectivity, fast rates, and great enzyme stability (Compton & Laszlo, 2002; Sweeny & Peters, 2001). The cationic property of modified MWNT-based sensors was developed by RIGP of vinyl monomers with ionic properties, such as 1-butylimidazole bromide (#8 in Fig. 6), 3-(butyl imidazol)-2-(hydroxyl)propyl methyl methacrylate and 1-[(4-ethenylphenyl)methyl]-3-buthyl-imidazolium chloride, in aqueous solution at room temperature (K. I. Kim et al., 2009; Ryu & Choi, 2010a). Subsequently, the *tyrosinase*-immobilized biosensor was fabricated by hand-casting the ionic property-modified MWNTs, *tyrosinase*, and chitosan solution as a binder onto the ITO glass surface. The biosensors were used to determine phenolic compounds in red wines or caffeine in commercial coffee. As a result, the amount of phenolics in commercial red wines has been determined to be in the range of 383.5-3,087 mg/L in a phosphate buffer solution (K. I. Kim et al., 2009), and the amount of caffeine in commercial coffee was in the range of 144.8 ~ 1765 mg/L in a phosphate buffer solution (Ryu & Choi, 2010a).

In addition, colloidal gold nanoparticles (Au-NPs) have been widely used as a model system because of their ease of synthesis and surface modification (Feng et al., 2007), good biocompatibility (Qu et al., 2006), as well as their ability to act as tiny conduction centers which facilitate electron transfer (Jia et al., 2002). Fabrication of a gucose oxidase (GODox) immobilized biosensor has been attempted by two methods (Piao et al., 2010). In one of the methods, gold nanoparticles (Au-NPs) prepared by γ-irradiation were loaded into the poly(MAn)-g-MWNT electrode via physical entrapment. In the other method, the Au-NPs were prepared by electrochemical reduction of Au ions on the surface of the poly(MAn)-g-MWNT electrode and then GODox was immobilized into the Au-NPs. The GODox immobilized biosensors were tested for electrocatalytic activity to sense glucose. The sensing range was from 30 μM to 100 μM for the glucose concentration, and the detection limit was 15 μM. Interference of ascorbic acid and uric acid were below 7.6%. The physically Au deposited poly(MAn)-g-MWNT paste electrodes appear to be good sensors in detecting glucose.

Hydroxyl group was introduced onto the surface of fullerene by RIGP of VPBA in a methanol/1,2-dichlorobenzene mixture solution. The obtained functionalized-fullerene, F-fullerene, was then used as a sensor support material. The enzyme electrode was prepared on the ITO electrode via hand-casting of the chitosan solution based on F-fullerene and tyrosinase. The sensing range of the biosensor was 0.1 ~ 0.6 mM for phenol in a phosphate buffer solution. Furthermore, the prepared biosensor was used to determine concentration of phenolics in commercial red wines (Chung et al, 2011).

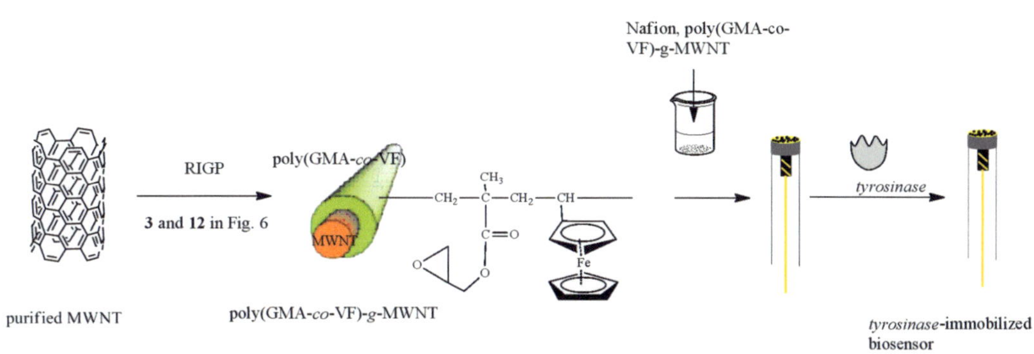

Fig. 7. Preparation of enzymatic biosensor based on poly(GMA-*co*-VF)-g-MWNT prepared by RIGP.

Ferrocene derivatives are widely used as electron transfer mediators for amperometric glucose biosensors since ferrocene meets the criteria of a good mediator, such as inert behavior with oxygen, stable in both redox forms, independent of pH, shows reversible electron transfer kinetics, and reacts rapidly with enzymes (Eggins, 1996). A polymeric mediator is necessary since polymers allow the incorporation of reagents to achieve reagentless sensing devices. Some examples of redox copolymers trialing the covalent attachment of ferrocene include poly(vinylferrocene-co-hydroxyethyl methacrylate),

poly(N-acryloylpyrrolidine-co-vinylferrocene) and ferrocene-containing polythiophene derivative (T. Saito & Watanabe, 1998; Koide & Yokoyama, 1999).
The electrochemical phenol biosensor was fabricated by immobilizing tyrosinase on poly(glycidyl methacrylate-*co*-vinylferrocene)/MWNT [poly(GMA-*co*-VFc)/MWNT] film, as shown in Fig. 7. A polymeric electron transfer mediator, containing copolymers of glycidyl methacrylate (GMA) and vinylferrocene (VFc) with different molar ratios, was prepared by RIGP. The prepared poly(GMA-*co*-VFc)/MWNT was confirmed via Fourier transform infrared spectrometer (FT-IR), thermogravimetric analysis (TGA), transmission electron microscopy (TEM) and X-ray photoelectron spectra (XPS). Also, the sensing efficiency of the fabricated electrochemical phenol biosensor was evaluated by cyclic voltametric (CV) (Lee & Choi, 2010).

3.2 ECL biosensor

Electrogenerated chemiluminescence (ECL) is a light emission produced from a high energy electron transfer (redox) reaction between electrogenerated species, which is usually accompanied by the regeneration of emitting species. In ECL, light emission is controlled by turning on/off the electrode potential. ECL has been receiving great attention as an important and valuable detection method in analytical chemistry. Application of ECL is widely found in chemical sensing (Knight, 1999), imaging (Wightman et al., 1998), and optical studies (Fan et al., 1998). Moreover, it is also used in chromatography (Noffsinger & Danielson, 1987) and capillary electrophoresis (Arora et al., 2001). Among the various ECL systems, $Ru(bpy)_3^{2+}$ is the most widely used complex due to its excellent intrinsic characteristics and capability to produce ECL with a wide range of analysis, such as oxalate, amines, and amino acid.
Chemiluminescence Sensor was fabricated based on conducting polymer@SiO_2/Nafion composite film (Jung et al., 2010). The Tris(2,2′-bipyridyl)ruthenium (II) ($Ru(bpy)_3^{2+}$) ECL sensor was fabricated by immobilization of $Ru(bpy)_3^{2+}$ complex on the functionalized MWNT-Nafion composite film coated glass carbon (GC) electrode. The functionalized MWNT was prepared by coating polythiophene (PTh), polyaniline (PANI), and poly(3-thiopheneacetic acid) [P(3-TAA)] on the surface of the carboxylic acid-modified MWNTs. The sensitivity and reproducibility of the prepared ECL sensor to tripropylamine (TPA) was evaluated. As a result, the carboxylic acid-modified MWNT composite electrode showed higher sensitivity and better reproducibility than that of other functionalized MWNT composite electrodes (S. H. Kim et al., 2008).
A SO_3H-F-MWNT-Nafion-$Ru(bpy)_3^{2+}$-ADH ECL electrode for ethanol sensing is shown in Fig. 8. The ECL sensor was fabricated by immobilization of $Ru(bpy)_3^{2+}$ on the SO_3H-functionalized MWNT (SO_3H-F-MWNT)-Nafion composite film coated on a GC electrode. Finally, ADH was immobilized on the electrode in a phosphate buffer solution at 4 °C. The SO_3H-F-MWNT ECL biosensor showed higher sensing efficiency for ethanol than that of the ECL biosensor prepared by purified MWNT. Experimental parameters affecting ethanol detection were also examined in terms of pH, and the content of SO_3H-F-MWNT in Nafion. Little interference of other compounds for assay of the ethanol was observed. Results suggest that the ECL biosensor could be applied for ethanol detection in real samples (Ryu & Choi, 2010b).
A COOH-F-MWNT-Nafion-$Ru(bpy)_3^{2+}$-Au-ADH ECL electrode using COOH-functionalized MWNTs (COOH-F-MWNT) and Au nanoparticles synthesized by γ-irradiation was fabricated for ethanol sensing (Piao et al., 2009). Here, Au atoms were produced in solution

by radiation-induced reduction of Au ion-precursors without chemical reducing agents. The species arising from the radiolysis of water, solvated electrons, e_{aq}^-, and H· atoms are the strongest reducing agents. They easily reduce Au ions to produce Au nanoparticles. A higher sensing efficiency for ethanol for the ECL biosensor prepared by Poly(AAc)*g*-MWNT (#1 in Fig. 6) was measured compared to that of the ECL biosensor prepared by Poly(Mac)-*g*-MWNT (#2 in Fig. 6), and purified MWNT. Experimental parameters affecting ethanol detection were also examined in terms of pH and the content of Poly(AAc)-*g*-MWNT in Nafion. The sensors can effectively avoid interference from the oxidation of citric acid, ascorbic acid, acetic acid and oxalic acid. The experimental results show that the ECL biosensor could be applied for ethanol detection in real samples (Piao et al., 2009).

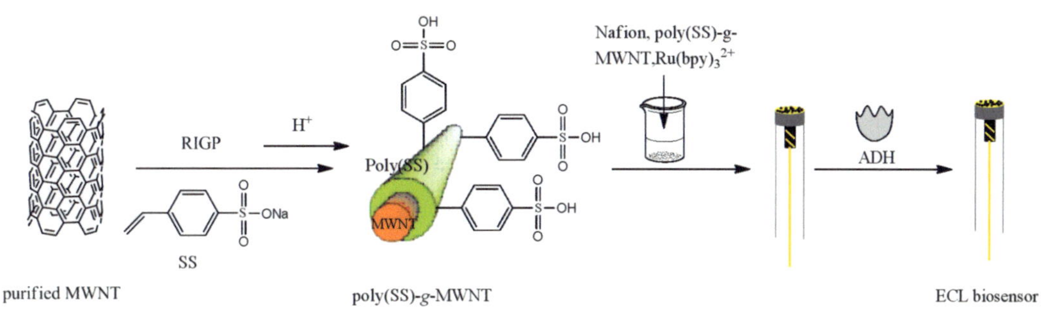

Fig. 8. Preparation of ECL biosensor based on poly(SS)-*g*-MWNT prepared by RIGP.

4. Bacteria biosensors based on polymer grafted MWNTs prepared by RIGP

Various bio-elements, including enzymes, antibodies, microorganism, organelles, tissues, and cells have been used in the fabrication of biosensors (Lei et al., 2006). Enzymes are the most widely used bio-element due to their unique specificity and sensitivity (D'Souza, 2001). However, the use of enzymes is often hampered by costly and time-consuming procedures in purification. Also, the enzyme activity could be decreased in *in vitro* operating environments (Byfield & Abuknesha, 1994). Microbes, such as algae, bacteria, and yeast can be alternatively used in the fabrication of biosensors since they can be massively produced by cell culturing. In addition, microbial cells are relatively easier to be manipulated and have better viability and stability *in vitro* compared to the cells from higher organisms such as plants, animals, and human beings (Byfield & Abuknesha, 1994).

Bacterial sensors using *Pseudomonas fluorescens* (*Pseudomonas putida* DSM 6521) and *P. putida* DSM 50026 cells entrapped with chitosan matrix onto the surface of graphite electrodes have been prepared (Odaci et al., 2008). The measurements were based on the respiratory activity of the cells. The sensor showed good linearity and repeatability with high operational stability. Also prepared were CNT-modified chitosan membranes to test the effect of nanoparticles on the biosensor performance. The results showed that combining the properties of carbon nanotubes and the versatility and biocompatibility of chitosan created chitosan surface coated carbon nanotubes.

As discussed earlier, nanomaterials have been used to improve the efficiency of electron transfer between the redox center of enzymes and electrodes (Li et al., 2006; Zhang & Fang, 2010; Guo et al., 2008). Owing to their unique properties, quantum dots (QDs) have generated considerable interest as electron transport nanomaterials for biodetection. The direct electron transfer of glucose oxidase (GOD) adsorbed on a CdS QDs modified pyrolytic graphite electrode has been reported, where the enzyme demonstrated significantly enhanced electron-transfer reactivity (Huang et al., 2007). The CdS QDs-coated electrode was displayed as a pair of well-defined redox peaks of GOD.

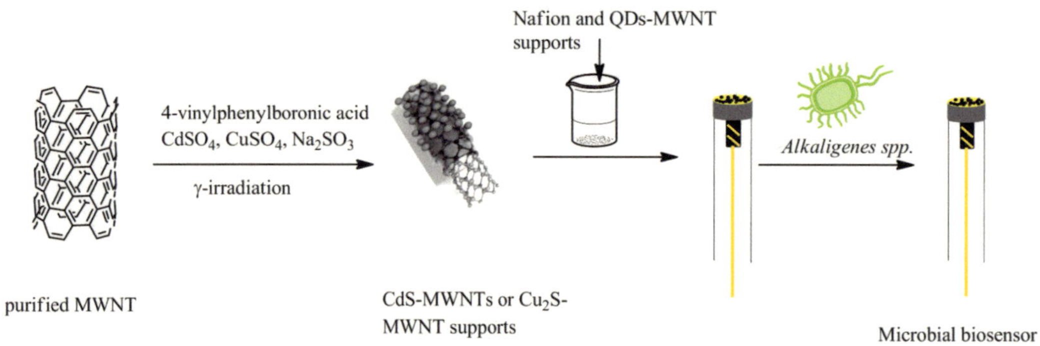

Fig. 9. Preparation of microbial biosensor based on QD-MWNT prepared by radiation reaction.

The *Acaligense sp.*-immobilized biosensor was fabricated based on QD-MWNT composites as an electron transfer mediate and a microbe immobilization support for sensing phenolic compounds in commercial red wines, as shown in Fig. 9 (S. K. Kim et al., 2011). First, the quantum dot-modified MWNT composite (QD-MWNTs) was prepared in an aqueous solution at room temperature. The successful preparation of the QD-MWNT composite was confirmed through XPS, TEM, and elemental analysis. Second, the microbial biosensor was fabricated by immobilization of *Acaligense sp.* on the surface of the GC electrode, which was prepared by hand-casting with the mixture of obtained composite and Nafion solution. The sensing ranges of the microbial biosensor based on CdS-MWNT and Cu_2S-MWNT supports were 0.5-5.0 mM and 0.7-10 mM for phenol in phosphate buffer solution, respectively. Total concentration of phenolic compounds contained in commercial red wines was also determined using the prepared microbial immobilized biosensor (S. K. Kim et al., 2011).
RIGP of the poly(GMA) onto MWNT surfaces in an aqueous solution at room temperature was performed to introduce an epoxy group (Shin et al, 2011). The epoxy group can be easily converted to alcohols, amines, phosphonic acid, and sulfonic acid. Subsequently, triethylene diamine (TEDA) was introduced onto the epoxy group of the grafted poly(GMA) to prepare MWNT supports with an amine group. Finally, the electrochemical microbial biosensor (EMB) was fabricated after immobilization of a microbe (*Alkaligenes spp.)* on the modified electrode. The EMB was evaluated for its sensing efficiency for phenol in a phosphate buffer solution. The total concentration of phenolic compounds in commercial red wines was determined using the EMB.

5. E-DNA biosensor based on polymer grafted MWNT prepared by RIGP

Currently, direct detection of nucleic acids is an area of tremendous interest, as it plays a major role in forensics (Jelly et al., 2008), pharmaceutical applications (Kranaster & Marx, 2007), medical diagnosis (Marras et al., 2006), food and agricultural analysis (Timko et al.,

2008), and environmental control (X. C. Shen et al., 2008). Electrochemical transducers offer many potential advantages that include sensitivity, accurate specificity, simplicity and low-cost, in converting nucleic acid hybridization events into useful analytical signals (Millan et al., 1994; Hashimoto et al., 1994; S. F. Wang et al., 2005). Electrochemical DNA (E-DNA) biosensors have been popularly developed for DNA sequence analysis with immobilization of single-stranded DNA (ssDNA) probes on various electrode surfaces (Niu et al., 2009).

Fabrication of E-DNA biosensors has been reported by the physical immobilization of probe DNA, 5'NH_2-GGA GCT GCT GGC ATT ATT GAA-3', on ionic-liquid (IL) modified MWNTs with ITO electrodes to detect *Salmonella typhi* (*S.* typhi), as shown in Fig. 10 (Chung et al., 2009). IL-MWNTs were prepared by the introduction of 1-butylimidazole bromide onto an epoxy group on poly(GMA)-grafted MWNTs, which were synthesized by RIGP of GMA onto MWNTs in aqueous solution. Subsequently, IL-MWNTs were coated onto the ITO electrode surface, and then the physical immobilization of the probe DNA performed in solution at room temperature for 1 h. The IL-MWNTs were characterized by elemental analysis, XPS, and TGA. The electron transfer resistance (R_{et}) of the E-DNA biosensor was evaluated after hybridization of the probe DNA and target DNA using electrochemical impedance spectroscopy (EIS). The R_{et} increased after the hybridization of probe DNA and target DNA. The target DNAs used were: (1) Complementary DNA, 5'-TTC AAT AAT GCC AGC AGC TCC-3', (2) Single-base mismatch DNA, 5'-TTC AAT AAT GGC AGC AGC TCC-3 ' and (3) Three-base mismatch DNA, 5'-TTC ATT AAT GGC AGC ACG TCC-3' (Chung et al. 2009).

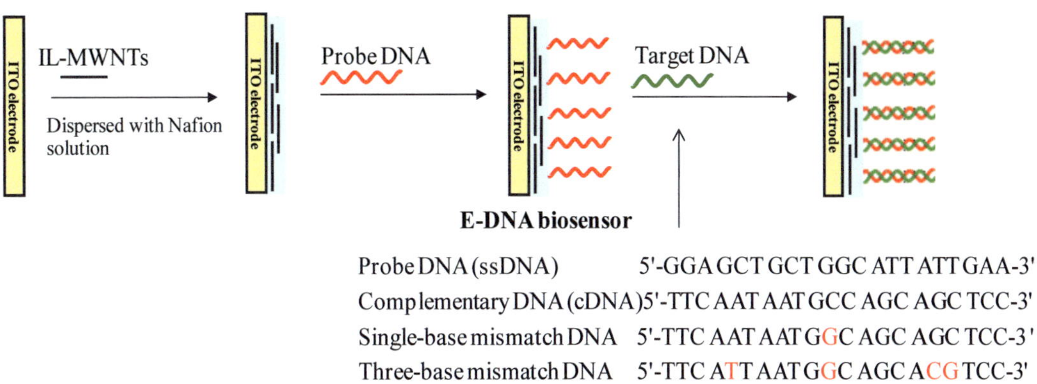

Fig. 10. Preparation of E-DNA biosensor based on IL-MWNTs prepared by RIGP.

6. Conclusion

This chapter has discussed fabrication of biosensors using vinyl polymer-grafted carbon nanotubes prepared by RIGP. To fabricate a biosensor, biomolecules should be immobilized on transducers or support matrices either by chemical methods or by physical methods. Nanostructured materials have been applied in biosensing due to their good biocompatibility, enhanced electron transfer property, and high surface area. Immobilization of bio-elements on nanostructured electrodes could potentially improve the sensitivity of biosensors

The small size and electronic properties of CNTs make them ideal for use in electrochemical biosensors and nanoscale electronic devices. However, the insolubility of CNTs in most solvents is a major barrier for developing such CNT-based biosensing devices. Therefore, surface modification is necessary for CNT materials to be biocompatible and to improve solubility in common solvents and selective binding capability to biotargets. Various vinyl monomers have been used to functionalize CNTs since they possess both hydrophobic and hydrophilic properties. The vinyl group of the monomer comes to the surface of CNTs because of a hydrophobic-hydrophobic interaction, while the functional group of monomer comes to the surface in an aqueous solution because of a hydrophilic-hydrophilic interaction.

When irradiated by γ-rays, the radical polymerization of the monomer on the surface of CNT occurs. RIGP is a useful method for the introduction of functional groups into polymer *matrices* using specially selected vinyl monomers. Two active species such as a free radical and a hydrated electron generated during γ-irradiation are used in preparing polymer nanocomposites. Various polymer–CNT nanocomposites using RIGP of the desired vinyl monomers can be prepared in a one-step process at room temperature and ambient pressure. The obtained vinyl polymer-grafted CNTs are used as biosensor supporting materials to increase sensitivity and affinity for biomolecules.

Catalyst dispersion and utilization have been shown to improve supporting Pt-Ru nanoparticles on high-surface area carbon materials. The metal (Ag or Pd) and alloy (Pt-Ru) nanoparticles have been deposited on the polymer-wrapped MWNT supports using γ-irradiation without anchoring agents. Non-enzymatic glucose sensors employing PVP modified-MWNTs with highly dispersed Pt-M (M = Ru and Sn) nanoparticles were fabricated by radiolytic deposition. The biosensor with Pt-Ru nanoparticles for glucose shwed good sensitivity, linear range, and a lower detection limit in NaOH electrolyte.

The obtained vinyl polymer-grafted CNTs have been successfully used as biosensor supporting materials for various types biosensors, including enzyme-free biosensors, enzymatic biosensors, bacterial biosensors, and E-DNA biosensors. Poly(VPBAc)-grafted MWNTs were prepared and used in enzyme-free glucose sensors for the detection of glucose without enzymes. The electrode displayed an excellent linear response to glucose concentration in the range 1.0–10 mM. The *tyrosinase*-immobilized biosensor was fabricated by a hand-casting of the modified MWNTs, *tyrosinase*, and chitosan solution as a binder onto ITO glass surface. The sensing ranges of the *tyrosinase*-biosensor for phenol in phosphate buffer solution was in the range of 0.005 ~ 0.2 mM. The biosensors were used to determine phenolic compounds in red wines or caffeine in commercial coffee. The *Acaligense sp.*-immobilized biosensor was also fabricated based on QD-MWNTs composites as an electron transfer mediator and a microbe immobilization support for sensing phenolic compounds in commercial red wines. E-DNA biosensor has been fabricated by physical immobilization of probe DNA on IL-MWNTs modified glassy carbon (GC) electrode in order to detect *Salmonella typhi* (S. typhi).

7. References

Arora, A., Eijkel, J. C. T., Morf, W. E. & Manz, A. (2001). A Wireless Electrochemiluminescence Detector Applied to Direct and Indirect Detection for Electrophoresis on a Microfabricated Glass Device. *Anal. Chem.*, Vol. 73, No. 14, (June 2001), pp. 3282–3288, ISSN 0003-2700

Arvinte, A., Sesay, A. M., Virtanen, V. & Bala, C. (2008). Evaluation of Meldola Blue-Carbon Nanotube-Sol-Gel Composite for Electrochemical NADH Sensors and Their Application for Lactate Dehydrogenase-Based Biosensors. *Electroanalysis*, Vol. 20, No. 21, (November 2008), pp. 2355-2362, ISSN 1521-4109

Badugu, R., Lakowicz, J. R. & Geddes, C. D. (2004a). Excitation and emission wavelength ratiometric cyanide-sensitive probes for physiological sensing. *Anal. Biochem.*, Vol. 327, No. 1, (April 2004), pp. 82–90, ISSN 0003-2697

Badugu, R., Lakowicz, J. R. & Geddes, C. D. (2004b). Noninvasive continuous monitoring of physiological glucose using a monosaccharide-sensing contact lens. *Anal. Chem.*, Vol. 76, No. 3, (February 2004), pp. 610–618, ISSN 0003-2700

Bae, H. B., Ryu, J. H., Byun, B. S., Jung, S. H. & Choi, S. H. (2010). Facile synthesis of a few novel Pt-Ru@PPy-MWNT electrocatalysts for direct methanol fuel cells. *Current Applied Physics*, Vol. 10, No. 2, (March 2010) pp. S44–S50, ISSN 1567-1739

Bahr, J. L., Mickelson, A. T., Bronikowski, M. J., Smalley, R. E. & Tour, J. M. (2001). Dissolution of small diameter single-wall carbon nanotubes in organic solvents. *Chem. Commun.*, Vol. 2001, No. 2, (January 2001), pp. 193-194, ISSN 1359-7345

Bai, Y., Sun, Y. & Sun, C. (2008). Pt–Pb nanowire array electrode for enzyme-free glucose detection. *Biosens. Bioelectron.*, Vol. 24, No. 4, (December 2008), pp. 579-585, ISSN 0956-5663

Byfield, M.P. & Abuknesha, R.A. (1994). Biochemical aspects of biosensors. *Biosens. Bioelectron.*, Vol. 9, No. 4-5, (May 1994), pp. 373–399, ISSN 0956-5663

Cesare, N. D. & Lakowicz, J. R. (2002a). New sensitive and selective fluorescent probes for fluoride using boronic acid. *Anal. Biochem.*, Vol. 301, No. 1, (February 2002), pp. 111–116, ISSN 0003-2697

Cesare, N. D. & Lakowicz, J. R. (2002b). Charge transfer fluorescent probes using boronic acids for monosaccharide signaling. *J. Biomed. Opt.*, Vol. 7, No. 4, (October 2002), pp. 538-545, ISSN 1083-3668

Chakraborty, S. & Raj, C. R. (2007). Mediated electrocatalytic oxidation of bioanalytes and biosensing of glutamate using functionalized multiwall carbon nanotubes-biopolymer nanocomposite. *J. Electroanal. Chem.*, Vol. 609, No. 2, (November 2007), pp. 155-162, ISSN 0022-0728

Choi, S. H., Nho, Y. C. & Kim, G. T. (1999). Adsorption of Pb^{2+} and Pd^{2+} on Polyethylene Membrane with Amino Group Modified by Radiation-Induced Graft Copolymerization. *J. Appl. Polym. Sci.*, Vol. 71, No. 4, (January 1999), pp. 643-650, ISSN 1097-4628

Choi, S. H. & Nho, Y. C. (1999a). Adsorption of Co^{2+} and Cs^{1+} by Polyethylene Membrane with Iminodiacetic Acid and Sulfonic Acid Modified by Radiation-Induced Graft Copolymerization. *J. Appl. Polym. Sci.*, Vol. 71, No. 6, (February 1999), pp. 999-1006, ISSN 1097-4628

Choi, S. H. & Nho, Y. C. (1999b). Adsorption of Co^{2+} by Styrene-g-polyethylene Membrane Bearing Sulfonic Acid Group Modified by Radiation-Induced Graft Copolymerization. *J. Appl. Polym. Sci.*, Vol. 71, No. 13, (March 1999), pp. 2227-2235, ISSN 1097-4628

Choi, S. H., Park, S. Y. & Nho, Y. C. (2000a). Electrochemical properties of polyethylene membrane modified with carboxylic acid group. *Radiat. Phys. Chem.*, Vol. 57, No. 2, (February 2000), pp. 179-186, ISSN 0969-806X

Choi, S. H., Lee, K. P., Lee, J. G. & Nho, Y. C. (2000b). Graft Copolymer-metal Complexes Obtained by Radiation Grafting on Polyethylene Film. *J. Appl. Polym. Sci.*, Vol. 77, No. 3, (July 2000), pp. 500-508, ISSN 1097-4628

Choi, S. H., Kang, H. J., Ryu, E. N. & Lee, K. P. (2001). Electrochemical Properties of Polyolefin Nonwoven Fabric Modified with Carboxylic Acid Group for Battery Separator. *Radiat. Phys. Chem.*, Vol. 60, No. 4-5, (March 2001), pp. 495-502, ISSN 0969-806X

Choi, S. H., Lee, S. H., Hwang, Y. M., Lee, K. P. & Kang, H. D. (2003a). Interaction between the surface of the silver nanoparticles prepared by γ-irradiation and organic molecules containing thiol group. *Radiat. Phys. Chem.*, Vol. 67, No. 3-4, (June 2003), pp. 517-521, ISSN 0969-806X

Choi, S. H., Lee, K. P. & Park, S. B. (2003b). Preparation and characterization of poly(ester)-silver and nylon-silver nanocomposites. *Proceedings of the 3rd International Materials Symposium*, ISBN 9780444514349, Jeju, Korea, July 2002

Choi, S. H., Lee, S., Kim, S. J., Sohn, S. H., Kang, H. D., Zhang, Y. P., Lee, K. P. & Chun, J. H. (2005). Preparation of Polymer-Stabilized Palladium-Silver Bimetallic Nanoparticles by γ-Irradiation and Their Catalytic Properties for Hydrogenation of *cis,cis*-1,3-Cyclooctadiene. *Catalysis Letters*, Vol. 105, No. 1-2, (November 2005), pp. 59-65, ISSN 1011-372X

Choi, S. H., Gopalan, A. I., Ryu, J. H. & Lee, K. P. (2010). Hollow Spherical Nanocapsules of Poly(pyrrole) as a promising support for PtRu nanoparticles - A New Strategy for catalyst preparation to Direct Methanol Fuel Cells. *Mater. Chem. Phys.*, Vol. 120, No. 1, (March 2010), pp. 18–22, ISSN 0254-0584

Chung, D. J., Kwon, S. Y. & Choi, S. H. (2009). Fabrication of E-DNA sensor based on Au nanoparticle and ionic liquid-modified MWNT, *Proceedings of the IUPAC 5th International Symposium*, shanghai, China, October 2009

Chung, D. J., Kim, K. I., Seong, M. K. & Choi, S. H. (2011). Radiolytic synthesis of -OH group functionalized fullerene structures and their biosensor application, *J. Appl. Polym. Sci.*, accepted on now (2011-01-19). ISSN 1097-4628

Clark, L. & Lyons, C. (1962). Electrode systems for continuous monitoring in cardiovascular surgery. *Ann. N.Y. Acad. Sci.*, Vol. 102, (October 1962), pp. 29-45, ISSN 1749-6632

Compton, D. L. & Laszlo, J. A. (2002). Direct electrochemical reduction of hemin in imidazolium-based ionic liquids. *J. Electroanal. Chem.*, Vol. 520, No. 1-2, (February 2002), pp. 71-78, ISSN 1572-6657

Crumbliss, A. L., Stonehuerner, J. G., Henkens, R. W., Zhao, J. & O'Daly, J. P. (1993). A carrageenan hydrogel stabilized colloidal gold multi-enzyme biosensor electrode utilizing immobilized horseradish peroxidase and cholesterol oxidase/cholesterol esterase to detect cholesterol in serum and whole blood. *Biosens. Bioelectron.*, Vol. 8, No. 6, (June 1993), pp. 331-337, ISSN 0956-5663

Cui, H. F., Ye, J. S., Zhang, W. D., Li, C. M., Luong, J. H. T. & Sheu, F. S. (2007). Selective and sensitive electrochemical detection of glucose in neutral solution using platinum–lead alloy nanoparticle/carbon nanotube nanocomposites. *Anal. Chim. Acta*, Vol. 594, No. 2, (July 2007), pp. 175–183, ISSN 0003-2670

D'Souza, S. F. (2001). Microbial biosensors. *Biosens. Bioelectron.*, Vol. 16, No. 6, (August 2001), pp. 337–353, ISSN 0956-5663

Domenecha, A. & Alarcon, J. (2002). Determination of hydrogen peroxide using glassy carbon and graphite/polyester composite electrodes modified by vanadium-doped zirconias. *Anal. Chim. Acta*, Vol. 452, No. 1, (January 2002), pp. 11-22, ISSN 0003-2670

Dzyadevych, S. V., Arkhypova, V. N., Soldatkin, A. P., El'skaya, A. V., Martelet, C. & Jaffrezic-Renault, N. (2008). Amperometric enzyme biosensors: Past, present and future. *Irbm*, Vol. 29, No. 2-3, (April-May 2008), pp. 171-180, ISSN 1959-0318

Eggins, B. (1996). *Biosensors: An Introduction*, Wiley & Teubner, London

Eitan, A., Jiang, K., Dukes, D., Andrews, R. & Schadler, L. S. (2003). Surface Modification of Multiwalled Carbon Nanotubes: Toward the Tailoring of the Interface in Polymer Composites. *Chem. Mater.*, Vol. 15, No. 16, (August 2003), pp. 3198-3201, ISSN 0897-4756

Fan, F.-R. F., Cliffel, D. & Bard, A. J. (1998). Scanning Electrochemical Microscopy. 37. Light Emission by Electrogenerated Chemiluminescence at SECM Tips and Their Application to Scanning Optical Microscopy. *Anal.Chem.*, Vol. 70, No. 14, (July 1998), pp. 2941-2948, ISSN 0003-2700

Feng, H., Wang, H., Zhang, Y., Yan, B. N., Shen, G. L. & Yu, R. Q. (2007). A Direct Electrochemical Biosensing Platform Constructed by Incorporating Carbon Nanotubes and Gold Nanoparticles onto Redox Poly(thionine) Film. *Anal. Sci.*, Vol. 23, No. 2, (February 2007), pp. 235-239, ISSN 0910-6340

Gavalas, V. G. & Chaniotakis, N. A. (2000). Polyelectrolyte stabilized oxidase based biosensors: effect of diethylaminoethyl-dextran on the stabilization of glucose and lactate oxidases into porous conductive carbon. *Anal. Chim. Acta*, Vol. 404, No. 1, (January 2000), pp. 67-73, ISSN 0003-2670

Gavalas, V. G. & Chaniotakis, N. A. (2001). Phosphate biosensor based on polyelectrolyte-stabilized pyruvate oxidase. *Anal. Chim. Acta*, Vol. 427, No. 2, (January 2001), pp. 271-277, ISSN 0003-2670

Guan, W. J., Li, Y., Chen, Y. Q., Zhang, X. B. & Hu, G. Q. (2005). Glucose biosensor based on multi-wall carbon nanotubes and screen printed carbon electrodes. *Biosens. Bioelectron.*, Vol. 21, No. 3, (September 2005), pp. 508-512, ISSN 0956-5663

Guo, C., Hu, F., Li, C. M. & Shen, P. K. (2008). Direct electrochemistry of hemoglobin on carbonized titania nanotubes and its application in a sensitive reagentless hydrogen peroxide biosensor. *Biosens. Bioelectron.*, Vol. 24, No. 4, (December 2008), pp. 819-824, ISSN 0956-5663

Habrioux, A., Sibert, E., Servat, K., Vogel, W., Kokoh, K. B. & Alonso-Vante, N. (2007). Activity of Platinum−Gold Alloys for Glucose Electrooxidation in Biofuel Cells. *J. Phys. Chem. B*, Vol. 111, No. 34, (August 2007), pp. 10329-10333, ISSN 1089-5647

Hashimoto, K., Ito, Y. & Ishimori, Y. (1994). Novel DNA sensor for electrochemical gene detection. *Anal. Chim. Acta*, Vol. 286, No. 2, (February 1994), pp. 219-224, ISSN 0003-2670

Hsu, N. Y., Chien, C. C. & Jeng, K. T. (2008) Characterization and enhancement of carbon nanotube-supported PtRu electrocatalyst for direct methanol fuel cell applications. *Appl. Catal., B: Environ.*, Vol. 84, No. 1-2, (October 2008), pp. 196-203, ISSN 0926-3373

Huang, C. P., Li, Y. K. & Chen, T. M. (2007). A highly sensitive system for urea detection by using CdSe/ZnS core-shell quantum dots. *Biosens. Bioelectron.*, Vol. 22, No. 8, (March 2007), pp. 1835–1838, ISSN 0956-5663

Hwang, C. G., Kim, S. H., Oh, J. H., Kim, M. R. & Choi, S. H. (2008). Reduction of Aromatic Nitro Compounds on Pd Colloids Prepared by γ-Irradiation. *J. Industr. Eng.Chem.*, Vol. 14, No. 6, (November 2008), pp. 864-868, ISSN 1226-086X

Hyeon, T., Han, S., Sung, Y., Park, K. & Kim, Y. (2003). High-Performance Direct Methanol Fuel Cell Electrodes using Solid-Phase-Synthesized Carbon Nanocoils. *Angew. Chem. Int. Ed.*, Vol. 42, No. 36, (September 2003), pp. 4352–4356, ISSN 0926-3373

Islam, M. F., Rojas, E., Bergey, D. M., Johnson, A. T. & Yodh, A. G. (2003). High Weight Fraction Surfactant Solubilization of Single-Wall Carbon Nanotubes in Water. *Nano Letters*, Vol. 3, No. 2, (February 2003), pp. 269-273, ISSN 1530-6984

Jelly, R., Lewis, S. W., Lennard, C., Lim, K. F. & Almog, J. (2008). Lawsone: a novel reagent for the detection of latent fingermarks on paper surfaces. *Chem. Commun.*, Vol. 2008, No. 30, (August 2008), pp. 3513-3515, ISSN 1364-548X

Jia, J. B., Wang, B. Q., Wu, A. G., Cheng, G. J., Li, Z. & Dong, S. J. (2002). A Method to Construct a Third-Generation Horseradish Peroxidase Biosensor: Self-Assembling Gold Nanoparticles to Three-Dimensional Sol-Gel Network. *Anal. Chem.*, Vol. 74, No. 9, (May 2002), pp. 2217-2223, ISSN 0003-2700

Jung, D. J., Piao, M. H., Oh, S. H., Woo, J. C. & Choi, S. H. (2010). Fabrication of Chemiluminescence Sensor Based on Conducting Polymer@SiO_2/Nafion Composite Film. *J. Nanosci. Nanotechnol.*, Vol. 10, No. 10, (October 2010), pp. 6855-6858, ISSN 1533-4880

Kang, Y. & Taton, T. A. (2003). Micelle-Encapsulated Carbon Nanotubes: A Route to Nanotube Composites. *J. Am. Chem. Soc.*, Vol. 125, No. 19, (April 2003), pp. 5650–5651, ISSN 0002-7863

Kim, K. I., Kang, H. Y., Lee, J. C. & Choi, S. H. (2009). Fabrication of MWNT ion liquid electrode and its application for sensing phenolics in red wines. *Sensors*, Vol. 9, No. 9, (August 2009), pp. 6701-6714, ISSN 1424-8220

Kim, K. I., Lee. J. C., Kevin, R. & Choi, S. H. (2010). Immobilization of tyrosinase in carboxylic- and carbonyl group-modified MWNT electrode and its application for sensing phenolics in red wines. *J. Nanosci. Nanotechnol.*, Vol. 10, No. 6, (June 2010), pp. 3790-3798, ISSN 1533-4880

Kim, M. R. & Choi, S. H. (2009). One-Pot Synthesis of Pd-M/ZnO (M = Ag, Cu, and Ni) Catalysts by γ-Irradiation and Their Use in Hydrogenation and Suzuki Reaction. *J. Nanomaterials*, Vol. 2009, (February 2009), pp. 1-7, ISSN 1687-4110

Kim, O. K., Je, J., Baldwin, J. W., Kooi, S., Pehrsson, P. E. & Buckley, L. J. (2003). Solubilization of Single-Wall Carbon Nanotubes by Supramolecular Encapsulation of Helical Amylose. *J. Am. Chem. Soc.*, Vol. 125, No. 15, (March 2003), pp. 4426–4427, ISSN 0002-7863

Kim, S. H., Oh, J. H., Yoo, B., Jung, D. J., Piao, M. H. & Choi, S. H. (2008). Fabrication of Chemiluminescence Sensor Based on the Funcinalized MWNT-Nafion Composite Film. *Adv. Mater. Res.*, Vol. 47-50, (June 2008), pp. 1474-1477, ISSN 1022-6680

Kim, S. J., Oh, S. D., Lee, S. & Choi, S. H. (2008). Radiolytic Synthesis of Pd-M (M = Ag, Ni, and Cu)/C Catalyst and Their Use in Suzuki-type and Heck-type Reaction. *J. Industr. Eng. Chem.*, Vol. 14, No. 4, (July 2008), pp. 449-456, ISSN 1226-086X

Kim, S. K., Ryu, J. H., Kwen. H. D. & Choi, S. H. (2010). Convenient Preparation of Ion-Exchange PVdF Membrane by Radiation-Induced Graft Polymerization for a Battery Separator. *Polymer(Korea)*, Vol. 34, No. 2, (March 2010), pp. 126-132, ISSN 0379-153X

Kim, S. K., Kwen, H. D. & Choi, S. H. (2011). Fabrication of microbial biosensor based on the QDs-MWNTs supports by one-step radiation reaction and detection of phenolic compounds in red wines. *Sensors*, vol. 11, (January 2011), pp. 2001-2012, ISSN 1424-8220

Kitano, H., Tachimoto, K. & Anraku,Y. (2007). Functionalization of single-walled carbon nanotube by the covalent modification with polymer chains. *J. Colloid Interface Sci.*, Vol. 306, No. 1, (February 2007), pp. 28-33, ISSN 0021-9797

Knight, A. W. (1999). A review of recent trends in analytical applications of electrogenerated chemiluminescence. *Trends Anal. Chem.*, Vol. 18, No. 1, (January 1999), pp. 47-62, ISSN 0165-9936

Koide, S. & Yokoyama, K. (1999). Electrochemical characterization of an enzyme electrode based on a ferrocene-containing redox polymer. *J. Electroanal. Chem.*, Vol. 468, No. 2, (June 1999), pp. 193–201, ISSN 0022-0728

Kooi, S. E., Schlecht, U., Burghard, M. & Kern, K. (2002). Electrochemical Modification of Single Carbon Nanotubes. *Angew. Chem. Int. Ed.*, Vol. 41, No. 8, (April 2002), pp. 1353-1355, ISSN 1521-3773

Kranaster, R. & Marx, A. (2007). Increased single-nucleotide discrimination in allele-specific polymerase chain reactions through primer probes bearing nucleobase and 2'-deoxyribose modifications. *Chem. Eur. J.*, Vol. 13, No. 21, (July 2007), pp. 6115-6122, 1521-3765

Kwon, S. Y., Whittaker, A. & Choi, S. H. (2011). Fabrication of non-enzymatic glucose sensor based on MWNTs with bimetallic Pt-M (M= Ru and Sn) catalysts by radiolytic deposition. *Biosens. Bioelectron.*, submitted for publication (2010-11-08), ISSN 0956-5663

Lee, Y. J., Kim, J. D. & Park, J. Y. (2009). CMOS-Integrable Enzyme-Free Amperometric Cholesterol Nano-Biosensor for U-Health and POC Applications. *Journal of the Korean Physical Society*, Vol. 54, No. 5, (May 2009), pp. 1769-1773, ISSN 0374-4884

Lee, Y. J. & Choi, S. H. (2010). Electrochemical phenol biosensor based on immobilization of tyrosinase on poly(GMA-co-VFc)/MWNT electrode. *Proceedings of the Korean society of analytical sciences*, Jeju, Korea, November 2010

Lei, Y., Chen, W. & Mulchandani, A. (2006). Microbial biosensors. *Anal. Chim. Acta*, Vol. 568, No. 1-2, (May 2006), pp. 200–210, ISSN 0003-2670

Li, Y., Kotzeva, V. P. & Fray, D. J. (2006). Electrochemical performance of CdS nanomaterials synthesized by microemulsion techniques. *Materials Letters*, Vol. 60, No. 21-22, (September 2006), pp. 2743-2746, ISSN 0167-577X

Lin, K. C., Tsai, T. S., & Chen, S. M. (2010). Performing enzyme-free H_2O_2 biosensor and simultaneous determination for AA, DA, and UA by MWNT–PEDOT film. *Biosens. Bioelectron.*, Vol. 26, No. 2, (October 2010), pp. 608–614, ISSN 0956-5663

Lin, M. S. & Leu, H. J. (2005). A Fe_3O_4-Based Chemical Sensor for Cathodic Determination of Hydrogen Peroxide. *Electroanalysis*, Vol. 17, No. 22, (November 2005), pp. 2068–2073, ISSN 1521-4109

Liu, H., Mao, G. & Meng, S. (1992). Preparation and characterization of the polymer-protected palladium—gold colloidal bimetallic catalysts. *J. Mol. Catal.*, Vol. 74, No. 1-3, (July-August 1992), pp. 275-284, ISSN 1381-1169

Liu, P. (2005). Modifications of carbon nanotubes with polymers. *Eur. Polym. J.*, Vol. 41, No. 11, (November 2005), pp. 2693-2703, ISSN 0014-3057

Male, K. B., Hrapovic, S. & Luong, J. H. T. (2007). Electrochemically-assisted deposition of oxidases on platinum nanoparticle/multi-walled carbon nanotube-modified electrodes. *Analyst*, Vol. 132, No. 12, (December 2007), pp. 1254-1261, ISSN 0003-2654

Marras, S. A. E., Tyagi, S. & Kramer, F. R. (2006). Real-time assays with molecular beacons and other fluorescent nucleic acid hybridization probes. *Clin. Chim. Acta*, Vol. 363, No. 1-2, (January 2006), pp. 48-60, ISSN 0009-8981

Men, X. H., Zhang, Z. Z., Song, H. J., Wang, K. & Jiang, W. (2008). Functionalization of carbon nanotubes to improve the tribological properties of poly(furfuryl alcohol) composite coatings. *Comp. Sci. Technol.*, Vol. 68, No. 3-4, (March 2008), pp. 1042-1049, ISSN 0266-3538

Millan, K. M., Saraullo, A. & Mikkelsen, S. R. (1994). Voltammetric DNA Biosensor for Cystic Fibrosis Based on a Modified Carbon Paste Electrode. *Anal. Chem.*, Vol. 66, No. 18, (September 1994), pp. 2943-2948, ISSN 0003-2700

Musameh, M., Wang, J., Merkoci, A. & Lin, Y. (2002). Low-potential stable NADH detection at carbon-nanotube-modified glassy carbon electrodes. *Electrochem. Commun.*, Vol. 4, No. 10, (October 2002), pp. 743-746, ISSN 1388-2481

Niu, S. Y., Wu, M. L., Hu, L. Z., Mei, Z. H. & Liu, S. F. (2009). Nucleic acid biosensor for DNA hybridization detection using rutin–Cu as an electrochemical indicator. *Electrochimica Acta*, Vol. 54, No. 5, (February 2009), pp. 1564–1569, ISSN 0013-4686

Noffsinger, J. B. & Danielson, N. D. (1987). Liquid chromatography of aliphatic trialkylamines with post-column chemiluminescent detection using tris(2,2'-bipyridine)ruthenium(III). *J. Chromatorgr.* A, Vol. 387, (March 1987), pp. 520-524, ISSN 0021-9673

Odaci, D., Timur, S. & Telefoncu, A. (2008). Bacterial sensors based on chitosan matrices. *Sens. Actuators B*, Vol. 134, No. 1, (August 2008), pp. 89–94, ISSN 0925-4005

Oh, S. D., So, B. K., Choi, S. H., Gopalan, A., Lee, K. P., Yoon, K. R. & Choi, I. S. (2005). Dispersing of Ag, Pd, and Pt–Ru alloy nanoparticles on single-walled carbon nanotubes by γ-irradiation, *Materials Letters*, Vol. 59, No. 10, (April 2005), pp. 1121–1124, ISSN 0167-577X

Oh, S. D., Choi, S. H., Gopalan, A., Lee, K. P. & Kim, S. H. (2006a). Radiolytic Functionalization of Single- and Multi-Walled Carbon Nanotubes. *J. Industr. Eng. Chem.*, Vol. 12, No. 1, (January 2006), pp. 156-160, ISSN 1226-086X

Oh, S. D., Yoon, K. R., Choi, S. H., Gopalan, A., Lee, K. P., Sohn, S. H., Kang, H. D. & Choi, I. S. (2006b). Dispersion of Pt–Ru alloys onto various carbons using γ-irradiation, *J. Non-Cryst. Solids*, Vol. 352, No. 4, (April 2006), pp. 355–360, ISSN 0022-3093

Oh, S. D., Kim, M. R., Choi, S. H., Chun, J. H., Lee, K. P., Gopalan, A. I., Hwang, C. G., Kim, S. H. & Oh, J. H. (2008). Radiolytic Synthesis of Pd-M (M = Ag, Au, Cu, Ni and Pt) Alloy Nanoparticles and Its Use in Reduction of 4-Nitrophenol. *J. Industr. Eng.Chem.*, Vol. 14, No. 5, (September 2008), pp. 687-692, ISSN 1226-086X

Park, K., Choi, J. H., Ahn, K. S. & Sung, Y. E. (2004). PtRu Alloy and PtRu−WO_3 Nanocomposite Electrodes for Methanol Electrooxidation Fabricated by a Sputtering Deposition Method. *J. Phys. Chem. B*, Vol. 108, No. 19, (May 2004), pp. 5989–5994, ISSN 1089-5647

Park, S. J., Chung, T. D. & Kim, H. C. (2003). Nonenzymatic Glucose Detection Using Mesoporous Platinum. *Anal. Chem.*, Vol. 75, No. 13, (July 2003), pp. 3046–3049, ISSN 0003-2700

Patolsky, F., Weizmann, Y. & Willner, I. (2004). Long-Range Electrical Contacting of Redox Enzymes by SWCNT Connectors. *Angew. Chem. Int. Ed.*, Vol. 43, No. 16, (April 2004), pp. 2113-2117, ISSN 1521-3773

Piao, M. H., Yang, D. S., Yoon, K. R., Lee, S. H. & Choi, S. H. (2009). Development of an Electrogenerated Chemiluminescence Biosensor using Carboxylic acid-functionalized MWNT and Au Nanoparticles. *Sensors*, Vol. 9, No. 3, (March 2009), pp. 1662-1677, ISSN 1424-8220

Piao, M. H., Son, P. S., Chang, C. H. & Choi, S. H. (2010). A glucose biosensor based on deposition of glucose oxidase onto Au nanoparticles poly(maleic anhydride)-grafted multiwalled carbon nanotube electrode. *Anal. Sci. Tech.*, Vol. 23, No. 2, (April 2010), pp. 165-171, ISSN 1225-0163

Qu, L. T., Dai, L. M. & Osawa, E. (2006). Shape/Size-Controlled Syntheses of Metal Nanoparticles for Site-Selective Modification of Carbon Nanotubes. *J. Am. Chem. Soc.*, Vol. 128, No. 16, (April 2006), pp. 5523-5532, ISSN 0002-7863

Reddy, A. L. M. & Ramaprabhu, S. (2007). Pt/SWNT−Pt/C Nanocomposite Electrocatalysts for Proton-Exchange Membrane Fuel Cells. *J. Phys. Chem. C*, Vol. 111, No. 44, (November 2007), pp. 16138–16146, ISSN 1932-7447

Ryu, H. N. & Choi, S. H. (2010a). Tyrosinase-immobilized Biosensor Based on Ionic Property-modified MWNTs Prepared by Radiation-induced Graft Polymerization. *Carbon Letters*, Vol. 11, No. 3, (December 2010), pp. 216-223, ISSN 1976-4251

Ryu, H. N. & Choi, S. H. (2010b). Fabrication of electrochemiluminescence (ECL) sensor based on sulfonic acid (-SO_3H) functionalized carbon nanotube. *Proceedings of the Korean society of analytical sciences*, Jeju, Korea, November 2010

Saito, T. & Watanabe, M. (1998). Characterization of poly(vinylferrocene-co-2- hydroxyethyl methacrylate) for use as electron mediator in enzymatic glucose sensor. *React. Funct. Polym.*, Vol. 37, No. 1-3, (June 1998), pp. 263–269, ISSN 1381-5148

Saito, Y., Yoshikawa, T., Okuda, M., Fujimoto, N., Sumiyama, K., Suzuki, K., Kasuya, A. & Nishina, Y. (1993). Carbon nanocapsules encaging metals and carbides. *J. Phys. Chem. Solids.*, Vol. 54, No. 12, (December 1993), pp. 1849-1860, ISSN 0022-3697

Seo, K. D., Oh, S. D., Choi, S. H., Kim, S. H., Park, H. G. & Zhang, Y. P. (2008). Radiolytic loading of the Pt–Ru nanoparticles onto the porous carbons. *Colloids Surf. A: Physicochem. Eng. Aspects*, Vol. 313–314, (February 2008), pp. 393–397, ISSN 0927-7757

Shen, J., Huang, W., Wu, L., Hu, Y. & Ye, M. (2007). Study on amino-functionalized multiwalled carbon nanotubes. *Mater. Sci. Eng. A*, Vol. 464, No. 1-2, (August 2007), pp. 151-156, ISSN 0921-5093

Shen, X-C., Zhang, Z-L., Zhou, B., Peng, J., Xie, M., Zhang, M. & Pang, D-W. (2008). Visible lightinduced plasmid DNA damage catalyzed by a CdSe/ZnS-photosensitized nano-TiO_2 film. *Environ. Sci. Technol.*, Vol. 42, No. 14, (July 2008), pp. 5049-5054, ISSN 0013-936X

Shin, S. R., Kwen, H. D. & Choi, S. H. (2011). Fabrication of Electrochemical Microbial Biosensor Based on MWNT Supports prepared by Radiation-Induced Graft Polymerization, Polymer(Korea), submitted for publication (2010-09), ISSN 0379-153X

Shumyantseva, V., Deluca, G., Bulko, T., Carrara, S., Nicolini, C., Usanov, S. & Archakov, A. (2004). Cholesterol amperometric biosensor based on cytochrome P450scc. *Biosens. Bioelectron.*, Vol. 19, No. 9, (April 2004), pp. 971-976, ISSN 0956-5663

Song, Y. Y., Zhang, D., Gao, W. & Xia, X. H. (2005). Nonenzymatic Glucose Detection by Using a Three-Dimensionally Ordered, Macroporous Platinum Template, *Chem. Eur. J.*, Vol. 11, No. 7, (March 2005), pp. 2177-2182, ISSN 1521-3765

Steigerwalt, E. S., Deluga, G. A. & Lukehart, C. M. (2002). Pt–Ru/Carbon Fiber Nanocomposites: Synthesis, Characterization, and Performance as Anode Catalysts of Direct Methanol Fuel Cells. A Search for Exceptional Performance. *J. Phys. Chem. B*, Vol. 106, No. 4, (January 2002), pp. 760–766, ISSN 0022-3654

Sun, Y., Buck, H. & Mallouk, T. E. (2001). Combinatorial Discovery of Alloy Electrocatalysts for Amperometric Glucose Sensors. *Anal. Chem.*, Vol. 73, No. 7, (April 2001), pp. 1599–1604. ISSN 0003-2700

Sweeny, B. K. & Peters, G. G. (2001). Cyclic voltammetric study of the catalytic behavior of nickel (I) salen electrogenerated at a glassy carbon electrode in an ionic liquid (1-butyl-3-methylimidazolium tetrafluoroborate, BMIM+BF4−). *Electrochem. Commun.*, Vol. 3, No. 12, (December 2001), pp. 712-715, ISSN 1388-2481

Tasis, D., Tagmatarchis, N., Georgakilas, V. & Prato, M. (2003). Soluble Carbon Nanotubes. *Chem. Eur. J.*, Vol. 9, No. 17, (September 2003), pp. 4000-4008, ISSN 0947-6539

Timko, M. P., Rushton, P. J., Laudeman, T. W., Bokowiec, M. T., Chipumuro, E., Cheung, F., Town, C. D. & Chen, X. F. (2008). Sequencing and analysis of the gene-rich space of cowpea. *BMC Genomics.*, Vol. 9, (February 2008), pp. 103-123, ISSN 1471-2164

Wang, J., Li, M., Shi, Z., Li, N. & Gu, Z. (2002a). Electrocatalytic Oxidation of Norepinephrine at a Glassy Carbon Electrode Modified with Single Wall Carbon Nanotubes. *Electroanalysis*,Vol. 14, No. 3, (February 2002), pp. 225-230, ISSN 1521-4109

Wang, J., Li, M., Shi, Z., Li, N. & Gu, Z. (2002b). Direct Electrochemistry of Cytochrome c at a Glassy Carbon Electrode Modified with Single-Wall Carbon Nanotubes. *Anal. Chem.*, Vol. 74, No. 9, (March 2002), pp. 1993-1997, ISSN 0003-2700

Wang, J. & Musameh, M. (2003a). Carbon Nanotube/Teflon Composite Electrochemical Sensors and Biosensors. *Anal. Chem.*, Vol. 75, No. 9, (March 2008), pp. 2075-2079, ISSN 0003-2700

Wang, J., Musameh, M. & Lin, Y. (2003b). Solubilization of Carbon Nanotubes by Nafion toward the Preparation of Amperometric Biosensors. *J. Am. Chem. Soc.*, Vol. 125, No. 9, (February 2003), pp. 2408-2409, ISSN 0002-7863

Wang, J., Jina, S. & Wang, B. (2005). A new boronic acid fluorescent reporter that changes emission intensities at three wavelengths upon sugar binding. *Tetrahedron Lett.*, Vol. 46, No. 41, (October 2005), pp. 7003–7006, ISSN 0040-4039

Wang, J., Thomas, D. F. & Chen, A. (2008). Nonenzymatic Electrochemical Glucose Sensor Based on Nanoporous PtPb Networks. *Anal. Chem.*, Vol. 80, No. 4, (February 2008), pp. 997–1004, ISSN 0003-2700

Wang, S. F., Wang, W. & Cai, H. C. (2005). Recognition and detection of dsDNA at a thionalid self-assembled monolayer modified gold electrode. *Sens. Actuator B: Chem.*, Vol. 104, No. 1, (January 2005), pp. 8-14, ISSN 0925-4005

Wang, Y., Huang, J., Zhang, C., Wei, J. & Zhou, X. (1998). Determination of Hydrogen Peroxide in Rainwater by Using a Polyaniline Film and Platinum Particles Co-Modified Carbon Fiber Microelectrode. *Electroanalysis*, Vol. 10, No. 11, (September 1998), pp. 776–778, ISSN 1521-4109

Wang, Z. H., Liu, J., Liang, Q. L., Wang, Y. M. & Luo, G. (2002). Carbon nanotube-modified electrodes for the simultaneous determination of dopamine and ascorbic acid. *Analyst*, Vol. 127, No. 5, (May 2002), pp. 653-658, ISSN 0003-2654

Wightman, R. M., Curtis, C. L., Flowers, P. A., Maus, R. G. & McDonald, E. M. (1998). Imaging Microelectrodes with High-Frequency Electrogenerated Chemiluminescence. *J. Phys. Chem. B.*, Vol. 102, No. 49, (December 1998), pp. 9991-9996, ISSN 1089-5647

Xiao, F., Zhao, F., Zhang, Y., Guo, G. & Zeng, B. (2009). Ultrasonic Electrodeposition of Gold−Platinum Alloy Nanoparticles on Ionic Liquid−Chitosan Composite Film and Their Application in Fabricating Nonenzyme Hydrogen Peroxide Sensors. *J. Phys. Chem. C*, Vol. 113, No. 3, (January 2009), pp. 849–855, ISSN 1932-7447

Yang, D. S., Jung, D. J. & Choi, S. H. (2010). One-step functionalization of multi-walled carbon nanotubes by radiation-induced graft polymerization and their application as enzyme-free biosensors. *Radia. Phys. Chem.*, Vol. 79, No. 4, (April 2010), pp. 434–440, ISSN 0969-806X

Yang, D. S., Sim, K. S., Kwen, H. D. & Choi, S. H. (2011). Radiolytic synthesis of Pt-Ru catalysts based on functional polymer-grafted MWNT and their catalytic efficiency for CO and MeOH. *J. Nanomaterials*, Vol. 2011, pp. 1-8, ISSN 1687-4110

Yang, J. H., Lee, J. C. & Choi, S. H. (2009). Tyrosinase-Immobilized Biosensor Based on the Functionalized Hydroxyl Group-MWNT and Detection of Phenolic Compounds in Red Wines. *J. Sensors*, Vol. 2009, (August 2009), pp. 1-9, ISSN 1687-725X

Yang, R., Qiu, X., Zhang, H., Li, J., Zhu, W., Wang, Z., Huang, X. & Chen, L. (2005). Monodispersed hard carbon spherules as a catalyst support for the electrooxidation of methanol. *Carbon*, Vol. 43, No. 1, (January 2005), pp. 11–16, ISSN 0008-6223

Yu, W., Liu, M., Liu, H. & Zheng, J. (1999). Preparation of Polymer-Stabilized Noble Metal Colloids. *J. Colloid Interf. Sci.*, Vol. 210, No. 1, (February 1999), pp. 218-221, ISSN 0021-9797

Zhang, L. & Fang, M. (2010). Nanomaterials in pollution trace detection and environmental improvement. *Nano Today*, Vol. 5, No. 2, (April 2010), pp. 128-142, ISSN 1748-0132

Zhang, Y. J., Shen, Y. F., Li, J. H., Niu, L., Dong, S. J. & Ivaska, A. (2005). Electrochemical Functionalization of Single-Walled Carbon Nanotubes in Large Quantities at a Room-Temperature Ionic Liquid Supported Three-Dimensional Network Electrode. *Langmuir*, Vol. 21, No. 11, (May 2005), pp. 4797-4800, ISSN 0743-7463

Zhao, Y., Zheng, W. D., Chen, H. & Luo, Q. M. (2002). Anodic oxidation of hydrazine at carbon nanotube powder microelectrode and its detection. *Talanta*, Vol. 58, No. 3, (September 2002), pp. 529-534, ISSN 0039-9140

13

Design and Fabrication of 3D Skyscraper Nanostructures and Their Applications in Biosensors

Guigen Zhang
Department of Bioengineering, Department of Electrical and Computer Engineering
Institute for Biological Interfaces of Engineering 301, Rhodes Engineering Research Center
Clemson University Clemson, SC 29634
USA

1. Introduction

Biosensors are analytical devices that combine a biologically sensitive element with a physical transducer to selectively and quantitatively detect the presence as well as the amount of a specific compound in biological environments. The biosensitive element is for target recognition and the physical transducer is for signal transduction. For the biosensitive element, molecular couples such as antibody-antigen, protein-ligand, protein-aptamer, paired-nucleotides and avidin-biotin are often used, and for the physical transducer electrochemical methods such as voltammetric, impedimetric and amperometric measurements are popular choices. For example, a sensing platform using the avidin-biotin couple as the biosensitive element and an electrochemical technique as the physical transducer has been widely explored to achieve rapid, specific and sensitive detections (Ding *et al.*, 2005; Hou *et al.*, 2006, 2007; Lee *et al.*, 2008).

Biosensors are important devices for monitoring biological species in various processes of environmental, food, pharmaceutical and biomedical concerns. The main challenges many biosensors face today include low sensitivity, poor specificity and proneness to fouling. The advent of nanotechnology presents some promising solutions for alleviating these problems. For example, improvements for the sensitivity and antifouling capability of biosensors have been explored through the incorporation of nanostructures into the electrodes of biosensors (Koehne *et al.*, 2004; Wang *et al.*, 2005; Anandan *et al.*, 2006, 2007). Nanostructures like gold nanotubes (Delvaux *et al.*, 2003), carbon nanotubes (Gao *et al.*, 2003; Wang *et al.*, 2003, 2004) and gold nanoparticles (Bharathi *et al.*, 2001) have been incorporated into electrodes and they exhibited much improved performance than conventional flat electrodes.

Biosensors using an electrochemical method as the underlying transducer offer a cost-effective and more specific means to measure the electrical responses resulted from electrochemical reactions between the sensitive element and the target analyte. In an electrochemical based biosensor, the sensitivity is related to the surface area of its electrode (Bard *et al.*, 2001; Delvaux *et al.*, 2003) because a large surface area is beneficial not only for enzyme immobilization but also for electron transfer. The surface area of the electrode can be increased by the use of nanostructures because the surface-to-volume ratio of a structure increases as its size decreases (Jia *et al.*, 2007; Anandan *et al.*, 2007, Gangadharan *et al.*, 2008). Since most of these nanostructures are made of inorganic materials, to use them as electrodes they have to be functionalized for biological recognition purposes (Gangadharan *et al.*, 2008; Lee *et al.*, 2008). To functionalize these electrodes, biosensitive elements need to be immobilized onto the electrode surface. In many situations, biosensitive molecules cannot be immobilized directly onto the surface of these inorganic materials, thus anchoring molecules are necessary. Therefore, the ability to improve the performance of these inorganic-based nanostructured electrodes relies on not only the morphological design of the nanostructures but also the selection of anchoring molecules, aside from the effects of electrode reactions and the underlying mass transport mechanisms (Anandan *et al.*, 2007).

To achieve high efficiency in enzyme immobilization on electrode surface, many techniques have been developed including the use of self assembled monolayer (Gooding *et al.*, 1998, 2000; Losic *et al.*, 2001a, 2001b; Berchmans *et al.*, 2003), conducting polymers (Uang *et al.*, 2002; Gao *et al.*, 2003) and sol-gels (Qiao *et al.*, 2005). Among these methods, the self-assembled monolayer (SAM) technique offers a better control for enzyme distribution at the molecular level and a high degree of reproducibility in enzyme immobilization (Losic *et al.*, 2001a, 2001b; Berchmans *et al.*, 2003). Physical entrapment of an enzyme in a porous conducting polymer film at electrode surface offers an attractive alternative. Conducting polymer like polypyrrole (PPy) can be electro- polymerized and deposited onto the electrode surface to form a porous film, providing pores large enough for efficient electron transfer (Ramanavicius *et al.*, 2001; Gangadharan *et al.*, 2008). Thus by mixing an enzyme in pyrrole solution, a porous polymeric film with the enzyme entrapped inside can be formed at electrode surface via electrodeposition.

However, the question remains unanswered is: how do these functionalization methods fare in enhancing the sensing performance of electrodes made of three dimensional (3D) nano structures? This chapter aims to seek an answer to this question. First, the design of high-surface-area 3D nanostructures in a skyscraper metaphor is proposed for producing structures with high surface on a limited projection area and the importance of having sufficient mechanical robustness for the 3D skyscraper structures is discussed. Then, methods to fabricate robust 3D skyscraper nanopillar structures in an aqueous process are presented. Following that, electrochemical evaluations of these 3D nanopillar structures having bare, molecularly treated, and functionalized surfaces are discussed. Finally, for comparing the two functionalization methods, two cases are discussed in which the 3D nanopillar structures are used as electrodes for glucose detection. In the first case, the 3D electrodes are functionalized through a SAM/enzyme approach in which the biosensitive enzyme (i.e., glucose oxidase, or GOx) is tethered to a SAM of anchoring molecules formed at the electrode surface, and in the second case, the 3D electrodes are functionalized through a PPy/enzyme approach in which GOx is entrapped in a porous film of PPy electrodeposited at the electrode surface.

2. Design of high-surface-area nanostructures

Nanostructures such as nanorods, nanowires, nanotubes and nanoparticles have been widely explored for application in biosensors because these structures offer large surface areas in addition to their unique optical, electrical and mechanical properties. For example, the use of carbon nanotubes (Wang *et al.*, 2003, 2004; Gao *et al.*, 2003), peptide nanotube (Yemini *et al.*, 2005) and nanoparticles (Bharathi *et al.*, 2001) in various biosensors resulted in increased signal measurements. Electrodes modified with peptide nanotubes showed a 2.5-fold increase in amperometric response when compared with non-modified electrodes. Similarly, electrodes incorporated with carbon nanotubes showed a significant increase in selectivity and sensitivity for glucose detection.

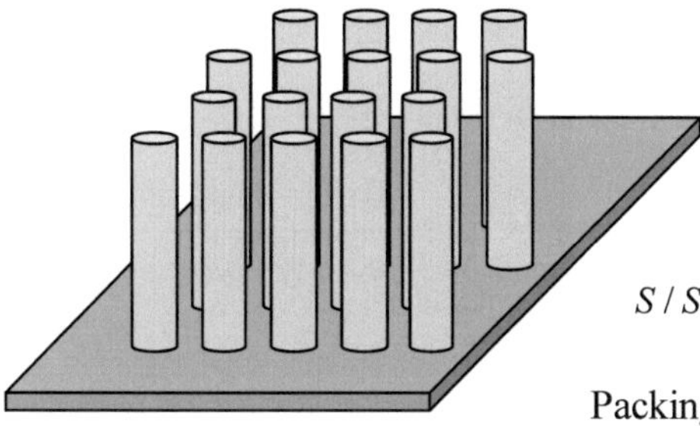

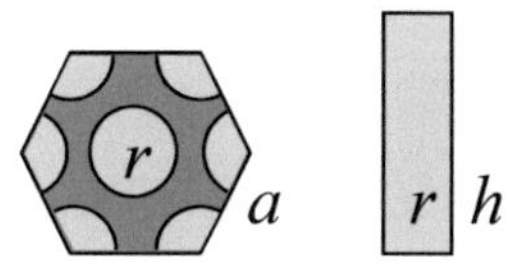

$$S/S_0 = \left(\frac{3\sqrt{3}}{2}a^2 + 6\pi rh\right) / \left(\frac{3\sqrt{3}}{2}a^2\right)$$

Packing density: $p = 2\pi r^2 / \sqrt{3}a^2$

For r = 100 nm, h = 5 μm and p = 50%: $S/S_0 = 1 + \frac{2h}{r}p = 51$

Fig. 1. Schematic illustration for increasing the overall surface area by building 3D skyscraper structures on a limited areal footprint.

One reason for the performance improvement when nanostructures are used is that these nanostructures provide large surface areas due to the fact that the surface-to-volume ratio of a structure increases as its size decreases. But when these nanostructures are formed on a planar substrate, the overall surface-area enhancement will be limited, to a certain extent, by the size of the underlying substrate. Then the question becomes: how can one achieve a higher surface area when the size of the planar area (or the 'real estate') is fixed? The answer lies in a "skyscraper" metaphor, that is, to build up within a limited areal footprint. Adding 3D skyscraper nanostructures onto a planar surface offers a significant increase in its overall surface area when compared with the planar surface. This fact can be illustrated by the example given in figure 1, where a 2D hexagonal array of vertically aligned nanorods or nanopillars is constructed on a planar substrate to form a 3D structure. At an aspect ratio ($h/2r$) of 25 and a packing density p= 50% for the nanopillars, a 51-fold increase in surface area can be achieved.

To date, various 3D skyscraper nanostructures have been fabricated using chemical vapor deposition (CVD) (Lau *et al.*, 2003), physical vapor deposition (PVD) (Fan *et al.*, 2004) and template based electrodeposition (Forrer *et al.*, 2000; Wang *et al.*, 2002; Xu *et al.*, 2004). Lately, evidence has emerged to reveal that the nanotubes and nanorods developed by the CVD and PVD techniques could not sustain the capillary forces generated by the nanostructure-liquid interaction (Lau *et al.*, 2003; Fan *et al.*, 2004). When vertically aligned 3D nanostructures are exposed to a liquid environment, capillary forces will develop between the vertically aligned nanostructures and the liquid medium (Kralchevsky *et al.*, 2000). If the forces are large, the nanostructures will deform or clump together. For example, the nanorods fabricated by the PVD technique in our lab deformed severely upon water exposure as shown in figure 2. Such a deformation in these 3D skyscraper nanostructures will reduce the total surface area, thus posing a serious problem for their application in functional biosensor devices because a majority of biosensors will have to be exposed aqueous environments. Therefore, to be useful as a component in a biosensor, these nanostructures need to have sufficient mechanical strength to overcome the capillary forces.

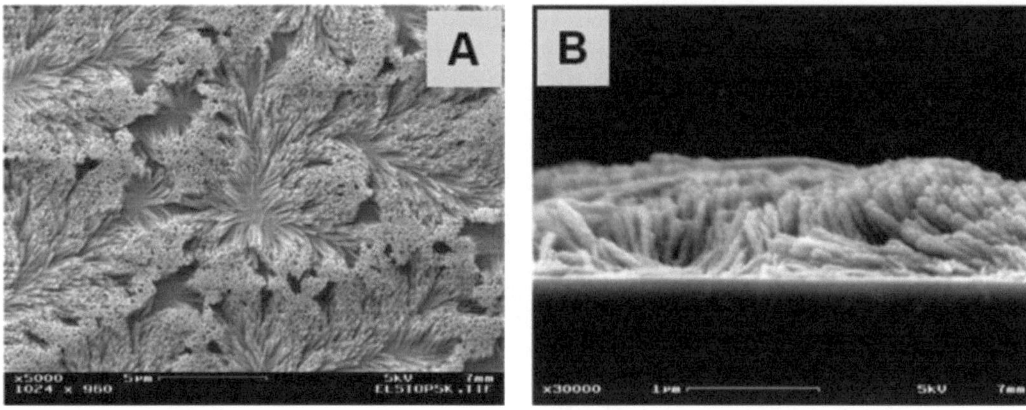

Fig. 2. Deformed 3D skyscraper silicon nanorod structures upon water exposure: (A) a top view and (B) a side view.

3. Fabrication processes for robust 3D skyscraper nanostructures

To overcome this problem, robust 3D skyscraper structures are necessary. One solution is to use an aqueous based fabrication technique instead of a vapor based method. We have developed a template based electrodeposition technique to fabricate 3D skyscraper nanostructures (Anandan *et al.*, 2006, 2007). In this aqueous based fabrication method, porous anodic alumina (PAA) discs are used as templates to guide the electrodeposition of conducting materials through the pores of the PAA templates in a three-electrode electrochemical cell, in which a gold-coated PAA disc is used as working electrode, a platinum (Pt) wire gauze as counter electrode and an Ag/AgCl electrode as reference electrode. In this fabrication process, a thin gold layer about 150 nm thick is first sputter-coated onto one side of a PAA disc to provide a conductive coating. Then a thicker gold layer (~3 μm) is electrodeposited on top of the sputtered gold film to form a strong supporting base in Orotemp24 gold plating solution (Technic Inc, Cranston, RI) at a deposition current of 5 mA/cm^2 for about two minutes. The supporting base is then masked with Miccrostop solution (Pyramid plastics Inc., Hope, Arkansas). After that, gold nanopillars are electrodeposited through the open pores of the PAA disc from the uncoated side at a deposition current of 5 mA/cm^2 at 65 °C in the same plating solution. The deposition time can be varied for achieving nanopillars of different heights. After nanopillar deposition, the PAA disc is dissolved in 2.0 M NaOH, resulting in a thin sheet structure with a 2D array of vertical gold nanopillars standing on a gold film.

To assess the mechanical robustness of these nanopillars, a water droplet test can be performed (Fan *et al.*, 2004). To do that, a water droplet is placed on a 3D nanopillar structure and is allowed to dry for several hours. After that, the morphology of the nanopillars is examined under scanning electron microscopy (SEM). Figure 3 shows two SEM images of 3D gold nanopillar structures. These nanopillars have a diameter of about 150 nm and a height approximately 4.5 μm. Clearly, the nanopillars exhibited slight clumping or bunching at their top ends. This bunching phenomenon, however, is different from the collapsing type of deformation shown in figure 2. Although this bunching deformation is due to the same capillary interaction between the nanopillars and water during the removal of PAA templates, the morphology of the 3D nanopillar structures after water exposure (Fig. 3A) is found to be almost identical to that before water exposure

(Fig. 3B). This fact indicates that exposing these nanopillar structures to water did not cause any further deformation, suggesting that the nanopillars fabricated by this aqueous based electrodeposition method are mechanically strong.

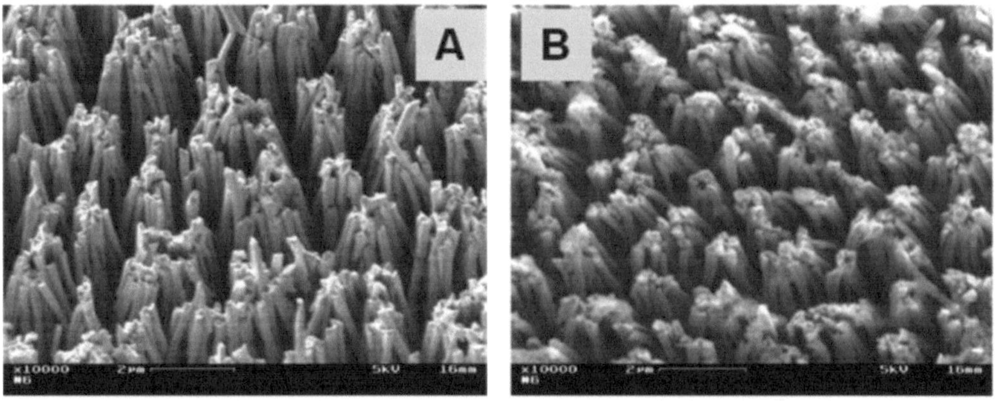

Fig. 3. 3D gold nanopillar (aspect ratio=30) structures developed using an aqueous based electrodeposition method: (A) as deposited, and (B) after water exposure.

The type of deformation shown in figure 3 is believed related to the high aspect ratio of these nanopillars. With an aspect ratio of 30, the bending resistance of the nanopillars will certainly be reduced. When silver nanopillar structures with an aspect ratio of 10 (Fig. 4A & 4B) and gold nanopillar structures with an aspect ratio of 5 (Fig. 4C & 4D) are tested, both cases show no bunching or clumping deformation in the nanopillars after water exposure (Fig. 4B & 4D) as compared with before water exposure (Fig. 4A & 4C). These results indicate that the nanopillar array structures developed using an aqueous electrodeposition method do possess sufficient mechanical robustness to resist the capillary interaction forces.
Since the 3D skyscraper nanopillar presented above are made of different materials and with different diameters, it raises a question: will such differences affect the resistance of these nanopillars to capillary interaction? By considering a standing nanopillar as a cantilever beam with a point load (P, representing the net equivalent capillary force) acting on it, the deflection of the nanopillar (δ) can be expressed as $\delta = PL^3/3EI$ (Beer *et al.*, 2002), where E is Young's modulus of the material, L is the height of the nanopillar and I is the second moment of inertia ($I = \pi \cdot D^4/64$, D is the diameter of the nanopillar). Obviously, the diameter of the nanopillar will affect the bending rigidity. However, according to Kralchevsky *et al.* (2000) the capillary force generated at the nanopillar is proportional to the diameter of nanopillar as $P = K(\gamma,\varphi,d_i)\cdot D$, where $K(\gamma,\phi,d_i)$ is a function of physical conditions such as the surface tension (γ), contact angle (ϕ) as well as the internanopillar distance (d_i). Thus, the deflection of the nanopillar upon capillary interaction is proportional to the aspect ratio to the third power and is inversely related to the Young's modulus as $\delta \propto (L/D)^3/E$. Therefore, aside from these physical conditions, the aspect ratio of the nanopillars and their mechanical properties are important factors influencing the resistance of these nanopillars to capillary interaction. Since the values of the Young's modulus of amorphous silicon, gold and silver are very close: 80 GPa for silicon (Freund *et al.*, 2003), 78 GPa for gold and 83 GPa for silver (Gardner *et al.*, 2002), only the physical conditions (the surface tension, contact angle and internanopillar distance) and the aspect ratio will have dominating effects on the resistance of these nanopillars to capillary interaction.

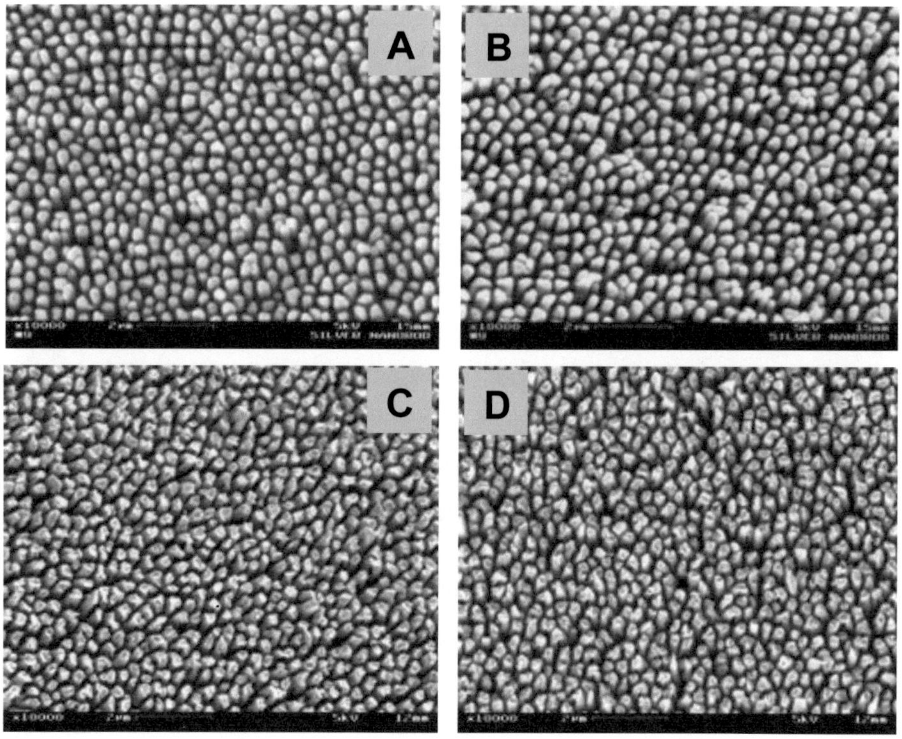

Fig. 4. 3D silver nanopillar (aspect ratio = 10) structures before (A) and after (B) water exposure and 3D gold nanopillar (aspect ratio = 5) structures before (C) and after (D) water exposure.

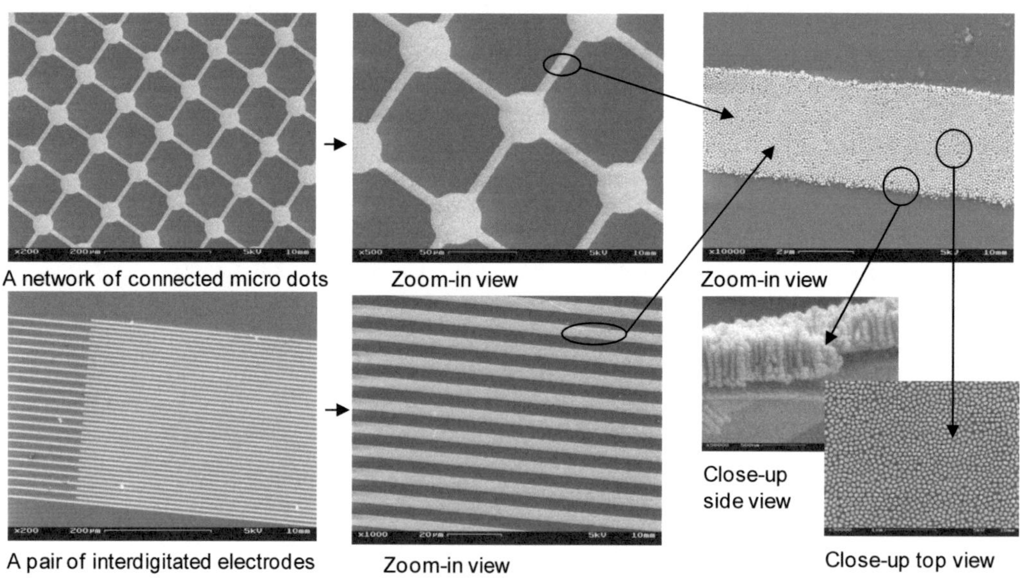

Fig. 5. SEM images showing a micro scale structure (a network of connected microdots) and a device (a pair of interdigitated electrodes) fabricated out of 3D skyscraper nanopillar structures.

Although robust, these 3D skyscraper nanostructures are formed on free-standing thin films. One drawback of such structures is that it is difficult to turn them into devices through further structural processing. To be able to process these 3D structures through conventional lithographical steps, it is ideal to have these 3D nanostructures formed on a supporting wafer substrate. To meet this need, we have developed a novel process to fabricate 3D skyscraper nanostructures on glass or wafer substrates (Zhang *et al.*, 2008). In this process, multiple layers of metallic films (e.g., 5 nm Titanium layer, 10 nm Gold layer and 10 μm Alumium layer) are first deposited onto the substrate. Then the top aluminum layer is anodized to form a porous Alumina template. After that, gold nanopillars are electrodeposited into the pores of the template. Finally, the porous alumia template is removed. With such nano structures formed on this surpporting substrate, we then pattern them into micro devices via conventional photolithographic processes. Figure 5 shows some examples of such integrated micro and nano structures on glass substrates: a network of connected micro dots and a pair of interdigitated electrodes fabricated out of 3D skyscraper nanopillar structures.

4. Electrochemical characterization of 3D skyscraper nanostructures

4.1 Bare surfaces

To characterize the 3D skyscraper nanostructures with bare surfaces, cyclic voltammetry (CV) analysis can be performed. To do that, the 3D nanostructures are used as working electrode in a three-electrode electrochemical cell. Figure 6 shows the CV curves for three nanopillar structures and a flat control structure measured in blank solution containing 0.3 M sulphuric acid as a supporting electrolyte. The inset in figure 6 shows the SEM images of a side-view of the three specimens. From these SEM images, it is estimated that the nanopillars in specimens A, B and C have a diameter of about 150.0 nm and a height approximately 1.0 μm, 2.5 μm and 6.0 μm, respectively.

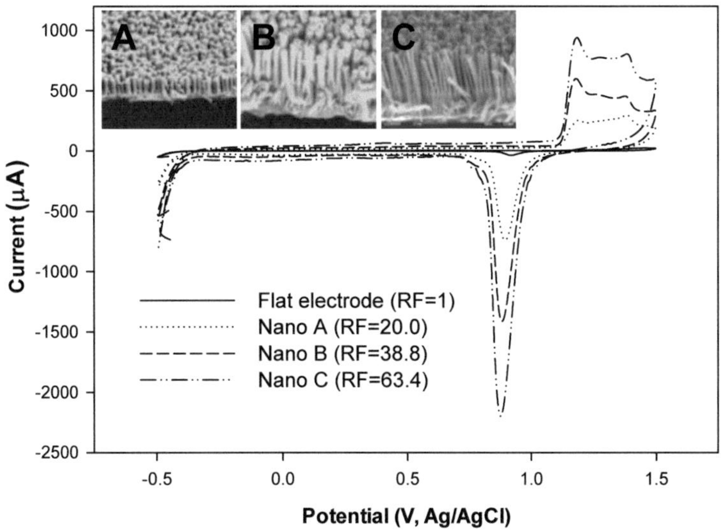

Fig. 6. CV curves for three 3D nanopillar structures and a flat structure with bare surfaces obtained in blank solution containing 0.3 M sulphuric acid as a supporting electrolyte. The inset shows the SEM images of a side-view of the three specimens.

All these CV curves show an Au-oxide reduction peak at around 0.85 V, as expected. To quantify the difference in the height of the nanopillars in these 3D skyscraper structures, a roughness factor is determined as the area under the reduction peak of a nanopillar electrode divided by that of the flat electrode. The roughness factor (RF) for specimens A, B and C is found to be 20.0, 38.8 and 63.4, respectively.

When a redox couple, $[Fe(CN)_6]^{4-}/[Fe(CN)_6]^{3-}$, is used along with a supporting electrolyte, more structural characteristics can be revealed from the CV curves. Figure 7 shows the CV curves for a 3D and a flat gold structures measured in solution containing 0.5 M Na_2SO_4 as a supporting electrolyte and 4 mM $K_4Fe(CN)_6$ as a redox probe. The CV curves show that the redox peak current increases with increasing scan rate. Furthermore, the peak currents for the 3D nanopillar structures are much higher than those for the flat one. Here each CV curve represents 10 cycles of repeated measurements, suggesting that the 3D nanopillar structures are very stable with no further deformation or change in morphology during the electrochemical processes. If these nanopillars are not strong enough to overcome the capillary forces in such an aqueous environment, they will deform during the electrochemical processes, which will subsequently lead to decreased active surface area and hence decreased current output.

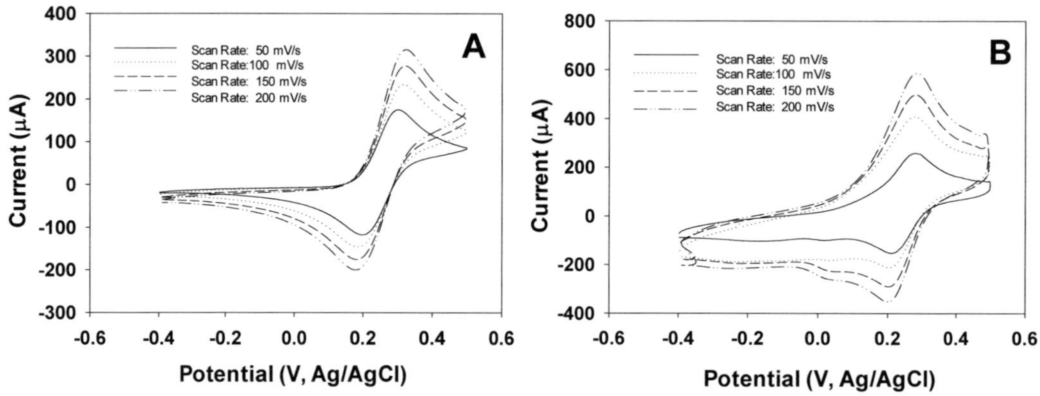

Fig. 7. CV curves for a gold flat (A) and 3D nanopillar (B) structures with bare surfaces obtained in solution containing 0.5 M Na_2SO_4 as a supporting electrolyte and 4mM $K_4Fe(CN)_6$ as a redox probe.

From these CV curves, a peak separation ΔE_p = 70 mV is found for the 3D nanopillar structure, which is much closer to an ideal Nernstian behavior (ΔE_p = 59 mV) as compared with that for the flat structure (ΔE_p = 110 mV), indicating that electron transfer at the surface of the 3D nanopillar structures is significantly enhanced.

4.2 SAM treated surfaces

As discussed earlier, most of these 3D skyscraper nanostructures are made of inorganic materials, thus for applications as electrodes in biosensors they have to be functionalized for biological recognition purposes. Since most biosensitive molecules cannot be immobilized directly onto the surface of these inorganic materials, anchoring molecules such as self assembled monolayer (SAM) molecules are necessary. We have evaluated the formation of two SAM molecules, i.e., (1) 3-mercaptopropionic acid or MPA: $HS-(CH_2)_2-COOH$ and (2)

11-mercaptoundecanoic acid or MUA: HS-$(CH_2)_{10}$-COOH at the surface of these 3D nanopillar structures (Anandan et al., 2009). To treat the 3D nanopillar structures with the SAM molecules, the structures are immersed in ethanol solution containing 10 mM of either the MPA or MUA molecules for 24 hours. SAM formation on these 3D structures is characterized by the CV and electrochemical impedance spectroscopy (EIS) techniques. The CV measurements are performed by scanning the potential from -0.2 V to 0.6 V at a scan rate of 100 mV/s and the EIS measurements are performed in a frequency range from 0.1 Hz to 100 KHz at a potential of 10 mV in 0.1 M phosphate buffered solution (PBS, pH7) containing 2 mM $Fe(CN)_6^{3-/4-}$ (ferri:ferro=1:1) mixture as a redox probe.

For assessing the percentage of defects in the SAM molecules, the voltammetric reduction peak associated with the uncovered area (i.e., the exposed gold oxide) in the SAM treated 3D structures is evaluated. The ratio of the uncovered area of a SAM treated 3D structure to that of a bare 3D structure is calculated and the percentage of defects in the SAM molecules is determined. To quantify the surface coverage (Γ) of the SAM molecules, the method reported in the literature (Walczak *et al.*, 1991; Sawaguchi *et al.*, 2001; Ding *et al.*, 2005) is used to evaluate the voltammetric reduction peak associated with SAM desorption. From the reduction peak, the amount of charge is determined by first integrating the reduction current under the peak over time and then offsetting the value by that of a bare 3D electrode. With the formula $\Gamma = Q/nFA$ (Walczak *et al.*, 1991), in which Q is the amount of charge, n (=1) is the number of electrons involved in the reaction, F (=96485 C/mol) is the Faraday constant and A (=0.04 cm^2) is the electroactive surface area, the surface coverage of SAM molecules is determined.

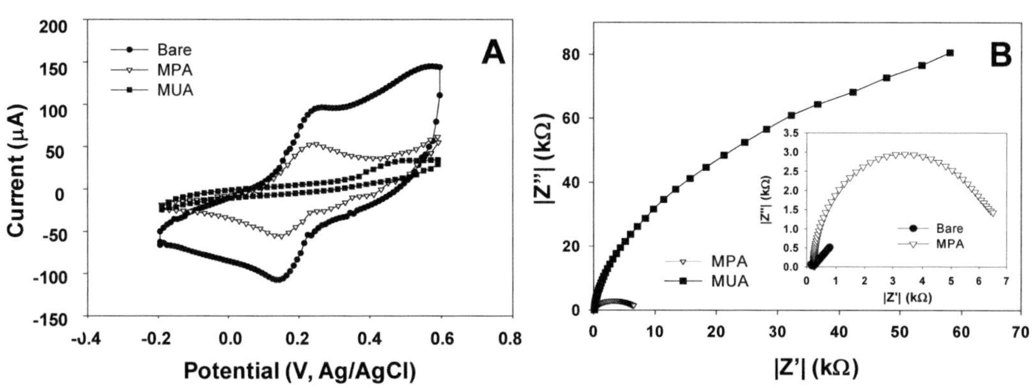

Fig. 8. (A) CV curves for a bare, MPA and MUA treated surfaces obtained in solution containing H_2SO_4 as a supporting electrolyte and $[Fe(CN)^6]^{4-}/[Fe(CN)^6]^{3-}$ as a redox probe at a scan rate of 100 mV/s. (B) The corresponding Nyquist plots from the EIS measurements with a close-up view of the low impedance range given in the inset.

In figure 8A the CV curves obtained for a bare, MPA and MUA treated 3D structures evaluated in the presence of the redox couple $[Fe(CN)_6]^{4-}/[Fe(CN)_6]^{3-}$ are shown. In comparison between the bare and SAM treated structures, the bare one exhibits much higher redox peak currents. Between the two SAM treated structures, the MUA treated one exhibits lower redox peak currents than the MPA treated one, suggesting a higher degree of blockage for electron transfer resulting from the MUA molecules than from the MPA molecules. For both the bare and the MPA treated 3D structures the CV curves show a reversible redox event occurring at the surface with the electron transfer limited by diffusional mass transport. By contrast, the CV curves for the MUA treated structure exhibits highly irreversible redox behavior, confirming a high degree of blockage at the surface for electron transfer. Taken together, the above results indicate that both the MUA and MPA molecules form SAM structures covering the surface of the 3D nanopillar structures and that there are more MUA molecules than MPA molecules blocking the pathways for electron transfer across the electrode-electrolyte interface, owing possibly to the longer chain length of the MUA molecules forming more lateral molecular bonds.

Figure 8B shows the corresponding impedance spectra (Nyquist plots) for these 3D structures. The two SAM treated structures show semicircular Nyquist plots whereas the bare one exhibits a straight line plot (see the lower inset plot in Fig. 8B). Since a semicircular feature is indicative of blockage for electron transfer across the electrode/electrolyte interface, this result confirms the formation of SAM molecules at the surfaces. Moreover, the MUA treated structure exhibits a larger semicircle than the MPA treated one, suggesting a high degree of SAM coverage for the MUA than for the MPA molecules. By using a Randles equivalent circuit to fit the obtained semicircular Nyquist plots, the resistance value for electron transfer (R_{et}) can be resolved. In this case, the R_{et} value obtained for the MUA treated structure is 27 times higher than that for the MPA treated structure. This result confirms that the MUA molecules indeed post a higher electron transfer resistance at the electrode surface than the MPA molecules.

The CV curves obtained from the Au-oxide reduction experiments (figure 9A) exhibit an Au-oxide reduction peak at around 0.78 V, indicating that all these 3D electrodes possess a certain amount of defects on the SAM treated surfaces. By the ratio of the area under the reduction peak (by integrating the CV curve under the peak) of the SAM treated 3D structure to that of the bare 3D structure, the percentage of defects is found to be approximately 87.3% and 37.8% for the MPA and MUA SAMs, respectively. These values are high when compared with flat structures: 52% for the MPA and 0% for the MUA SAMs (Campuzano *et al.*, 2002).

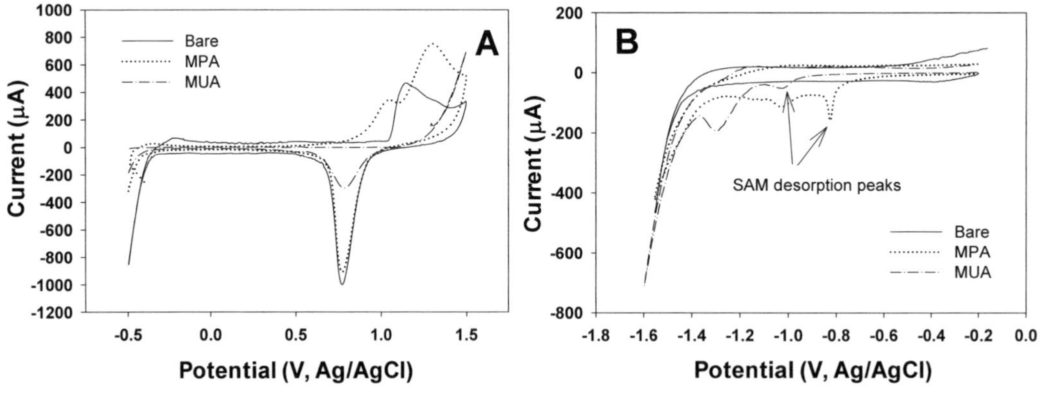

Fig. 9. (A) CV curves for a bare, MPA and MUA treated 3D structures obtained in quantifying the percentage of defects in SAM molecules in blank solution containing 0.1 M H_2SO_4 as a supporting electrolyte. (B) CV curves for the same structures obtained in evaluating SAM desorption in blank solution containing 0.1M NaOH as a supporting electrolyte.

Figure 9B shows the CV curves obtained for evaluating the voltammetric reduction peak associated with desorption of the MPA and MUA molecules. In the CV curves, two peak currents are visible for both the MPA and MUA treated 3D structures. The peak current at around -0.82 V for the MPA and around -1.03 V for the MUA are due to the cleavage of the gold-sulfur bond, according to the literature that a peak desorption current between -0.6 to -0.9 V is reported for short alkanethiols (n=2 to 6) and between -1.0 to -1.2 V for long alkanethiols (n=11 to 18) (Widrig *et al.*, 1991; Imabayashi *et al.*, 1997; Sawaguchi *et al.*, 2001; Ding *et al.*, 2005). Based on these desorption peak currents, the desorption charge is determined by integrating the reduction peak from -0.8 V to -0.9 V for the MPA treated structure and from -1.0 V to -1.2 V for the MUA treated structure. The surface coverage values are found to be 1.38×10^{-8} mol/cm^2 and 2.37×10^{-8} mol/cm^2 for the MPA and MUA treated electrodes respectively. Comparing with the reported values for the surface coverage for the MPA (5.12×10^{-10} mol/cm^2) and the MUA (8.30×10^{-10} mol/cm^2) on flat surfaces (Campuzano *et al.*, 2002), the values for the 3D nanopillar structures are roughly 27 and 28 times higher. This increase can be attributed to the increase in the electroactive surface area in the 3D electrodes.

4.3 Functionalized surfaces using SAM and avidin

Since these SAM molecules only serve as an anchoring layer, functional molecules are still needed to make these 3D skyscraper nanostructures functionally sensitive to analyte targets. Many biological couples such as antibody-antigen, protein-ligand, protein-aptamer, paired-nucleotides and avidin-biotin can be used for this purpose. Here we will discuss a case using the avidin-biotin couple as the biosensitive element for a biosensor. In using the avidin-biotin couple, one species, often avidin, has to be immobilized onto the active surface of the biosensor, and the other is usually tethered to a target molecule. As a demonstration, we will immobilize avidin and use biotin as the target.

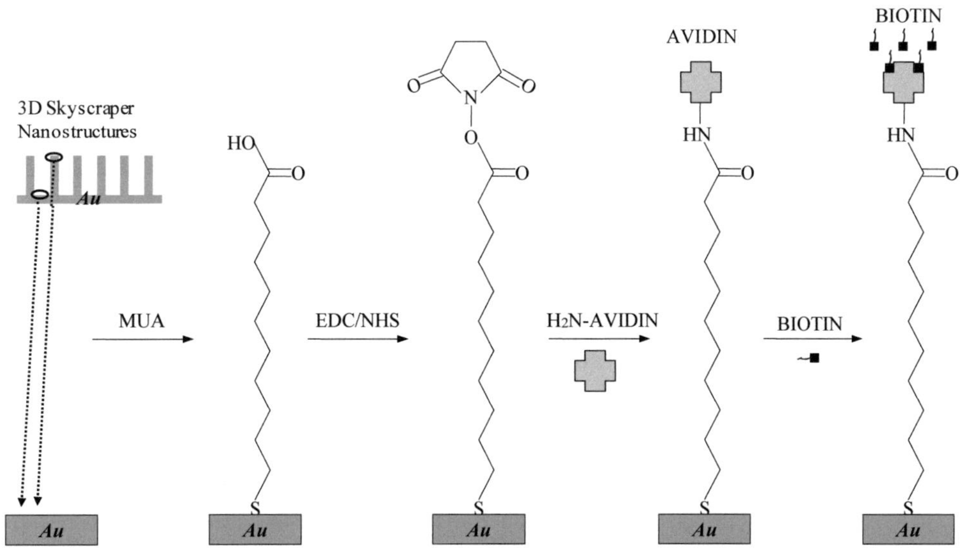

Fig. 10. Schematic illustration of a sequential procedure used to modify the surface of a 3D gold nanopillar structure.

A SAM of anchoring MUA molecules is first formed at the surface of a 3D nanopillar structure. The MUA is then activated (i.e., turning the COOH groups into reactive N-hydroxysuccinimice esters) by immersing the structure in PBS containing 30 mM 1-3-Dimethyl-amino-propyl-3-ethyl-carbodiimide hydrochloride and 15 mM N-hydroxy-succin-imide for 3 hours at 25°C. The 3D structure is then functionalized with avidin in PBS solution containing 300 µL of avidin at 200 µg/mL for 2 hours at 25°C. Figure 10 shows a schematic illustration of the stepwise procedures for the surface modification.

Figure 11A shows the CV measurements during the stepwise surface modification using MUA, avidin and biotin. Clearly, a bare 3D structure exhibits a peak-shaped CV curve, indicating a diffusion-controlled electrode process. Moreover, the CV curve has a peak-to-peak separation measured at ΔE_p = 59.8 mV, which is very close to an ideal Nernstian one-electron reaction having ΔE_p = 59 mV (Bard *et al.*, 2001). This fact suggests a highly efficient electron transfer mechanism across the electrode/electrolyte interface of the 3D nanopillar structure.

After the MUA layer is adsorbed to the electrode surface, the peak-shaped CV curve exhibits much reduced peak currents and increased peak-to-peak separation, suggesting blockage for electron transfer due to MUA adsorption. With more layers of molecular adsorption (i.e., avidin and biotin), the CV curve shows no obvious redox peaks. Instead, it looks more like a sigmoid having significant hysteresis between the forward and backward scans. This behavior implies that the electrons passing across the electrode/electrolyte interface are fulfilling two duties: to facilitate redox reaction and to charge the electrical double layer. Also, a lack of peak currents in these CV curves suggests that the adsorption of molecules to the surface has significantly lowered the electron transfer rate such that the electrode process is no longer controlled by a diffusion process as in the case of a bare electrode. Instead, it is now a kinetics-controlled process, meaning that it is limited by the rate of electron transfer.

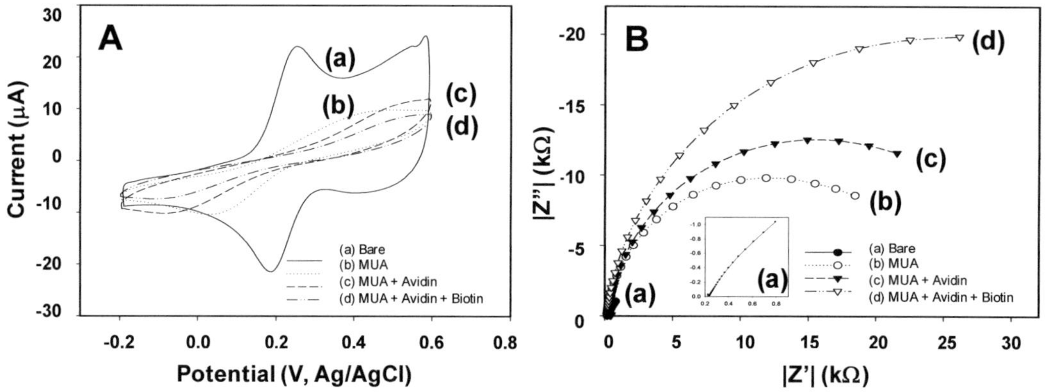

Fig. 11. (A) CV curves for examining the electrode/electrolyte interface during stepwise surface modification. (B) The corresponding Nyquist plots with a close view of the trace (a).

As shown in figure 11A, the peak current (or the limiting current) of these CV curves decreases as more layers of molecules are adsorbed to the surface. This is because the increase in the thickness of the adsorbed molecular layer at the surface has caused further reduction in electron transfer, thus slowing down the redox activity of $[Fe(CN)_6]^{4-}/[Fe(CN)_6]^{3-}$.

The observed sequential change in the CV curve corresponds very well with the stepwise adsorption of MUA, avidin and biotin at the surface.
From the EIS measurements shown in figure 11B, it is seen that the Nyquist plot for the bare 3D structure (see inset) is nearly a straight line with its slope close to one. This fact confirms a diffusion-controlled electrode process occurring at the surface of the bare 3D structure. For the other cases, semicircular Nyquist impedance spectra are observed. The diameter of these Nyquist semicircles increases as the sequential adsorption of MUA, avidin and biotin proceeds at the surface. This fact indicates that the resistance to electron transfer at the electrode/electrolyte interface increases as more layers of molecules are added to the surface. Moreover, these Nyquist plots do not possess a linear part at low frequency, confirming that after the adsorption of various molecules the electrode process is no longer a diffusion-controlled process but a kinetics-controlled one.

4.4 Functionalized surfaces using PPy and GOx

In many biosensors, the functionalization of electrodes made of 3D skyscraper structures is often aimed at a specific target. In a glucose biosensor, for example, its electrode should be reactive to glucose. Very often, glucose specific enzyme - glucose oxidase (GOx) - is immobilized onto the surface of the electrode with the use of anchoring molecules such as SAM molecules. One drawback of using SAM molecules is that they always get in the way of electron transfer across the electrode/electrolyte interface as demonstrated in section 4.3 (see figure 11), thus affecting the detection performances. In contrast, physical entrapment of GOx in a porous polymer film near the electrode surface offers an attractive alternative. Conducting polymer like polypyrrole (PPy) can be electro- polymerized and deposited onto electrode surfaces to form a porous film, providing pores large enough for efficient electron transfer. Thus by mixing GOx in pyrrole solution, a porous polymeric film with GOx entrapped inside can be formed at the electrode surface via electrodeposition.

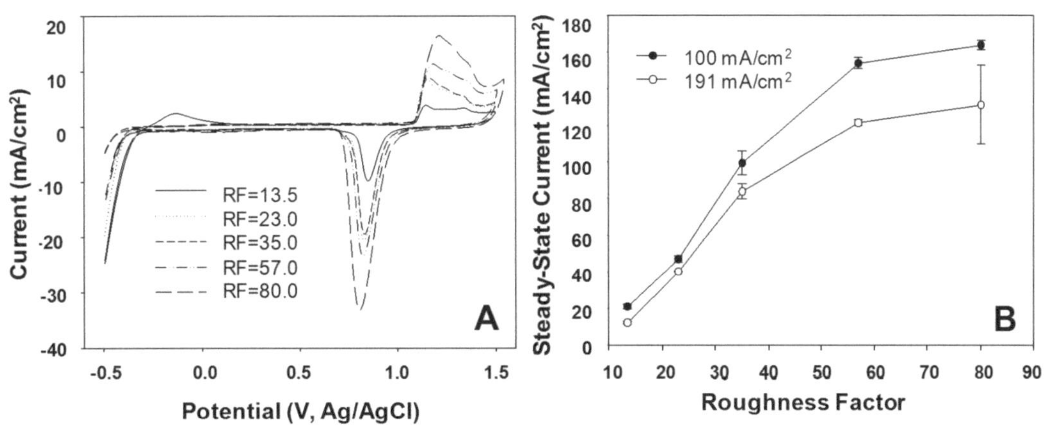

Fig. 12. (A) CV curves for five 3D nanopillar structures with different roughness factors obtained in blank solution containing 0.5 M H_2SO_4 as a supporting electrolyte. (B) Variation of amperometric steady-state current with roughness factor in response to glucose for the five 3D electrodes. Note N=3 for each data point.

We have applied the functionalization procedure using PPy and GOx to 3D skyscraper nanopillar structures and investigated the effect of various parameters, such as the height of nanopillars, the electrodeposition current and the total charge passed, on the performance of the 3D electrodes in glucose detection. Figure 12A shows the CV curves obtained in blank solution containing 0.5 M H_2SO_4 for five 3D structures with different nanopillar heights. All the CV curves exhibit an Au-oxide reduction peak at around 0.85 V. From these reduction peaks, the roughness factor for the five 3D structures is found ranging from 13.5, 23.0, 35.0 and 57.0 to 80.0.

Figure 12B shows the amperometric steady-state current in response to glucose at a fixed concentration of 4 mM for the five 3D structures functionalized at two deposition currents (100 μA/cm² and 191 μA/cm²) with the total charge set at 150 mC/cm². Clearly, the steady-state current increases as the roughness factor increases and it appears to saturate when the roughness factor goes beyond 57. The same phenomenon is seen for both current cases. This current-saturation behavior at a higher roughness factor is believed due to the difficulty encountered by glucose in diffusing down to the sides and roots of the nanopillars for oxidation as the height of the nanopillars reaches a certain level. This result is consistent with our previous observation (Anandan *et al.*, 2007), and it may suggest that for glucose detection using the present method it is not necessarily beneficial to have 3D structures with nanopillars that are too tall. Figure 12B also shows that the steady-state current for the structures functionalized under a lower deposition current is higher than that under a higher deposition current, owing to a more uniform thickness for the PPy/GOx film formed under a lower deposition current.

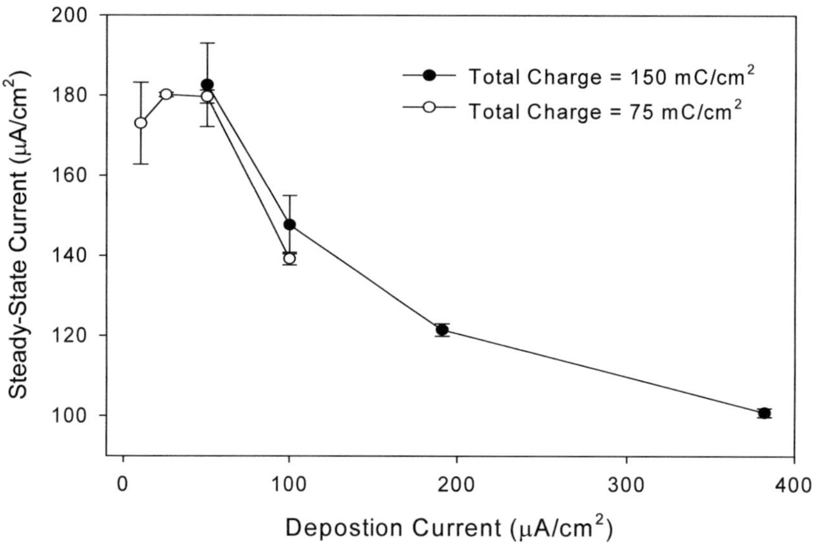

Fig. 13. Variation of the amperometric steady-state current with deposition current obtained under two different total charges. Note N=3 for each data point.

Figure 13 shows the variation of stead-state current with deposition current for 3D structures with a roughness factor around 60. At a total charge of 150 mC/cm² the steady-state current increases as the deposition current decreases but with no obvious peak current performance within the range of the applied deposition currents (i.e., from 50 to 573 μA/cm²). When the deposition current is lowered below 50 μA/cm² (achieved at a reduced total charge of 75 mC/cm²) it became obvious that the steady-state current reached at the deposition current of 50 μA/cm^2 is a peak value. From the overlap region of the two curves it is seen that these two curves are not only very close to each (the one under a lower charge density is slightly lower than the one under a higher charge density, as expected) but also following the same varying trend. Based on these results, the deposition current of 50 μA/cm^2 is deemed as an optimal value, which is quite different from that obtained for flat electrodes (382 μA/cm^2).

This difference is attributed to the presence of the nanopillars. Because of these closely packed skyscraper nanopillars, the mass transport of the electroactive species (including pyrrole during electrodeposition and glucose during detection) to and from the functionalized surface will be different from the case without nanopillars. This is evident from the SEM images. Under a lower deposition current of 50 μA/cm^2 all nanopillars are covered with a thin uniform layer of PPy/GOx (see Fig.14A). However, under a higher deposition current of 573 μA/cm^2, the space between nanopillars close to the tips is all clogged up by the PPy/GOx (Fig.14B). This thick film formed under high deposition currents will surely pose a diffusion barrier for glucose, thus leading to low current responses (Fortier *et al.*, 1990). Therefore, in the presence of closely packed skyscraper nanopillars, a much lower deposition current (e.g., 50 μA/cm^2 instead of 382 μA/cm^2) is necessary for forming a uniform functionalization layer at the surface of these 3D nanopillar structures.

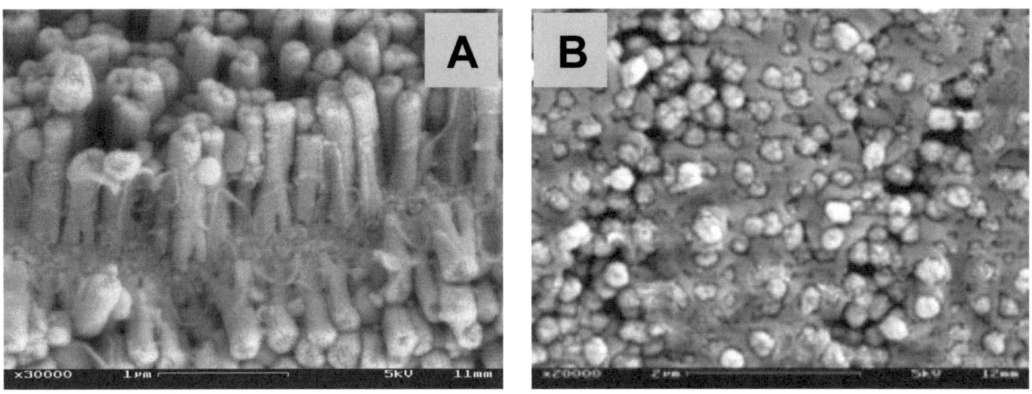

Fig. 14. SEM images of 3D nanopillar structures functionalized with PPy/GOx through an electrodeposition process when the total charge is controlled at 150 mC/cm^2 under a deposition current of 50 μA/cm^2 (A) and 573 μA/cm^2 (B).

Figure 15A shows the variation of steady-state current with total charge measured in response to glucose for the 3D nanopillar structures (with a roughness factor around 60) functionalized at a fixed deposition current of 50 μA/cm^2. As the total charge increases from 50 to 600 mC/cm^2, the steady-state current increases a little bit in the beginning and then decreases after reaching a peak value at 150 mC/cm^2. Figure 15B shows the steady-state currents for the 3D nanopillar structures measured in response to ascorbic acid. Ascorbic acid, uric acid and acetaminophen are the common electroactive species coexisting in blood, and they tend to affect the accuracy of a glucose sensor (Cho *et al.*, 1996). Thus for a better performance, a glucose sensor should have negligible responses to these nonspecific species. In general, ascorbic acid is considered as a representing endogenous interfering agent (Moatti *et al.*, 1992), thus for this reason we choose ascorbic acid as a representative interfering species. These results show that the interference also reaches a peak value at a total charge of 150 mC/cm^2. But the current value in response to ascorbic acid is much lower (14.3 $\mu A/cm^2$) than that to glucose (138.3 $\mu A/cm^2$). With a signal-to-noise ratio of about 9.7, the specificity of the functionalized 3D nanopillar structures to glucose is considered to be reasonably good.

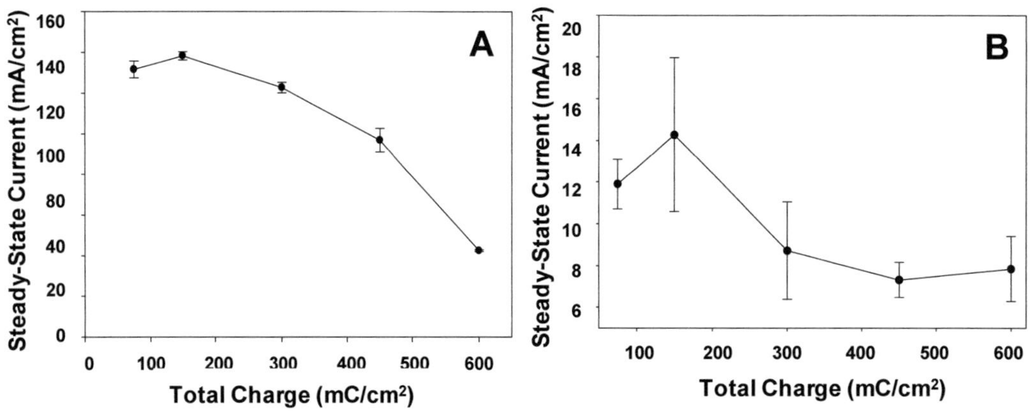

Fig. 15. Variation of amperometric steady-state current with total charge obtained for the functionalized 3D nanopillar structures (under a deposition current of 50 $\mu A/cm^2$) in response to glucose (A) and to ascorbic acid (B). Note N=3 for each data point.

Based on these results we believe that an electro-process with a deposition current of 50 $\mu A/cm^2$ and a total charge of 150mC/cm^2 will provide an optimal condition for functionalizing the 3D nanopillar structures using PPy/GOx. These electro-processing parameters are quite different from those obtained for the flat electrodes (Uang *et al.*, 2002), and it can be attributed to the added surface area provided by the cylindrical walls of the nanopillars as well as the added difficulty for the active species in reaching the tiny space between these nanopillars (Anandan *et al.*, 2007).

5. Application of 3D skyscraper nanostructures as electrodes in biosensors

Now let us compare the two functionalization methods by examining the detection sensitivity when these functionalized 3D nanopillar structures are used as electrodes for glucose detection. In the first case, the 3D nanopillar structures functionalized with SAM and GOx (in which GOx is tethered to the SAM) are used as electrodes, and in the second case the 3D nanopillar structures functionalized with PPy and GOx (in which GOx is entrapped in a porous film of PPy) are used as electrodes. In both cases, the amperometric steady-state current responses of these functionalized electrodes are measured in response to glucose at different concentrations. With the amperometric measurements, the relationship between the steady-state current and glucose concentration is calibrated in each case. From the calibration curves the detection sensitivity of the 3D nanopillar electrodes functionalized with two different methods is evaluated and compared.

5.1 Electrode reactions in Gox catalyzed glucose detection

For GOx catalyzed glucose detection, glucose first reacts with GOx to form gluconic acid and reduced-GOx. The reduced-GOx will then be converted back to its original form by reacting with p-benzoquinone (BQ), a mediator having better solubility than most other popular mediators (Cooper *et al.*, 1993). In a cascade of electrode reactions, the mediator gets reduced and then converted back to its original state at the electrode surface by giving away electrons. Figure 16 shows a cascade of events occurring in a mediator based glucose detection scheme.

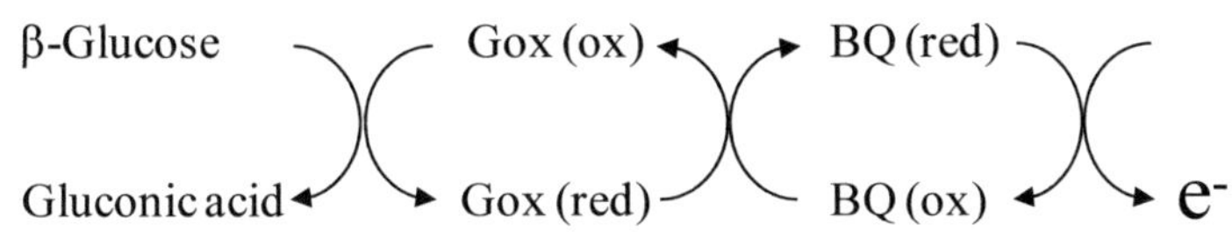

Fig. 16. A cascade of events in a mediator-based glucose detection scheme.

5.2 Glucose detection using electrodes functionalized with SAM and GOx

By using 3D nanopillar structures treated first with a SAM of MPA molecules followed by GOx as electrodes, amperometric measurements are made in PBS containing 3mM p-benzoquinone and certain amount of glucose at a constant electrode potential of 0.35 V (vs. Ag/AgCl). During amperometric experiment, the solution is stirred constantly for ensuring instant equilibrium for mass transport. During each test run, the background current is allowed to stabilize before a drop of glucose is added to the solution. After the amperometric current response reaches a steady-state, another drop of glucose is added and the corresponding current response is measured until a new steady state is reached. In this experiment each incremental drop of glucose is controlled to cause an equivalent increase in glucose concentration of approximately 2.5 mM.

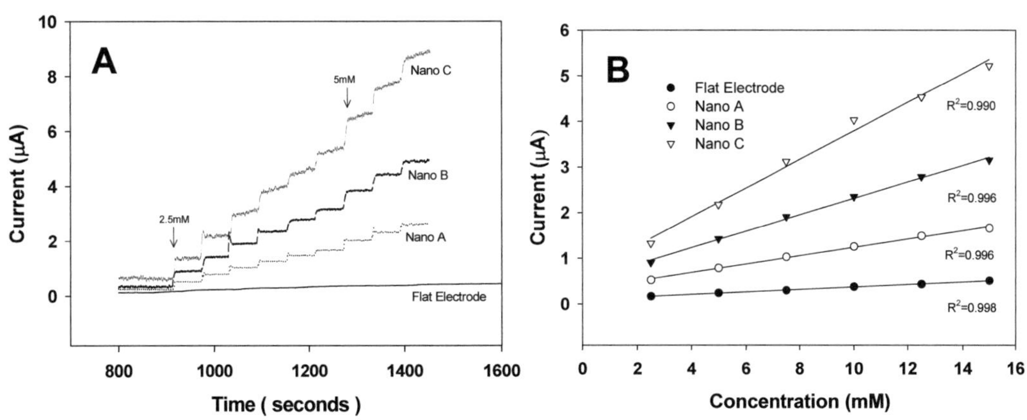

Fig. 17. (A) Amperometric current responses obtained for 3D electrodes functionalized with SAM and GOx when incremental drops of glucose are added to the solution. (B) Calibration curves along with linear-regression analyses for the relationship between the steady-state current and glucose concentration (from 2.5mM to 15mM).

Figure 17A shows the amperometric current responses for three 3D nanopillar electrodes and a flat control electrode functionalized with MPA SAM and GOx. These three 3D electrodes have different surface roughness factors as characterized in figure 6. All three electrodes exhibit a higher current response than the flat control case at each glucose level. Figure 17B shows the variations of steady-state current with glucose concentration (from

2.5mM to 15mM) along with the corresponding linear regression lines. By taking the slope of each regression line and normalizing it with respect to the geometric area of the electrode in each case, the sensitivity measurement for the functionalized electrodes is evaluated. In this case, the highest sensitivity value is found as 3.13 $\mu A \cdot mM^{-1} \cdot cm^{-2}$ (for specimen C) which is about 12 times higher than that of the flat electrode. This sensitivity value is much higher than the value reported for a gold nanotube electrode (0.4 $\mu A \cdot mM^{-1} \cdot cm^{-2}$, Delvaux *et al.*, 2003).

5.3 Glucose detection using electrodes functionalized with PPy and GOx

By using 3D nanopillar structures coated with a mixture of PPy and GOx as electrodes, amperometric measurements are made under the same conditions as described in section 5.2. Figure 18 shows some measurements of the amperometric current responses when the concentration of glucose is increased in an increment of 2.5 mM. By taking the steady-state current at each glucose level, a scatter plot calibrating the relationship between the steady-state current and the glucose concentration is made. As shown in the inset in figure 18, the calibration curve shows a fairly good linear relationship (R^2=0.9998) between the steady-state current and glucose concentration in a glucose concentration range from 2.5 to 15 mM. Based on the slope of this calibration curve, the sensitivity value is determined as 36 $\mu A \cdot mM^{-1} \cdot cm^{-2}$. This value is about twelve times higher than that in the case presented in section 5.2. This sensitivity value is the highest ever achieved for gold electrodes functionalized with PPy and GOx.

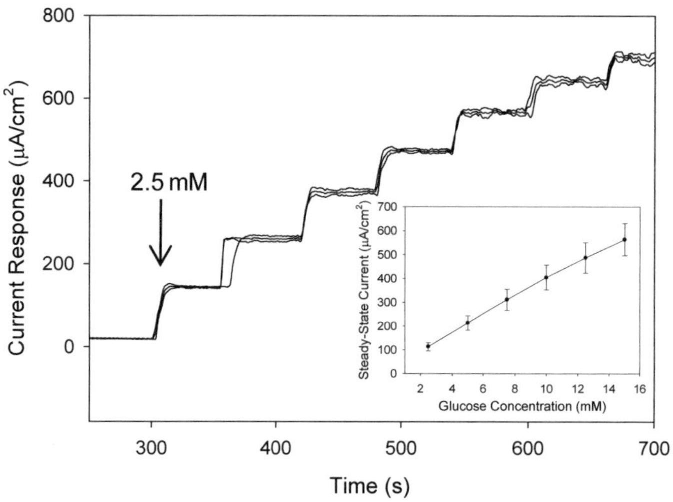

Fig. 18. Amperometric current responses to successive addition of glucose in the amount of 2.5 mM. The insert shows the calibration curve for the relationship between the steady-state current and glucose concentration.

6. Conclusion and future perspective

Nanotechnology holds great promises for improving the performance of many biosensors. In this chapter, we have domenstrated that the use of 3D electrodes having skyscraper nanopillar structures as electrodes in biosensors can drastically improve the sensitivity of glucose biosensors as compared with the use of flat electrodes. Of course, such improvement can only be achieved when the 3D skyscraper nanostructures are robust to overcome the capillary forces encountered in various solid-liquid interactions. The 3D skyscraper nanopillar structures fabricated by the electrodeposition technique described in this chapter have sufficient mechanical robustness to resist the capillary interaction forces.

To utilize these 3D nano structures in various fluidic systems, we have developed a novel process to fabricate 3D skyscraper nanostructures on wafer substrates. This development allows the formed 3D nano structures to be further processed through conventional lithographical steps such that they can be easily incorporated into various micro devices.

In addition to the 3D skyscraper morphological design, the sensing performance of these inorganic-based nanopillar electrodes is also affected by the type of functionalization methods used. For example, the 3D nanopillar electrodes functionalized with MPA SAM and GOx showed a detection sensitivity value of 3.13 $\mu A \cdot mM^{-1} \cdot cm^{-2}$, which is about 12 times higher than that for a flat electrode. By contrast, the 3D nanopillar electrodes functionalized with PPy and GOx exhibited an even higher sensitivity value of 36 $\mu A \cdot mM^{-1} \cdot cm^{-2}$. This fact suggests that using physical entrapment of GOx near the 3D electrode surface within porous PPy indeed provides an efficient means for electron transfer. In comparison, using a uniform layer of short chain SAM (i.e., the MPA) to tether GOx may still post a barrier to electron transfer across the electrode/electrolyte interface thus lowering the detection performance.

In the coming years it is anticipated that nanotechnology based biosensors will continue to evolve and expand their use in many areas of biological, pharmaceutical and biomedical concerns. These biosensors are expected to possess some ideal features such as high sensitivity, high specificity, fast response, low detection-limit, continuous and long-term functionality, and passively operational. As for the use of 3D nano structured electrodes in fluidic sensors, further efforts are needed in optimizing the geometric parameters of the 3D nano structures in terms of fluidic flow rates and channel geometries and dimensions.

7. Acknowledgement

I would like to thank my students V. Anandan, Y.L. Rao, R. Gangadharan and postdoctoral fellow S.J. Lee for their contributions to the work discussed here and the financial supports from the National Science Foundation, the Faculty of Engineering at the University of Georgia, and the Institute for Biological Interfaces of Engineering at Clemson University.

8. References

Anandan V, Gangadharan R, and Zhang G. (2009) The role of SAM chain length in enhancing the sensitivity of nanopillar modified electrodes for glucose detection. Sensors, 9(3): 1295-1305.

Anandan V, Yang X, Kim E, Rao Y and Zhang G (2007) Role of reaction kinetics and mass transport in glucose sensing with nanopillar array electrodes. Journal of Biological Engineering. 1, 1, 5.

Anandan V, Rao YL. and Zhang G. (2006) Nanopillar array structures for high performance electrochemical sensing. International journal of nanomedicine. 1, 73 - 79.

Bard AJ and Faulkner LR. (2001) Electrochemical Methods: Fundamentals and Applications. 2nd Edition, John Wiley & Sons, New York.

Beer FP, Johnston ER, Deworf JT. (2002) Mechanism of materials. *McGraw-Hill*. 3rd edition.

Berchmans S, Sathyajith R, Yegnaraman V. (2003) Layer-by-layer assembly of 1,4-diaminoanthraquinone and glucose oxidase. *Materials Chemistry and Physics*. 77: 390-396.

Bharathi S, Nogami M. (2001) A glucose biosensor based on electrodeposited biocomposites of gold nanoparticles and glucose oxidase enzyme. *Analyst. 126*, 1919-1922.

Campuzano, S.; Galvez, R.; Pedrero, M.; de Villena, F.J.M.; Pingarron, J.M. (2002) Preparation, characterization and application of alkanethiol self-assembled monolayer modified with tetrathiafulvalene and glucose oxidase at a gold disk electrode. *J. Electroanal. Chem.* 526(1-2), 92-100.

Cho JH, Shin MC, Kim HS. (1996) Electrochemical adsorption of glucose oxidase onto polypyrrole film for the construction of a glucose biosensor *Sensors and Actuators B: Chemical* 30(2) 137-141.

Cooper JC, Hall EAH. (1993) Catalytic reduction of benzoquinone at polyaniline and polyaniline enzyme films. *Electroanal*. 5(5-6), 385-397.

Delvaux M, Demoustier-Champagne S. (2003) Immobilisation of glucose oxidase within metallic nanotubes arrays for application to enzyme biosensors. *Biosensors & Bioelectronics* 18: 943-951.

Ding SJ, Chang BW, Wu CC, Lai MF, Chang HC. (2005) Impedance spectral studies of self-assembly of alkanethiols with different chain lengths using different immobilization strategies on Au electrodes. *Anal. Chim. Acta*. 554(1-2), 43-51.

Fan JG, Dyer D, Zhang G, Zhao Y. (2004) Nanocarpet effect: pattern formation during wetting of vertically aligned nanorod arrays. *Nanoletters. 4*, 2133-2138.

Forrer P, Schlottig F, Siegenthaler H. (2000) Electrochemical preparation and surface properties of gold nanowire array formed by template technique. *J. Appl. Electrochem. 30*, 533-541.

Fortier G, Brassard E, and Bélanger D. (1990) Optimization of a polypyrrole glucose oxidase biosensor *Biosensors and Bioelectronics* 5(6) 473-490.

Freund LB, Suresh S. (2003) Thin Film Materials. Cambridge University Academic Press.

Gangadharan R, Anandan V, Zhang G. (2008) Optimizing the functionalization process for nanopillar enhanced electrodes with GOx/PPY for glucose detection. *Nanotechnology*. 19, 395501.

Gao M, Gordon LD, Dai L, Wallace G. (2003) Biosensor based on vertically aligned carbon nanotubes coated with inherently conducting polymers. *Electroanalysis. 15*, 13, 1089-1094.

Gardner JW, Varadan VK, Awadelkarim OO. (2002) Microsensors MEMS and smart deices. New York. Wiley.

Gooding JJ, Erokhin P, Hibbert DB. (2000) Parameters important in tuning the response of monolayer enzyme electrodes fabricated using self-assembled monolayers of alkanethiols. *Biosensors & Bioelectronics*. 15: 229-239.

Gooding JJ, Praig VG, Hall EAH. (1998) Platinum-catalyzed enzyme electrodes immobilized on gold using self-assembled layers. *Analytical Chemistry*. 70: 2396-2402.

Gooding JJ, Erokhin P, Losic D, Yang W, Policarpio V, Liu J, Ho F, Situmorang M, Hibbert DB, Shapter JG. (2001) Parameters important in fabricating enzyme electrodes using self-assembled monolayers of alkanethiols. *Analytical Science*. 17: 3-9.

Hou Y, Helali S, Zhang A, Nicole JR, Martelet C, Minic C, Gorojankina T, Persuy MA, Edith PA, Salesse R, Bessueille F, Samitier J, Errachid A, Akimov V, Reggiani L, Pennetta C, Alfinito E. (2006) Biosensors and Bioelectronics. 21, 1393–1402.

Hou Y, Nicole JR, Martelet C, Zhang A, Jasmina MV, Gorojankina T, Persuy MA, Edith PA, Salesse R, Akimov V, Reggiani L, Pennetta C, Alfinito E, Ruiz O, Gomila G, Samitier J, Errachid A. (2007) Biosensors and Bioelectronics. 22, 1550–1555.

Imabayashi S, Iida M, Hobara D, Feng ZQ, Niki K, Kakiuchi T. (1997) Reductive desorption of carboxylic-acid-terminated alkanethiol monolayers from Au(111) surfaces. *J. Electroanal. Chem.* 428, 33-38.

Jia F, Yu C, Ai Z and Zhang L. (2007) Fabrication of Nanoporous Gold Film Electrodes with Ultrahigh Surface Area and Electrochemical Activity *Chem. Mater* 19(15) 3648-3653.

Koehne J, Li J, Cassell A M, Chen H, Ye Q, Ng H T, Han J and Meyyappan M. (2004) The fabrication and electrochemical characterization of carbon nanotube nanoelectrode arrays. *Journal of Materials Chemistry* 14(4) 676-684.

Kralchevsky PA, Nagayama K. (2000) Capillary interactions between particles bound to interfaces, liquid films and biomembranes. *Advances in colloid and interface science.* 85, 145-192.

Lambrechts M and Sansen WMC. (1992) Biosensors: Microelectrochemical Devices *CRC Press.*

Lau KKS, Bico J, Teo KBK. (2003) Superhydrophobic carbon nanotube forests. *Nanoletters. 3,* 1701-1705.

Lee SJ, Anandan V, Zhang G. (2008) Electrochemical fabrication and evaluation of highly sensitive nanorod-modified electrodes for a biotin/avidin system. *Biosens. Bioelectron.* 23(7), 1117-1124.

Losic D, Gooding JJ, Shapter JG, Hibbert DB, Short K. (2001) The influence of the underlying gold substrate on glucose oxidase electrodes fabricated using self-assembled monolayers. *Electroanalysis* 13: 1385-1393.

Losic D, Shapter JG, Gooding JJ. (2001) Influence of surface topography on alkanethiol SAMs assembled from solution and by microcontact printing. *Langmuir.* 17(11), 3307-3316.

Moatti SD, Velho G, Reach G. (1992) Evaluating in vitro and in vivo the interference of ascorbate and acetaminophen on glucose detection by a needle-type glucose sensor Biosensors and Bioelectronics 7(5) 345-352.

Qiao CS, Tuzhi P, Yunu Z, Yang CF. (2005) An Electrochemical Biosensor with Cholesterol Oxidase/ Sol-Gel Film on a Nanoplatinum/Carbon Nanotube Electrode. *Electroanalysis.* 17: 857-861.

Ramanavicius A, Kausaite A, and Ramanaviciene A. (2005) Polypyrrole-coated glucose oxidase nanoparticles for biosensor design. *Sensors and Actuators B: Chemical* 111-112 532-539.

Sawaguchi T, Sato Y, Mizutani F. (2001) In situ STM imaging of individual molecules in two-component self-assembled monolayers of 3-mercaptopropionic acid and 1-decanethiol on Au(111). *J. Electroanal. Chem.* 496(1-2), 50-60.

Trasatti S and Petrii OA. (1991) Real Surface Area Measurements in Electrochemistry *Pure and applied chemistry* 63(5) 711-734.

Uang YM, Chow TC. (2002) Criteria for Designing a Polypyrrole Glucose Biosensor by Galvanostatic Electropolymerization. *Electroanalysis.* 14: 1564-1570.

Wang J, Musameh M. (2003) Carbon Nanotube/Teflon Composite Electrochemical Sensors and Biosensors. *Anal. Chem.* 75: 2075-2079.

Wang J, Mustafa M. (2004) Carbon nanotube screen-printed electrochemical sensors. *Analyst.* 129, 1-2.

Wang Z, Su YK, Li HL. (2002) AFM study of gold nanowire array electrodeposited within anodic aluminum oxide template. *Applied Physics A. 74,* 563-565.

Wang J, Nosang M, Minhee Y, Harold M. (2005) Glucose oxidase entrapped in polypyrrole on high-surface-area Pt electrodes: a model platform for sensitive electroenzymatic biosensors. *Journal of Electroanalytical Chemistry.* 575: 139-146.

Walczak MM, Popenoe DD, Deinhammer RS, Lamp BD, Chung C, Porter MD. (1991) Reductive desorption of alkanethiolate monolayers at gold: a measure of surface coverage. *Langmuir.* 7(11), 2687-2693.

Widrig CA, Chung C, and Porter M D. (1991) The electrochemical desorption of n-alkanethiol monolayers from polycrystalline Au and Ag electrodes. *J. Electroanal. Chem.* 310, 335-359.

Xu J, Huang X, Xie G. (2004) Study on the structures and magnetic properties of Ni, Co-Al_2O_3 electrodeposited nanowire arrays. *Materials Research Bulletin. 39,* 811-818.

Yemini M, Reches M, Rishpon J. (2005) Novel electrochemical biosensing platform using self assembled peptide nanotube. *Nanoletters. 5,* 183-186.

Zhang G, Anandan V and Rao YL. (2008) Fabrication of microstructures integrated with nanopillars along with their applications as electrodes in sensors. US PTO patent pending, the University of Georgia.

14

Screen Printed Electrodes with Improved Mass Transfer

Jan Krejci, Romana Sejnohova,
Vitezslav Hanak and Hana Vranova
*BVT Technologies, a.s., Hudcova 533/78c, 612 00 Brno,
Czech Republic*

1. Introduction

Electrochemical sensors in contrast to many other analytical methods enable possibility of their production at low price and their miniaturization. The first feature leads to their possibility massive application in industry, home products and as input devices of computers. The possibility of electrochemical sensor preparation in micro-scale enables creation of arrays and fields of sensors on chips of size of some square of mm. Despite of these excellent properties the electrochemical sensors are not widely spread in practice. Despite of their massive research and development, their penetration into the practise is slow. They suffer by some weaknesses namely in reproducibility. Only very skilled experts obtain reliable and reproducible results by their use. The survey of patent literature, scientific and economical literature prove that the advantages of electrochemical sensor are without discussion however the journey to use their advantages in practise is more difficult and complicated than it can be supposed after first positive experiments. This can by approved by examples. The development of glucose chips for diabetic patients took more 20 years. In early 90ties the lost from their production was in millions of GBP per year. The development of colourometric diagnostic strips takes significantly less time than 10 years dry chemistry. They were used as diabetic strips till middle of 90ties. The advantage of electrochemical sensors wins but it was very difficult and expensive development. In end of 70ties many companies stated (Krejčí, 1988) that implantable sensor of glucose will be in market in months. After 30 years does not exist reliable implantable sensor of glucose on market. Ten years ago it was stated that electrochemical DNA sensor array will be important analytical tool but only optical arrays are routinely used now. Generally after first results which can be obtained in very easy manner in electrochemical sensors the development to final device is at least two times longer than optical methods or other methods where the first experiments are quite complicated e.g. Surface Plasmon Resonance (SPR) (Frost & Sullivan, 1994; Sethi et al., 1989, 1990).There are many reasons which are behind low robustness of electrochemical sensors. One of them is mass transport between bulk of sample and active sensor area. The background of this phenomenon is in fig. 1.
On the surface of an electrochemical sensor there are three layers defining its response. The first layer of specially adsorbed ions and molecules is called the compact Helmholz layer (sometimes Stern layer). This is defined by centres of atoms "sitting" on the electrode

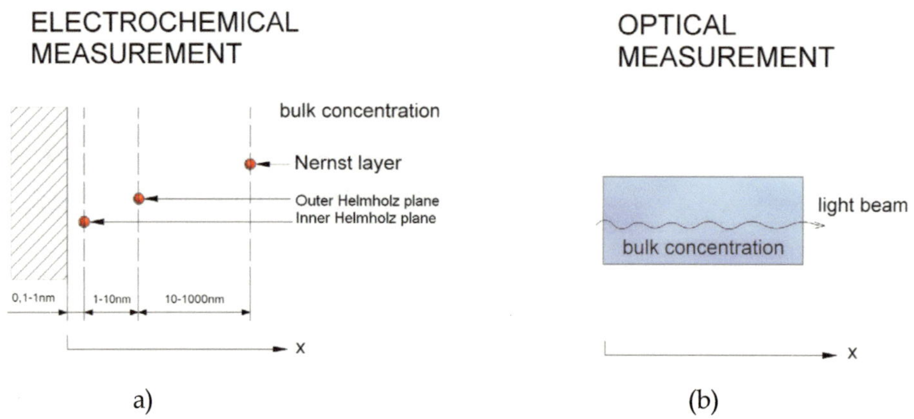

Fig. 1. Difference between electrochemical (a) and optical (b) measurement.

surface. The locus of electrical centres of ions adsorbed in the Helmholz layer (more precisely centres of symmetry of ion electrical field) is called the inner Helmholz plane. The outer Helmholz layer is formed by the space charge region which is created by interaction between electrode and charged ions in solutions. The outer Helmholz plane is the locus of centres of the nearest solvated ions with respect of to the electrode surface (Bard & Faulkner, 1980). The third layer is created by Nernst layer where the concentration differs from the bulk concentration due to the diffusion of electro active compounds to the electrode surface. The response of the sensor will depend on the structure of each of these layers and on the chemical reactions which run in each of these layers. There are also fluctuations of properties of each of this layer. It is obvious that these fluctuations will be averaged on the electrode surface but not in the distance x. The electrochemical biosensor is prepared from electrochemical sensor by immobilization of bioactive compound (Macholán, 1991; Turner et al., 1987). The immobilized layer lies in the outer Helmholz layer and in the Nernst layer. It assures not only the run of reaction which is responsible for sensor selectivity but it influences the structure of inner Helmholz layer. The process of immobilization significantly changes the specific adsorption on the active electrode. The influence of bioactive layer on the structure of outer Helmholz layer and Nernst layer is dramatic. The bioactive membrane changes the space distribution of the charge, solvation processes, pH equilibration in outer Helmholz layer. The bioactive layer also changes the concentration distribution in Nernst layer. The interactions are mutual. The presence of electrode and reactions on its surface influences the bioactive membrane. The local changes of pH can move the reaction out of pH optimum. Local changes of ionic strength can influence the reaction in bioactive membrane (Kotyk et al., 1977). The situation with optical sensor is quite different. The beam of light goes trough the analyzed solution and interacts with molecules. It interacts directly with each molecule and there is no subsequent interaction in layer as in the case of electrochemical sensors. Fluctuations in optical measurement also occur however these will be averaged not only on the optical detector surface but also along the distance x along, the path of beam. It assures better robustness of optical measurement. This demonstrates the important role played by mass transport in electrochemical measurements and in electrochemical biosensors (Dvořák & Koryta, 1983; Rieger, 1993; Riley, et al. 1987). The role of mass transport can be shown experimentally. It is possible to measure the surface of screen printed electrodes by SEM and confocal microscopy and compare the result with electrochemical measurement. This procedure is in detail described in (Schröper et al., 2008). The importance of this measurement consists not only in the fact of obtaining the active area of the sensor but experiments these can be considered as model of typical amperometric measurement. The result is in fig. 2 and fig. 3.

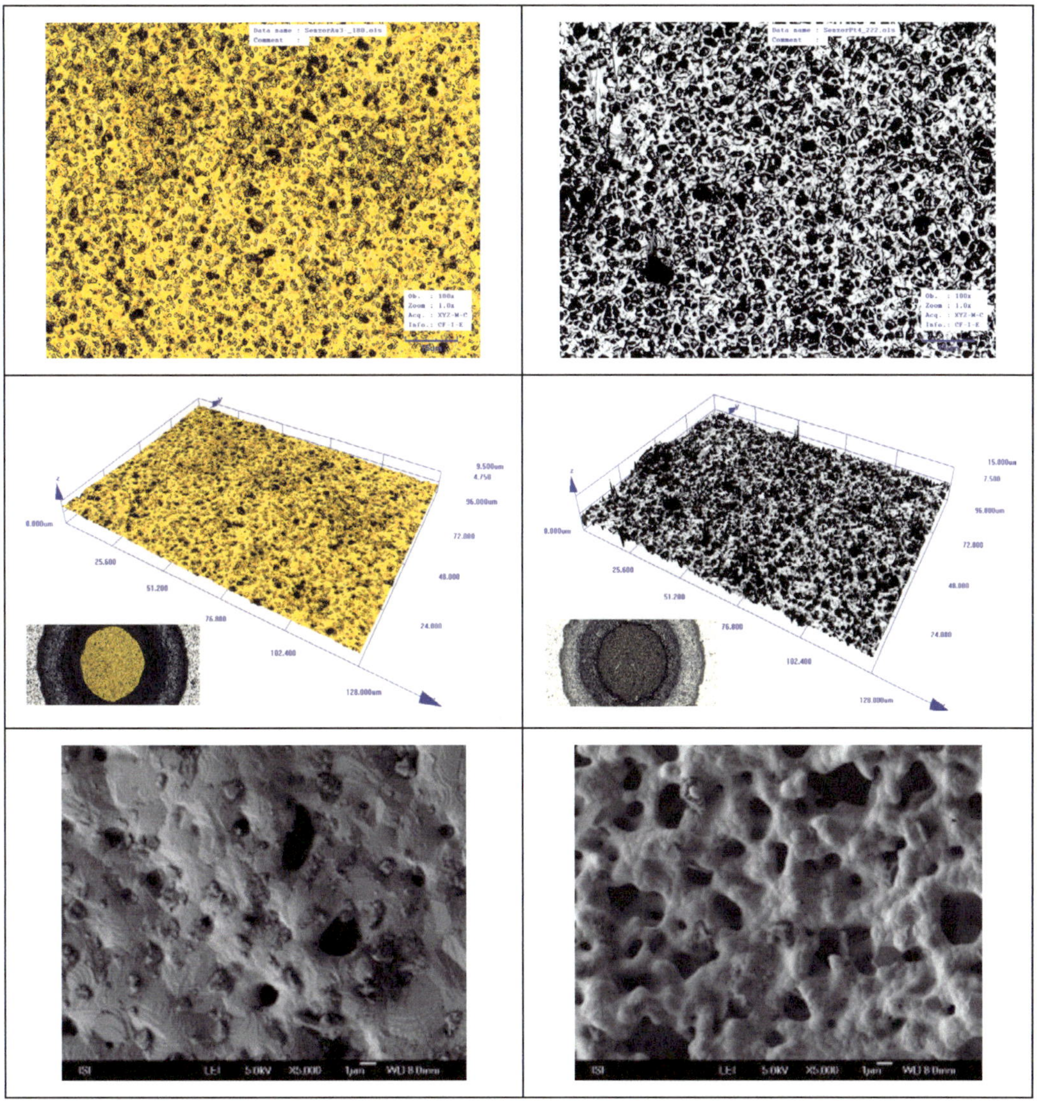

Fig. 2. The surface structure of AC1.W1.RS (left panel) and AC1.W2.RS (right panel) recorded by optical (upper and middle part) and scanning electron microscopy (bottom part).

Fig. 2 shows the anaysis of gold and platinum active surface of electrodes by optical microscopy and scanning electron microscopy. The comparison with electrochemical measurement is in fig. 3. Independent methods show the active surface significantly bigger as electrochemical measurement.

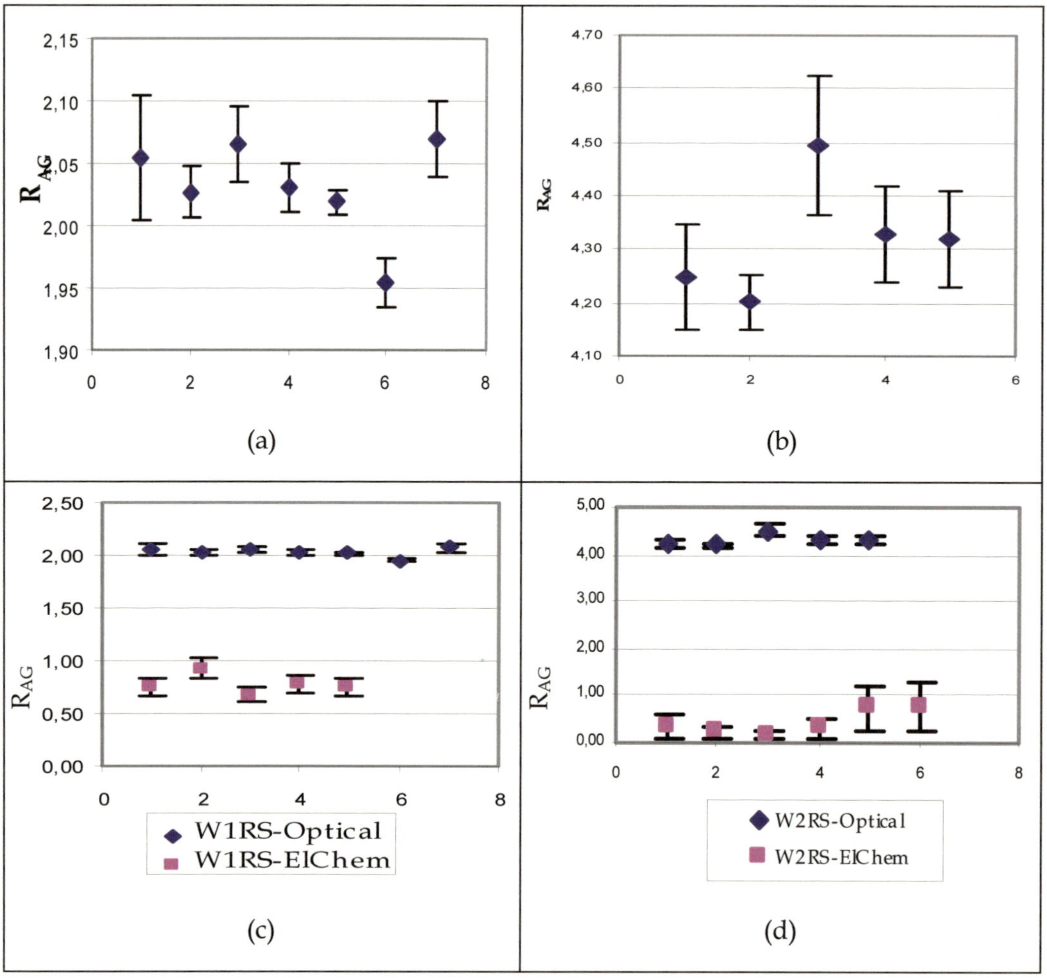

Fig. 3. The results of confocal microscope relation of active area to geometrical area (R_{AG}) measurement, a) (R_{AG}) for the sensor AC1.W1.RS (Au) b) (R_{AG}) for the sensor AC1.W2.RS (PT). Comparison with electrochemical measurement c) Sensor AC1.W1.RS (Au) d) Sensor AC1.W2.RS (Pt).

The surface properties of Au and Pt working electrodes prepared by screen printing (BVT Technologies, a.s.) were studied on statistical data sets. The mean ratio of active to geometrical surface (R_{AG}) obtained by optical measurement is in Tab. 1.

Type of sensor	Working electrode	R_{AG}	Number of measurements
AC1.W1.RS	Au	2.03 ± 0.04	(n = 7)
AC1.W2.RS	Pt	4.35 ± 0.08	(n = 5)

Table 1. Optical measurement

(R_{AG}) obtained by electrochemical measurement of the same sensors. Results for AC1.W1.RS and AC1.W2.RS are as follows (Tab. 2).

Type of sensor	Working electrode	R_{AG}	Number of measurements
AC1.W1.RS	Au	0.61 ± 0.06	(n = 5)
AC1.W2.RS	Pt	0.34 ± 0.20	(n = 6)

Table 2. Electrochemical measurement

Electrochemical results are approximately an order of magnitude lower than optical measurement data (3x, 12x).
The simplest explanation for this difference can be explained by insufficient mass transport and its poor reproducibility. The electrochemical reaction runs only on the upper edges of the complicated electrode surface. This reaction shields the lower layers of the electrode where no reaction takes place (see fig. 4). It is obvious that mass transport under such conditions will be very sensitive to experimental arrangement namely stirring of the solution. This also explains the difference between electrochemical determinations of active surface measurement in the literature where results can differ in range by one order. This shielding explains the low efficiency of nanostructures on the electrode surface (Fig. 4) which was indirectly confirmed by experiments in (Maly et al., 2005). These results are valid not only for special measurement as mentioned above but more generally for all measurements based on the electrochemical principle.

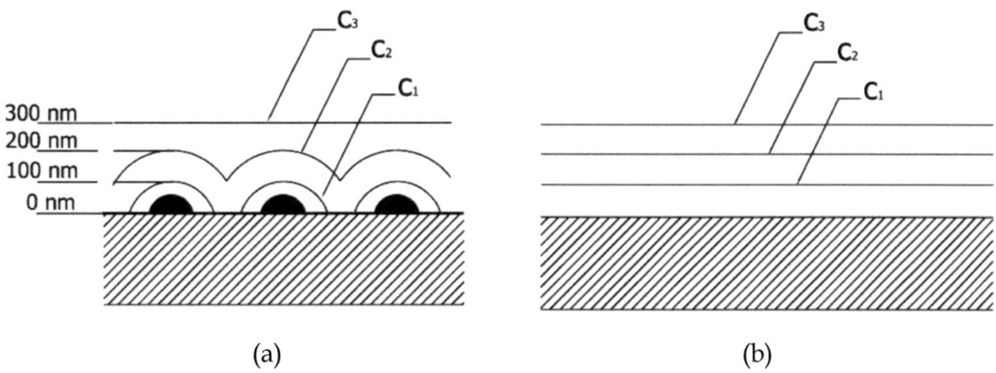

Fig. 4. Nanostructured (a) and planar (b) electrode of electrochemical sensor.

2. Properties by controlled mass transport

In the next section the improvement of screen printed electrochemical sensors and biosensor will be demonstrated and wall jet cell by three techniques

- Microfluidic arrangement which uses a thin layer cell
- Rotated disc microelectrode
- Thermodiffusion

The improvement is based on controled and amplified mass transport from bulk of solution to the active surface of electrode.

2.1 Microfluidic arrangement

The experimental arrangement of the microflow system (MFS) is illustrated in figure 5.

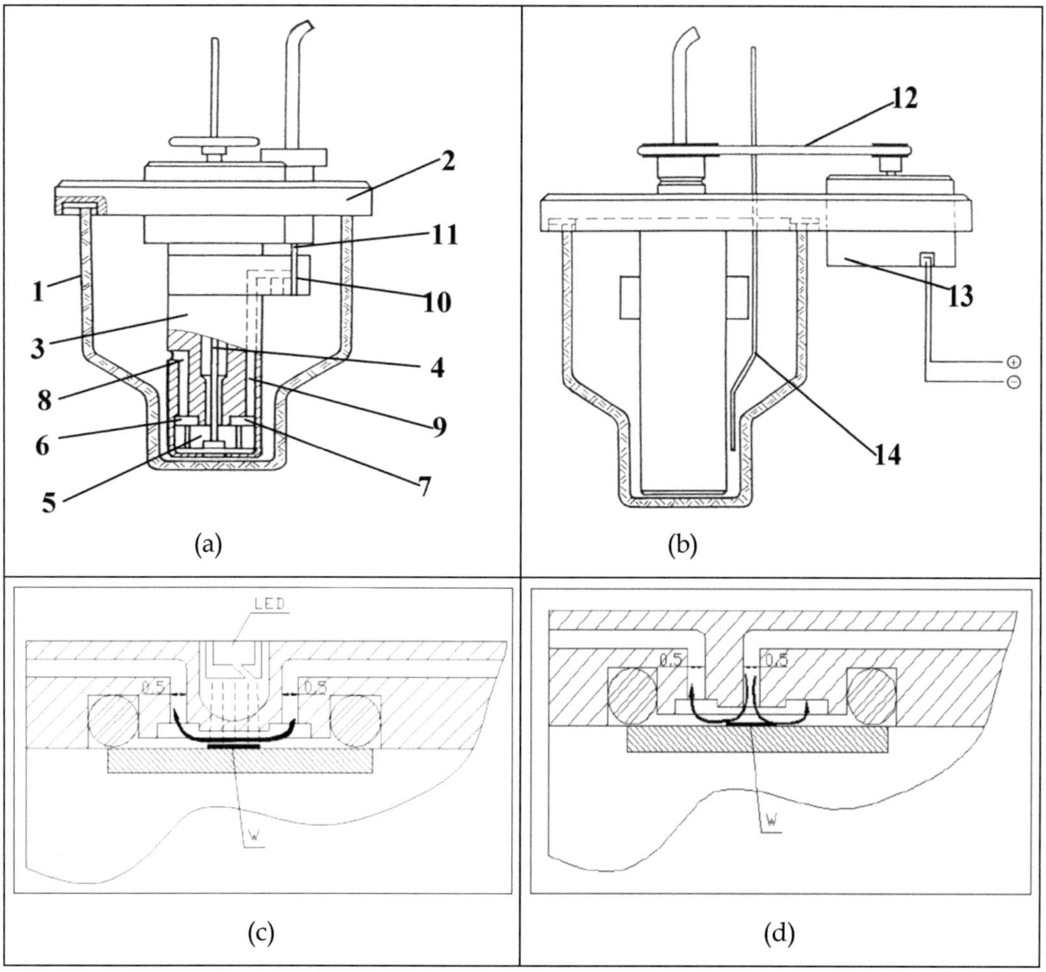

Fig. 5. a,b) Experimental arrangement of the Microflow system (Patent CZ 287676); 1) electrochemical vessel, 2) modified lid, 3) body of microflow insert, 4) driving shaft, 5) pump rotor, 6) sample mixing chamber, 7) sample pumping chamber, 8) mixing channel outlet, 9) capillary, 10) microflow chamber, 11) thick film sensor, 12) mixing channel inlet, 13) driving belt, 14) motor, 15) inert gas input. c) Flow cell arranged in thin layer format. d) Flow cell arranged in wall-jet format (Krejci et al., 2008).

A conventional electrochemical vessel (Rieger, 1993) (1) in figure 5 (TC1) (BVT Technologies, a.s., Czech Republic) is covered by a modified lid (2) carrying the body of the microflow insert (3). The driving shaft (4) located in the centre of the microflow insert is connected to the pump rotor (5) immersed in the electrolyte/sample fluid. The electrolyte/sample fluid comes to the pump rotor (5) via mixing channel inlet (12). The two chambers located above the rotor fulfil two different functions. The first of the chambers (6) is connected via mixing channel outlet (8) to the bulk of electrolyte/sample solution inside the electrochemical vessel. The portion of the liquid being pumped through this passageway provides for sufficient stirring of the solution inside the electrolyte vessel. The second chamber (7) helps to guide the fluid coming from the rotor into the capillary (9) and into the electrode cell (10).

The function of the narrow capillary is to stabilize the flow of the liquid before it enters into the electrode cells. The overall design of the insert is such that only 1 - 5% of the liquid is flowing through the chamber (7) and capillary (9), while bout 95 - 99% of it is pumped through the chamber (6): and channel (8), ensuring intensive stirring of the solution. The electrode cell (10) contains the integrated three-electrode amperometric sensor (11) (AC1.W2.R1, BVT Technologies, a.s., Czech Republic; Fig. 6b). Following its passage past the sensor, the liquid is returned from the electrode cell directly into the bulk of the electrolyte/sample solution inside the vessel. The driving shaft (4) is connected by means of an elastic belt (13) to the external motor (14). The entire electrochemical vessel with the microflow insert immersed in the electrolyte/sample solution is placed in a thermostat bath and the temperature is kept constant at 25 ± 0.1 °C. The tube (15) can be used for inert gas introduction for work under inert atmosphere. A few other openings in the lid (2) are provided for sample additions, insertion of a thermometer and for other accessories. The arrangement is mainly destined for batch injection analysis. The principle was integrated into the device MFS (BVT Technologies, a.s.) (Fig. 6a) (Krejci et al., 2008).

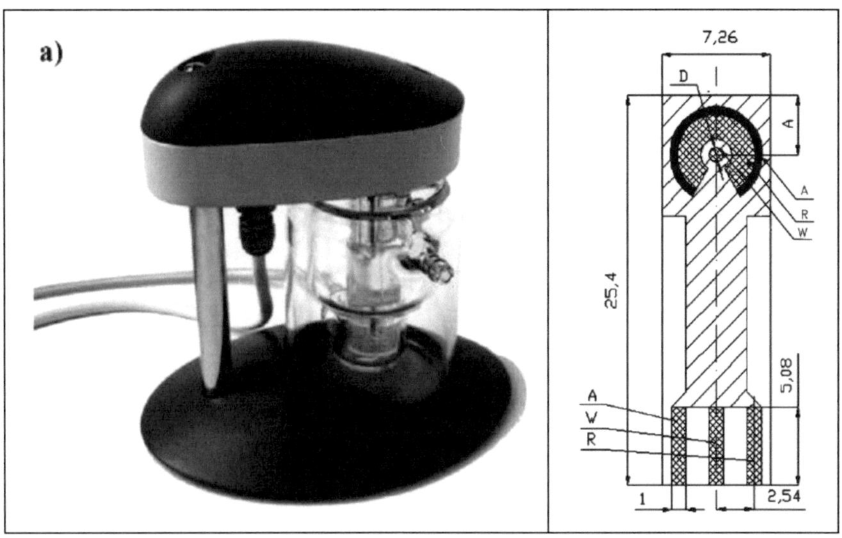

Fig. 6. a) Photo of the microflow system (MFS) device (BVT Technologies, a.s., Czech Republic). b) Integrated three-electrode amperometric sensor (Patent CZ 291411) (A: auxiliary electrode, R: reference electrode, W: working electrode) (Krejci et al., 2008).

The device can be equipped with two types of electrode cells (fig. 5, 10). The wall jet cell and thin layer cell (fig. 5 c, d). In case of wall jet cell the stream of analyte flows from small orifice of diameter a perpendicularly to the active surface of electrode. The current of electrode in wall jet arrangement where the diameter of electrode active area is bigger than jet opening is described by equation (1) (Painton & Mottola, 1983). The theory of wall-jet hydrodynamic arrangement was originally derived by Matsuda (Matsuda, 1967; Yamada & Matsuda, 1973). The more detailed description of jet flow is in excellent monography of Polyanin (Polyanin et al., 2002).

$$I = 1{,}15\ n\ F\ R^{3/4}\ a\ D^{2/3}\ \upsilon^{-5/12}\ U^{3/4}\ c_0 \qquad (1)$$

where
n-Number electrons in reaction; F-Faraday constant [96 485 $C.mol^{-1}$]; R-Radius of electrode [m]; a-Diameter of jet [m]; D-Diffusion coefficient [$m^2.s^{-1}$]; υ-Kinematic viscosity [$m^2.s^{-1}$]; U-Velocity in the jet [$m.s^{-1}$]; c_0-Concentration [$mol.l^{-1}$]; I-Current [A]
The important characterization of the cell is its conversion efficiency η. This quantity describes the relation of actual current with respect of current produced by all electroactive (active in case of biosensor) compounds entering the cell. Using data from Polyanin (Polyanin et al., 2002) it can be evaluated as

$$\eta = \frac{4 \times 1.15}{\pi^{3/4}} R^{3/4} D^{2/3} \upsilon^{-5/12} Q^{-1/4} a^{-1/2} \quad (2)$$

where
Q-volume flow of sample trough cell [$m^3.s^{-1}$]
The thin layer arrangement is characterized by electrode active surface placed in channel with very small height. Important characterization of thin layer arrangement is that channel height h is significantly smaller than channel width b (h << b) (see fig. 5c). There are many different equations in literature which describes thin layer hydrodynamic arrangement. They can by summarized as equation (4a) where different authors found different value of constant k (Brunt & Bruins, 1979; Hanekamp & Nieuwkerk, 1980; Levich, 1947; Wranglén et al., 1962). If the flow around electrode is stable and laminar then Matsuda derived equation (4b) (Matsuda, 1967). More recent and excellent discussion namely concentrated on was made by (Squires, 2008). Comprehensive analysis is also in (Polyanin et al., 2002). If the length of electrode in the channel is higher than l (equation 3) then the sensor measures in coulometric mode with 100% conversion. All electrochemical compounds are reacted/converted at the electrode. In summary the current in case of thin layer cell is described by equation (4c).

$$l \geq \frac{3}{8}\frac{h}{b}\frac{Q}{D} \quad (3)$$

where
D-Diffusion coefficient [-]; b-width of the channel [m]; h-channel height [m]; l-length of electrode [m]

$$I = k\, n\, F\, D^{2/3}\, b\, l^{1/2}\, \upsilon^{-1/6}\, U^{1/2}\, c_0 \quad (4a)$$

$$I = 1{,}47\, n\, F\, D^{2/3}\, A\, b^{-2/3}\, U^{1/3}\, c_0 \quad (4b)$$

$$I = n\, F Q c_0 \quad (4c)$$

where
k-lies in the range 0.68 – 0.83; b-width of the channel and electrode covering the wall of the channel [m]; U-the linear velocity with laminar flow [$m.s^{-1}$]; A-electrode area [m^2]; Q-volume flow of electro-active material [$m^3. s^{-1}$]
The meaning of rest of symbols is same as in previous equations.
The conversion efficiency in above three cases is in equation (5)

$$\eta = k\, D^{2/3} \left(\frac{Qh}{lb}\right)^{-1/2} \upsilon^{-1/6} \quad \text{for (4a)} \tag{5a}$$

$$\eta = 1.47\, D^{2/3} \left(\frac{Q}{h}\right)^{-2/3} \quad \text{for (4b)} \tag{5b}$$

$$\eta = 1 \quad \text{for (4c)} \tag{5c}$$

2.2 Rotated disc microelectrode

A rotating disc electrode (RDE) is one exceptional example where the hydrodynamics (Navier stokes equations) and convective mass transport can be solved in analytical approximation. This means that relatively simple formulas exist that describe the electrode response with sufficient precision. (Some authors states that the hydrodynamics and convective diffusion at RDE can be analytically solved but this is not true.) The main principles of RDE are theoretically described in the literature (Bard & Faulkner, 1980; Riger 1993; Riley et al., 1987) for example. However the exact and comprehensive description of RDE physics can be found in Levich's works (Levich, 1942, 1944, 1944, 1947). The results are summarized in (Levich, 1962). The Levich derivation is based on results of Karman (Karman, 1921). These results are used not only in Levich's derivation but in many recent works. Comprehensive analysis of RDE principle is in literature (Sajdlová, 2010; King et al., 2005). An example of a RDE is shown in fig. 7. Classical RDE involve a platinum wire within glass tubing sealed in the plastic body of the RDE. The shape of the insulating mantle has an important role for the RDE function. It is obvious from the fact that Levich equation (6) describing RDE response is valid for disc of infinite radius in semi infinite homogenous media. This condition can not be fulfiled in real experimental conditions. However the thickness of hydrodynamic boundary layer (δ0) is significantly lower than electrode diameter. If the electrode is placed in distance from bottom of reaction vessel which is at least 1 order bigger than (δ0) then Levich equation will be very good approximation of RDE function. It means if the low angular speed is used the active surface of electrode is placed at least 10 mm above bottom of reaction vessel (see tab. 3). Corruption of this condition leads to hydrodynamic instability (Sajdlová, 2010). The electrical connection on the opposite end is made by the means of a brush contact. The noise of electrode significantly depends on the contact material and its construction. Will be had best experience with gold contact and precious metal brush. The RDE can be prepared also as disposable insert (fig. 7) where the active surface is made by screen-printing. The main advantage of RDE consists of possibility to control the mass transport by rotation speed. If the experiments are done at different velocities then the response can be extrapolated to infinite rotation speed where the mass transport is eliminated and the response is determined by electrode kinetic only or by immobilized enzyme kinetic if RDE is used as biosensor. It enables the optimization of immobilization procedure including precise measurement of membrane properties including enzyme biosensor membrane characterization. The RDE is characterized by two most important parameters: δ0 – thickness of the hydrodynamic boundary layer and thickness of Nernst diffusion layer (δ), where the maximum changes of concentration with respect of bulk concentration take place. Both parameters depend on angular velocity and they can be expressed, as is shown in equations (6) and (7) (Levich, 1962).

$$\delta_0 = 3.6 \sqrt{\frac{\upsilon}{\omega}} \tag{6}$$

$$\delta = 0.5 \sqrt[3]{\frac{D}{\upsilon}} \delta_0 \tag{7}$$

where
υ- kinematics viscosity; ω-angular velocity; D-diffusion coefficient of analyte
Due to power 1/3 the dependence on υ is small. The typical values of δ_0 and δ for H2O and glycerol are shown in table 3.

ω [s-1]	H2O δ0 [μm]	H2O δ [μm] (D = 10-10 m2.s-1)	glycerol δ0 [μm]	glycerol δ [μm] (D = 10-10 m2.s-1)	Time resolution [s]
1	1000	50	33000	33	16
10	330	16.5	10000	10	2.2
100	100	5	3300	3.3	0.16
1000	33	1.6	1000	1	0.022

Table 3. Typical values for H2O and glycerol.

The knowledge of the diffusion boundary layer enables to estimate the time resolution of measurement as with RDE $\tau \doteq \frac{\delta^2}{D}$. The typical values are in table 3 too.

The output current of RDE is derived from the Levich equation.

$$I = 0.620\, n\, F\, A\, D^{2/3}\, \upsilon^{-1/6}\, \omega^{1/2}\, c_0 \tag{8}$$

where
n-Number of electron in the reaction,; F-Faraday constant [96 485 C.mol^{-1}]; A-Area of Electrode [m^2]; D-Diffusion coefficient [m^2.s^{-1}]; υ-Kinematic viscosity [m^2.s^{-1}]; ω-Angular velocity [s^{-1}]; c_0-Concentration [mol.l^{-1}]; I-Current [A]
The conversion efficiency of RDE is

$$\eta = 0{,}697 \left(\frac{D}{\upsilon} \right)^{2/3} \tag{9}$$

The conversion efficiency does not depend on electrode rotation speed and electrode diameter. It values for small molecules in water is $\eta_{H2O} \sim 0.01$ and for glycerol $\eta_{glycerol} \sim 10^{-4}$. Equations (1, 4 and 8) are confirmed in the literature (King et al., 2005; Masavať et al., 2008; Painton & Mottola, 1983; Tóth et al., 2004). Nearly all publications use these equations with improper description of quantities, and improper coefficients. We have checked these equations in the original literature and confirmed their validity. The fact, that majority of publications which uses the equations (1, 4 and 8) for evaluation of electrode parameters or membrane parameters, uses wrong equations; introduce some doubts about their reliability and reliability of published data where these equations were used for calculation of diffusion coefficient or other parameters. In analytical practice the use of wrong formulas does not play much important role because the measurement is calibrated and all equation (1, 4 and 8) has a general structure I = konst c_0. On the other hand it proves that the results are not comparable between different experimental arrangements without cross calibration. Implicitly the above low reliability of measurement is nothing else than insufficient definitions of mass transport. All equations (1, 4 and 8) are nothing else than solution of mass transport to the electrode under special conditions.

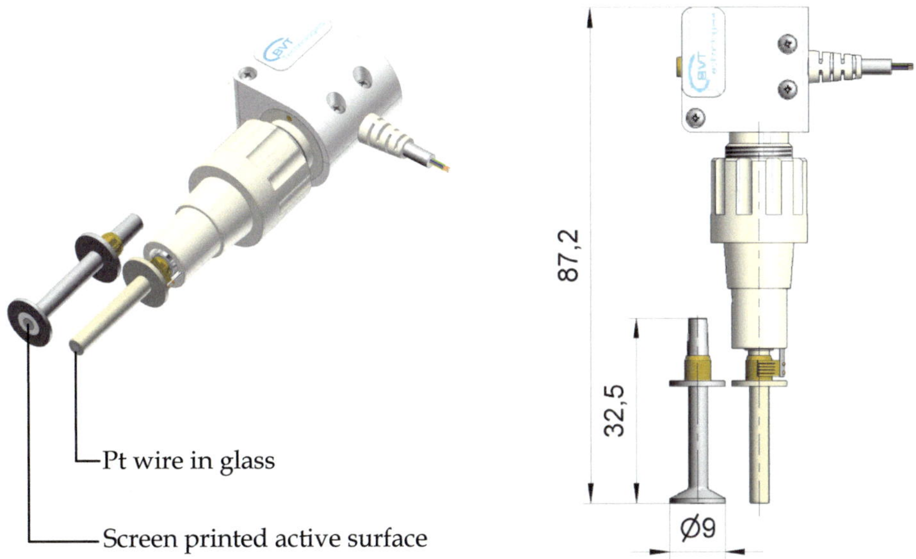

(a) (b)

Fig. 7. a, b) Mini-rotated disc electrode

The principle of RDE can be enhanced to move complicated hydro-dynamical arrangement. It can be used for elimination of cross talk of array of electrodes (Dock et al., 2005; Sajdlová, 2010).

The comparison of conversion efficiencies for typical parameters used in measurement in experimental part are summarized in tab. 4.

The parameters are:

diameter of jet nozzle a = 0.5 mm; radius of electrode R = 1 mm; height of channel h = 0.3 mm; width of channel b = 1 mm; length of electrode l = 2 mm; diffusion coefficient D = 10^{-9} m^2 s^{-1}; kinematics' viscosity of water $\upsilon = 10^{-6}$ m^2 s^{-1}; angular speed of RDE $\omega = 60$ s^{-1}

ηw (equation 2)	5 . 10-2
η5a (equation 5a)	3 . 10-2
η5b (equation 5b)	1 . 10-3
ηRDE (equation 9)	1 . 10-2
Hchannel (equation 3)	100 mm

Table 4. Comparison of different conversion efficiencies for typical parameters of cell listed in text.

2.3 Thermodiffusion

Electrochemical measurements are generally done under isothermal conditions. Thermal gradient can be also used to improve the mass transport. The application of a controlled temperature gradient between the working electrode surface and the solution, using electrochemical sensors prepared on ceramic materials with extremely high heat conductivity, enables that applied thermal gradient creates a the second driving force of mass transport. This application of the Soret phenomenon increases the mass transfer in the Nernst layer and enables more accurate control of the electrode response enhancement by a combination of diffusion and thermodiffusion. The key physical phenomenon is difference of thermal conductivity of ceramic and water solutions. The thermal conductivity of Al_2O_3 ceramic is about 35 $Wm^{-1}K^{-1}$. The thermal conductivity of water is 0.6 $Wm^{-1}K^{-1}$. If the active electrode is printed on the ceramic where on its opposite side just under working electrode is placed heating then the thermal gradient can be significantly higher than concentration gradient. The thermodiffusion coefficient is about 1-3 % of diffusion coefficient but at high temperature gradients the thermodiffusion mass flow can be comparable with mass flow driven by concentration gradient. It is important that thermodiffusion driving force can be adjusted independently on the concentration by temperature of sensor. Cotrell-Soret equation (10) has been derived in the literature (Krejčí, 2010).

$$I = n\,F\,A\,C_0\,\frac{D}{1+\theta(T_1)}\,s_T\,\alpha\left(T_1 - T_2\right) \tag{10}$$

where

$$\theta(T_1) = e^{\left(\frac{nF\left(E-E^0\right)}{RT_1}\right)}$$

$\theta(T_1)$ stresses the fact that due to high temperature conductivity of ceramic substrate of the sensor, the temperature T_1 of the electrode surface is known. The Cotrell-Soret equation has significant advantage with respect to Cotrell equation as it does not depend on the time. The derived the Cotrell-Soret equation describing the steady-state response with an applied temperature difference enables the measurement of electrode equilibrium potential at given temperature.

The termodiffusion can remove the accumulation of reduced/oxidised compounds at closed neighbourhood of electrode which is responsible for the hysteresis and complicated form of cyclic voltametry (CV) response. The example of use of thermodiffusion for sensor response improvement shows the ability of use of microelectronic technologies in electrochemical sensor production. The screen-printed active electrode together with screen-printed heaters and integrated thermometer Pt 1000 creates the electrochemical device which does not have classical analogy.

2.4 Experimental

The above discussion about mass transport will be demonstrated on four examples which demonstrate that screen-printed electrochemical sensor is very precise and sensitive device. These examples are amperometric measurement of H_2O_2, which is important for biosensors application where H_2O_2 is product of enzymatic reaction (oxydases); measurement of glucose oxidase by electrochemical sensor with immobilized enzyme; fast measurement of enzyme activity; cyclic voltammetry at temperature gradient.

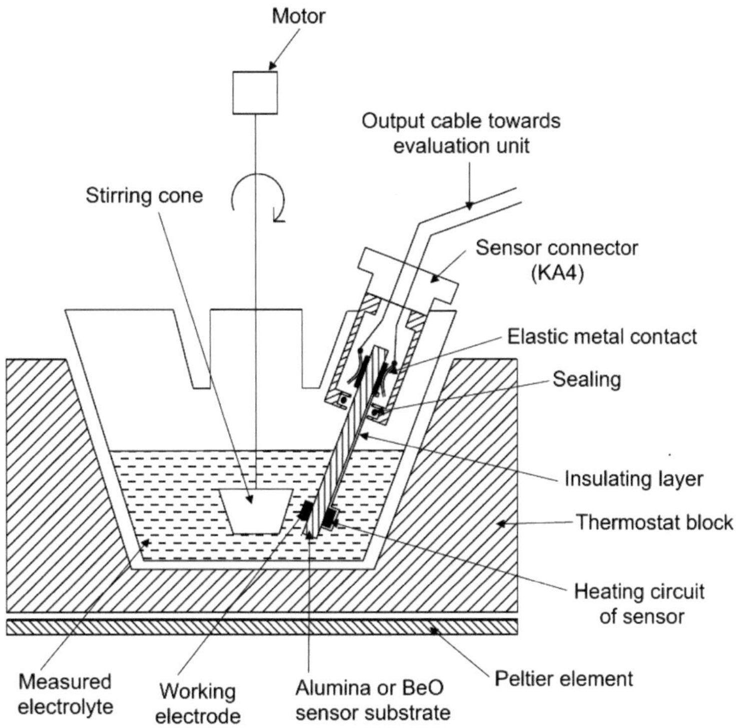

Fig. 8. Schematic of the Soret system (the gap between the cone and electrode surface is 1 mm)

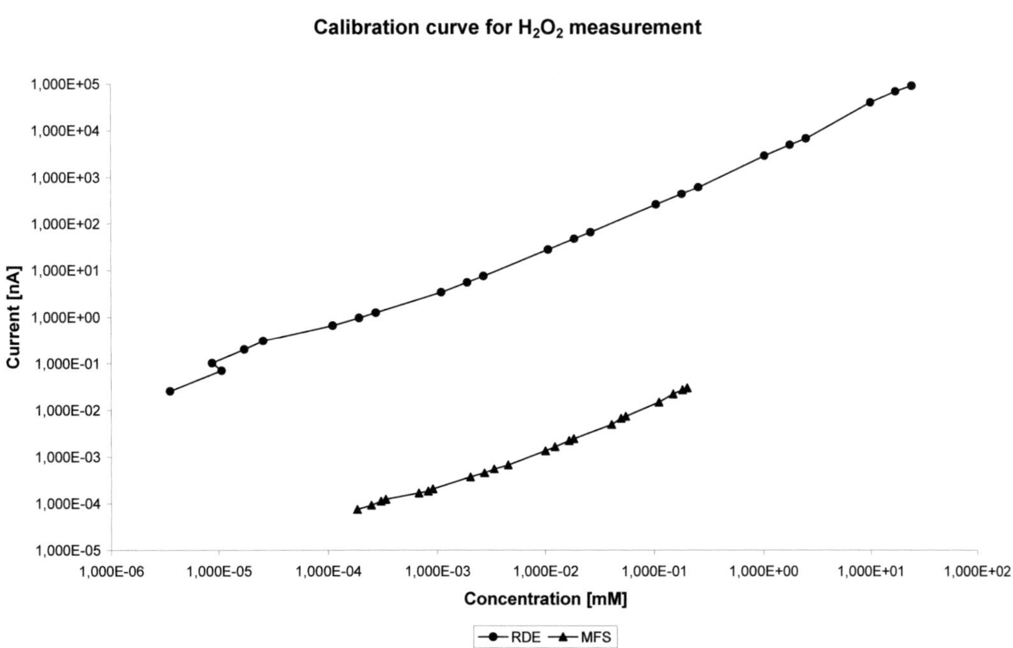

Fig. 9. Calibration curve for H_2O_2 measurement (Krejci et al., 2008).

2.4.1 Amperometric measurement of H_2O_2

The standard solution of hydrogen peroxide was prepared from a 3% stock solution (Lachema, Brno, Czech Republic). The electrochemical vessel filled with 5.00 ml of the working electrolyte (50 mM phosphate buffer, pH 7.0). The measurement was initiated by recording the background current in the absence of an analyte. After its stabilization, addition 50 μl aliquots of analytes (hydrogen peroxide) the changes in the current were recorded. Detection of hydrogen peroxide was carried out by amperometric measurement at the platinum working electrode of the AC1.W2.R1 sensor. The reaction chamber was wall-jet (see fig 5). Figure 9 shows the response to stepwise concentration changes of hydrogen peroxide spanning the range between 1.1×10^{-9} to 8×10^{-3} M. The extremely wide measurement range and very low limit detection is result of working electrode nanostructure (see fig. 2) and optimized mass transport in MFS device. The electrode is sintered from Pt grains of size 100 - 1000 nm, which assures extremely large active area as it is seen in fig. 2. Measurement was carried out with RDE under the same conditions. The angular velocity was $\omega = 60\ s^{-1}$. Experiments were done in 5 ml solution of phosphate buffer and 50 μl aliquots of different concentrations of H_2O_2 were added. The results are in the fig. 9 too. Under this condition the time the time resolution of RDE is 200 ms. The time resolution of current recorder is 100 ms. It enables to follow the homogenization of concentration in reaction vessel after analyte addition. The result can be seen in fig. 10.
The result on the fig. 10 demonstrates the dependence of the RDE response on its geometry. It shows typical response of classical RDE and RDE with wider disk. In both cases the material of electrode was polished platinum wire of 2 mm diameter melted in glass. The angular velocity was the same 62 s^{-1}. The response time of both electrodes was 200 ms at sampling time 100 ms electronic recorder.
The electrode with a 3 mm diameter (Fig. 10a) has significantly lower noise (0.1 nA - inserted noise analysis). The noise was analyzed when fluctuations of the signal disappeared. These fluctuations are caused by homogenization of the concentration in the bulk of solution. The homogenous concentration is reached after 180 s (3 min.). The electrode with a 10 mm (additional disk but the active area is same as in case of previous one) stabilizes significantly faster but with greater noise (7 nA - inserted noise analysis). The fluctuation of signal differs significantly from the previous arrangement and the concentration is homogenous in 15 s. Similar influence can be seen in dependence of signal on the distance of RDE and bottom of reaction vessel (Sajdlova, 2010).

2.4.2 Measurement of glucose oxidase by electrochemical sensor with immobilized enzyme

The measurement was done by the same procedure as in case of H_2O_2 only the sensor with immobilized glucose oxidase on the AC1.W2.RS was used in microfluidic system (MFS) with wall-jet reaction chamber. In Fig. 11 there is the calibration curve. The flattening of the calibration curves at higher concentrations is dictated by Michaelis-Menten kinetics. It is possible to see that at lower levels the enzyme reaction approximates the first order kinetics whereas at highest concentrations the reaction order approaches zero and the measured current becomes independent of glucose (enzyme substrate) concentration (Mell & Maloy, 1974)
The wide measured concentration range and extremely low limit of detection is the result of nanostructure as mentioned in section 1. The immobilization is made by this manner that

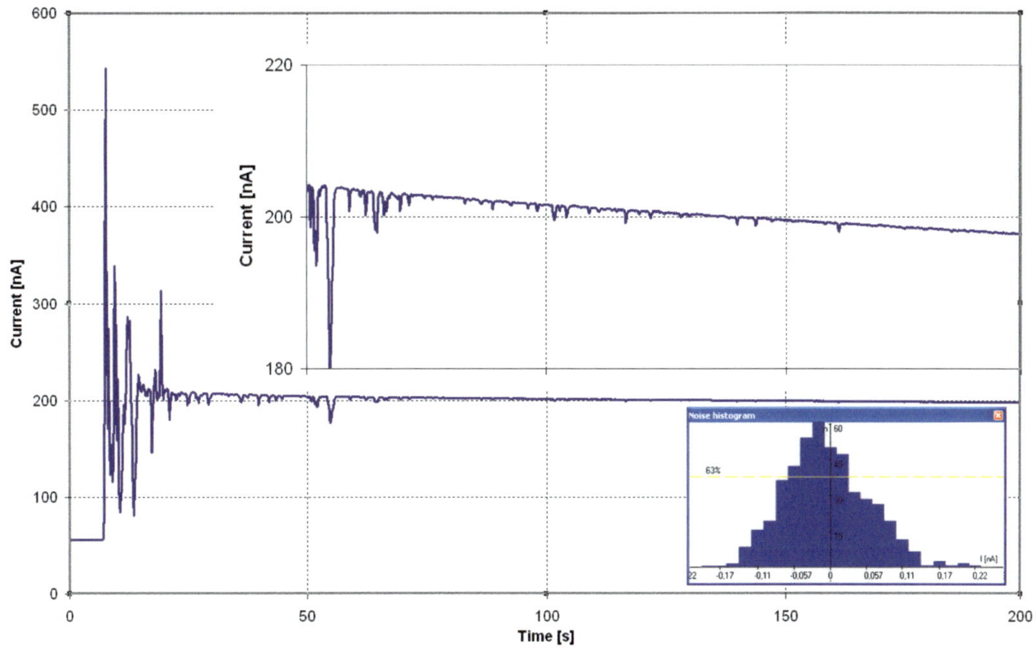

(a)

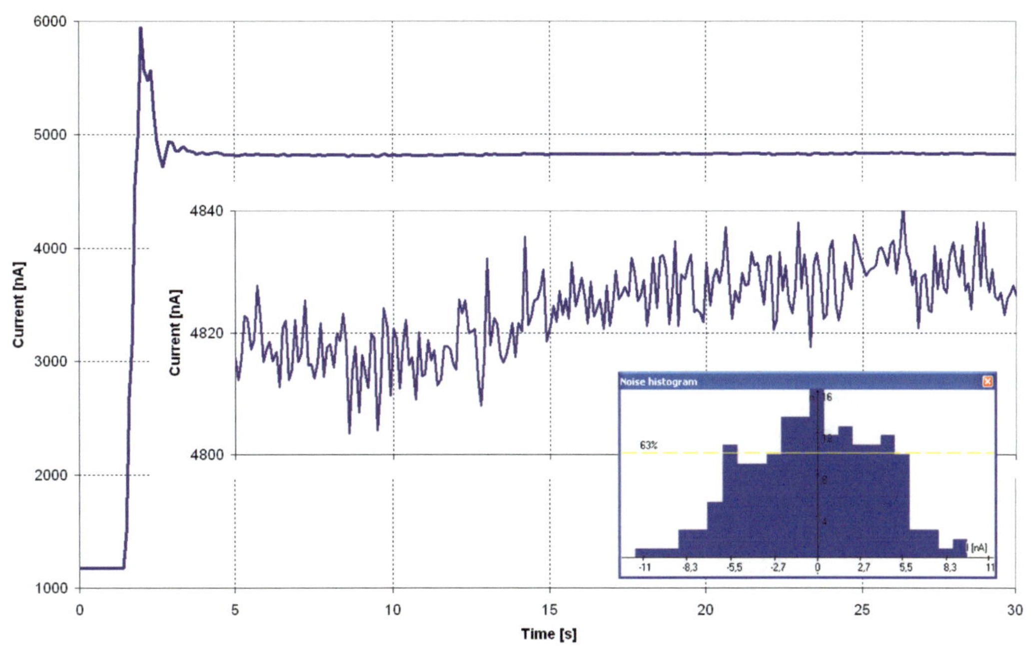

(b)

Fig. 10. The response to addition of analyte of the RDE of diameter a) 3 mm in 5 ml buffer and b) 10 mm diameter in 5 ml buffer.

the bioactive layer fills the free space between grains of Pt. It assures very tight connection between immobilized enzyme and active Pt surface. The overall active layers thickness (Pt and immobilized enzyme) is about 5 x 10^{-3} mm. This assures the respond time less than 1 s.

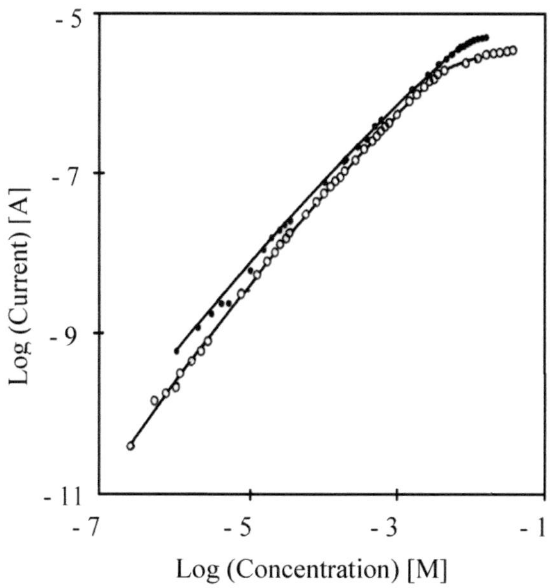

Fig. 11. Calibration curves of glucose biosensor in stirred vessel (•) and in the microflow system (○)

2.4.3 The measurement of soluble enzyme activity

The measurement of soluble enzymes activity is based on simplified Michaelis-Menten equation (Macholán, 1991). It can be written on condition [S] > 100 K_M i.e., the initial slope of the record of reaction of substrate with enzyme is proportional to the enzyme activity. The precision of approximation is better than 1 %. The absolute H_2O_2 production in mols can be recalculated for known volume of reaction vessel. It enables to calculate the activity of GOD sample addition. The same experiment was done with RDE at same conditions (ω = 60 s^{-1}), see section 2.4.1. The measurement principle has been depicted in the fig. 12a on an example of GOx. After the reaction vessel was filled with 5 ml of glucose solution of concentration 0.5 M ([S] ≈ 100 K_M) the observation was started and the background current measurements were recorded (A). The current response of the sensor was calibrated trough addition of aliquot of product, i.e., H_2O_2 (B). Then the solution of enzyme (GOx) was added (C). With the reaction initiation the current started rising linearly (D). The slope of current rising describes production of H_2O_2. The international unit of enzyme activity is defined for GOx as an amount of enzyme which oxidized 1 μmol of D-glucose to gluconolacton and H_2O_2 per 1 minute, at temperature 35 °C and at pH 5.1. The resulting calibration curve is in fig. 12b for MFS and RDE. The results of RDE are significantly better (lower limit of detection) which is caused by better time resolution of RDE and better long term stability of RDE current. Better long term stability enables higher resolution of extremely small changes of current slope.

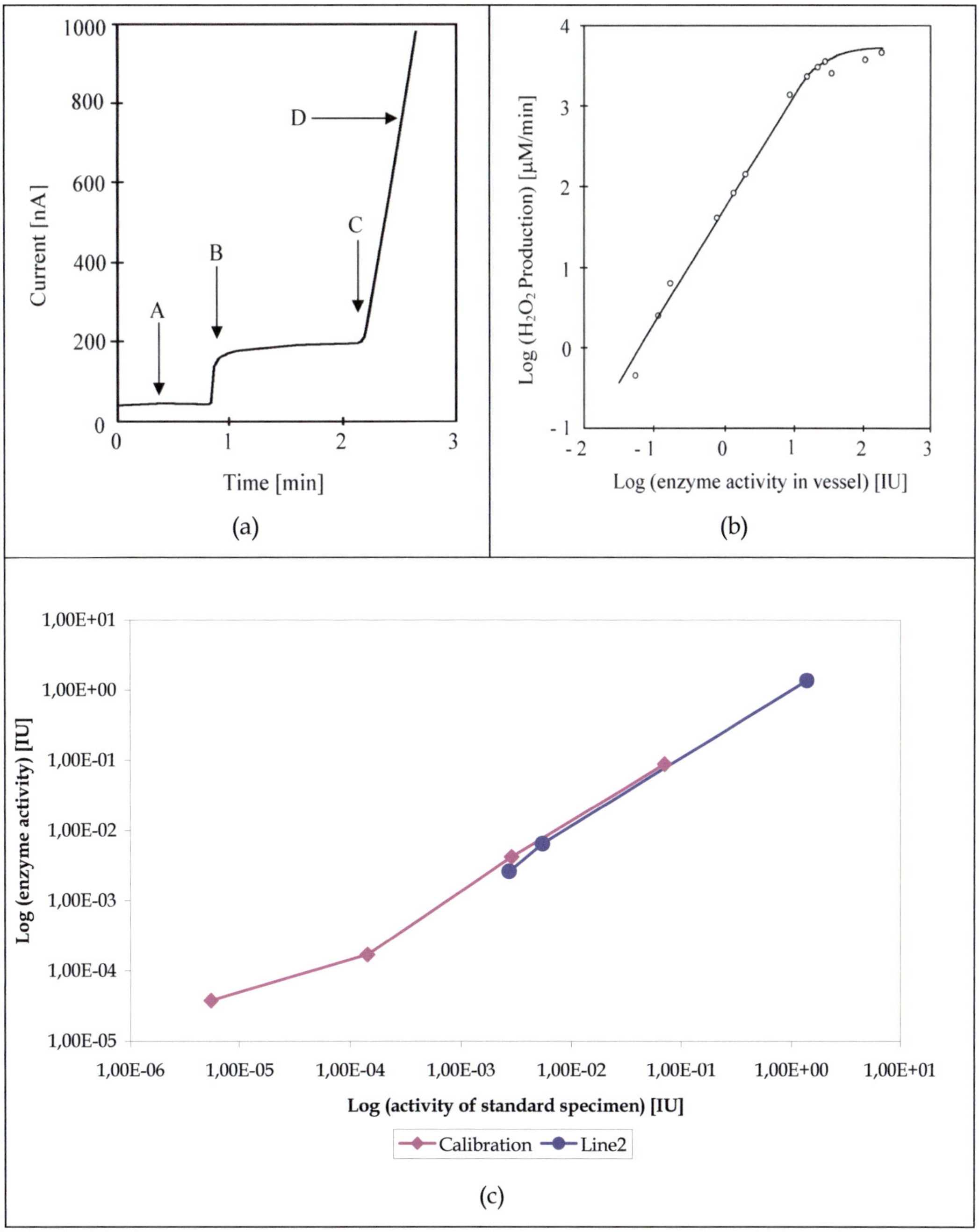

Fig. 12. a) Schematic view of enzyme activity measurement; A) addition of glucosse concentration in vessel c_{vessel} = 500 mM; B) addition of H_2O_2 for calibration c_{vessel} = 20.2 μM; C) injection of GOx solution of unknown activity; D) H_2O_2 production (478 μM/min).
b) Calibration curve for enzyme activity measurement using MFS (Krejci et al., 2008).
c) Calibration curve for enzyme activity measurement using RDE.

2.4.4 Cyclic voltammetry (CV) at temperature gradient

Measurements were performed in a device consisting of a glass cell TC1, conic stirrer and connector KSA1 and electrochemical sensor AC1.W2.RS (H, T) (BVT Technologies, Czech Republic). The AC1.W2.RS (H) electrochemical sensor bears platinum working and auxiliary electrodes, a pseudo-reference silver electrode and a heating circuit. The cell TC1 was placed in a small thermostat TK-1 (KEVA, Czech Republic). The whole system schematic is shown in figure 8 (Krejci et al., 2010).

CV is the most common electrochemical method used to investigate the electrochemical behaviour of an analyte. It enables the investigation of electrode reaction which occurs in the proximity of electrode (Bard & Faulkner, 1980; Riger, 1993; Riley & Tomlinson, 1987). On the other hand the hysteresis of cyclic voltammety curves which is related to mass transport (one compounds is cumulated at the electrode during reduction scan which is reoxidized under oxidation scan) makes the evaluation of CV quite difficult and more or less dependent on the experience of evaluator. The improvement by the string does not work because of causing noise. However the improving of mass transport by thermo diffusion significantly improves the CV and facilitates its evaluation. The improvement can be seen in fig 13.

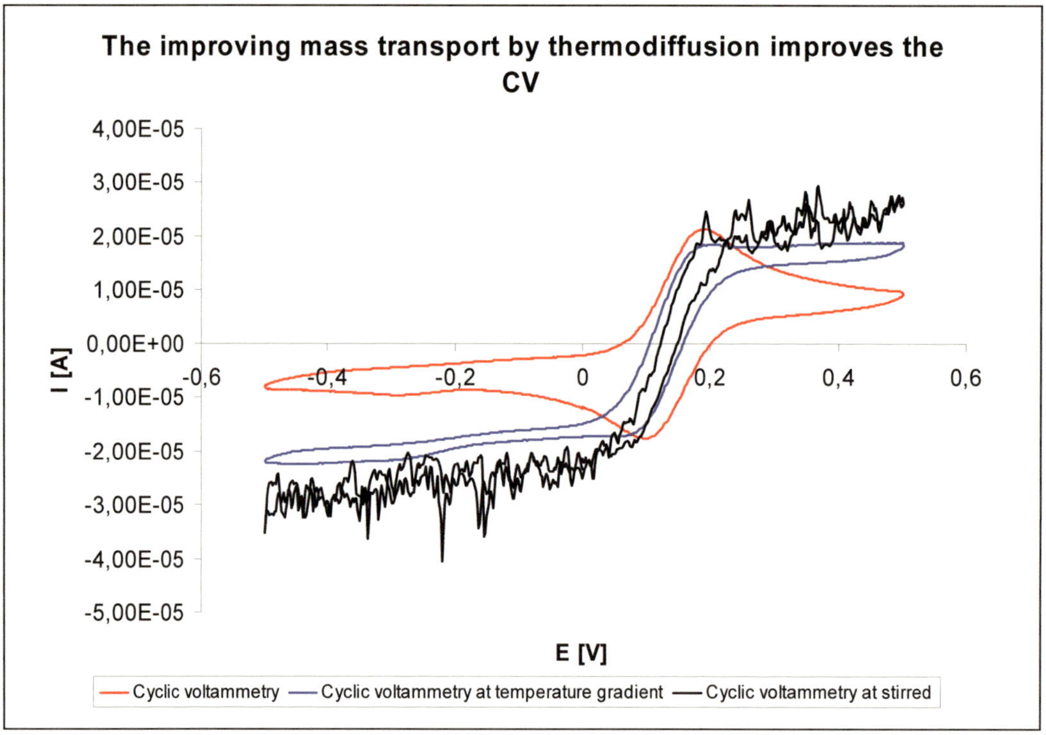

Fig. 13. The improving of mass transport by thermo diffusion

The samples of CV with thermo diffusion mass transport agree with equation (10) and it can be used to measurement of E_0 at given temperature. Due to high thermal conductivity of ceramic sensor base and precise temperature measurement using Pt 1000 thermometer integrated in the proximity of working electrode the dependence of $E_0(T)$ can be measured. The temperature difference about 10 - 40 °C significantly improves the mass transport and measured current.

3. Conclusion

The importance of mass transport has been discussed, namely with respect to screen printed electrodes. The technology of screen printing and more general application of microelectronic technologies open new area for electrochemical sensor application. However their effective use relies on a clear and comprehensive understanding of mass transport between electrode surface and bulk of solution. Advances with micro fluidics can significantly help, as demonstrated using the micro fluidic system (MFS) with wall-jet and thin layer micro fluidic arrangement. The classical arrangement of RDE can be miniaturized and produced at significantly lower cost. Consequently disposable RDE can be used as highly efficient tools for immobilized enzyme investigation, for optimization of the immobilization process and enzymatic membrane kinetic measurement as well as other parameters important for the immobilization process. Screen printing is a subset of Thick Film Technology used in microelectronics. This enables the integration not only of the sensor active electrodes but also heating elements and thermometers. Such complicated integrated sensors offer new possibility to improve mass transport form the bulk of solution to the active electrode surface. An example is thermo diffusion which may simplify the evaluation of CV. The importance of mass transport was discussed, namely with respect of screen printed electrodes. The technology of screen printing and more generally application of microelectronic technologies opens new area of electrochemical sensor application.

4. Acknowledgment

This work was supported by the EU 7th Framework Programme 230749, EU 7th Framework Programme 262007 and Czech Science Foundation KAN200520702. I would like to thank Mark O'Connell from Probe Scientific for help with English text.

5. References

Bard, A.J.; Faulkner, L.R. (1980). Electrochemical Methods-Fundamentals and Applications. John Wiley & Sons. New York. USA

Brunt K.; Bruins C.H.P. (1979). Evaluation of the characteristics of the differential amperometric detector in combination with anion-exchange chromatography, using l-ascorbic acid as test compound. Journal of Chromatografy A, Vol.172, Issue 1, pp. 37-47

Clark, L.C.; Lyons, C. (1962). Ann.N.Y. Acad.Sci., Vol.102, pp. 29-45.

Dock, E.; Christenson, A.; Sapelnikova, S.; Krejci, J.; Emnes, J.; Ruzgas, T. (2005). A steady-state and flow-through cell for screen-printed eight-electrode arrays. Analytica Chimica Acta, Vol. 531, pp. 165–172.

Dvořák, J.; Koryta, J. (1983). Elektrochemie. Academia, nakladatelství ČSAV, Praha

Frost and Sullivan. (1994). Technnical insights, A.D.Litlle in Transducer aspects of biosensors, Sethi, R.S., Biosensors and Bioelectronics 9, 243-264

Hanekamp H.B.; Nieuwkerk H.J. (1980). Anal. Chim., Acta 121, pp. 13-22. http://www.lorentzcenter.nl/lc/web/2008/317/presentations/Baltruchat.pdf

Chan, F.-L.; Chang,W.-Y.; Kuo, L.-M.; Lin, Ch.-H.; Wang, S.-W.; Yang,Y.-S.; Lu, M. S-C. (2008). IOP publishing journal of micromechanic and microengineering. Vol.18, No.12.

Karman, T. (1921); Uber laminare and turbulente Reibung. Zeitschrift fur angewandte Mathematik und Mechanik, Vol.1, No.4, pp. 233-252.

King, P.; Prasard,V. S. R. K.; Rao, G. H. (2005). Indian Journal of Chemical Technology, pp. 455-461.

Kotyk, A.; Horák, J. (1977) Enzymová kinetika. Academia, Praha

Krejci, J. (1988). Glucose sensor - Internal report. Research institute of medical engineering, Brno

Krejci, J.; Lacina, K.; Vránová, H.; Grosmanová, Z. (2008). Microflow Vessel Improvning Reproducibility and Sensitivity of Electrochemical measurements. Electroanalysis 20, No.23, pp. 2579-2586.

Krejci, J.; Sajdlová, Z.; Krejci, J., Jr.; Marvanek, T. (2010). Voltammetry under Controlled Temperature Gradient. Sensors, Vol.10, pp. 6821-6835.

Levich, V.G. (1962) Physicochemical Hydrodynamics. Prentice Hall, Inc. Englewood Cliffs, N.J.

Levich, V.G. (1947). Discuss. Faraday Soc. 1, Vol.37.

Levich, V.G. (1944). Acta Physicochem. USSR 19, Vol.113.

Levich, V.G. (1944). Acta Physicochem. USSR 19, Vol.117.

Levich, V.G. (1942). Acta Physicochem. USSR 17, Vol.257.

Levich, V.G. (1947). Disc. Faraday Soc. 1, Vo.37.

Macholán, L. (1991) Biocatalytic Membrane Electrodes in. Bioinstrumentation and Biosensors. Wise, L. D. (ed.); Dekker, M. New York-Basel-Honkong

Maly, J.; Krejci, J.; Ilie, M.; Jakubka, L.; Masojidek, J.; Pilloton, R.; Sameh, K.; Steffan, P.; Stryhal, Z.; Sugiura, M. (2005). Analytical and Bioanalytical Chemistry, Vol.381, pp. 1558-1567.

Masavať, P.; Liawruangrath, S. (2008). Chiang Mai J. Sci., Vol.35, pp. 355-369.

Matsuda H. (1967). J. Electroanal. Chem., Vol.15, pp. 325-336.

Matsuda H. (1967). J. Electroanal. Chem., Vol.15, pp. 109.

Mell, L.D.; Maloy, J.T. (1974). Anal. Chem., Vol.47, pp. 299-307.

Painton, C.C.; Mottola, H.A. (1983). Anal. Chim. Acta 154, pp. 1-16.

Polyanin, A.D.; Kutepov, A.M.; Vyazmin, A.V.; Kazenin, D.A. (2002). Hydrodynamics, Mass and Heat Transfer in Chemical Engineering. London and New York, Taylor & Francis

Riger, P.H. (1993). Electrochemistry. Chapman & Hall, New York

Riley, T.; Tomlinson, C. (1987) Principles of Electroanalytical Methods. New York: John Wiley & Sons

Sajdlová, Z. (2010). Ph.D. thesis, Elactrochemical detector with electrodes array and rotating disk

Sethi, R. S.; Gray Stephens, L. D.; Bruce, N. C.; Lowe, C. R.. An Improved Silicon Chip Based Biosensor in "Proc.Third International Meeting on Chemical Sensors" Cleveland, Ohio, USA, 116-117, 24/26 September (1990).

Sethi, R. S. Silicon Processing in the Fabrication of Biosensors. Semiconductor International, NEC, Birmingham, UK, 14-16 March (1989).

Todd M. Squires; Robert J. Messinger & Scott R. Manalis. (2008) Nature Biotechnology

Tóth, K.; Štulík, K.; Kutner, W.; Fehér, Z.; Lindner, E. (2004). Pure Appl. Chem., Vol.76, No.6, pp. 1119-1138

Turner, A.P.F.; Karube, I.; Wilson, G. S. (1987) eds.: "Biosensors: Fundamentals and Applications", Oxford Press, Oxford

Updike, S.J.; Hicks, G. P. (1986). The Enzyme Electrode. Nature 214, pp. 986-988

Wranglén G.; Nilsson O. (1962). Electro chim., Acta 7, pp. 121-137.

Yamada J.; Matsuda H. (1973). J. Electroanal. Chem., Acta 44, pp. 189-198.

15

CMOS, Delta-Sigma pH-to-Digital Converter as New Integrated Device for Potentiometric Biosensors Applications

Chung-Yuan Chen[1], Tai-Ping Sun[2] and Hsiu-Li Hsieh[2]
[1]*Sitronix Technology, Hsinchu County,*
[2]*National Chi Nan University, Nantou Hsien Country,*
Taiwan

1. Introduction

The explosive growth in the healthcare and lifestyle application has fueled recent research efforts to increase both integration and adaptability in biosensor readout design. Potentiometric sensor is emerging as important sensing devices in the areas of biomedical applications since the pioneer work on pH sensor has been introduced (Bergveld, 1970). It has appreciable advantages over traditional glass-electrode sensors on the basis of its small size, robustness, simplicity in fabrication and low cost (Yin et al., 1999). Moreover, many research works have exploited different circuit architectures of readout circuits, which usually play the role in translating the values to voltage domain presentation, with the goal to obtain good sensitivity as well as linearity (Chan et al., 2007). However, the conventional readout circuitry of pH sensor comprises multiple chips and discrete components which are fabricated in different technologies. The goal of this research is to propose a novel pH sensor readout circuitry onto a single chip in standard CMOS technology. Such fully integrated solution results in pH sensor readout devices with lower cost and higher performance.

New architectures and circuit techniques need to be explored in the design of fully integrated potentiometric sensor readout circuit. The wide dynamic range and low power are necessitated by the elimination of discrete high Q filters in traditional potentiometric sensor readout channel. In addition, readout circuits need to adapt to the different dynamic range, linearity, and signal bandwidth requirements of multiple potentiometric sensors. This programmability can be easily achieved by performing signal processing in the digital domain. Moreover, the reliability of signal processing in digital form can readily permit sensor systems to combine with other instruments.

In moving the signal response of pH sensor to the digital domain, a high dynamic range, low power analog-to-digital converter (ADC) is needed to quantize a small desired signal. Delta-sigma modulators are uniquely suited to this application because the high pass shaped quantization noise falls into the same band as the environment noise (Kuo et al., 2001). This implies that a single programmable digital decimation filter following the delta-sigma analog-to-digital modulator can attenuate both the quantization and environment noise.

2. Delta-Sigma pH-to-digital converter

The delta-sigma modulator is an attractive candidate for the sensor applications due to its robust capability to process variations and high-resolution performance (Lemkin et al., 1999). Furthermore, delta-sigma modulator can trade time for improvements of the resolution and signal to noise ratio.

Direct sensor signal-to-digital converter provides digital output without the need for its intermediate processing circuit. Direct capacitance-to-digital converters (Petkov et al., 2005) and magnetic-to-digital converters (Kuo et al., 2001), based on the principles of the delta-sigma technique, are suitable for sensors signal processing. In this study, direct pH-to-digital converter based on delta-sigma modulator in fully integrated pH sensor readout circuitry is proposed.

2.1 Conventional pH sensor readout system

The sensor readout system shown in Fig. 1 is the conventional approach to pH sensor receiver architecture. With high Q off-chip filters (shaded in Fig. 1), this conventional architecture is not amenable to a highly integrated solution. The off chip filters also must be specific to a particular sensor.

Consider the propagation of a desired pH sensor signal through the readout path as shown in the frequency plan. The pH sensor signal at the sensing membrane passes through an off-chip filter and is amplified by the pre-amplifier or low-noise amplifier (LNA). Amplification of the pH sensor signal is required to achieve adequate sensitivity by reducing the noise contributions of environment noise in the receive path. After the pre-amplifier or LNA, the sensor signal goes off-chip through the filter. The combination of the pH sensor signal and filters rejects environment noise which is out off pH sensor signal bandwidth that must be attenuated prior to offset cancellation circuit. The offset cancellation circuit is constructed by a digital-to-analog converter and a differential amplifier with low gain. The general correction method used in readout channel is successive approximation. The variable gain amplifier (VGA) is used to reduce the dynamic range (DR) requirement of subsequent stages. The most important design factor of variable gain amplifier is the total harmonic distortion (THD). The variable gain amplifier must amplify the sensor signal without distortion. Finally, anti-aliasing and analog-to-digital conversion (ADC) are performed. ADC is required so that output bits can be recovered in the digital domain. The filter can be performed in the analog domain using either continuous time or discrete time (switched-capacitor) filters or in the digital domain. The choice of analog or digital selection impacts the dynamic range requirements of the ADC and the programmability of the sensor readout system.

Analog filter in front of the ADC must band-limit the incoming signal with enough stop band rejection to remove the environment noise prior to sampling by the ADC. In alternate way, the ADC must oversample enough so that the environment noise does not alias into the desired frequency band and can be removed by a subsequent digital filter. Thus, from the ADC design view, the bandwidth selection of sensor signal reduces to providing adequate anti-aliasing in either the analog or digital domain. The analog filter must have enough dynamic range and linearity to select the desired bandwidth in the presence of pH sensor signal. Since all bandwidth select filtering is performed prior to the ADC, only a low resolution ADC with enough bandwidth to digitize the desired bandwidth is required. One implementation of the pass band processing block would employ a continuous time low pass analog filter in front of the ADC. This filter would be implemented by switched-capacitor technology since the pH sensor signal is DC-like signal. Linearity considerations dictate the signal-handling capability of the filter. Moreover, bandwidth selection can be performed in the digital domain using an oversampled delta-sigma modulator followed by a digital decimation filter.

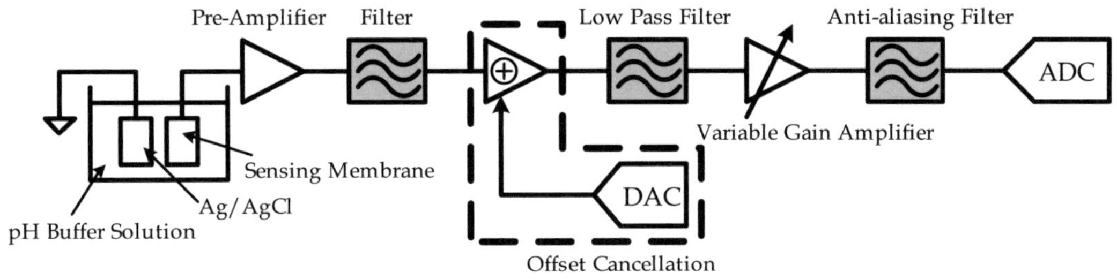

Fig. 1. Block diagram of conventional pH sensor readout circuit

2.2 EGFET-operational amplifier

Ion sensitive field effect transistors (ISFETs) are emerging as important sensing devices in the areas of environmental monitoring applications and biomedical applications (Bergveld, 1970). The ISFET used as a pH sensor is an integrated device composed of a conventional ion selective membrane and a metal oxide semiconductor field effect transistor (MOSFET). Extended gate field effect transistor (EGFET) is another structure to isolate field effect transistor (FET) from chemical environment, in which a sensitive membrane is fabricated on the end of the signal line extended from the gate electrode of FET (Spiegel et al., 1983). EGFET has advantages over ISFET such as low cost, simple structure and ease to package (Chin et al., 2001). Behavior of surface ion adsorption effect of the ISFET and EGFET are the same (Chou et al., 2009). The much difference between ISFET and EGFET is the impedance of sensing film. The gate electrode of EGFET must be high conductivity material to be a sensing electrode that can transmit sensing signals easily.

The EGFET can be represented by a model as depicted in Fig. 2. It consists of a chemical part and an MOS transistor part. In chemical part, two series capacitances and represent the equivalent Gouy-Chapman and Helmholtz capacitance (Grattarola et al., 1992), which has been developed by site-binding model and the electrical double-layer theory (Fung et al., 1986). Two voltage sources and are connected in series to denote the voltage components of chemical threshold voltage of EGFET. The chemical threshold voltage consists of two potentials $-\Psi_{eo}+\chi^{sol}$, χ^{sol} in which is a constant with respect to the pH value, and Ψ_{eo} is the only chemical parameter that is responsible for pH sensitivity of EGFET. χ^{sol}, with a typical value of 50 mV, is the surface dipole potential of the solvent being independent of pH (Chan et al., 2007). The sensitivity of Ψ_{eo} , which is defined as the change of Ψ_{eo} with respect to a change of the pH value of the solution $\Delta\Psi_{eo}/\Delta pH$, has already been explained by the Hal and Eijkel's theory (Van Hal et al., 1995). This is elaborated by using the general accepted site-binding model and the Gouy-Chapman-Stern model to yield on:

$$\frac{\Delta\psi_{eo}}{\Delta pH} = -2.303 \cdot \frac{KT}{q} \cdot \alpha \tag{1}$$

where K is the Boltzmann constant, T is the absolute temperature, q is the magnitude of the electron charge, α is a dimensionless sensitivity parameter, with the value ranging between 0 and 1.

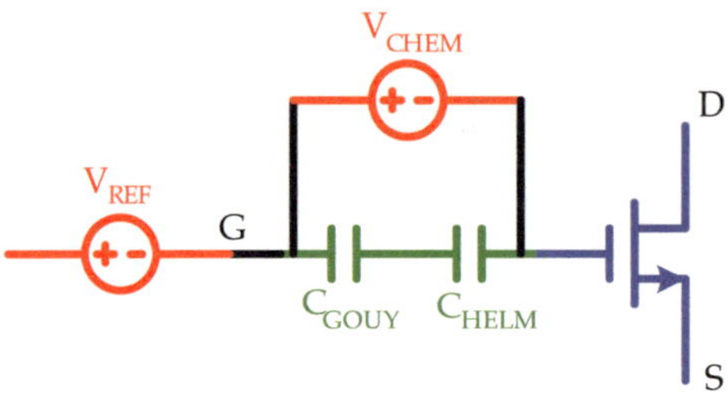

Fig. 2. EGFET modeling components

The other physical constants have their usual meanings. Therefore, the voltage source becomes:

$$V_{CHEM} = 2.303\frac{KT}{q}\alpha \cdot pH + (\chi^{sol} - C) \tag{2}$$

where the first term is pH-dependent and the constant terms in the parentheses are pH-independent.
Like the standard MOSFET, for a long-channel EGFET operating in a saturation region, the drain current can be expressed as

$$I_{DS} = \frac{1}{2}\frac{W}{L}\mu C_{OX}\left(V_{GS} - V_{TH(EGFET)}\right)^2 \tag{3}$$

where μC_{ox} is the process transconductance parameter, W/L is the aspect ratio. Moreover, the EGFET threshold voltage combined with the MOS transistor counterpart which includes body effect in a four-terminal device can be unified as

$$V_{TH(EGFET)} = V_{CHEM} + V_{TH} \tag{4}$$

where V_{TH} is the threshold voltage of the MOS transistor.
As this potential is pH-independent, it can be viewed as a common-mode input signal for an EGFET interface circuit in any pH buffer solution and can be nullified during system calibration and measurement procedures. The SnO_2/ITO glass, fabricated by sputtering SnO_2 on the conductive ITO glass, was used as a pH-sensitive membrane of EGFET-operational amplifier. The SnO_2 thin films were formed by the radio frequency sputtering system at a substrate temperature of 150°C. Mixed sputtering gases included O_2 and Ar. Thickness of the SnO_2 thin film was about 2000 Å. The ITO glasses were supplied by the Wintek corporation. The coating thickness of ITO was about 230 Å. The sheet resistance of ITO is 50-100 Ω/□. The conducting line was bound from the ITO layer and packaged by epoxy after the thin film was deposited. The commercial buffer solutions were used as the test solutions. The micro slide glass and corning 7059 glass were purchased from Kimax Glass Instrument and Tekstarter corporation. The deposition parameters are summarized as follows:

1. Deposition rate is 20 Å/s.
2. Deposition pressure is 20 e-3 Torr.
3. Background pressure is 2×e-6 Torr.
4. The Ar/O_2 ratio is 4:1.
5. Substrate temperature is 150°C.

The fabrication processes of sensing structure were summarized as follows and its cross-section is shown in Fig. 3.

1. Clean the silicon substrate.
2. SnO_2 was deposited on ITO about 3000Å by sputtering method.
3. Bounding and packaging by epoxy.

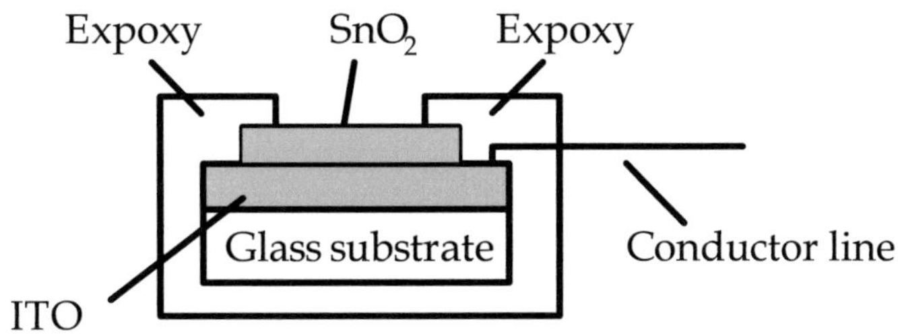

Fig. 3. Cross-section of SnO2/ITO glass sensing membrane

The operation of the extended-gate field effect transistor is very similar to that of a conventional MOS, except that an additional sensing structure is dipped in the buffer solution. In the study of pH sensitivity of the SnO_2/ITO glass, the SnO_2/ITO glass sensing membrane was connected to an instrumentation amplifier (Yin et al., 2000). The instrumentation amplifier was used to measure output response of the SnO_2/ITO glass in the pH buffer solutions, and the result shows that the sensing membrane, SnO_2/ITO glass, has a linear pH sensitivity of approximately 59.3mV/pH in the ion concentration ranging between pH 2 and 10. To evaluate the hysteresis characteristic of the SnO_2/ITO glass sensing membrane, we measured the output offset voltage after solution change such as pH7→pH4→pH7 and pH 7→pH10→pH7. The results show that the hysteresis of the SnO_2/ITO glass sensing membrane is about 4.2mV. For the sensor signal measurement, we need an interface circuit that tracks the threshold voltage (or the flat-band voltage) of the EGFET as the electrolyte pH is varied. A more practical solution to monitor the sensor signal with electronics is to view the EGFET as a circuit component in an integrated circuit rather than as an add-on sensor whose output signal is further processed. In this work, we adapt the EGFET-operational amplifier approach of utilizing the EGFET as one of the input transistors in the differential stage of an operational amplifier shown as in Fig. 4.

Circuit functions of the EGFET-operational amplifier as follows: when the EGFET-operational amplifier is configured as a voltage follower (β=1), the output voltage is equal to the input voltage; any difference in threshold voltages and bias currents between the two input transistors at the differential input stage will also appear at the output. Writing out the terms of the threshold voltages of the MOSFET and the EGFET explicitly, the output of the EGFET-operational amplifier is as followings:

$$V_{OUT} = \Delta V_{TH} = V_{CHEM} \quad (5)$$

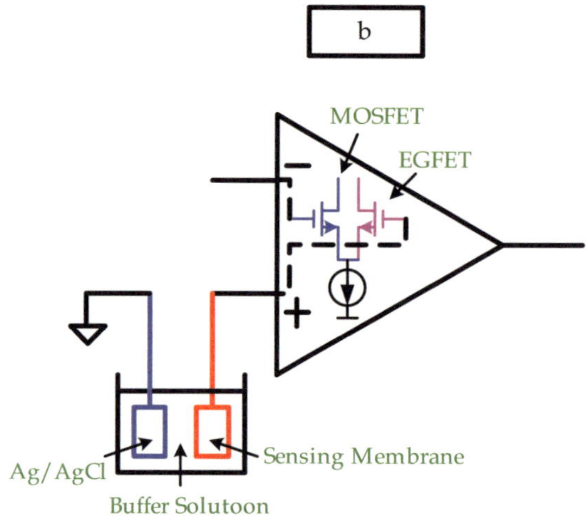

Fig. 4. Block diagram of the EGFET modeling components

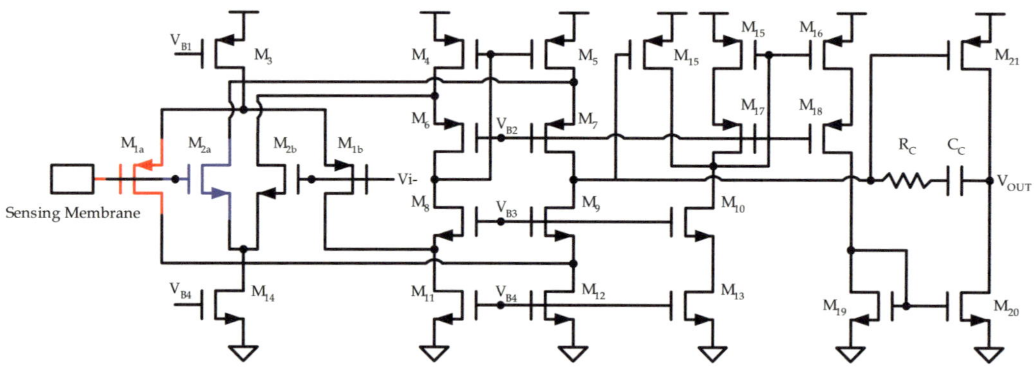

Fig. 5. EGFET operational amplifier

For the realization of pH sensor readout systems, low power and high dynamic range interface circuits are indispensable building blocks. EGFET operational amplifier shown in Fig. 5 is investigated to track the output response caused by the H^+ ion concentration. To improve the input dynamic range, the n-p complementary EGFETs differential stage was adopted as the input stage of the EGFET operational amplifier. The EGFETs were biased in the suitable operating point by the reference electrode. It is important to keep the total transconductance variation small if n-p complementary differential input stage of the amplifier was adopted. The gain of the amplifier used in the negative feedback must be large enough to keep the transconductance variation small instead of adding compensation structure. For this purpose, the voltage gain of the amplifier was chosen to be higher than 75 dB for 12-bits application. The first stage of the EGFET-operational amplifier is a folded cascode structure which provides most of the overall DC gain. The second stage is a slew rate enhancement circuit to provide a high driving capability. The output stage senses the PMOS driver current of the first stage and subtracts this current from a reference current source M_{13}. The difference is then mirrored to the NMOS output device M_{20}. Thus, the output stage works in a push-pull fashion and results in significantly improved slew rate performance. This output stage must be able to drive loads up to 2pF for the discrete time pH-to-digital converter application. Moreover, the MOSFETs of the EGFET-operational amplifier were integrated in one process to enable a more stable operation. A nulling resistor R_C in series with the compensation capacitor C_C was inserted to move the right half-plane zero into the left half-plane to improve the phase margin of the amplifier.

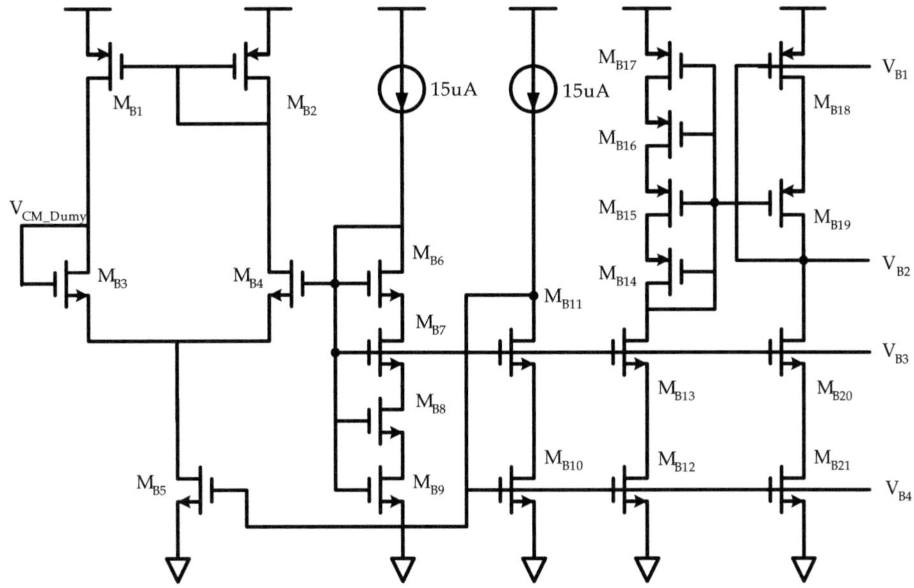

Fig. 6. Bias network for EGFET operational amplifier

Fig. 6 shows the biasing scheme for the prototype chip. High-swing cascade biasing circuit is generated by stacking a number of triode-region devices. The PMOS portion of the biasing is slaved off the NMOS portion for better matching and tolerance toward process shifts. To provide good isolation between circuits on the chip, the EGFET operational amplifier (where performance is the most critical) has its own bias network while the other three amplifiers designed for reference regulator share another bias network. The master bias currents shown in Fig. 6 are generated on chip by mirroring the current from an external master current source, as shown in Fig. 7. The master bias is distributed to local bias networks as a current so that IR drops in routing do not affect the biasing.

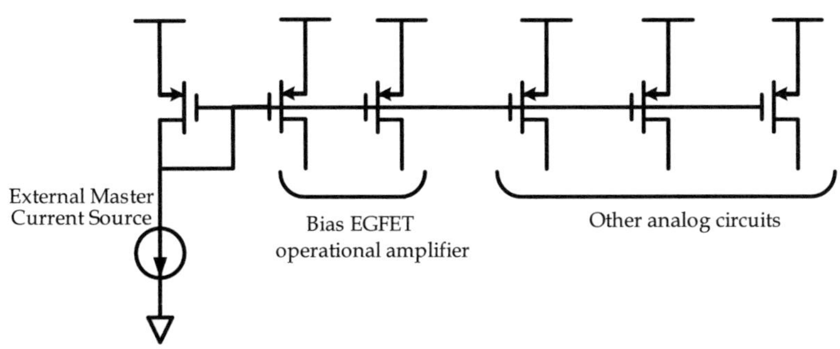

Fig. 7. Master bias circuit

2.3 Direct pH-to-digital converter

Delta-sigma analog-to-digital converter is another important sensor readout technology. Modern sensor instrumentation systems become favorable in digital form due to its excellent user interface and anti-noise performance (Ezekwe et al., 2008). Moreover, digital signal processing can readily permit sensor systems to combine with other instruments. Delta-sigma converters achieve high resolution by transferring the quantization noise into high frequency and removing it with a digital filter. Fig. 8 shows the block diagram of a delta-sigma analog-to-digital modulator.

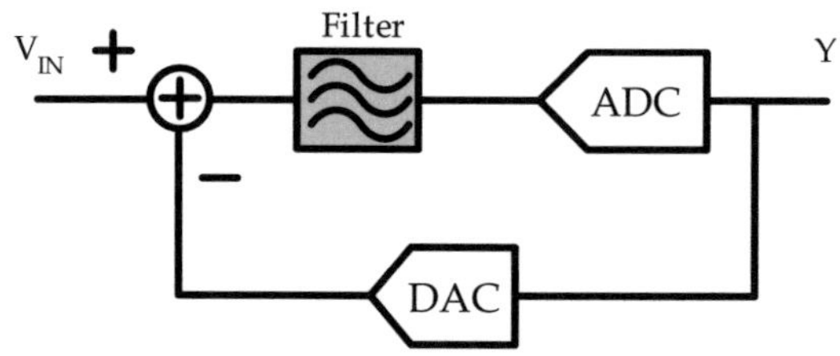

Fig. 8. Block diagram of delta-sigma analog-to-digital modulator

Intuitively, the negative feedback loop causes the output of the DAC to on average equal the input voltage V_{IN} (Ezekwe et al., 2008). Therefore the output bits of the ADC are a rough, low frequency representation of the analog input V_{IN}. If the signal bandwidth is sufficiently smaller than the sampling frequency then the high frequency quantization noise can then be digitally separated and removed with a low pass filter to yield the final digital output signal Y. The transfer function from V_{IN} to Y is a pure delay. If the quantizer is modeled as white quantization noise, the converter can be treated as a linear system. Now the transfer function of the quantization noise Q to the output Y is a high-pass (Boser et al., 1988). Thus the quantization noise at low-frequencies is suppressed as shown in Fig. 9. The remaining high-frequency quantization noise can then be removed with the digital low-pass filter. From equation (6), the power of quantization noise is independent of the sampling rate. And the quantization noise power in oversampled converters is the same as that for Nyquist rate converters, but is now distributed over a wider band (Norsworthy et al., 1997).

$$P_{Q,Oversampled} = \int_{-f_{BW}}^{f_{BW}} \frac{\Delta^2}{12} \cdot \frac{1}{f_S} df = \frac{P_{Q,Nyquist}}{\frac{f_S}{2f_{BW}}} = \frac{P_{Q,Nyquist}}{M} \tag{6}$$

where oversampling ratio, $M = f_S / 2f_{BW}$

Increasing the sampling rate therefore reduces the quantization noise power by a fraction M, which is the oversampling ratio. Let $Z=e^{jwT}=e^{jw/fs}$ and rewrite the noise transfer function as following (Johns et al., 1997)

$$N_{TF}(f) = 1\text{-}e^{-jw/f_S} = \sin\left(\frac{\pi f}{f_S}\right) \cdot 2j \cdot e^{-j\pi f/f_S} \tag{7}$$

Assuming the maximum signal power is the same as the quantization noise of Nyquist rate converters, the maximum SNR for the first order sigma-delta modulator is given by

$$SNR_{MAX} = 6.02N + 1.76 - 5.17 + 30\log(M) \tag{8}$$

The benefits increase as the sampling rate is increased relative to the input signal bandwidth. The ideal output SNR increases 9dB per octave in oversampling ratio (Johns et al., 1997). Thus, delta-sigma converters can achieve very high resolution for small signal bandwidths, such as bio-sensor and audio applications. By using a high oversampling ratio, an inherently linear, single-bit quantizer can be used which is beneficial because it does not require any precision, matched components. Finally a high oversampling ratio is also an advantage because it relaxes the roll-off characteristics of the anti-alias filter preceding the ADC. Furthermore, more integrators may be added to increase the noise-shaping characteristics of the system. This dramatically reduces the in-band quantization noise. Adding too many integrators, however, introduces loop stability problems. Delta-sigma applications usually make heavy use of switched-capacitor circuits. Switched-capacitor integrators usually used in the forward path, and switched capacitor comparators and DACs are also used in the loop. It is the settling time of the integrators, however, that typically limits the sampling rate of the system.
By oversampling the input and then averaging the output, we can predict the input signal. The signal transfer function, $S_{TF}(Z)$, and noise transfer function, $N_{TF}(Z)$, can be derived as following (Norsworthy et al., 1997)

$$S_{TF}(Z) = \frac{Y(Z)}{V_{IN}(Z)} = \frac{H(Z)}{1+H(Z)} \tag{9}$$

$$N_{TF}(Z) = \frac{Y(Z)}{E(Z)} = \frac{1}{1+H(Z)} \tag{10}$$

where $H(z)=1/(Z-1)$
The output signal function can be derived by the combination of the input signal and the noise signal. The transfer function is given by

$$Y(Z) = S_{TF}(Z) \cdot V_{IN}(Z) + N_{TF}(Z) \cdot E(Z) \tag{11}$$

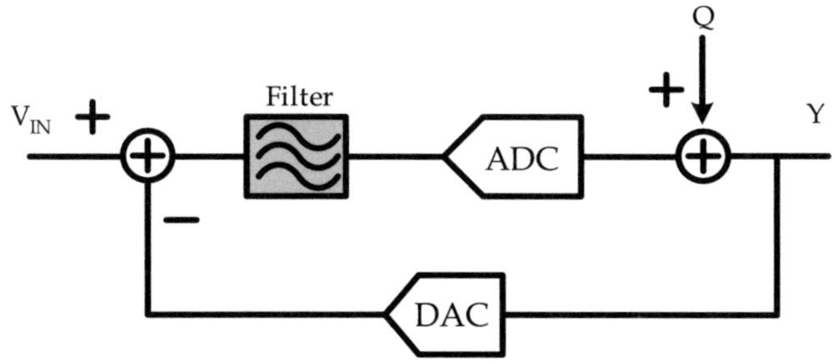

Fig. 9. Quantization noise model

The signal transfer function is simply a delay. Since the transfer function from the quantization error source to the output is given by $(1-Z^{-1})$ the noise is shaped by a high-pass characteristic. The switched-capacitor (SC) technique is used to realize the first-order delta-sigma modulator. A first-order modulator where a 1-bit quantizer is used in the feedback loop is shown in Fig. 10. The delta-sigma modulator consists of both analog and digital circuitry. The integrator of delta-sigma modulator needs a two-phase non-overlapping clock (with delays) to minimize signal-dependent charge-injection errors. Shown in Fig. 11 is the waveform of the two-phase clock. Φ1d are the delayed versions of Φ1. The rising edges of the delayed clocks should be lined up with the rising edges of the non-delayed versions to increase the amount of available settling time for the integrator. A simple dynamic comparator shown in Fig. 12 is used to perform a single bit conversion.

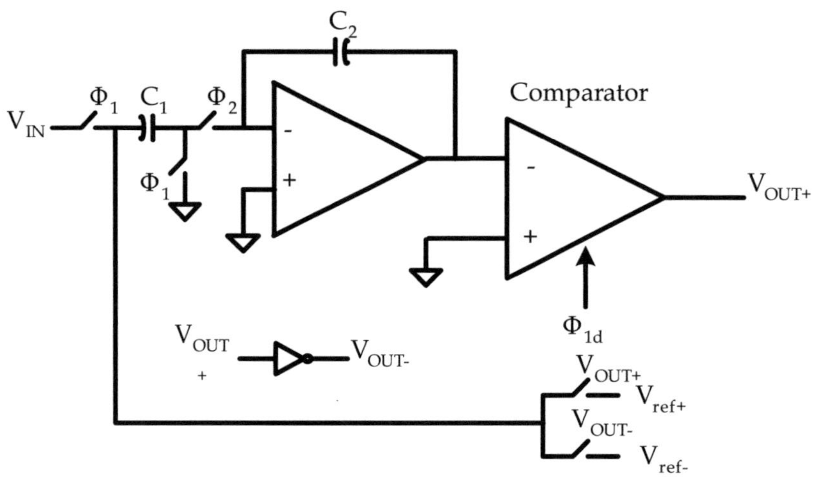

Fig. 10. First-order delta-sigma modulator

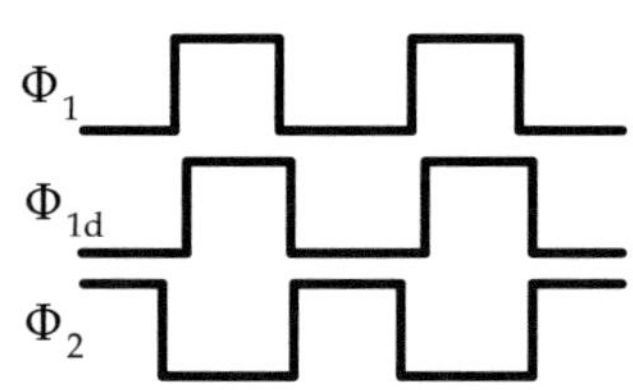

Fig. 11. Clock timing for the first time delta-sigma modulator

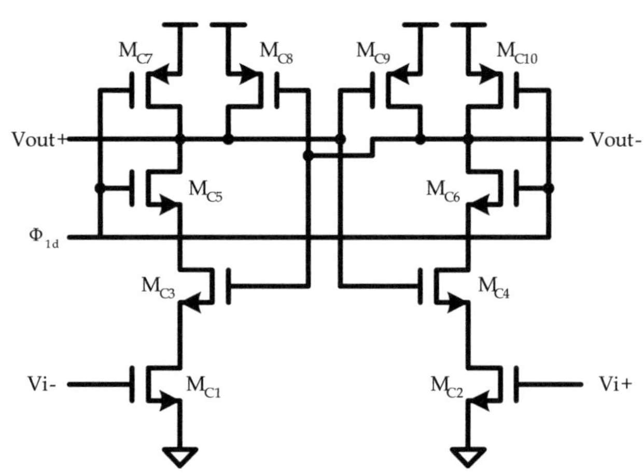

Fig. 12. Dynamic comparator circuit

The dynamic comparator in Fig. 12 is simplified to perform a comparison with zero standby current (Kuo et al., 2001). The differential signal varies the resistance of triode region devices M_{C1} and M_{C2}. When the latch signal (Φ_{1d}) is low, the comparator output is pre-charged to positive power by devices M_{C7} and M_{C10}. On the rising edge of the latch signal, the outputs of the cross-coupled inverters formed by M_{C3}, M_{C4}, M_{C7} and M_{C8} flip in the appropriate direction based on the differential resistance of the triode region input devices.

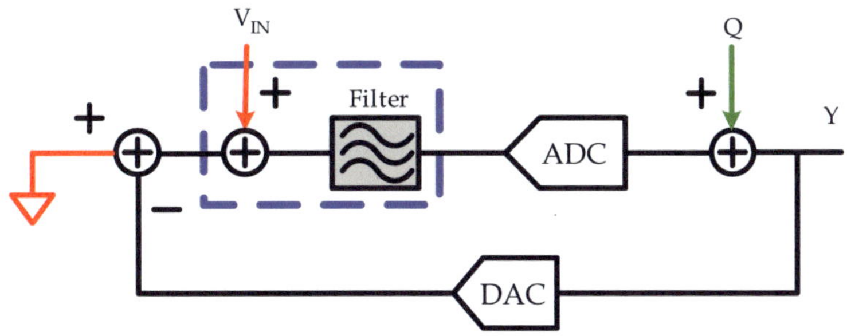

Fig. 13. Modified delta-sigma modulator

Adding analog ground in the input stage of the delta-sigma modulator will not affect the behavior function of original delta-sigma modulator. Redrawing the linear model shown in Fig. 13, we can transfer the location of the input signal into the filter block without changing the system behavior. The redrawing block diagram is shown in Fig. 14. Integrator can be used to replace the filter if the behavior of filter type is low pass filter. In other words, we can implant a direct pH-to-digital modulator based on delta-sigma technology if we can design an integrator and its output is dependent on the pH value. The direct pH-to-digital modulator is shown in Fig. 15. Following the modulator, a simple digital low pass filter can be used to remove the quantization and environment noise. For integrated pH sensor, the extended-gate field effect transistor (EGFET) operational amplifier was investigated to track the threshold voltage of the EGFET. The sensing part used in EGFET operational amplifier (EGFET-OP) is SnO_2/ITO glass. The commercial buffer solutions were used as the test solutions. First order switched capacitor low pass delta-sigma modulator constructed using EGFET-OP, shown in Fig. 15, was used to transfer the pH signal into digital. The H^+-ion induced voltage V_{pH} can be regarded as the voltage difference between two input nodes of the EGFET-OP in the switched-capacitor integrator.

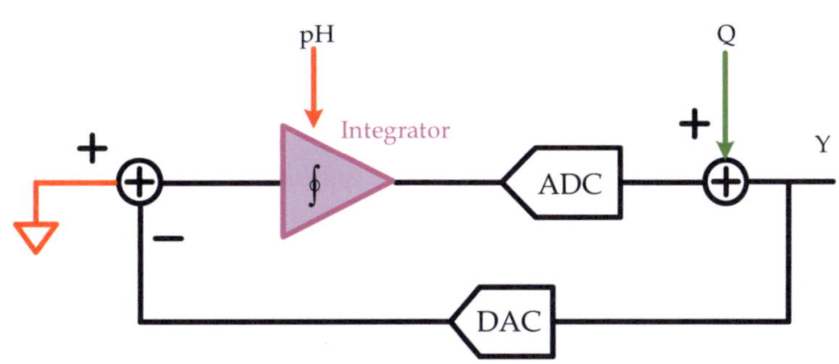

Fig. 14. Direct pH-to-digital modulator

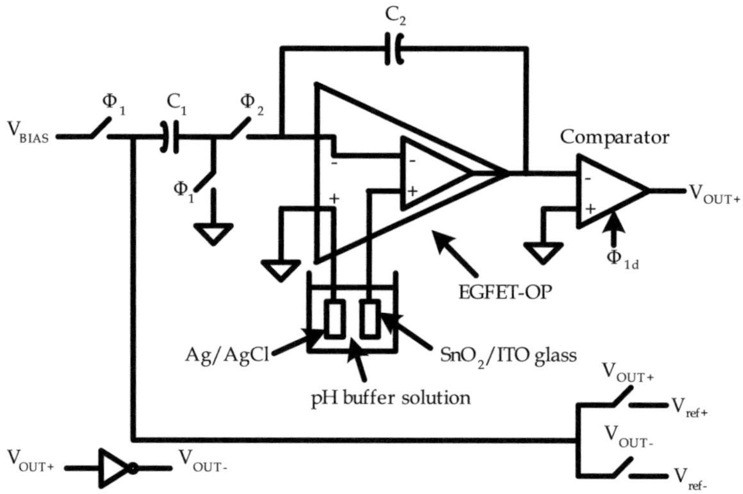

Fig. 15. Implementation of the pH-to-digital modulator

The transfer function of the pH-to-digital converter can be derived as follows:

$$Y = \left(1 + \frac{C_1}{C_2}\right) \cdot V_{pH} + \frac{1 - z^{-1}}{1 + \left(\frac{C_1}{C_2} - 1\right) z^{-1}} \cdot E \tag{12}$$

where Y denotes the average digital output of the quantizer, and E indicates the quantization noise. When choosing $C_1 = C_2$, the expression will be simplified to:

$$Y = 2 \cdot V_{pH} + (1 - z^{-1}) \cdot E \tag{13}$$

Furthermore, the quantization noise is first-order shaped as expected. Through an on-chip simple digital filter realized by 14-bits up-down counter, the digital average value of the comparator was obtained after shifting the bits of the output code depending on the sampled numbers. The high frequency quantization noise was filtered out. The general regenerative latch comparator shown in Fig. 12 was employed as the quantizer in the delta-sigma modulator.

The direct pH-to-digital converter derived is used to measure the pH response. The chip has been encapsulated in a standard dual inline package. The sensing art has been exposed to test solutions in the ion concentration range between pH 2 and 12. The measurements were performed under a 1.8V power supply, and the sampling frequency of the converter was 6.25 MHz. Through an on-chip simple digital filter realized by 14-bits up-down counter, the digital average value of the comparator was obtained after shifting the bits of the output code depending on the sampled numbers. Layout microphotograph of the pH-to-digital converter circuit is shown in Fig. 16. The circuit (without pad) occupied an area of 0.66mm × 0.43mm. The input range of the delta-sigma modulator is 1.2V since the positive and negative reference voltages of the delta-sigma modulator are 0.3V and 1.5V, respectively. The sensitivity of the pH-to-digital converter is 197 digital counts/pH. The plot of the digital output versus pH value is shown in Fig. 17. Deviation between measured points and the linear regression line of sensitivity shown in Fig. 18 is under ±0.02pH. The performance of this pH-to-digital converter was summarized in Table 1.

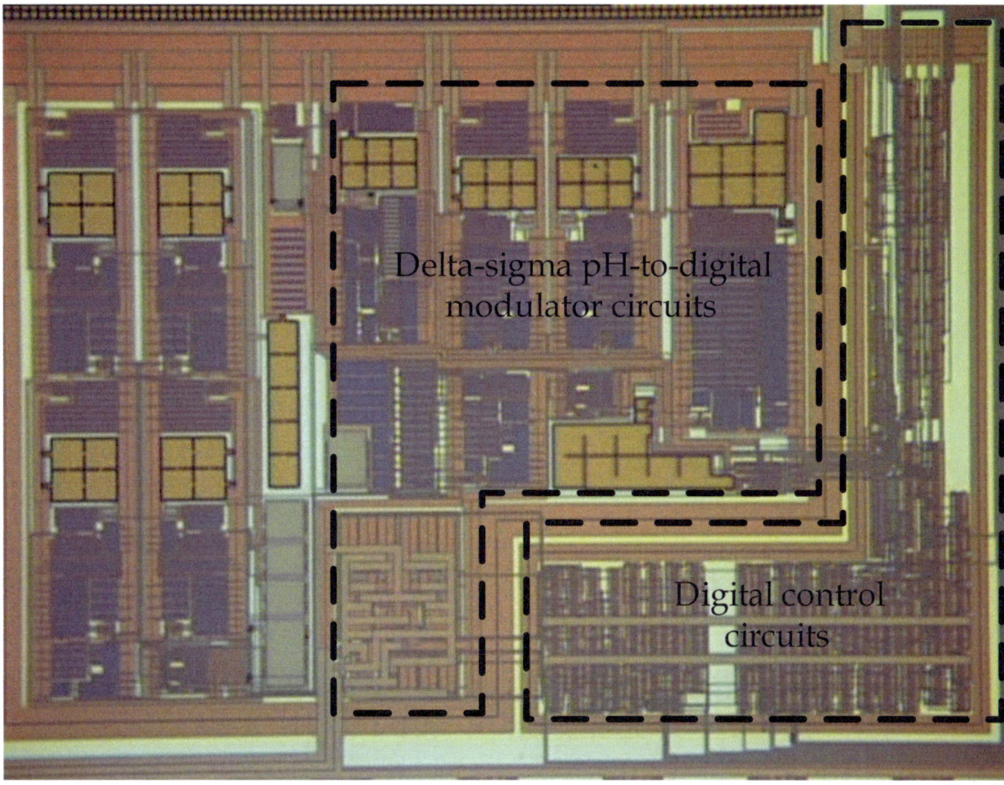

Fig. 16. Layout microphotograph of the pH-to-digital converter circuit

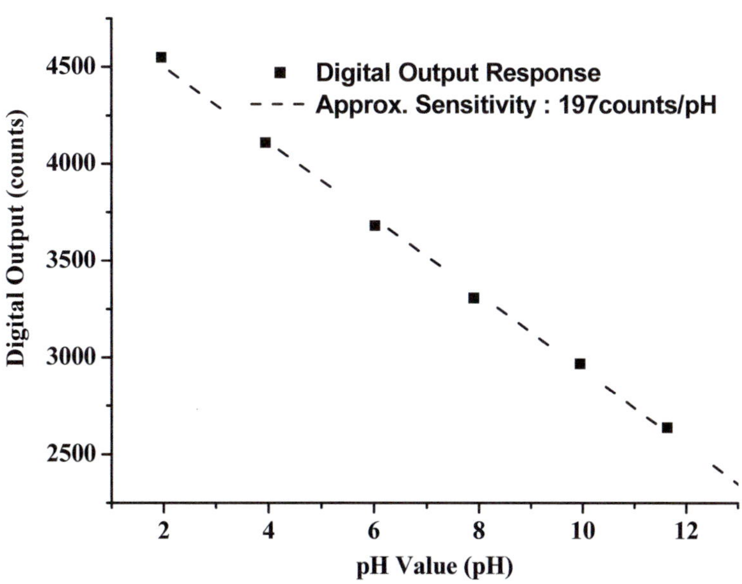

Fig. 17. Plot of the digital output versus pH value

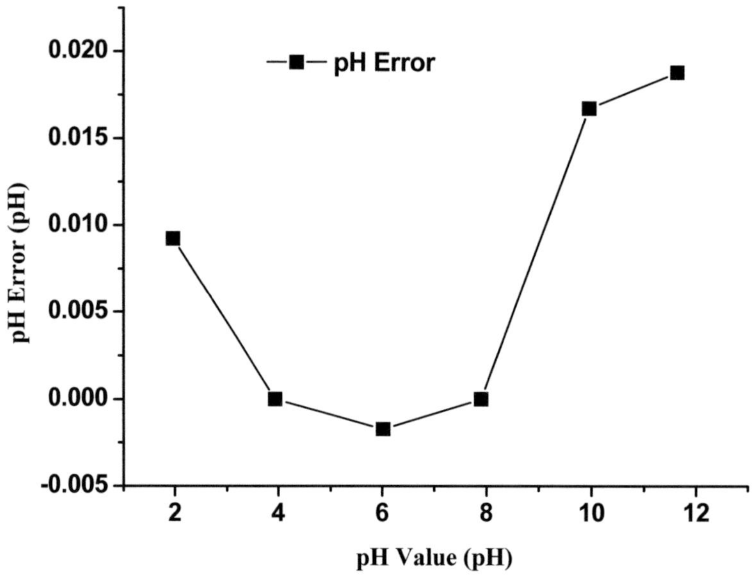

Fig. 18. pH error of the proposed pH-to-digital converter

Parameter	pH-to-Digital Converter
Supply Voltage	1.8V
Power Consumption	9.8mW
Dynamic Range	pH2 - pH12
Sensitivity	197 digital counts/pH
Gain Error	2%
pH Error	±0.02pH
Sampling Frequency	6.25MHz

Table 1. Performance summary

3. Conclusion

A CMOS ΣΔ pH-to-digital converter has been developed for continuous monitoring of H^+-ion concentrations in this research. The ΣΔ pH-to-digital converter, constructed using EGFET-OP to realize switched-capacitor (SC) ΣΔ converter, converted directly the H^+-ion concentration into digital form. First order low pass ΣΔ modulator constructed using EGFET-OP was used to transfer the signal into digital. Through an on-chip simple digital filter realized by 14-bits up-down counter, the digital average value of the comparator was obtained after shifting the bits of the output code depending on the sampled numbers. The high frequency quantization noise was filtered out. The circuit (without pad) occupied an area of 0.66mm × 0.43mm. The sensitivity of the pH-to-digital converter is about 197 digital counts/pH. This chip, fabricated in a 0.18-um CMOS 1P6M process, operated at a 1.8V supply voltage and normal sampling rate of 6.25MHz. The linearity errors of the converter in the H^+-ion concentration range between pH 2 and pH 10 is less than 2%, and the minimum detectable pH value can reach as small as ±0.02pH.

4. Acknowledgment

The authors would like to thank the Sitronix Technology and Chip Implementation Center (CIC) of the National Science Council, Taiwan, for fabricating the chips.

5. References

Bergveld, P. (1970). Development of an Ion-Sensitive Solid-State Device for Neurophysiological Measurements. *IEEE Transactions on Biomedical Engineering*, Vol. 17, No. 1, (January 1970), pp. 70-71, ISSN 0018-9294

Yin, L. T.; Chou, J. C.; Chung, W. Y.; Sun, T. P., & Hsing, S. K. (2000). Separate Structure Extended Gate H^+-Ion Sensitive Field Effect Transistor on a Glass Substrate. *Sensors and Actuators B*, Vol. 71, (November 2000), pp. 106-111, ISSN 0925-4005

Chan, P. K. & Chen, D. Y. (2007). A CMOS ISFET Interface Circuit with Dynamic Current Temperature Compensation Technique. *IEEE Transactions on Circuits System I*, Vol. 54, (January 2007), pp. 119-129, ISSN 1057-7122

Kuo, C. H.; Wu, Chen, S. L.; Ho, L. A., & Liu, S. I. (2001). CMOS Oversampling Magnetic to Digital Converters. *IEEE Journal of Solid-State Circuits*, Vol. 36, (October 2001), pp. 1582-1586, ISSN 0018-9200

Lemkin, M. & Boser, B. E. (1999). A Three-Axis Micromachined Accelerometer with a CMOS Position-Sense Interface and Digital Offset-Trim Electronics. *IEEE Journal of Solid-State Circuits*, Vol. 34, (April 1999), pp. 456-468, ISSN 0018-9200

Petkov, V. P. & Boser, B. E. (2005). A Fourth-Order ΣΔ Interface for Micromachined Inertial Sensors. *IEEE Journal of Solid-State Circuits*, Vol. 40, (August 2005), pp. 1602-1609, ISSN 0018-9200

Spiegel, J. V. D.; Lauks, I.; Chan, P., & Babic D. (1983). The Extended Gate Chemical Sensitive Field Effect Transistor as Multi-Species Microprobe. *Sensors and Actuators*, Vol. 4, (October 1983), pp. 291-298, ISSN 0250-6874

Chin, Y. L.; Chou, J. C.; Chung, W. Y.; Sun, T. P., & Hsing, S. K. (2001). A Novel SnO_2/Al Discrete Gate ISFET pH Sensor with CMOS Standard Process. *Sensors and Actuators B*, Vol. 75, (April 2001), pp. 36-42, ISSN 0925-4005

Chou, J. C. & Chen, C. W. (2009). Fabrication and Application of Ruthenium-Doped Titanium Dioxide Films as Electrode Material for Ion-Sensitive Extended-Gate FETs. *IEEE Sensor Journal*, Vol. 9, (April 2009), pp. 277-284, ISSN 1530-437X

Grattarola, M.; Massobrio, G., & Matinoia S. (1992). Modeling H+-Sensitive FET's with SPICE. *IEEE Transactions on Electron Devices*, Vol. 39, (April 1992), pp. 813-819, ISSN 0018-9383

Fung, C. D.; Cheung, P. W., & Ko, W. H. (1986). A Generalized Theory of an Electrolyte-Insulator-Semiconductor Field-Effect Transistor. *IEEE Transactions on Electron Devices*, Vol. 33, (January 1986), pp. 8-18, ISSN 0018-9383

Van Hal, R. E. G.; Eijkel, J. C. T., & Bergveld, P. (1995). A Novel Description of ISFET Sensitivity with the Buffer Capacity and Double-Layer Capacitance as Key Parameters. *Sensors and Actuators B*, Vol. 24, (March 1995), pp. 201-205, ISSN 0925-4005

Pezekwe, C. D. & Boser, B. E. (2008). A Mode-Matching ΣΔ Closed-Loop Vibratory Gyroscope Readout Interface with a 0.004°/s/√Hz Noise Floor over a 50 Hz Band. *IEEE Journal of Solid-State Circuits*, Vol. 43, (December 2008), pp. 3039-3048, ISSN 0018-9200

Boser, B. & Wooley, B. (1988). The Design of ΣΔ Modulation Analog-to-Digital Converters. *IEEE Journal of Solid-State Circuits*, Vol. 23, (December 1988), pp. 1298-1308, ISSN 0018-9200

Norsworthy, Ed. S.; Schreier, R., & Temes, G. (1997). *Delta-Sigma Data Converters: Theory, Design, and Simulation*, IEEE Press, ISBN 0780310454, New York

Johns, D., & Martin, K. (1997). *Analog Integrated Circuit Design*, Wiley, ISBN 0471144487, Cloth

Part 2

Biosensors for Health

16

Design and Preparation of Nanostructured Prussian Blue Modified Electrode for Glucose Detection

Wanqin Jin, Zhenyu Chu and Yannan Zhang
State key laboratory of Materials-Oriented Chemical Engineering,
Nanjing University of Technology
China

1. Introduction

High sensitivity and anti-interference ability are critical parameters in glucose biosensor design, because of the complexity of blood composition. Prussian blue (PB) is a hexacyanoferrate with two different iron valences (+2 and +3) and was initially developed as a blue pigment in the 1700s (Bartoll, 2008). Recently researchers found that PB is an excellent material for use in the fabrication of glucose biosensors, because of its non-toxicity, high electrocatalytic activity, and low overpotential detection (Ricci & Palleschi, 2005; Karyakin et al., 2007; Wang, 2008). During glucose detection, hydrogen peroxide (H_2O_2) is produced via the enzymatic oxidation of glucose. Subsequently, PB reduces the H_2O_2 and transfers the electrons to generate a current response on the electrode surface. Thus, PB is the mediator of electron transfer in the detection process, making the electron sensitivity of PB - a key component of biosensor performance.

Chemical deposition and electrodeposition are the main processes used to synthesize a PB film on the electrode surface (Itaya et al., 1982; Zakharchuket al., 1995). However, the sensitivity of the electrode modified with a PB film cannot be controlled, because of difficulties in film construction. Millward et al. (2001) used a self-assembly approach to deposit a PB film on a gold electrode, which greatly accelerated the development of PB-based biosensors. The advantages of applying nanostructured materials for improving biosensor performance have been recognized in recent years, especially for improving sensitivity (Cella et al., 2010; Cao et al., 2010). The utilization of nanoparticles can enhance electrode performance, even if the same materials are used. We developed a PB nanostructure to produce a high sensitivity biosensor for glucose detection, which can be directly grown on the electrode surface.

We previously synthesized PB nanoparticles on a platinum (Pt) electrode surface using a self-assembly approach (Liu et al., 2009). We found that the size and quantity of PB particles greatly affected H_2O_2 detection performance. After immobilization of the glucose enzyme, this type of biosensor was sensitive to trace concentrations of glucose in solution (Liu et al. 2009). However, it was difficult to form a regularly structured PB particle film, when synthesis was conducted via self-assembly. Thus, we further developed the self-assembly approach to deliver a novel method for obtaining a regular film of PB crystals, are thereby improving biosensor sensitivity and effectiveness.

2. Mechanism of H_2O_2detection

PB is typically produced from a reaction between two compounds, $K_4[Fe(CN)_6]$ and $FeCl_3$ (see equation 1).

$$\begin{aligned} &3K_4[Fe(CN)_6] + 4FeCl_3 \rightarrow Fe_4[Fe(CN)_6]_3 + 12KCl \\ &K_4[Fe(CN)_6] + FeCl_3 \rightarrow KFe[Fe(CN)_6] + 3KCl \end{aligned} \quad (1)$$

$KFe[Fe(CN)_6]$ and $Fe_4[Fe(CN)_6]_3$ are soluble and insoluble PB, respectively, and both species are required. The unit cell of PB is a face-centered cubic structure with lattice parameters, a = b = c = 10.143 Å. It is interesting that neighboring iron ions have different valences. The Fe^{2+} ion, in the $Fe(CN)_6^{4+}$ complex, is readily reduced to the Fe^{3+} ion. The signal generated by electron transfer from $Fe(CN)_6^{4+}$ is generally used in electrochemical detection to characterize the properties of the PB film.

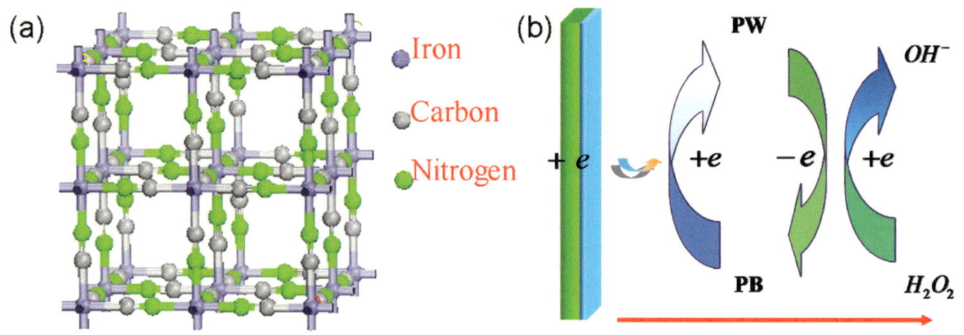

Fig. 1. (a) The structure of the PB unit cell. (b) Mechanism of H_2O_2 detection.

PB has two functions when used as a material in biosensor fabrication, i.e., electrocatalysis and electron transfer: When a potential (typically - 0.05 V) is imposed on a PB modified electrode, the PB will acquire electrons and move into its reduced state, Prussian White (PW). If H_2O_2 is present in the detection system, PW rapidly reduces H_2O_2 to OH^-. After donating electrons, PW reverts back to PB (Fig. 1). The direction of electron transfer during this process is from the electrode surface to H_2O_2. Thus, electrocatalysis and electron transfer determine overall electrode performance.

Regular crystalline structure is a morphological feature that has been widely demonstrated to enhance catalytic ability (Liu et al., 2010; Prevot et al., 2011). However, it is difficult to control regular PB crystal growth using conventional preparative methods, because of its rapid reaction rate during crystal formation. Consequently, novel methods are required to facilitate the regular crystal structure growth in the PB film.

3. PB crystal formation using a self-assembly approach

Self-assembly is a common approach for production of PB-modified electrodes. Scheme 1 shows the process of PB synthesis, which starts with a pre-coating layer of polyelectrolyte, to provide electrostatic adsorption sites, followed by dipping the electrode into a reactive solution for PB formation. Poly(diallyldimethylammonium chloride) (PDDA) is typically applied as the cation polyelectrolyte layer (Hornok & Dékány, 2007; Li et al., 2008). This layer provides a foundation for further layer deposition, which means that its properties are essential for regular PB growth. The regular structure of PB is not readily formed *via* self-assembly, but this approach has been successfully applied to regular crystal growth for other materials (Wang et al., 2009; Guang et al., 2009). The PB self-assembly problem might be attributable to first layer selection, and temperature can greatly affect polymer properties. We determined the optimum method for regular crystal formation in a PB film by controlling PDDA load temperature.

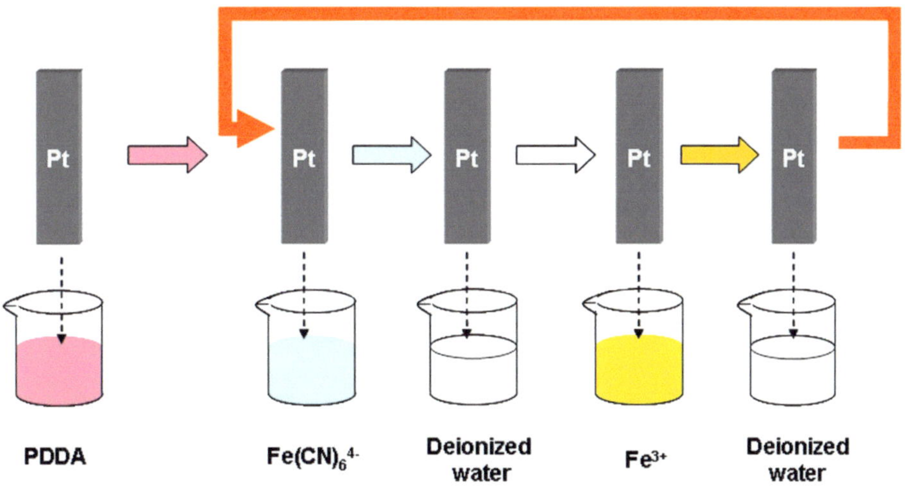

Scheme 1. Production of a PB-modified electrode using a self-assembly method.

We investigated the properties of PDDA layer with respect to changes in temperature, prior to the self-assembly of PB. Electrochemical impedance spectroscopy (EIS facilitates observation of the structure and charge transfer behavior of polymer films. We compared the impedances of bare Pt and the electrodes loaded by PDDA at different temperatures. Electron transfer is essential for sensitivity in the detection of H_2O_2. However, PDDA is not an excellent mediator for electron transfer, but we were more concerned with the resistance provided by the PDDA layer. Fig. 2 shows the results of impedance experiments, illustrating the electrode property at high frequencies due to the electron transfer kinetics of redox species at the electrode surface. The linear region is dominated by the mass transfer of probe species from the bulk solution to the interface region. We found that increasing the adsorption temperature led to a reduction in interface resistance. We compared the exact resistance values using a classical Randles circuit (inset of Fig. 2), the results of which were applied to fitting the EIS curves. The values of R_{ct} which resulted in electron transfer ability were calculated as 4.741, 5.932, 9.722, 11.47, and 13.03 Ω respectively, for the bare Pt electrode, and the electrode with PDDA adsorbed at 35, 30, 25, and 20 °C. The resistance of the unmodified Pt electrode was the lowest, and the addition of PDDA gradually decreased the electron transfer ability. The impedance was enhanced by a reduction of the PDDA adsorption temperature. The fluidity of the polymer was very poor at low temperatures, which led to severe surface aggregation of the substrate with detrimental effects on PB assembly. This prompted the investigation of surface coverage. The fractional electrode coverage rate (θ) of PDDA was estimated according to equation 2.

$$\theta = 1 - \frac{R_{ct}^{bare}}{R_{ct}^{PDDA}} \quad (2)$$

Where R_{ct}^{bare} is the charge transfer resistance value for the bare Pt electrode, and R_{ct}^{PDDA} is the same value for the PDDA modified electrode at different adsorption temperatures.
The calculated results were 0.2062, 0.5123, 0.5867, and 0.6361 for 35, 30, 25, and 20 °C, respectively. By combining these results with the resistance results, we determined why resistance did not decrease as a function of temperature increase. PDDA did not cover the whole Pt surface and electrons preferred to transfer in areas without polymer because of the lower resistance. Local preferences for electron transfer resistance were consistent with variations in polymer coverage.

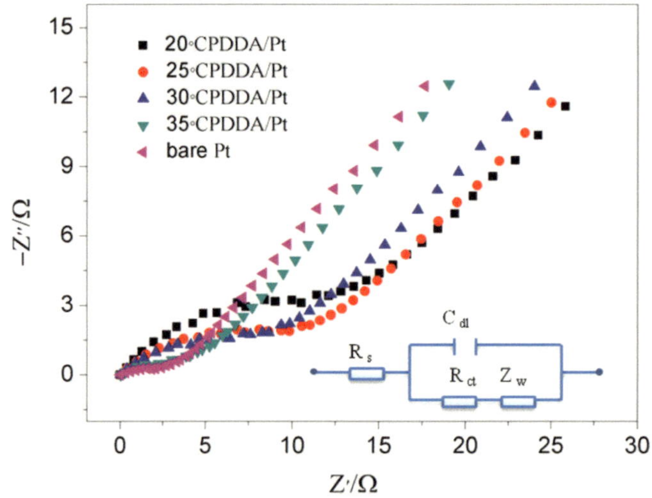

Fig. 2. The EIS diagram for the bare electrode and the electrodes loaded with a PDDA layer at 20, 25, 30, and 35 °C. The inset shows the equivalent circuit used for PDDA modified electrodes, where R_{ct} is the charge transfer resistance, R_s is the solution resistance, Z_w is the Warburg impedance due to the mass transfer from the redox probe to the electrode, and C_{dl} is the double layer capacitance.

Thus, the improvement of electron transport, demands that PDDA is loaded as sparingly as possible. This is because a high loading of PDDA further hinders assembly of PB, which means that a correct loading balance must be achieved.
The affect of PDDA adsorption temperature on PB morphology, and performance, were evaluated to determine the optimum production temperature, and provide a higher electrode performance via the synthesis of a regular PB structure. We investigated whether a regular PB morphology could be achieved by adjusting the PDDA adsorption temperature. Fig. 3 (a) to (d) shows the great differences in surface morphology of PB on modified electrodes, when the PDDA layer was adsorbed at different temperatures. When the PDDA was deposited at 20 °C, the film surface was covered with irregular particles, but the particles grew bigger as the temperature increased to 25 °C. As the temperature increased, the whole surface changed and, instead of irregular particles, an abundance of nanocubes was observed on the electrode surface, with each nanocube measuring ~100 nm. These

regular crystals formed the film and although some nanocubes remained on the surface, the amount decreased. We also measured the PB concentrations on the electrodes. Fig. 3 (e) shows that the PB concentration was 6.059, 6.771, 7.03, and 4.827 nmol cm^{-2} at temperatures of 20, 25, 30, and 35 °C, respectively. At the low temperature, the amount of PDDA covering the Pt surface was so large that it caused the aggregation of PB particles. Thus, an excess of crystal nuclei might lead to imperfect growth of PB crystals.

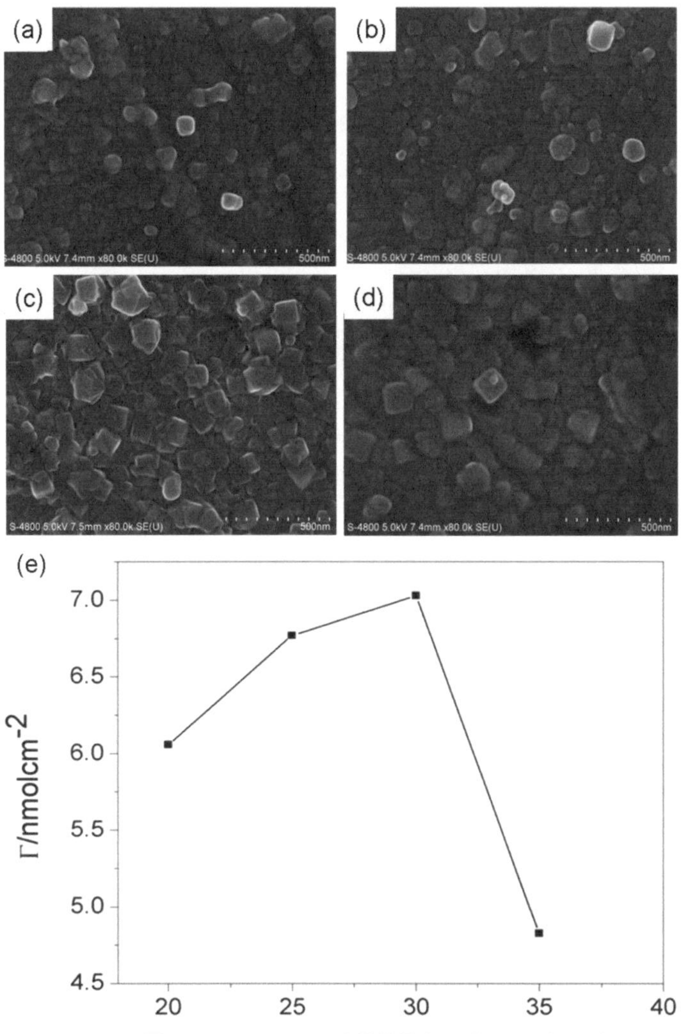

Fig. 3. The FESEM images of PB modified electrodes, where PDDA were adsorbed at different temperatures: (a) 20 °C; (b) 25 °C; (c) 30 °C; (d) 35 °C. (e) Shows the PB concentrations on electrodes at different PDDA adsorption temperature.

The film was comprised of small PDDA particles, which provided adsorption sites for PB assembly. The PB concentration was low at high temperature, because of low PDDA coverage. We showed that a PDDA layer adsorbed at low temperature resulted in a strong

impedance to electron transfer, so we selected 30 °C as the optimal temperature for PDDA adsorption. According to the performance detection procedure, the sensitivity of an electrode prepared at 30 °C was 1179.6 mA M^{-1} cm^{-2}, which was much higher than electrodes prepared with no control over PDDA adsorption temperature (Liu et al., 2009).
This improved self-assembly approach to PB film formation successfully produced nanocubic PB crystals and enhanced the sensitivity of H_2O_2 detection. This study demonstrated the constraints on electron transfer impedance imposed by the PDDA layer so we next determined the factors affecting the regular growth of PB in the absence of a polyelectrolyte.

4. Aerosol deposition (AD) for synthesis of PB nanocubes

4.1 Synthesis mechanism

Synthesis of a PB film with a regular morphology, in the absence of polyelectrolyte, demands control of the formation rate during regular PB film growth. Current approaches require PB formation in reactive solutions. However, the concentration of molecules in solution is very high, and PB is produced in seconds when solutions of K4[Fe(CN)6] and $FeCl_3$ are mixed. Thus, it is desirable to achieve PB formation with lower concentration solutions
Aerosols are composed of tiny droplets, which are so small that they are readily suspended in the air. There has been a recent growth in interest in the application of aerosols (Boissiere et al., 2010). The advantages of aerosols are as follows: small volumes lead to micro-reactions and the production of small particles; fewer molecules per unit are required in controlled reactions; the suspension of aerosols avoid the influence of gravity on preparation and promotes uniform growth. We aimed to produce regular PB crystals, without polyelectrolyte, by adopting the AD approach instead of conducting the reaction in solution.
If aerosols are to be used to deposit PB directly onto a Pt electrode, it was essential that an interaction occurred between Pt and reactive aerosols. Before we conducted the experiments, we confirmed that aerosols can be deposited on the electrode surface by virtue of Van der Waals force between the carbon and Pt atoms, according to the results of a Density Functional Theory (DFT) simulation (Chu et al., 2009). This simulation helped us to define the deposition order, i.e., the $K_4[Fe(CN)_6]$ aerosol should be initially attracted onto the Pt surface, because of the carbon conformation. The deposition time of the two aerosols was the same.

4.2 Morphology control

As shown in Fig. 4, aerosols of $Fe(CN)_6^{4-}$ and Fe^{3+} were deposited on the Pt surface to form the PB film. The deposition time was a controlled parameter that determined the concentration of aerosols. The small size of liquid used meant that aerosols were more readily affected by environmental temperature, which affected the growth of crystals. Thus, deposition time and temperature were the main controlled factors in the whole process (Chu et al., 2010).
Cyclic voltammetry (CV) experiment showed that the PB concentration on the modified electrode directly correlated with deposition time. Fig. 5 shows the maximal and minimal current values of each curve for the redox peaks of Fe^{2+}/Fe^{3+}, caused by electron transfer from PB to PW and PW to PB. PB concentrations can be calculated using the data by following equation 3 (Grundler, 2007).

$$\Gamma_T = \frac{Q}{nFA} \tag{3}$$

Where Γ_T represents the concentration of PB, Q is a single peak (either a reduction or oxidation peak), n is the average transfer of electrons calculated by 57/ΔE (ΔE is the difference in potential between the redox potentials), F is the Faraday constant, and A is the area of the electrode.

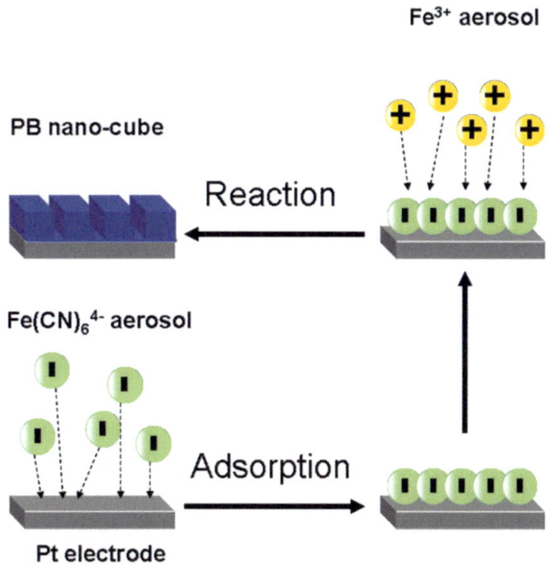

Fig. 4. PB film preparation using the aerosol deposition method.

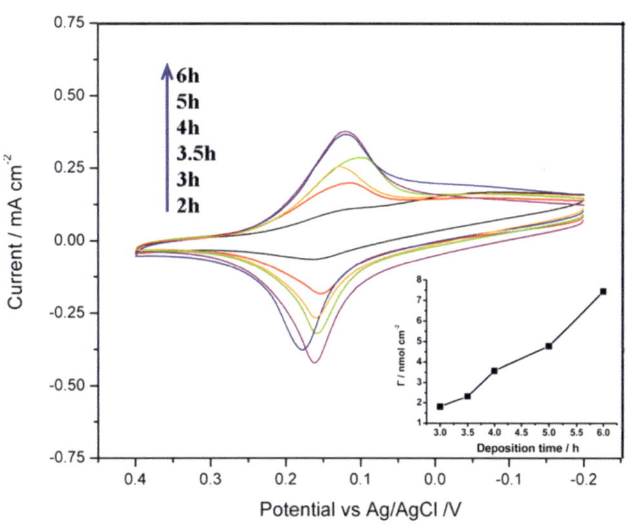

Fig. 5. The CV results for PB-modified electrodes produced for 2, 3, 3.5, 4, 5, and 6 hours. The preparation temperature was kept at 25 °C. The inset shows the diagram of calculated PB concentrations.

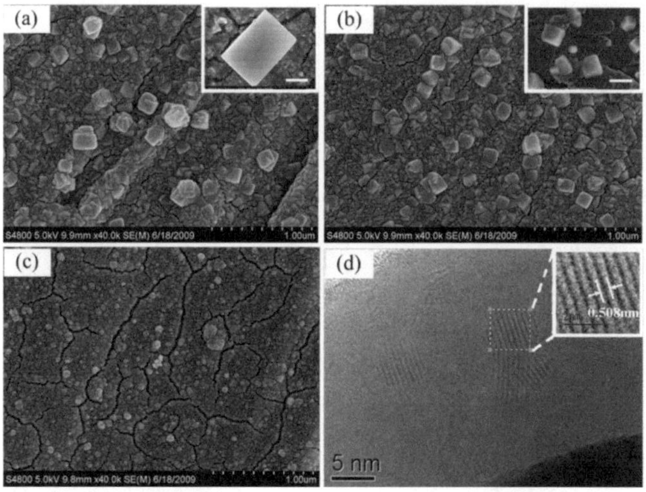

Fig. 6. (a) to (b) Field emission scanning electron microscopy (FESEM) images of PB modified electrodes prepared at 25, 35, and 45 °C. The insets show partial magnified images, where the bar is 250 nm. (d) High resolution transmission electron microscopy (HRTEM) image of an electrode prepared at 35 °C.

The Fig. 5 inset shows the calculated results for PB concentration. Concentration was an approximately linear function of increased deposition time. Thus, the amount of PB on the electrode surface can be finely controlled by the deposition time. The perfect growth of crystals demanded an adequate availability of substrate, so 6 hours was selected as the deposition time constant when investigating the influence of temperature on morphology. We investigated the PB crystal morphology for electrodes prepared at 25, 35, and 45 °C. Fig. 6 shows that regular nanocrystals formed on the electrode surface at 25 and 35 °C. When the film was prepared at 25 °C, the shape of crystal was cuboid-like with a size of ~500 nm, whereas at 35 °C, the crystals were smaller and possessed a more obviously cubic structure. Thus, it was determined that 35 °C was appropriate for the synthesis of larger volumes of crystals with a regular structure. A further increase of the temperature to 45 °C, led to the surface being populated with small particles with an undesirable morphology. Higher temperature also caused serious cracks in the film due to differences of thermal expansion between the PB film and the metal of the Pt electrode. Fig. 7(d) shows an HRTEM image of the growth of crystals produced in one direction, where the d-spacing of the lattice fringes was measured as 0.500 nm, which is consistent with the (200) lattice plane of PB in the PDF card (JCPDS card no.73-0687).

Temperature strongly affects PB morphology, because deposition of aerosols can reduce the amount of molecules available to participate in the reaction. Thus, the driving force of chemical equilibrium is reduced compared to reactions in solution, thereby slowing down the reaction product formation rate. High temperature might accelerate the formation of nuclei for further growth, but the availability of more growth cores could lead to an increase in the amount, but a decrease in the size, of PB crystals. Further problems occur if the temperature is increased further, because the interaction between PB and Pt is governed by the van der Waals force, which is a weak force. Thus, if the temperature is too high molecules will escape from the restraint of interaction due to high thermal motion activity. This can lead to inadequate and imperfect PB crystal growth.

Regular crystals with perfect edges lead to higher sensor performance, because they increase the catalytic activity of biosensors. Thus, a PB electrode with nano-cubic structure is expected to show enhanced sensitivity in the detection of H_2O_2.

4.3 Performance in H_2O_2 detection

Chronoamperometry is often used in the performance measurement of electrochemical biosensor detection performance. We tested the detection performance of three electrode systems; the Pt electrode we developed as described above, a counter Pt electrode, and an Ag/AgCl electrode. The process was conducted in a phosphate buffer solution (pH = 6.5) to ensure system stability. The potential imposed on the PB modified electrode was - 0.05 V. The stirring was provided to ensure the uniform dispersion of H_2O_2. After running the baseline, 10 μM H_2O_2 was repeatedly added into the buffer solution at a standard time interval.

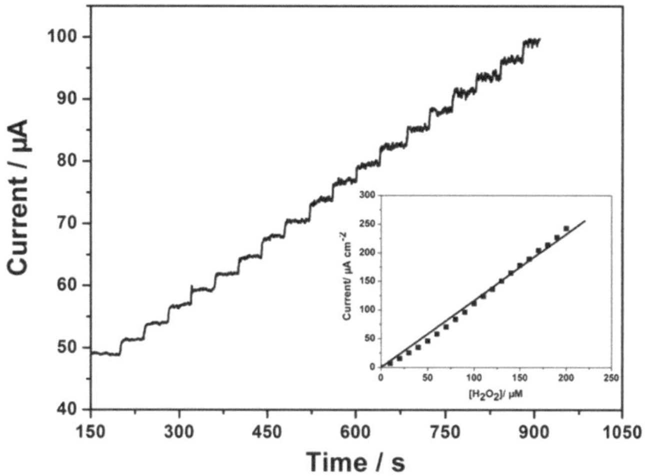

Fig. 7. Current response during H_2O_2 detection. The inset shows a simulation diagram of current versus H_2O_2 concentration.

Fig. 7 shows the change in current after the introduction of H_2O_2. After 19 treatments of H_2O_2 addition, the step of the current signal remained clear and stable. This shows that the PB construction maintains good stability with an increase of H_2O_2 concentration. The current response data had a linear relationship with the H_2O_2 concentration, which we simulated. The slope of this linear function indicated the H_2O_2 detection sensitivity of the PB modified electrode. The best sensitivity was calculated as 1163 mA M^{-1} cm^{-2}. This performance of an electrode prepared using the AD method was higher than traditional preparation methods. The enhancement of sensitivity was attributed to the formation of nanocubic PB crystals. The nanocubes possessed perfect edges, which provided strong electrocatalytic sites for the H_2O_2 reduction. High crystallinity might also provide more PB sites to participate in detection per unit area. Electrons transfer from Fe^{2+} and Fe^{3+} proceeds along a linear pathway $Fe-C\equiv N-Fe$ in the PB unit cell. Thus, the synthesized cube structure matches the PB cell construction of a face-centered cubic lattice, which means that we produced a regular path for electron transport that might decrease the resistance, in terms of geometry.

This production method for performance enhancement was based on the formation of regular structures by decreasing the reaction rate. A common approach for performance improvement depends on the introduction of other compounds with high catalytic ability or favorable conductivity. We confirmed that the AD approach can produce the regular nanocubes of PB, but we futher investigated whether the incorporation of other compounds during the production process might further increase the sensitivity. The inclusion of other compounds might affect the growth of PB, and the structure of the film, and further sensitivity improvements might accrue from cooperation between the two materials.

5. Codeposition of a PB-TiO_2 composite film using the AD method

Material selection during biosensor design demands attention to several critical requirements, i.e., non-toxicity, biocompatibility, stability, and cost. Codeposited compounds must also be compatible with PB. Titanium dioxide (TiO_2) is a common material, which satisfies all the required properties and is particularly suited to nanoparticle production, because it is very light. This allows the mixing of powdered TiO_2 with PB aerosols prior to suspension in the air. Synergistic reaction between semiconductors can increase performance, and both of PB and TiO_2 are semiconductors, with energy gaps of 1.58 and 3.2 eV, respectively. The main catalytic function of TiO_2 results from electron excitation of its valence bond to a conduction bond. However, 3.2 eV is a large gap which requires UV light to provide the energy for electron transit. The gap of PB is much lower than that of TiO_2. Combination of these two semiconductors means that they can pad each gap and make excitation easier (Yamamoto, 2009). Thus, doping TiO_2 nanoparticles into the PB film could improve the catalytic ability. This composite design might enhance the H_2O_2 detection sensitivity of the prepared PB electrode.
We next tested the effect of TiO_2 nanoparticle doping into deposition aerosols.

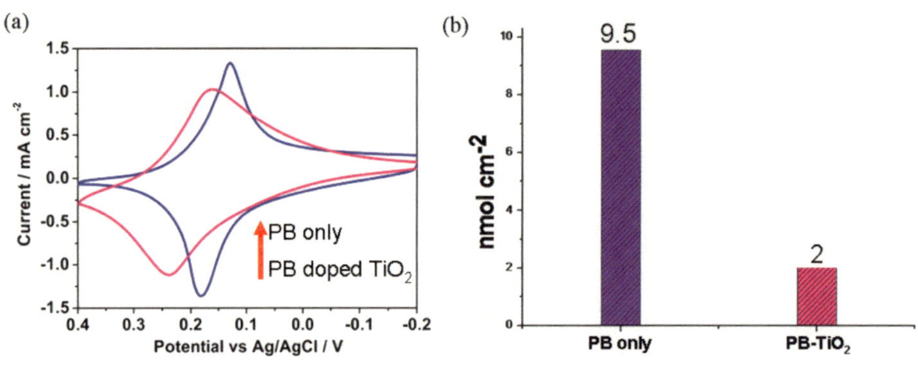

Fig. 8. (a) The comparison of CV diagrams for electrodes with only PB and PB doped with TiO_2. The electrode coating was conducted for 6 hours, at 35 °C. (b) Comparison of calculated PB surface concentrations for both electrodes.

We added 0.1 mmol TiO_2 to the 0.01 mol/L $FeCl_3$ solution to achieve co-deposition of TiO_2 during the preparation process. The mixed solution was converted to aerosols using an ultrasonic nebulizer. The concentration of TiO_2 was very low because of its poor solubility. Higher amounts would interfere with the ultrasonic method used to produce aerosols. Fig. 8

(a) shows that redox peaks for the electrode with a composite film was lower than that with a PB film. After doping with TiO_2, the difference between the potentials of oxidation and reduction was larger. The PB concentration was reduced approximately four-fold, according to the calculation results shown in Fig. 8 (b).The deposition of TiO_2 particles in the reactive aerosols, led to them becoming highly packed on the electrode surface, which meant they occupied many growth sites that might have been occupied by PB, after electrode surface adsorption. The interaction between Pt and TiO_2 was very weak. Thus, without the packing of PB particles, TiO_2 particles might easily fall off and detach PB crystals growing around them. This would reduce the concentration of PB on the electrode surface. The widening of the distance between peaks was caused by an increase in electron transfer resistance. Electron transfer through TiO_2 is much harder compared with PB, due to the larger bond gap. The change of concentration might also affect the surface morphology so we investigated the micro-scale surface morphology using FESEM. Fig. 9 (a) shows that the film did not grow fully over the surface. There were numerous flaws on the film surface, making the film discontinuous. The lack of adequate PB prevented correct growth. Compared to the surface morphology shown in Fig. 6(b), the ground film was smooth instead of rough, under the same preparation conditions. However, we found that some nanocubes grew on the ground film, which was very different from the PB-only modified electrode. Nanocubes only grew in the ground film, when the film was only formed of PB crystals, but because of the large size of TiO_2 particles, the PB crystals rapidly aggregated around TiO_2. PB might struggle to form a regular shape, because of interference form TiO_2 particles, and regular crystals only formed freely on the ground film. The low PB concentration and defects in the film limits any synergistic functionality of PB with TiO_2, thereby decreasing electrode performance. We prolonged the deposition time in order to form a uniform film and, after increasing the time to eight hours, surface concentration was found to be 5.4 nmol cm^{-2}. Fig. 9 (b) shows that the ground film was uniform and contained no defects. More nanocubes were apparent on the surface and the size increased to ~2 μm. This was an obvious improvement on electrodes prepared for less than six hours. We compared H_2O_2 detection sensitivity with an electrode prepared under 35 °C for six hours.

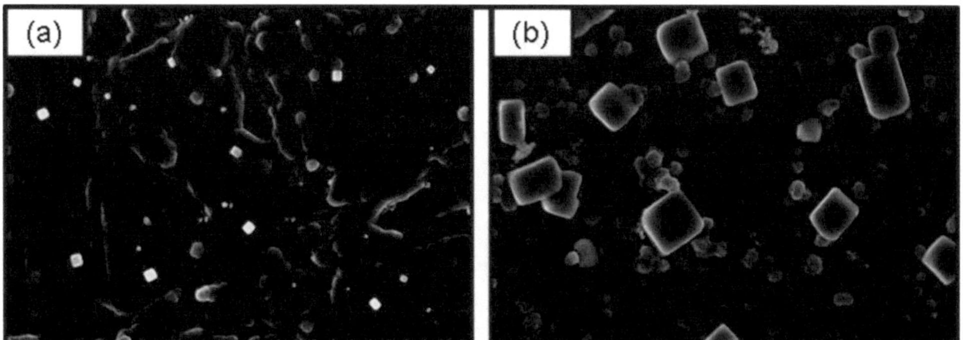

Fig. 9. FESEM images of PB-modified electrodes prepared at 35 °C for (a) 6 h, and (b) 8 h.

The introduction of TiO_2 decreased the PB surface concentration and resulted in significant changes in film morphology, particularly the PB crystal shape. This meant that the performance of the prepared PB-TiO_2 composite film was expected to be no improvement on the PB-only film. However, based on the results of H_2O_2 detection (Fig. 10), the sensitivity was calculated to be 1300 mA M^{-1} cm^{-2}, which was a little higher than the PB-only film. This sensitivity is based on a PB concentration that was half that of the PB-only film. The catalytic function of TiO_2 was confirmed. The reductive ability of PB was weakened due to lower PB coverage, but TiO_2 particles contribute to overall catalytic function.

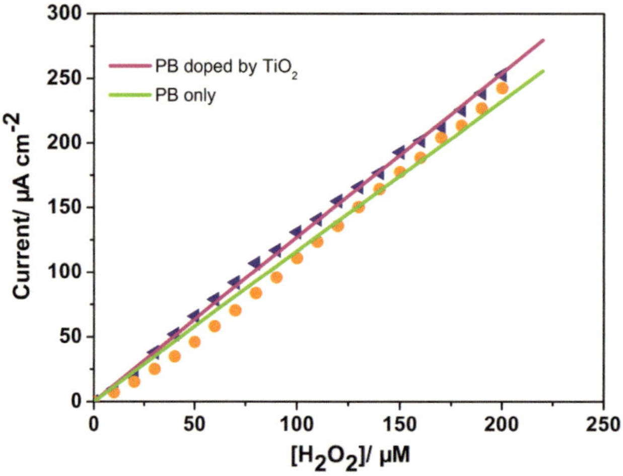

Fig. 10. H_2O_2 detection sensitivity comparison of electrodes with PB-only film and PB-TiO_2 composite film.

This preliminary work confirms that this approach can be applied to the production of regular structures PB and improve the performance of electrodes. Further research includes adjusting the ratio of the doping content and identifying other compounds with better solubility to substitute for TiO_2.

6. Conclusions and future prospects

Regular nanostructured PB can be synthesized using three methods: self-assembly with temperature controlled polyelectrolyte adsorption, the aerosol deposition approach, and the aerosol co-deposition approach. The regular structured PB film increased detection sensitivity of electrodes. Electron transfer direction in solution is from H_2O_2 to the electrode, and provision of a regular structured pathway for electron transport enhanced the detection efficiency of the modified electrode. This might require the production of oriented structures in the PB film, such as nanotubes or nanowires. However, if this assumption is to be satisfied a template or external force must be applied to set the PB growth direction. An alternative method is to identify compounds to dope the PB film and exploit their synergistic functionality, as we found with TiO_2. Such methods are not confined to PB fabrication and they may be appropriate in other fields requiring regular crystal synthesis.

7. Acknowledgement

This work was supported by the National Basic Research Program of China (No. 2009CB623406), National Nature Science Foundation of China (No.20990222), The "Six Kinds of Important Talents" Program of Jiangsu province (No.2007007), Innovation Foundation for Doctoral Dissertation of Jiangsu Province (CX09B-133Z).

8. References

Bartoll, J. (2008). The early use of Prussian blue in paintings, 9th International Conference on NDT of Art, NDT, Jerusalem Israel, pp. 1.

Boissiere, C., Grosso, D., Chaumonnot, A., Nicole, L. & Sanchez, C. (2010). Aerosol Route to Functional Nanostructured Inorganic and Hybrid Porous Materials, *Advanced Materials*, in press.

Cao, L., Liu, Y., Zhang, B. & Lu, L. (2010). In situ controllable growth of Prussian Blue nanocubes on reduced graphene oxide: facile synthesis and their application as enhanced nanoelectrocatalyst for H_2O_2 reduction, ACS Applied Materials & Interfaces, Vol. 2: 2339–2346.

Cella, L. N., Chen, W., Myung, N. V. & Mulchandani, A. (2010). Single-walled carbon nanotube-based chemiresistive affinity biosensors for small molecules: ultrasensitive glucose detection, *Journal of the American Chemical Society*, Vol. 132: 5024-5026.

Chu, Z., Liu, Y., Jin, W., Xu, N., Tieke, B. (2009). Facile fabrication of a Prussian Blue film by direct aerosol deposition on a Pt electrode, *Chemical Communications*, 3566-3567.

Chu, Z., Zhang, Y., Dong, X., Jin, W., Xu, N., Tieke, B. (2010). Template-free growth of regular nano-structured Prussian blue on a platinum surface and its application in biosensors with high sensitivity, Vol. 20: 7815-7820.

Grundler, P. (2007). Chemical Sensors: An Introduction for scientists and Engineers, Springer-Verlag, Berlin, 2007, ch. 2, pp. 64.

Guan, N., Sun, D. & Xu, J. (2009). Self-assembly of iron oxide nanoparticles into oriented nanosheets by one-pot template-free synthesis at low pH, *Materials Letters*, Vol. 63: 1272–1274.

Hornok, V. & Dékány, I. (2007). Synthesis and stabilization of Prussian blue nanoparticles and application for sensors, *Journal of Colloid and Interface Science*, Vol. 309: 176–182.

Itaya, K., Ataka, T. & Toshima, S. (1982). Spectroelectrochemistry and electrochemical preparation method of Prussian blue modified electrodes, *Journal of the American Chemical Society*, Vol. 104: 4767-4772.

Karyakin, A. A., Puganova, E. A., Bolshakov, I. A. & Karyakina, E. E. (2007). Electrochemical sensor with record performance characteristics, *Angewandte Chemie International Edition*, Vol. 46: 7678-7680.

Li, F., Shan, C., Bu, X., Shen, Y., Yang, G. & Niu, L. (2008). Fabrication and electrochemical characterization of electrostatic assembly of polyelectrolyte-functionalized ionic liquid and Prussian blue ultrathin films, *Journal of Electroanalytical Chemistry*, Vol. 616: 1-6.

Liu, M., Piao, L., Lu, W., Ju, S., Zhao, L., Zhou, C., Li, H. & Wang, W. (2010). Flower-like TiO2 nanostructures with exposed {001} facets: Facile synthesis and enhanced photocatalysis, *Nanoscale*, Vol. 2: 1115–1117.

Liu, Y., Chu, Z. & Jin, W. (2009). A sensitivity-controlled hydrogen peroxide sensor based on self-assembled Prussian Blue modified electrode, *Electrochemistry Communications*, Vol. 11: 484-487.

Liu, Y., Chu, Z., Zhang Y. & Jin, W. (2009). Amperometric glucose biosensor with high sensitivity based on self-assembled Prussian Blue modified electrode, *Electrochimica Acta*, Vol. 54: 7490-7494.

Millward, R. C., Madden, C. E., Sutherland, I., Mortimer, R. J., Fletcher, S. & Marken, F. (2001). Directed assembly of multilayers—the case of Prussian Blue, *Chemical Communications*, 1994-1995.

Prevot, V., Forano, C., Khenifi, A., Ballarin, B., Scavetta, E. & Mousty, C. (2011). A templated electrosynthesis of macroporous NiAl layered double hydroxides thin films, *Chemical Communications*, in press.

Ricci, F. & Palleschi, G. (2005). Sensor and biosensor preparation, optimisation and applications of Prussian Blue modified electrodes, *Biosensors and Bioelectronics*, Vol. 21: 389-407.

Wang, D., Choi, D., Li, J., Yang, Z., Nie, Z., Kou, R., Hu, D., Wang, C., Saraf, L. V., Zhang, J., Aksay, I. A. & Liu, J. (2009). Self-Assembled TiO2–Graphene Hybrid Nanostructures for Enhanced Li-Ion Insertion, *ACS Nano*, Vol. 3: 907-914.

Wang, J. (2008). Electrochemical glucose biosensors, *Chemical Review*, Vol. 108: 814-825.

Yamamoto, T., Saso, N., Umemura, Y. & Einaga Y. (2009). Photoreduction of Prussian Blue Intercalated into titania nanosheet ultrathin films,

Zakharchuk, N. F., Meyer, B., Hennig, H., Scholz, F., Jaworksi, A. & Stojek Z. (1995). Comparative study of Prussian-Blue-Modified graphite paste electrodes and solid graphite electrodes with mechanically immobilized Prussian Blue., *Journal of Electroanalytical Chemistry*, Vol. 398: 23-35.

17

Detection of Oxidative Stress Biomarkers Using Novel Nanostructured Biosensors

Maria Hepel and Magdalena Stobiecka
State University of New York at Potsdam, Potsdam, NY 13676
USA

1. Introduction

The oxidative stress is associated with the diminished capacity of a biological system to counteract an overproduction or invasion of reactive oxygen species and other radicals. Since oxidative stress is the leading cause of DNA damage, genetic disorders, cancer, and many environmental pollution related diseases, there is an urging need for oxidative stress screening and its prevention. There is growing evidence that oxidative stress may cause autism in children. The oxidative stress has also been implicated in the development of diabetes. Several biomarkers of oxidative stress have been identified, including glutathione (GSH), 3-nitrotyrosine (NT), homocysteine (Hcys), and cysteine (Cys). The tripeptide glutathione and its oxidized form, glutathione disulphide (GSSG), form a redox potential maintenance system in all eukaryotic cells. Since glutathione efficiently protects the DNA, proteins and lipid membranes from radical attacks, its diminished level is signaling an oxidative stress and the increased vulnerability of a biological entity to the environmental influences. An increased level of 3-nitrotyrosine, which is formed under oxidative stress in the presence of nitric oxide, has been found in diabetic patients. Homocysteine is a biomarker and an active agent leading to cardiovascular deterioration. While these biomarkers can be accurately determined using advanced instrumental assays, a wide screening would require the development of small, inexpensive, rapid, and simple in operation platforms for biomarker analysis. In this Chapter, the detection methods for the oxidative stress biomarkers based on their interactions with monolayer-protected gold nanoparticles (AuNP) are described. The nanoparticle utilization in a solution-phase analysis as well as in a multifunctional sensory film preparation is presented. The interactions of AuNP with glutathione and homocysteine have been investigated using resonance elastic light scattering (RELS) and plasmonic UV-Vis spectroscopy. The high sensitivity of the RELS measurements enables monitoring of ligand exchanges and the biomarker-induced AuNP assembly. The viability of designing simple and rapid assays for the detection of glutathione and homocysteine is discussed. The surface plasmon band broadening and bathochromic shift are consistent with the biomarker-induced AuNP assembly and corroborate the RELS measurements and HR-TEM imaging. The results of molecular dynamics and quantum mechanical calculations support the mechanism of the formation of GSH- and Hcys-linkages in the interparticle interactions and show that multiple H-bonding can occur. In contrast to homocysteine and glutathione that induce gold nanoparticle assembly in specific pH ranges, no aggregation of nanoparticles has been found in the presence of nitrotyrosine. The interactions of nitrotyrosine with gold nanoparticles and two fluorescent dyes with different spectral characteristics have also been investigated. These interactions result in changes in the resonance elastic light scattering (RELS) and fluorescence quenching that can be utilized in designing assays for the biomarker. The adsorption measurements of nitrotyrosine and coumarin 120 on a QC/Au quartz crystal piezoelectrode corroborate the observed RELS and static fluorescence quenching effects. Next, the novel molecularly-templated conductive polymer films are described. These films, utilized for the detection of various biomolecules, are mimicking the biorecognition processes occurring in nature, such as in the antibody-antigen interactions, or biotin-streptavidin binding. We have found that the functionalized gold nanoparticles enhance the response of molecularly-templated conductive polymer films for the detection of biomolecules and amplify the analytical signal through AuNP labeling. Novel designs of molecularly imprinted poly(orthophenylenediamine) sensor films are presented. The oxidative stress biomarker-induced assembly of monolayer-protected gold nanoparticles is evaluated in view of prospective applications of gold nanoparticles in designing inexpensive nanostructured sensors and microsensor arrays for field-deployable and point-of-care utilization.

2. Redox-potential homeostasis and protection against oxidative-stress

Glutathione and its oxidized disulfide form (GSSG) constitute the main redox regulation system in living organism's homeostasis. GSH protects cells against organic peroxides and damaging radicals, and is involved in signaling processes associated with cell apoptosis. The diminished active GSH levels in cells and body fluids lead to the reduced antioxidation capacity (Noble et al., 2005) to protecting against radicals and have been found to increase susceptibility to autism (Bernard et al., 2001, Clark-Taylor et al., 2004), diabetes (Beard et al., 2003), and other diseases (Almazan et al., 2000, Beard et al., 2003, Clark-Taylor et al., 2004, Clarkson, 1992, Noble et al., 2005, Polidoro et al., 1984, Repetto et al., 1996, Upadhya et al., 2004). The low GSH levels have been found to be caused by oxidative stress and exposure to toxic heavy metals (Hg, Cd, Pb). GSH and phytochelatines with general structure (γ-Glu-Cys)$_n$Gly participate as the capping agents (Barbas et al., 1992, Dameron et al., 1989) in heavy-metal sulfide nanoparticles formed in living organisms in natural detoxification processes (Inouhe, 2005, Mehra et al., 1991, Vatamaniuk et al., 2000, Vatamaniuk et al., 2001). While the kinetics of a systemic response to an oxidative stress is basically dependent only on the GSH level, the *redox potential* depends on both the GSH and GSSG. Still, the sensitivity of the redox potential to GSH level change is twice as high as that corresponding to the GSSG level change. This follows from the Nernst equation:

$$E = E^0 + 0.02958 \log [GSSG] - 0.05916 \log [GSH] - 0.05916\, pH \qquad (1)$$

relating to the reaction equation for the redox process: $GSSG + 2H^+ + 2e^- = 2GSH$. In other words, the redox potential depends on the ratio: $(\sqrt{[GSSG]})/[GSH]$ rather than on the straight ratio: [GSSG]/[GSH]. The *redox buffering capacity* to both the oxidative and reductive stresses can be defined by the sum of concentrations: [GSH]+2[GSSG]. The factor 2 in this expression is due to the stoichiometry of the redox reactions in which GSSG can accept 2 electrons whereas GSH can give up 1 electron. If we consider the effectiveness of bodily response only to the oxidative stress then the *oxidative stress buffering capacity* would be better expressed by [GSH] alone rather than the concentration sum of GSH and

GSSG. Commonly used is also the *redox ratio* defined as: [GSH]/[GSSG] which is more convenient than the square root ratio discussed above.

3. Gold nanoparticle-based colorimetric assays for biomarkers of oxidative stress

The biomolecule-induced gold nanoparticle assembly process can be monitored using surface plasmon (SP) absorbance and SP band shifts. The oscillation frequency of the local surface plasmon is very sensitive to the changes in dielectric environment of nanoparticles and distance between nanoparticles. The collective oscillation of local surface plasmons is excited when the distance d between AuNP is: $d < 5r$, where r is the AuNP radius. Theoretical studies of plasmonic oscillations (Brioude et al., 2005, Draine et al., 1994, Gonzales et al., 2007, Jain et al., 2006, Kooij et al., 2006, Lee et al., 2005, 2006, Prescott et al., 2006, Ungureanu et al., 2009, Yang et al., 1995, Yin et al., 2006) and SP absorbance spectra (Alvarez et al., 1997, Etchegoin et al., 2006, Johnson et al., 1972, Kamat, 2002, Link et al., 1999a, Link et al., 1999b, Mishchenko et al., 2002, Perez-Juste et al., 2005, Ping et al., 2008) have enabled the understanding of mechanisms leading to the absorbance maximum shifts associated with the assembly processes. Extensive studies of the surface plasmon absorbance for various AuNP systems have been carried out by several groups (Alivisatos et al., 1996, Elghanian et al., 1997, Hostetler et al., 1998, Hostetler et al., 1999, Kamat, 2002, Kariuki et al., 2004, Kelly et al., 2003, Lim et al., 2009, Maye et al., 2005, Park et al., 2002 , Reynolds et al., 2000, Storhoff et al., 1998, Taton et al., 2000, Taton et al., 2001, Zheng et al., 2000). In this work, the formation of networks of fluorosurfactant ZONYL-capped spherical AuNP's mediated by Hcys, and glutaraldehyde molecules have been investigated (Scheme 1).

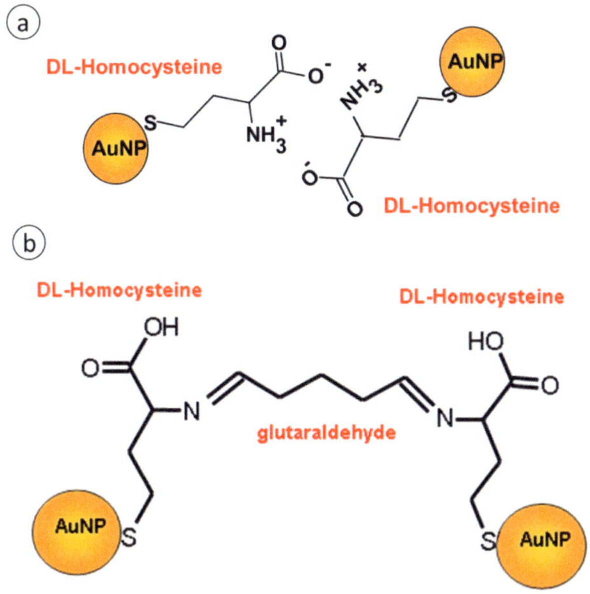

Scheme 1. Mechanisms of assembly of the gold nanoparticles: (a) Interparticle zwitterion-type electrostatic interactions between Hcys-capped AuNP; (b) Covalently-bonded glutaraldehyde nanobridge, linking Hcys-capped gold nanoparticles.

Fluorosurfactants provide similar advantages to other surfactants but, in addition, show high degree of chemical inertness. The ZONYL fluorosurfactant is known to form self-assembled monolayers on gold surfaces rendering the surface more hydrophobic and significantly retarding the gold oxide formation processes (Li et al., 2004). Although this surfactant forms water-tight shells, its bonding to a gold surface is not as strong as that of thiolates. Therefore, in presence of homocysteine, ZONYL is replaced in a ligand exchange process by thiol. The ligand exchange process taking place upon addition of homocysteine to ZONYL-capped AuNP solution can be monitored using SP band absorbance of AuNP (Figure 1 a). The UV–Vis spectra 1–9 were recorded for increasing concentrations of Hcys, from 0 to 22.2 μM and constant concentration of $AuNP_{5nm}$ (6 nM). It is seen that the SP band shifts toward longer wavelengths and the maximum absorbance increases with increasing C_{Hcys}. These observations are consistent with ligand exchange process:

$$AuNP/\ FES_x + yHcys = AuNP\ /Hcys_y + xFES \qquad (2)$$

where FES denotes a fluorosurfactant molecule and $x \approx y$, followed by interparticle molecular linking of AuNP/Hcys through direct Hcys-Hcys interactions. At the pH =6.0, homocysteine exists as a zwitterion with α-amino group protonated ($-NH_3^+$) and carboxylic group dissociated (COO^-). Therefore, the zwitterionic interparticle binding between Hcys-capped AuNP is playing a predominant role, as recently discussed by Zhong et al. (Lim et al., 2007). The bathochromic shift of the surface plasmon peak ($\Delta\lambda_{max}$ = 36 nm, for 16 μM Hcys) corresponds to the formation of small Hcys-linked AuNP ensembles. The increase of SP absorbance by 21% (from 0.253 to 0.305) indicates on the collective oscillations of local surface plasmons in AuNP that form these ensembles. The absorbance maximum increases with C_{Hcys} and reaches the saturation value at $C_{Hcys} > 7$ μM, with the half-absorbance change appearing at $C_{Hcys} = 3.38$ μM. The value of λ_{max} also reaches saturation at $C_{Hcys} > 7$ μM (Figure 1b). Therefore, we can assume that above 7 μM Hcys concentration the ligand exchange process has completed and nanoparticle shells are saturated with Hcys.

At neutral solutions, Hcys-capped AuNP do not assemble. In the following, we present a method for Hcys-capped AuNP assembly by interparticle crosslinking using glutaraldehyde as the linker (Scheme 1b). The linking is achieved through the condensation reaction between aldehyde groups of glutaraldehyde and amine groups of Hcys, with the formation of covalent amide bonds. The UV-Vis spectra were recorded for increasing concentrations of Hcys, from 0 to 30 μM, while maintaining the concentration of $AuNP_{5nm}$ constant (2.53 nM), as illustrated in Figure 2a. The concentration of glutaraldehyde was also maintained constant (1.12 %). These spectra show a bathochromic shift of the SP peak from 517.4 to 562.3 nm for 0 and 20 μM Hcys, respectively, with $\Delta\lambda$ = 44.9 nm (Figure 2b). It corresponds to the formation of glutaraldehyde-linked Hcys-capped AuNP ensembles. The surface plasmon band shift toward longer wavelengths is consistent with the assembly of Hcys-capped gold nanoparticle networks by glutaraldehyde interparticle linker. The increase of SP absorbance by 21% (from 0.24 to 0.29 for 20 μM Hcys) indicates on the excitation of collective oscillations of local surface plasmons in AuNP that form these ensembles.

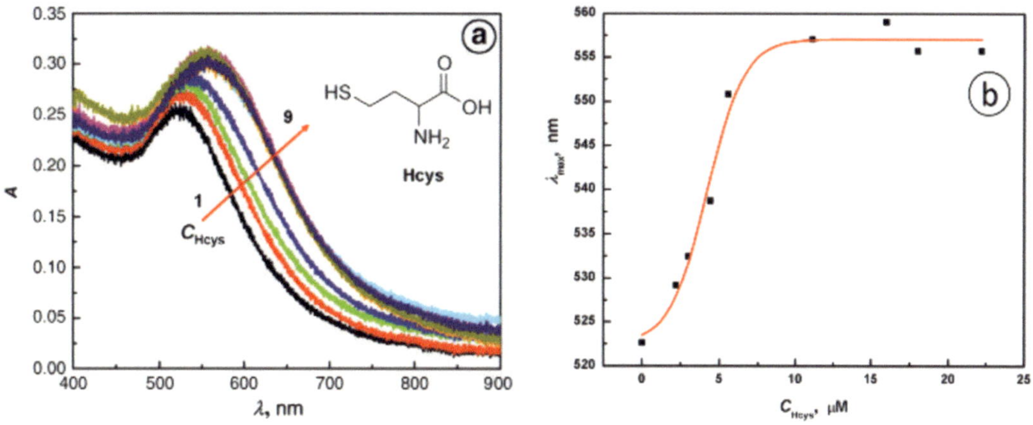

Fig. 1. (a) Absorbance spectra for ZONYL-capped AuNP for different concentrations of homocysteine, C_{Hcys} [µM]: (1) 0, (2) 2.22, (3) 3, (4) 4.44, (5) 5.56, (6) 11.11, (7) 16, (8) 18, (9) 22.22; C_{AuNP} = 6 nM, C_{ZONYL} = 0.22 %, pH = 6; (b) dependence of λ_{max} vs. C_{Hcys}.

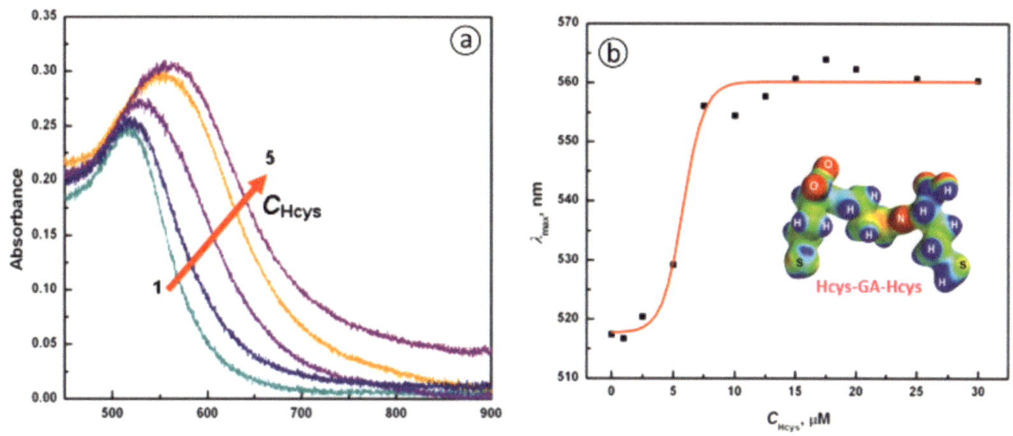

Fig. 2. (a) Absorbance spectra for glutaraldehyde linked homocysteine-capped AuNP for different concentration of DL-homocysteine, C_{Hcys}, µM: (1) 0, (2) 2.5, (3) 5, (4) 10, (5) 15. C_{AuNP} = 2.53 nM, C_{GA} = 1.12%, pH = 7; (b) Dependence of λ_{max} vs. C_{Hcys} for glutaraldehyde-linked AuNP@Hcys.

4. Biomolecule-induced gold nanoparticle assembly studied by RELS

The oxidative stress has been suggested as the causative factor in aging (Carlo et al., 2003) and many diseases such as cardiovascular, cancer, autism spectrum disorders (ASD) (James et al., 2006), and others. Among the biomarkers of oxidative stress are small biomolecules such as: ubiquinol (Yamamoto et al., 2002) which is very labile in the oxidation of low-density lipoprotein (LDL), glutathione (GSH) which is depleted in the presence of organic radicals and peroxides (Droge, 2002), homocysteine (Carmel et al., 2001, Jacobsen, 2000) which has been found at elevated levels in atherosclerosis (Boushey et al., 1995, Graham et al., 1997, Lentz et al., 2004, Refsum et al., 1989, Welch et al., 1998, Zhang et al., 2000),

Alzheimer disease (Seshadri et al., 2002, Varadarajan et al., 2001), dementia (Seshadri et al., 2002), and poses an increased risk of birth defects (Mills et al., 1996). Some biomarkers of oxidative stress are necessary to maintain healthy homeostasis (e.g. glutathione), while others participate in the development of diseases (e.g. homocysteine). There is now mounting evidence that oxidative and nitrosative stress resulting from hyperglycemia is involved in the development of diabetes and is implicated in the micro- and macrovascular complications of the disease. Such biomarkers of oxidative stress as nitrotyrosine and homocysteine show elevated levels and glutathione shows a decreased level in a progressing disease. In this study, the interactions of nitrotyrosine, homocysteine and glutathione with gold nanoparticles have been investigated. These interactions result in changes in the resonance elastic light scattering (RELS) that can be utilized in designing assays for the biomarker. Since the RELS spectroscopy offers an exceptional sensitivity to the AuNP assembly, we have employed the RELS measurements to determine if there is any aggregation of AuNP taking place in the presence of NT and Hcys. In Figure 3a, the synchronous full-scan RELS spectra recorded after addition of NT to cysteamine-capped AuNP are presented.

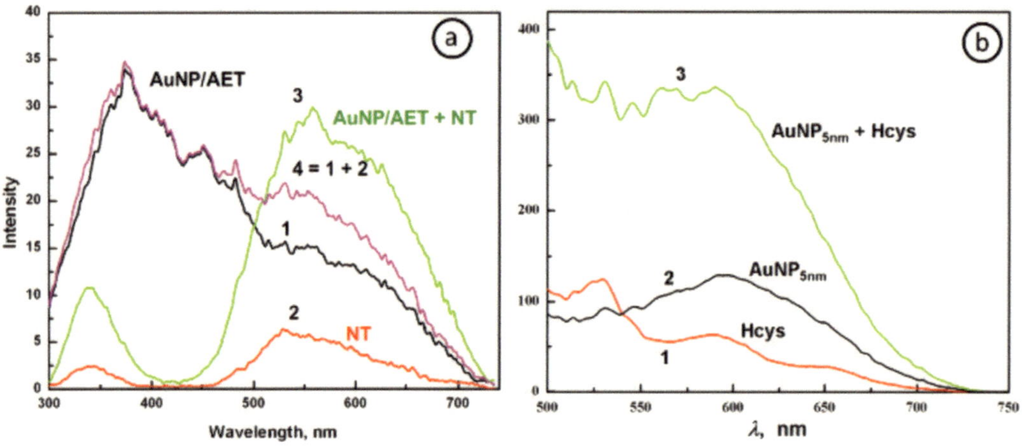

Fig. 3. Synchronous scan RELS spectra for: (a) (1) 0.95 nM cysteamine-capped $AuNP_{5nm}$, (2) 0.33 mM NT, (3) 0.95 nM cysteamine-capped $AuNP_{5nm}$ + 0.33 mM NT, (4) sum of spectra (1) and (2); 20 mM TrisHCl buffer, pH = 7.4. (b) (1) 20 μM Hcys, (2) 3.8 nM $AuNP_{5nm}$ and (3) 3.8 nM $AuNP_{5nm}$ + 20 μM Hcys recorded after 60 s reaction time.

The spectrum in curve 3 shows a decrease of RELS intensity upon addition of NT in the short wavelength region (300 - 500 nm) and an increase of RELS intensity in the long wavelength range (500 - 700 nm) in comparison with the spectrum of cysteamine-capped gold nanoparticles (Figure 3a, curve 1). The quenching of the light by NT molecules at shorter wavelengths indicates that a screening of gold nanoparticles by amino acid occurs. Curve 4 represents the theoretical sum of spectra for nanoparticles and NT (curve 1 and 2, respectively). This spectrum can be directly compared with spectrum which was recorded for 0.33 mM NT in the presence of 0.95 nM cysteamine-capped AuNP (curve 3). It is clear that the spectra for AuNP and for NT are not additive. This indicates on the formation of supramolecular assemblies. For AuNP@Hcys (Figure 3b), well resolved RELS spectra were obtained for excitation wavelengths in the range: λ_{ex} = 500 – 650 nm. The full-scan RELS spectra for citrate capped gold nanoparticles and Hcys mixture show the increase of RELS intensity of AuNP@Cit upon addition of homocysteine in the entire range of scanned wavelength. The increase of scattering intensity is due to the dependence of scattering cross-section on particle diameter a and the dielectric function (or refractive index) of the medium.

$$I_{sc} = I_0 N \frac{\left(1+\cos^2\theta\right)}{2R^3}\left(\frac{2\pi}{\lambda}\right)^4 \frac{\left[\left(n_p - n_s\right)^2 - 1\right]^2}{\left[\left(n_p - n_s\right)^2 + 2\right]}\left(\frac{a}{2}\right)^6 \tag{3}$$

where n_p and n_s are the refractive indices for the particles and the solution, respectively, λ is the wavelength of incident light beam, R – the distance from source, θ - the scattering angle, N - the number of particles, and I_0 is the constant.

The addition of NT to the cysteamine-capped $AuNP_{5nm}$ nanoparticles results in the enhancement of Rayleigh scattering for the excitation wavelength λ_{ex} = 560 nm, as indicated in Figure 4a, curves 2-5, obtained for 0.95 nM $AuNP_{5nm}$ + x μM NT, where x = 0 ... 333 μM. This confirms that supramolecular assemblies are formed. At 7.4, citrate ions stabilize gold colloids by forming tight negatively charged shells around nanoparticles cores ($pK_{a,1}$ = 3.09, $pK_{a,2}$ = 4.75, $pK_{a,3}$ = 5.41). After the addition of cysteamine to the solution of citrate-capped AuNP, citrates are replaced in a ligand exchange process by thiols. At pH 7.4 α-amino group of cysteamine are protonated ($-NH_3^+$) and form positively charged shells around the gold nanoparticles cores. At pH > 6.8, the deprotonation of hydroxyl group of NT is observed and NT exists as an anion (pK_{a1} = 2.20, pK_{a2} = 6.8, pK_{a3} = 9.11). Hence, the NT molecules are electrostatically attracted to AuNP@AET and supramolecular structure by electrostatic interactions and hydrogen bonding between $-COO^-$ and $-NH_3^+$ of NT molecules and cysteamine-capped gold nanoparticles AuNP@AET can be formed. Upon addition of homocysteine to citrate-capped AuNP, an increase in resonance elastic light scattering is also observed (Fig. 4b). The RELS spectra were obtained at pH = 5.0 for λ_{ex} = 560 nm, for increasing concentrations of Hcys from C_{Hcys} = 0 to 15 μM. The pK_a values for Hcys are: pK_1 = 2.22 (-COOH), pK_2 = 8.87 ($-NH_2$) and pK_3 = 10.86 (-SH)) making it a zwitterion at pH = 5. As the ligand exchange process progresses, the citrate ions are being replaced by the neutral Hcys molecules. The progression is accelerated at higher Hcys concentrations. The switching begins at C_{Hcys} = 4μM and ends at C_{Hcys} = 6μM with a sharp transition from the background scattering level of AuNP@Cit to that characteristic of the AuNP@Hcys. Similar RELS experiments carried out for other aminoacid ligands and glutathione show that the RELS response is highly selective to Hcys leading for analytical determinations of homocysteine in a matrix of aminoacids and glutathione. In the presence of GSH, at pH = 3.24 ± 0.03, the light scattering from $AuNP_{5nm}$ nanoparticles is also strongly enhanced (Fig. 4c). The RELS signal, measured within 1 min of reaction time, depends on GSH concentration and increases monotonously with C_{GSH} from $I_{sc,0}$ = 7.34 for the 0 mM to $I_{sc,max}$ = 66.14 for the 5 mM concentration of the glutathione solution. At this pH, the GSH is predominantly neutral (zwitterionic) form and may caused aggregation of AuNP. pKa values for GSH are: pK_1 = 2.04 (glutamate –COOH), pK_2 = 3.4 (glycine -COOH), pK_3 = 8.72 (–SH group), pK_4 = 9.49 ($-NH_2$ group). The enhancement of RELS from $AuNP_{5nm}$ by GSH molecules is attributed to the size increase of AuNP due to the ligand exchange (i.e. replacing short-chain citrate molecules in the nanoparticle shell with longer-chain GSH molecules) and interparticle interactions leading to AuNP assembly.

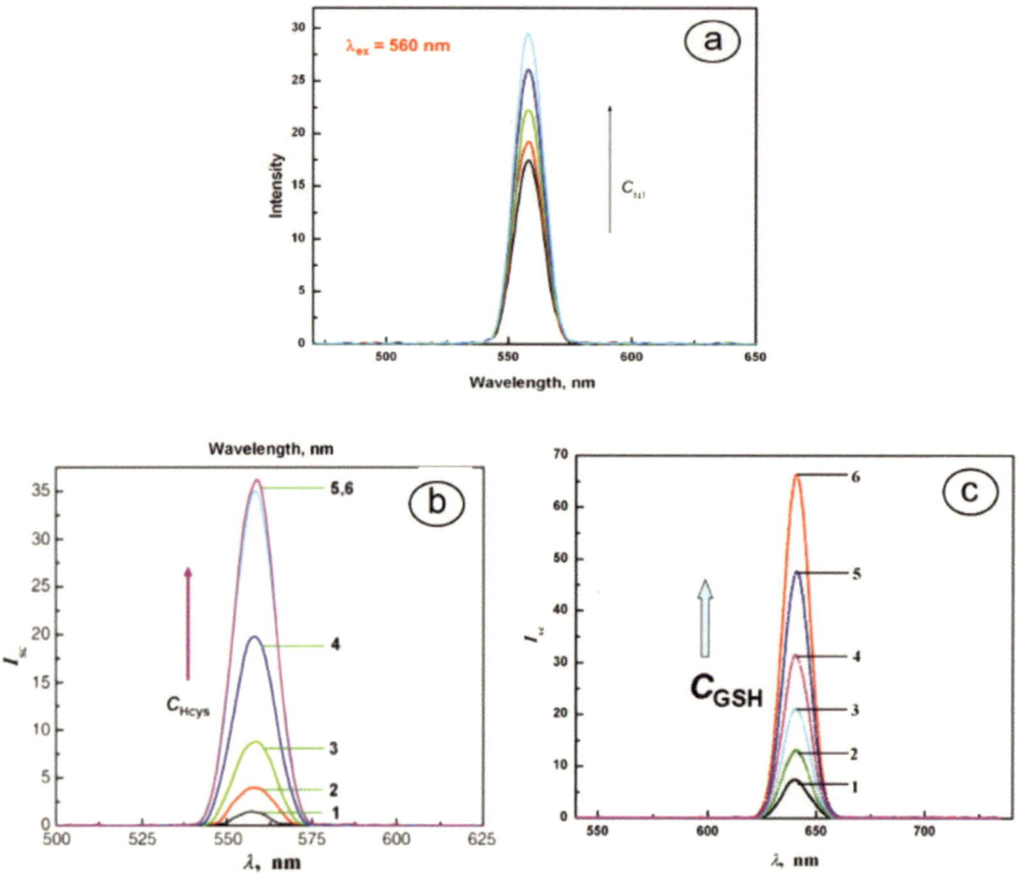

Fig. 4. (a) Dependence of RELS spectra for 0.95 nM cysteamine-capped $AuNP_{5nm}$ + x μM NT, x [μM]: (1) 0, (2) 83.3, (3) 166.7, (4) 250, (5) 333; λ_{ex} = 560 nm; 20 mM TrisHCl buffer, pH = 7.4; (b-c) Resonance elastic light scattering spectra for citrate-capped $AuNP_{5\,nm}$ for different concentrations of (b) homocysteine and (c) glutathione, C_{Hcys} [μM]: (1) 0, (2) 5, (3) 5.5, (4) 5.75, (5) 6.75, (6) 15, C_{AuNP} = 3.8 nM, pH = 5, λ_{ex} = 560 nm; C_{GSH} [mM]: (1) 0, (2) 2.67, (3) 3.0, (4) 3.17, (5) 3.33, (6) 5, C_{AuNP} = 10.1 nM.

In contrast to the behavior of NT, Hcys and GSH, replace nonthiolated AuNP shell and in the proper pH range induce assembly of gold nanoparticles (Figure 5) (Lim et al., 2007, Lim et al., 2008, Stobiecka et al., 2010a, Stobiecka et al., 2010b). Large increase of the RELS signal was reported for both GSH and Hcys confirming the assembly process (Stobiecka et al., 2010a, Stobiecka et al., 2010b). While in the Hcys-induced assembly, the main forces are H-bonding, in the case of GSH-induced assembly, the zwitterionic forces are dominant, although the H-bonding plays also a role (Lim et al., 2007, Lim et al., 2008). No aggregation of nanoparticles has been found in the presence of nitrotyrosine.

Taking into account the decrease in particle concentration due to assembly and assuming λ = const, the increase of the effective particle diameter a_{rel} can be estimated using the formula:

$$a_{rel} = \frac{a_1}{a_0} = \sqrt[3]{\frac{I_{sc,1}}{I_{sc,0}}} \quad (4)$$

where indices 0 and 1 stand for the particles before and after NT addition, respectively. From the data of Figure 4a, the scattering intensity increase is: $I_{sc,1}/I_{sc,0} = 1.695$ and, hence, $a_{rel} = 1.192$. This increase in a_{rel} is relatively small and indicates that aggregates of AuNP are not formed, otherwise the value of $a_{rel} \geq 2$ should be obtained (Stobiecka et al., 2010a, Stobiecka et al., 2010b). Therefore, the increase in particle diameter observed upon interactions of AuNP with NT is due to the attachment of NT to the outer interface of the AET-capped AuNP shell. The increase in scattering intensity upon addition of 15 μM Hcys is $I_{sc,1}/I_{sc,0} = 36.2/1.91 = 19.0$ (mean of 5 measurements) (Fig 4b). The 19-fold increase in scattering intensity clearly indicates on the homocysteine-induced assembly of AuNP. Utilizing Eq. (4), we obtain for the increase of particle diameter: $a_{rel} = 2.7$. From the data of Figure 4c, the scattering intensity increase after addition of the 5 mM GSH is: $I_{sc,1}/I_{sc,0} = 9.01$ and, hence, $a_{rel} = 2.08$. This means that most likely small aggregates composed of only few nanoparticles (e.g 2-6) are formed.

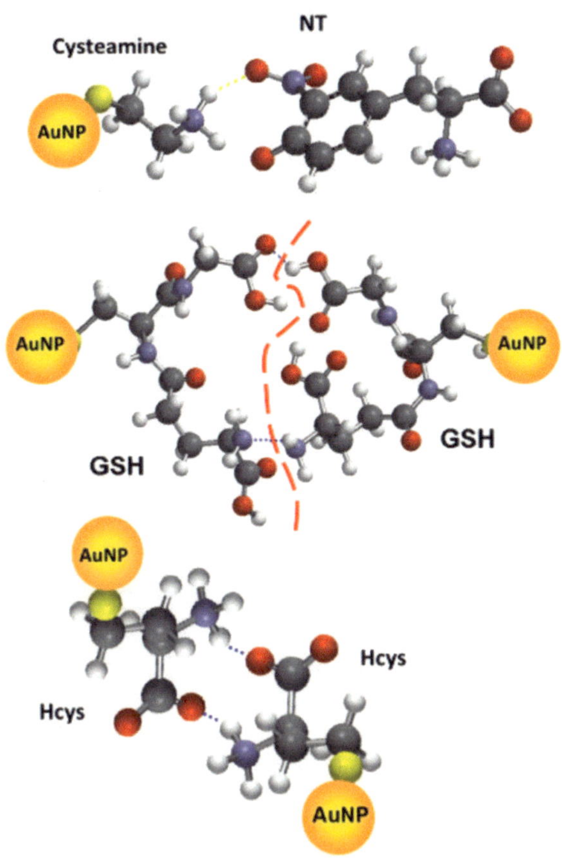

Fig. 5. Hydrogen bonding between AuNP@AET and NT, two glutathione/homocysteine molecules from shells of two interacting AuNP and ; H-bonds marked with a dotted line; atoms: yellow - sulfur, red -oxygen, blue - nitrogen, gray - carbon, light gray - hydrogen).

5. Ligand-exchange processes in core-shell nanoparticle systems

Growing interests in bioassays providing transduction of bioinformation to optical and electronic signals have recently been observed in conjunction with stimulating developments in synthesis of highly efficient quantum-dots and functionalized gold nanoparticles (AuNP) (Bain et al., 1989, Hostetler et al., 1999). Kinetic studies show that ligand-exchange process in a self-assembled monolayer (SAM) film is basically a Langmuirian pseudo-first-order process and is based on the random place-exchange proceeding evenly on the entire surface of AuNP. This process may be influenced by such slow steps as surface diffusion, hydrogen bond breaking, or slow desorption. The improvement of the rate of metal nanoparticle functionalization is then highly desired. In this work, we have described phenomena which are the key factors for the design of biosensors with fabrication of nanoparticle-enhanced sensory film and other applications such as the photodynamic cancer therapy or colorimetric assays for heavy metals. These phenomena relate to the speed of the film formation and modification of the film composition. In the proposed methodology, we have employed a biomolecule, homocysteine (Hcys), as the ligand replacing citrate capping of $AuNP_{5nm}$ and glutathione (GSH) which can act as the moderator for one-step ligand-exchange processes. The ultra-fast functionalization of gold nanoparticles process was monitored using RELS spectroscopy. It proceeds through the nucleation and avalanche growth of ligand-exchange domains in the self-assembled monolayer film on a gold nanoparticle surface (Scheme 2).

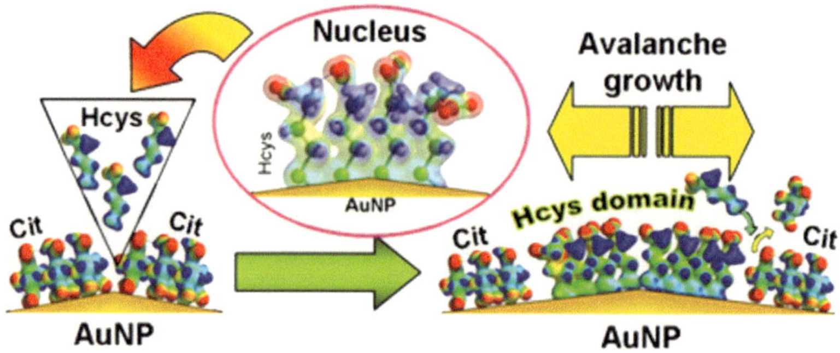

Scheme 2. Schematic view of the hydrogen bonded citrate SAM basal film and the nucleation and growth of a hydrogen bonded Hcys-ligand domain on an edge of a citrate-capped AuNP.

To distinguish between Hcys-dominated AuNP and GSH-dominated AuNP, the pH dependence of RELS was analyzed. By carefully selecting pH, it is possible to keep Hcys in the form of zwitterions, which leads to the AuNP assembly (Figure 6). In solution at pH = 5, we have predominantly zwitterionic Hcys and negatively charged GSH. Therefore, a high RELS intensity can be ascribed to the Hcys-dominated AuNP shells (due to Hcys-induced aggregation of AuNP's) and low RELS intensity to the GSH-dominated AuNP shells (due to repulsions between AuNP's).

The ability to control the SAM composition in the fast ligand-exchange process is the key element to the nanoparticle functionalization. The mechanism of action of the moderator molecules is not well understood but it likely involves the competition for the nucleation sites and/or tuning the exchange processes at ligand-exchange wave-front, i.e. at the perimeter of the growing domains of the incoming ligand. To control the SAM composition in the fast ligand-exchange process, GSH-moderator molecules able to influence the nucleation and growth processes in the short time-scale of the functionalization process have been used. A series of experiments has been performed in which the concentration ratios C_{GSH}/C_{Hcys} were changed in a wide range from 0.002 to 160. In Figure 7, the RELS intensity for 3.8 nM $AuNP_{5nm}$ solutions is plotted vs. C_{Hcys} for different concentration levels of GSH.

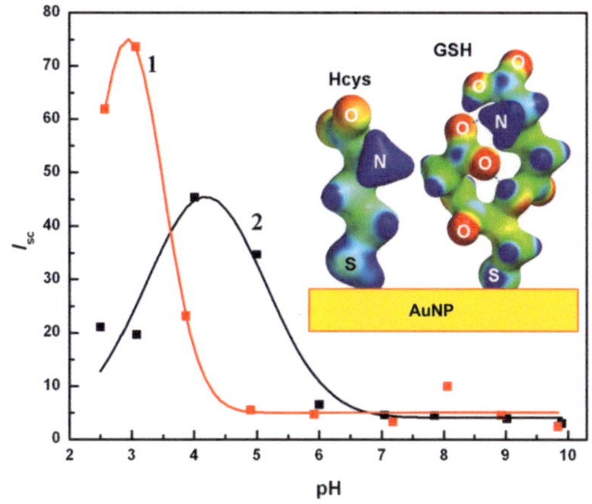

Fig. 6. Dependence of I_{sc} on pH for: (1) 20 μM GSH solutions and (2) 20 μM Hcys solutions; τ = 60s; C_{AuNP} = 3.8 nM; AuNP diameter: 5 nm, C_{Cit} = 0.46 mM.

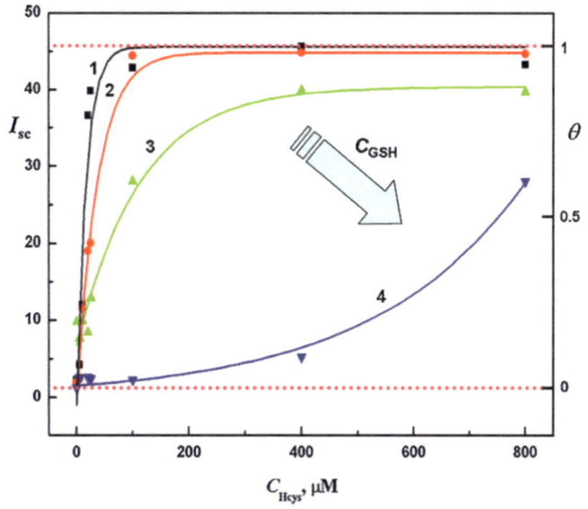

Fig. 7. Tuning the speed of ligand-exchange and SAM shell composition in fast AuNP functionalization; dependence of RELS intensity I_{sc} on C_{Hcys} for different C_{GSH} [μM]: (1) 5, (2) 20, (3) 100, (4) 400; C_{AuNP} = 3.8 nM, citrate buffer, C_{Cit} = 0.46 mM, pH= 5, λ_{ex} = 640 nm, τ = 60 s; all curves are fitted with sigmoidal Boltzmann function.

The average composition of the film is approximately given by:

$$\theta = \frac{(I - I_{\min})}{(I_{\max} - I_{\min})} \tag{5}$$

where θ is the content of the linker ligand (Hcys) in the SAM shell and I_{min}, I_{max} are the minimum and maximum scattering intensities corresponding to AuNP@GSH and AuNP@Hcys, respectively. This dependence enables a quick estimate of the average film composition.

The changes in film composition, are useful in several approaches in sensory film fabrication, such as in the process of: (i) embedding two, or more, different functionalities, (ii) introducing spacers for the attachment of large bioorganic molecules, or (iii) controlling the range of sensor response. On the other hand, no morphological changes in nanoparticle cores are encountered unless the system is heated to higher temperatures, which would result in AuNP core enlargement.

The aggregation of AuNP may also be caused by other factors, such as the addition of higher salt concentrations or injection of small amounts of multivalent metal cations able to coordinate to the ligands of nanoparticle shells, however, neither the salt or metal cations have any chance to replace a SAM film that protects AuNP. The affinity of thiols to a Au surface (Whitesides et al., 2005) enables such thiols as GSH and homocysteine to readily replace citrates from the nanoparticle shell (Lim et al., 2007, Lim et al., 2008, Stobiecka et al., 2010b). While GSH can form intermittently some weakly bound intermediate interparticle linking structures (Stobiecka et al., 2010a), these only help to isolate a citrate ion from its neighbors and remove that citrate from the film.

6. Bio-inspired molecularly-templated polymer films for biomarker detection

The strong affinity observed in host-guest recognition systems in biology, such as the antibody-antigen, receptor-protein, biotin-streptavidin, or DNA-polypeptide, has been widely utilized in designing various biosensors and assays for analytical determination of biomolecules of interest. The recently developed methods for bioengineering of aptamers based on oligonucleotides or polypeptides (Hianik et al., 2007, Tombelli et al., 2005) as ligands mimicking host molecules in biorecognition systems shows that aptamers can be used in sensors for various target (guest) molecules. The bioengineered aptamers provide some advantages over natural host-guest systems, including higher packing density and improved structural flexibility. Another bio-inspired host-guest system studied extensively is based on molecular imprinting of polymer films (Greene et al., 2005, Levit et al., 2002, Perez et al., 2000, Piletsky et al., 2001, Priego-Capote et al., 2008, Yan et al., 2005, Ye et al., 2000) whereby the polymerization of a polymer is carried out in the presence of guest molecules. The latter are then released from the template, e.g. by hydrolysis. The templated polymer films specific toward the target molecules are inexpensive and offer enhanced scalability, flexibility, and processibility. Hence, the molecularly-imprinted polymers are good candidates for sensor miniaturization and the development of microsensor arrays. The templated polymers show recognition properties resembling those found in biological receptors but they are more stable and considerably less expensive than biological systems (Malitesta et al., 2006).

A range of molecularly-imprinted polymer-based sensors have been investigated using different transduction techniques, including: acoustic wave (Kikuchi et al., 2006, Kugimiya et al., 1999, Liang et al., 2000, Matsuguchi et al., 2006, Percival et al., 2001, Tsuru et al., 2006, Yilmaz et al., 1999), potentiometry (Javanbakht et al., 2008), capacitance (Panasyuk et al., 1999), conductometry (Kriz et al., 1996, Sergeyeva et al., 1999), voltammetry (Prasad et al., 2005), colorimetry (Stephenson et al., 2007), surface plasmon spectroscopy (Tokareva et al.,

2006), and fluorescence (Chen et al., 2004, Chen et al., 2006, Jenkins et al., 2001, Moreno-Bondi et al., 2003) detection. Moreover, the molecularly-imprinted polymers can also be utilized for selective solid-phase separation techniques (Mahony et al., 2005, Masque et al., 2001), including electrophoresis and chromatography. Furthermore, it has been found that the analytical signal can often be enhanced by employing nanoparticle labeling of guest molecules (Stobiecka et al., 2009).

The key role in accomplishing the desired target recognition level is played by the synthesis of templated-polymer films. A polymer with appropriate functionalities has to be selected to provide effectively multiple binding sites for a target molecule. Therefore, the target molecules should interact with monomers during the polymerization stage and act as a template around which the polymer grows. Following the release of templating molecules, the high affinity sites should remain in the polymer matrix, constituting the host architecture for supramolecular interactions of the host with the guest molecules. The methods of molecular imprinting mainly utilize a non-covalent imprinting which is more versatile and easier than the covalent imprinting. Various forms of non-covalent binding have been explored, including hydrogen bonding, Van der Waals forces, electrostatic or hydrophobic interactions.

As an example of the design of a molecularly-imprinted sensor film, we describe in this section a sensor for the biomarker of oxidative stress, glutathione. The molecular imprinting of GSH has been performed by electropolymerization of orthophenylenediamine (oPD) in the presence of the target molecules. The templated polymer films of poly(orthophenylenediamine), or PoPD, was formed in situ on a gold-coated quartz crystal resonator wafer (QC/Au) which enabled using the Electrochemical Quartz Crystal Nanobalance (EQCN) for monitoring the polymerization process, as well as for testing the sensor response to the target analyte. The EQCN technique (Hepel, 1999) can serve as a very sensitive technique to monitor minute changes in the film mass and has recently been applied in a variety of systems to study the film growth (Hepel et al., 2002, Stobiecka et al., 2011) and dissolution (Hepel et al., 2006, Hepel et al., 2007), as well as ion dynamics and ion-gating (Hepel, 1996, Hepel et al., 2003) in intercalation process allowing one to distinguish between moving ions on the basis on their molar mass differences.

The design of a GSH-templated polymer film is presented in Figure 8.

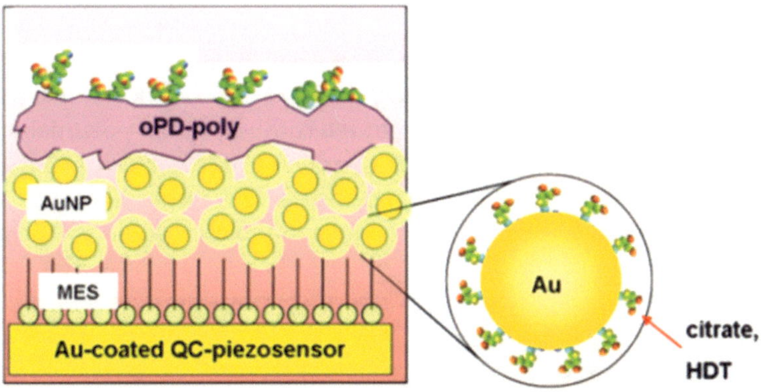

Fig. 8. Schematic of GSH-templated sensor design: GSH embedded in a PoPD film electrode-posited on a layer of AuNP network assembled on a SAM of MES on a Au piezoelectrode.

The sensor, QC/Au/AuNP/PoPD(GSH), was synthesized by direct electropolymerization of oPD in the presence of GSH, on a QC/Au substrate that was coated with a SAM of MES and a layer of HDT-capped AuNP network assembled on top of the SAM. The GSH molecules attached to the polymer surface at the end of the oPD polymerization stage leave impressions in the film which can be utilized for GSH detection. The disassociation of the templating GSH molecules is usually done by hydrolysis of GSH in 0.1-0.5 M NaOH solution.

Typically, the electropolymerization of PoPD is carried out either by successive potential scans from E_1 = 0 to E_2 = +0.8 V and back0020to E_1, or by potential pulses with E_1 = 0 to E_2 = +0.8 V and E_3 = 0, with pulse widths τ_1 = 1 s, τ_2 = 300 s.

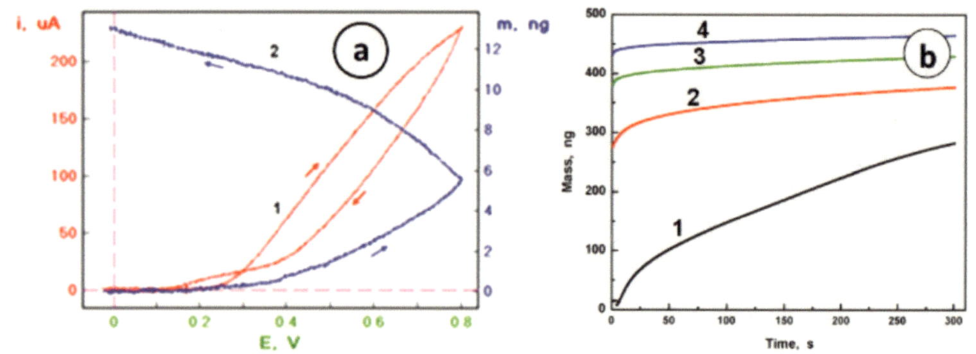

Fig. 9. (a) LSV and EQCN characteristics (first cycle) for a QC/Au electrode in 5 mM oPD + 10 mM GSH in 10 mM phosphate buffer solution: (1) current-potential, (2) mass-potential; v = 100 mV/s; (b) Apparent mass gain recorded in consecutive cycles of a potential-step electropolymerization of a GSH-templated poly(oPD) films from 5 mM oPD solutions containing 10 mM GSH; substrate: QC/Au/MES/AuNP; medium: 10 mM $HClO_4$; potential program: step from E_1 = 0 to E_2 = +0.8 V *vs* Ag/AgCl and back to E_1, pulse duration τ_1 = 1 s, τ_2 = 300 s; curve numbers correspond to the cycle number.

In simultaneous linear potential scan voltammetry (LSV) and nanogravimetry, we have found that the instant of the oPD oxidation is at E = 0.25 V vs. Ag/AgCl, followed by almost linear current increase in the potential range from E = +0.3 to +0.6 V. The apparent mass has been found to increase during the anodic potential scan. Further mass gain is also noted after the potential scan reversal. Moreover, we have found that the mass keeps increasing even after the current cessation at the end of the cathodic-going potential scan, at potentials E < +0.15 V. This clearly indicates on the formation of oPD radicals which are able to attach to the PoPD film after the oPD oxidation has ended. This mechanism is corroborated by the observed low Faradaic efficiency of the polymer formation caused by the diffusion of oPD intermediates and oligomeric radicals out of the electrode surface. The Faradaic efficiency can be investigated using the mass-to-charge analysis using the plots of apparent mass m versus charge Q. The experimental slope, $p_{exp} = \partial m/\partial Q$, is then compared to the theoretical slope p_{th} calculated for a given reaction as follows:

$$m = M\frac{Q}{nF} \tag{6}$$

$$p_{th} = \frac{\partial m}{\partial Q} = \frac{M}{nF} \tag{7}$$

where M is the *reaction molmass* reflecting the molar mass gain or loss of the electrodic film, F is the Faraday constant (F = 96,485 C/equiv) and n is the number of electrons transferred. For the reaction of electro-oxidation of oPD, we have:

$$C_6H_4(NH_2)_2(aq) - 4e^- = [\bullet N\text{-}C_6H_4\text{-}N\bullet] + 4H^+ \tag{8a}$$

$$C_6H_4(NH_2)_2(aq) - 4e^- = [\bullet N\text{-}C_6H_4\text{-}NH\bullet^+] + 3H^+ \tag{8b}$$

$$C_6H_4(NH_2)_2(aq) - 4e^- = [\bullet NH^+\text{-}C_6H_4\text{-}NH^+\bullet] + 2H^+ \tag{8c}$$

$$C_6H_4(NH_2)_2(aq) - 2e^- = [\bullet N\text{-}C_6H_4\text{-}NH_2\bullet] + 2H^+ \tag{8d}$$

oPD *PoPD unit*

where polymer chains with either closed phenazine moieties (8*a*-8*c*) or open phenazine (or quinoid) rings (8*d*) are formed. Assuming that the former dominate, we have the average molmass M_{ave} = 105 g/mol (i.e. the molar mass of species deposited on the electrode minus molar mass of species detached from the electrode surface; M ranges from 104 to 106 depending on the degree of nitrogen protonation) and n = 4. Equations (8) describe the oxidized PoPD units cross-linked to the electrodic polymer film. Under these conditions, the theoretical value of p is: p_{th} = 262 ng/mC (525 ng/mC for reaction (8d)). In comparison to that, the experimental values of p are much lower: p_{exp} = 7.1 ng/mC. This means that a large majority of the oxidized oPD radicals can escape to the solution before being able to bind to the electrode surface and become part of it. The polymerization efficiency does not increase in subsequent potential cycles.

In the potential step experiments, the potential program included 3 stages: E_1 = 0, E_2 = +0.8 V, and E_3 = 0, with pulse widths τ_1 = 1 s, τ_2 = 300 s. Generally, the current decayed monotonically and the apparent mass was increasing from the first moment of the step to E_2, as expected. The total mass increase observed in these experiments was much larger than that in the potential scan experiments and the analysis of p_{exp} indicates that the Faradaic efficiency ε is also higher (p_{exp} = 13.7 ng/mC) although still very low.

The number of PoPD monolayers deposited during the polymerization procedure can be estimated by calculating an equivalent monolayer mass of PoPD. Since the definition of the equivalent monolayer is rather ambiguous because the benzene rings of oPD may not be in plane or stacked parallel to each other in the PoPD (Stobiecka et al., 2009), we define the equivalent PoPD monolayer as a densely packed layer of flat oPD molecules. The calculated surface area for a unit oPD A = 27.1 Å^2 is assumed on the basis of quantum mechanical calculation of the electronic structure of the polymer (Stobiecka et al., 2009). Then, the maximum surface coverage is: Γ = 3.69 × 10^{14} molec/cm^2 and γ = 0.61 nmol/cm^2. The monolayer mass is then: m_{mono} = 65.0 ng/cm^2 and for our quartz resonator: $m_{mono,QC}$ = 16.6 ng/QC. Therefore, in a single potential scan experiment only a fraction of the equivalent PoPD monolayer is being formed.

Recent studies have shown that the polymer is mainly constituted by phenazinic and quinonediimine segments with different protonation levels (Sestrem et al., 2010). The formation of different crosslinks is illustrated in Scheme 3

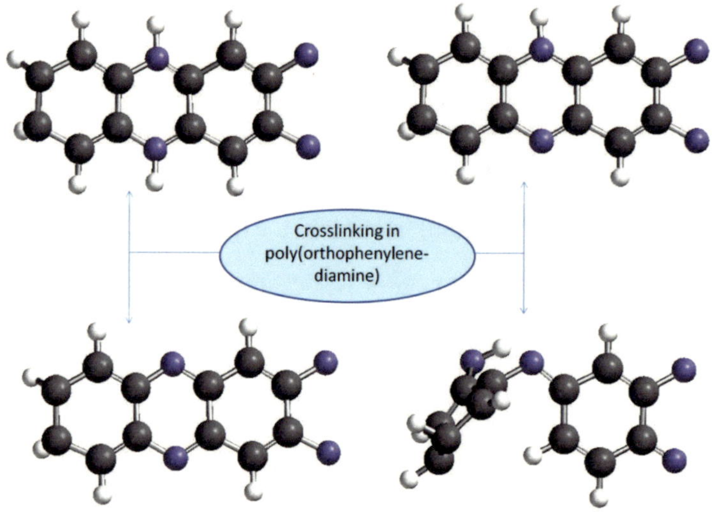

Scheme 3. Crosslinking in PoPD (adapted from (Sestrem et al., 2010)).

These experiments confirm that the GSH-templated films can be grown step by step under different conditions with straightforward control of the film thickness and its conductance by a simple choice of the pulse parameters and the number of applied potential pulses. This method is also faster than the potential scanning method in which only very thin films are obtained.

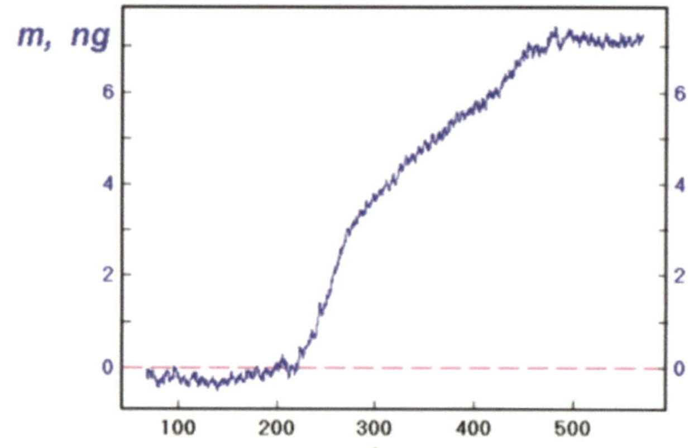

Fig. 10. Apparent mass vs. time response of a GSH-templated poly(oPD) film after injection of a free GSH solution (5 mM).

The process of molecular imprinting of a PoPD(GSH) film synthesized in-situ on a QC/Au/SAM/AuNP substrate is illustrated in Figure 10. The total mass deposited was Δm = 265 ng. After the template removal from the $PoPD_{GSH}$ polymer film, the piezosensor was tested in a solution of 5 mM GSH. Typical time transient recorded upon injection of GSH is presented in Figure 10. The total mass change Δm = 7 ng was observed.

Further improvement of the mass gain can be attained by templating GSH-capped gold nanoparticles in PoPD (Stobiecka et al., 2009). The nanoparticle labeling enhances the nanogravimetric biosensor response because of the larger mass of the AuNP-labeled analyte.

7. Piezoimmunosensors for glutathione

The analysis of biomarkers of oxidative stress, such as glutathione (GSH), glutathione disulfide (GSSG), 3-nitrotyrosine, homocysteine, nonenal, etc., becomes the key factor for preventive treatments (Knoll et al., 2005, Kohen et al., 2002, Malinski et al., 1992, Reddy et al., 2004 , Stobiecka et al., 2009, Stobiecka et al., 2010a). Since the main redox potential maintaining system in eukaryotic cell homeostasis is the GSH/GSSG redox couple (Noble et al., 2005), we have focused on the design of GSH immunosensor.

The pioneering works in developing immunosensors for GSH have been done by Cliffel and coworkers (Gerdon et al., 2005). They have immobilized the anti-GSH antibody on a protein A layer adsorbed nonspecifically on a gold electrode. The response to GSH-conjugates was monitored by recording the oscillation frequency of the quartz piezoresonator substrate. An extensive review of immunosensors including evaluation of instrumental methods has been published by Skladal et al. (Pohanka et al., 2008, Skládal, 2003).

In this work, the immunosensor design is based on the biorecognition principle with an anti-GSH monoclonal antibody immobilized covalently on a AHT basal SAM through a EDC activated reaction. The anti-GSH Ab molecules were immobilized on a thiol SAM via amide bonds between carboxylic groups of the Fc stem of an Ab and amine groups of the thiol. To control nonspecific binding, the electrodes were incubated with 0.001% BSA solution (Scheme 4).

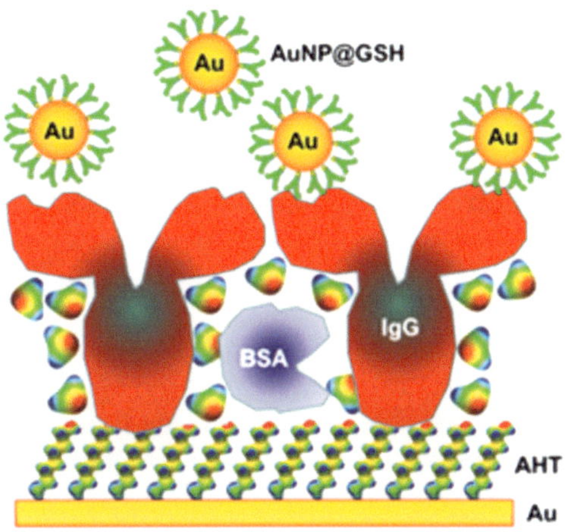

Scheme 4. The design of a nanogravimetric immunosensor for the detection of glutathione-capped AuNP.

The construction of sensory films was carefully monitored by EQCN in each step of the modification of a gold piezoelectrode to confirm binding of molecules and the structure build up on a gold electrode. The resonance frequency response of the AuQC/AHT/Ab_{mono} piezoresonator showed higher affinity towards glutathione-capped gold nanoparticles than to glutathione molecules alone. From the nanogravimetric mass transients, recorded after the injection of 0.95 nM glutathione capped AuNP (Figure 11a), the total resonant frequency shift Δf = 81.45 Hz (Δm = 70.64 ng) was observed. The resonant frequency shift transient, Δf, for a sensory film AHT/Ab_{mono}, formed on a gold-coated quartz crystal piezoresonator, recorded following an injection of 1.25 mM GSH (final concentration) as the analyte was Δf = 22.99 Hz (Δm = 19.94 ng). The lower immunoreactivity of Ab toward GSH alone indicates that GSH itself does not have the sufficient size to induce the very high affinity with Abmono (Amara et al., 1994). In Figure 11b, the apparent mass change vs. AuNP@GSH concentration is presented. The experimental data were fitted by the least-square fitting routine to give a straight line: $\Delta m = a + b\, C_{AuNP@GSH}$, with intercept a = 2.97 ng, slope b = 63.8 ng/nM (the nanoparticle concentration is given in nM) and the standard deviation σ = 6.74 ng. The limit of detection (LOD) for immunosensor, based on the generalized 3σ method is 0.3 nM.

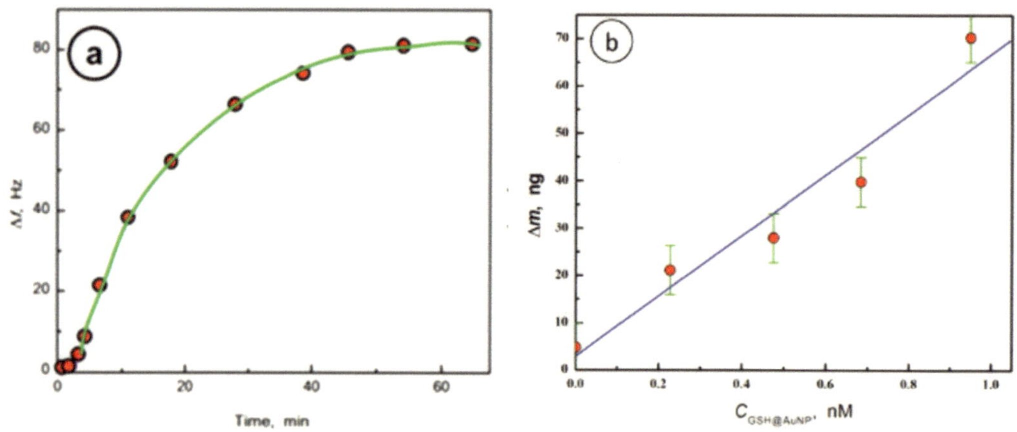

Fig. 11. (a) Resonant frequency transient for a QC/Au/AHT/Ab,BSA piezoimmunosensor recorded after addition of 0.95 nM AuNP@GSH; (b) calibration plot of the apparent mass vs. concentration of AuNP@GSH for a QC/Au/AHT/Ab_{mono} sensor in 50 mM PBS, with surface regeneration in 0.2 M glycine solution, pH = 3, after each test.

8. Label-less redox-probe voltammetric immunosensors

The oxidative stress has been implicated in a wide spectrum of disorders, including cardiovascular and Alzheimer's diseases, accelerates the aging process (Noble et al., 2005), and contributes to the development of autism in children (James et al., 2006). It has also been known that under oxidative stress, serious damage to DNA (formation of 8-oxoguanine, lesions, strand breaks) and to the membrane lipids by overoxidation may occur (Kohen et al., 2002). Therefore, considerable interests in the development of rapid assays for biomarkers of these diseases, such as biological thiols: homocysteine and glutathione have recently surfaced.

We have tested two types of sensors: one with of a positive and one with a negative potential-barrier SAM for the detection of GSH capped AuNP, on the voltammetric signals of ferricyanide $[Fe(CN)6]^{3-}$ redox probes. The anti-GSH antibody molecules were immobilized directly on the short carbon chain thiols (aminohexanethiol or GSH) used for the formation of basal film SAM. The influence of electrostatic interactions in designing sensory films has been well established, including multilayer films with layer-by-layer deposition of oppositely charged polyelectrolytes. In Figure 12, presented are voltammetric characteristics for a ferricyanide redox probe recorded after each step of the sensory film modification.

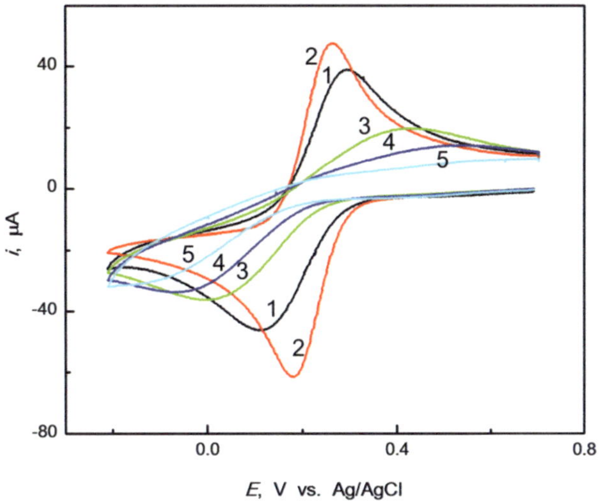

Fig. 12. Cyclic voltammograms for a 1 mM $K_3Fe(CN)_6$ test solution recorded after subsequent steps of the positive potential barrier immunosensor construction: (1) bare gold piezoelectrode and (2-5) gold piezoelectrode after immobilization of successive layers of: (2) 6-amino-1-hexanethiol, (3) monoclonal anti-GSH antibody, (4) bovine serum albumin, (5) glutathione-capped AuNP; v = 100 mV/s.

For a bare gold electrode, a couple of well-developed redox peaks (E_{pc} = 0.111 V and E_{pa} = 0.294 V) was observed (curve 1). The immobilization of AHT on the gold electrode surface results in the increase of the redox marker reaction reversibility (Figure 12, curve 2) since at pH = 7.4 of the test solution, the -NH_2 groups of a AHT film are protonated and attract negatively charged ferricyanide ions. This interaction results in a dramatic decrease of the peak separation of the redox probe, from ΔE = 183 mV for a bare gold electrode, to ΔE = 84 mV for a AuQC/AHT electrode. Thus, the strong electrostatic effect overcomes the thiol-SAM blocking effect leading to the enhancement of the redox probe voltammetric signal. After the immobilization of antibody, the electron transfer of $Fe(CN)_6{}^{3-/4-}$ couple has been found to decrease due to the formation of a blocking protein layer, reduced surface accessibility, and steric hindrance. Considerable increase of the redox peak separation, from ΔE = 84 mV in the absence of IgG, to ΔE = 408 mV, was observed. The antibody molecules are negatively charged at physiological pH since their isoelectric point (pI) is within the interval 4.6-7.2 (Brynda, 2006). Therefore, in addition to the blocking effect, the repulsion of negatively charged redox marker should occur. The GSH recognition process taking place during the incubation of the immunosensor in glutathione-capped AuNP solution leads to the decrease in the redox reaction reversibility of the ferricyanide probe (Figure 12, curve 5). This is consistent with the expected increase of the accumulation of negative charge brought in with GSH-capped AuNP. On the other hand, this behavior contrasts with the expectation of an increased redox activity of a sensor with added metal nanoparticle layer, observed in other systems. The observed effect is then largely dominated by the electrostatic interactions between the probe ions and GSH-capped AuNP bound to the anti-GSH antibody.

The testing of negative potential-barrier immunosensors shows generally weaker responses during the sensory film construction than those observed for positive potential-barrier films (Figure 13).

The GSH-SAM was used as the supporting film for the attachment of an antibody. After forming the GSH-SAM on a gold electrode, the repulsion of $[Fe(CN)_6]^{3-/4-}$ ions from the film was observed and the peak separation in the redox probe voltammetric characteristics increased from ΔE_p = 115 mV for bare gold electrode to ΔE_p = 294 mV for GSH-modified gold electrode. The attachment of an antibody counteracts this behavior and results in an increase of the redox response of the electroactive marker and a decrease in the peak separation for ferricyanide ions to ΔE = 214 mV. The addition of an analyte, GSH-capped AuNP, leads to further increase in the marker signal and a decrease in the peak separation for ferricyanide ions to ΔE = 188 mV. The increase of the ferricyanide probe signal after the immobilization of IgG is expected since a part of the negatively charged GSH-SAM underlayer is covered by IgG which is positively charged on top of the Fab arms thus enhancing the interactions of the sensor with the marker ions. However, the change of the probe signal upon binding the GSH-capped AuNP cannot be explained on the ground of electrostatic interactions since the expected change would be a decrease of the signal due to repulsions between AuNP@GSH and ferricyanide ions, which is not observed. Most likely, the effect of gold nanoparticle addition to the film is playing the dominant role. Therefore, the presence of the interacting conductive Au spheres with coupled surface plasmon oscillations is likely to act as to increase the charge transfer rate of the redox probe ions. The control experiments carried out using sensors without Ab as the recognition layer show no significant changes in the ferricyanide redox probe signal after addition of glutathione-capped gold nanoparticles. They have shown that the glutathione-capped gold nanoparticles can penetrate the blocking BSA film, increasing the conduction pathways and promoting the electron transfer between the redox marker and electrode surface. It is evident that the immobilization of antibody onto the surface of a gold electrode causes a blocking effect and hinders the electron transfer process of the marker ions (Stobiecka et al., 2011).

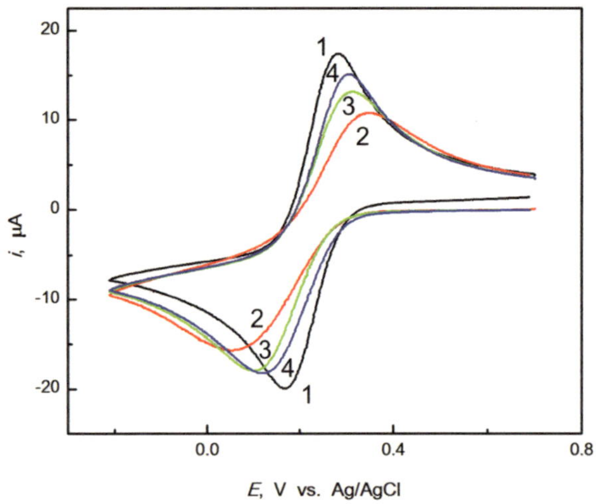

Fig. 13. Cyclic voltammograms of 1 mM $K_3Fe(CN)_6$ in 1 M KNO_3 solution for: (1) bare gold piezoelectrode and (2-4) gold piezoelectrode after immobilization of successive layers: (2) 5 mM glutathione (AuQC/GSH), (3) polyclonal rabbit anti-GSH antibody (AuQC/GSH/Ab_{poly}), (4) glutathione-capped AuNP (AuQC/GSH/Ab_{poly}/AuNP-GSH).

9. Microsensor arrays

Although the accurate advanced instrumental techniques can be used for the analysis of glutathione oxidative stress biomarker (Chiang et al., 2010), there is a need for the development of inexpensive, field-deployable analytical platforms for disease screening and protection against environmental exposure (Noble et al., 2005),(James et al., 2006).
The application of microsensors for screening of biomarkers of oxidative stress has been explored. The responses of sensors operating in the form of a microsensor array have been analyzed by an artificial neural network. The design of microsensor arrays developed in this work is presented in Figure 14. Each of the microsensors consisted of interdigitated electrodes and one reference electrode. The entire chip surface was isolated with the exception of small exposed areas for contact with electrolyte. The sensors were arranged in a group of six sensors in one chip. One of the electrodes of each interdigitated pair was connected to the common and the other had an independent connection. This arrangement enabled measurements of voltammetric characteristics, as well as monitoring of lateral conductance independently in each sensory film with reduced number of interconnections. The experimental setup was configured for the use of a single counter electrode and a single reference electrode reducing the number of electrodes for a six-cell array chip from 18 to 8.

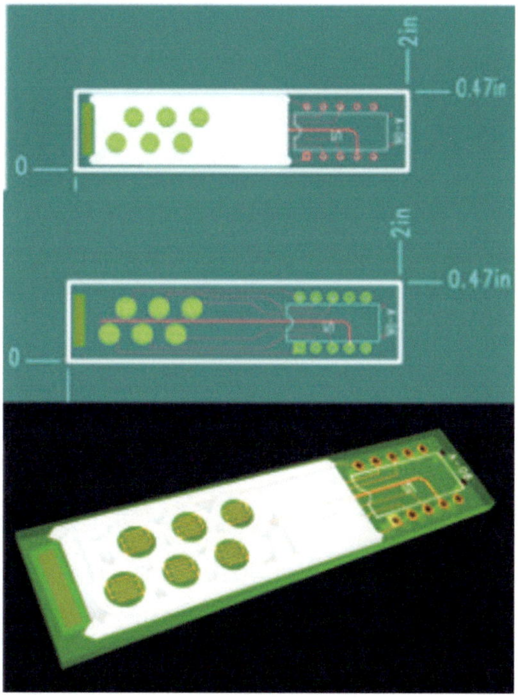

Fig. 14. Design of a microsensor array with pairs of interdigitated electrodes.

In the detection of low level analyte signals superimposed on varying matrix background, the calibration curves have to be constantly adjusted. Also, there are always interfering species which influence the analytical signal. To solve these problems, we have explored the use of artificial neural networks (ANN) that could be designed for a set of input sensors having different responses to the changing matrix, the analyte, and interferences.

The model ANN considered for the analysis of our sensor-array outputs consisted of a basic 4-layer Hopfield neural net presented in Figure 15. The analysis of incoming signals at each node *j* was accomplished using the logistic activation function of the form:

$$g(s_j) = \frac{1}{1+\exp(-s_j)} \tag{9}$$

where s_j is the sum of inputs to the node *j*:

$$s_j = \sum_{i=1}^{n} w_{ij} y_j + \theta_j \tag{10}$$

where w_{ij} is the weight of the *j*-node connection to the *i*-node in previous layer and θ_j is the bias.

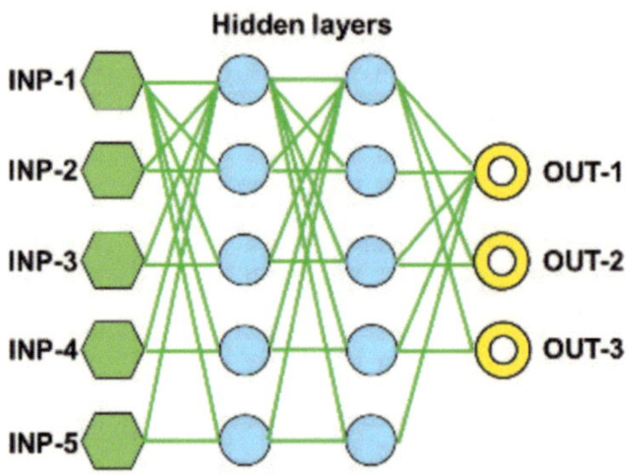

Fig. 15. Scheme of a neural network with input nodes, two hidden layers and an output layer; complete set of connections shown only for the first row of nodes for clarity.

The network was trained using Hopfield backpropagation routines. The artificial neural network approach enables adjusting the network responses to different types of samples, with different background matrix and interferences.
In future developments, the use of microsensor arrays and microfluids will help designing robust and inexpensive point-of-care deployable sensor arrays for oxidative stress biomarkers monitoring.

10. Conclusions

We have demonstrated that RELS and UV-Vis spectroscopy can provide a wealth of information about the interactions of biomarkers of the oxidative stress with gold nanoparticles (AuNP) and can be applied to monitor the ligand-exchange processes followed by AuNP assembly. The interactions of small biomolecules, such as glutathione, homocysteine, or nitrotyrosine with multifunctional gold nanoparticles are important in view of novel biomedical applications of nanoparticles for diagnostic and therapeutic purposes, as well as for the development of biosensors with metal nanoparticle-enhanced responsiveness. The potential application of AuNP in cancer treatment involves targeted drug delivery and photodynamic therapy (PDT). GSH and Hcys interact strongly with the monolayer-protected gold nanoparticles through the thiolate bonding results in an easy

replacement of a self-assembled protecting monolayer on a core-shell gold nanoparticle with the biomarker SAM. By carefully controlling the solution pH, it is possible to fine-tune the biomarker-induced nanoparticle assembly mediated by interparticle zwitterionic interactions and hydrogen bonding. The fine-tuning of the film composition is achieved by utilizing moderator molecules able to control the composition of the monolayer-shell. This process is based on a new paradigm of the ligand-exchange process through the nucleation and growth of 2D ligand domains. The functionalized gold nanoparticles have also been shown to enhance the design of molecularly-templated conductive polymer films for the detection of GSH. The molecular imprinting technique can be applied in polymer sensor designs based on biorecognition principles with piezoelectric transduction. We have also demonstrated that a buried potential barrier, introduced to an immunoglobulin-based sensory film, results in the improvement of voltammetric signals of a redox ion probe. The tests performed with monoclonal anti-glutathione antibody-based sensors using ferricyanide ion probe have shown stronger sensor response to the layer components for films with buried positive potential barrier than for films with negative barrier.
Novel sensing platforms have been explored for the detection of oxidative stress biomarkers. New microsensor arrays have been developed and tested for possible wide scale use in screening autistic children for GSH depletion which has been found to be associated with some phenotype sensitivity to develop autism. The artificial neural network protocol designed for analysis of microsensor array signals has been employed for the assessment of GSH level testing for synthetic solutions and plasma samples of autistic children.

11. Acknowledgement

This work was supported by the U.S. DoD Research Program "Idea", Grant No. AS-73218.

12. References

Alivisatos, A.P.; Johnsson, K.P.; Peng, X.; Wilson, T.E.; Loweth, C.J.; Bruchez, J.M.P. & Schultz, P.G. (1996). Organization of 'Nanocrystal Molecules' Using DNA." Nature, Vol.382, pp. 609-611.

Almazan, G.; Liu, H.N.; Khorchid, A.; Sundararajan, S.; Martinez-Bermudez, A.K. & Chemtob, S. (2000). Exposure of developing oligodendrocytes to cadmium causes HSP72 induction, free radical generation, reduction in glutathione levels, and cell death. Free Radical Bio Med, Vol.29, pp. 858-869.

Alvarez, M.M.; Khoury, J.T.; Schaaff, T.G.; Shafigullin, M.N.; Vezmar, I. & Whetten, R.L. (1997). Optical absorption spectra of nanocrystal gold molecules. J. Phys. Chem. B, Vol.101, pp. 3706-3712.

Amara, A.; Coussemacq, M. & Geffard, M. (1994). Antibodies to reduced glutathione. Brain Res., Vol.659, pp. 237-242.

Bain, C.D.; Evall, J. & Whitesides, G.M. (1989). Formation of monolayers by the coadsorption of thiols on gold: variation in the head group, tail group, and solvent. J. Am. Chem. Soc., Vol.111, pp. 7155-7164.

Barbas, J.; Ellis, W.R.; Santhanagopalan, V.; Blaszczynski, M. & Winge, D.R. (1992). Conversion in the peptides coating cadmium:sulfide crystallites in *Candida glabrata*. J Inorg Biochem, Vol.48, pp. 95-105.

Beard, K.M.; Shangari, N.; Wu, B. & O'Brien, P.J. (2003). Metabolism, not autoxidation, plays a role in alpha-oxoaldehyde- and reducing sugar-induced erythrocyte GSH depletion: relevance for diabetes mellitus. Mol. Cell. Biochem, Vol.252, pp. 331-338.

Bernard, S.; Enayati, A.; Redwood, L.; Roger, H. & Binstock, T. (2001). Autism: a novel form of mercury poisoning. Med Hypotheses, Vol.56, pp. 462-471.

Boushey, C.J.; Beresford, S.A.A.; Omenn, G.S. & Motulsky, A.G. (1995). A quantitative assessment of plasma homocysteine as a risk factor for vascular disease. Probable benefits of increasing folic acid intake. JAMA, Vol.274, pp. 1049-1057.

Brioude, A.; Jiang, X.C. & Pileni, M.P. (2005). Optical properties of gold nanorods: DDA simulations supported by experiments. J. Phys. Chem. B, Vol.109, pp. 13138-13142.

Brynda, E. (2006). Methods for attachment of antibodies onto optical biosensors, In: Optical Chemical Sensors, F. Baldini, (Eds), 387–401, Springer.

Carlo, M.D. & Loeser, R.F. (2003). Increased oxidative stress with aging reduces chondrocyte survival: correlation with intracellular glutathione levels. Arthritis Rheum, Vol.48, pp. 3419-3430.

Carmel, R. & Jacobsen, D.W. (2001). Homocysteine in Health and Disease, Cambridge, U.K.

Chen, Y.-C.; Brazier, J.J.; Yan, M.; Bargo, P.R. & Prahl, S.A. (2004). Fluorescence-based optical sensor design for molecularly imprinted polymers. Sensor Actuator B, Vol.102, pp. 107-116.

Chen, Y.-C.; Wang, Z.; Yan, M. & Prahl, S.A. (2006). Fluorescence anisotropy studies of molecularly imprinted polymers. Luminescence, Vol.21, pp. 7-14.

Chiang, C.-K.; Lin, Y.-W.; Chen, W.-T. & Chang, H.-T. (2010). Accurate quantitation of glutathione in cell lysates through surface-assisted laser desorption/ionization mass spectrometry using gold nanoparticles. Nanomedicine: Nanotechnology, Biology, and Medicine, Vol.6, pp. 530-537.

Clark-Taylor, T. & Clark-Taylor, B.E. (2004). Is autism a disorder of fatty acid metabolism? Possible dysfunction of mitochondrial β-oxidation by long chain acyl-CoA dehydrogenase Med Hypotheses, Vol.62, pp. 970-975.

Clarkson, T.W. (1992). Mercury: Major Issues in Environmental Health. Environ Health Persp, Vol.100, pp. 31-38.

Dameron, C.T.; Reese, R.N.; Mehra, R.K.; Kortan, A.R.; Carroll, P.J.; Steigerwald, M.L.; Brus, L.E. & Winge, D.R. (1989). Biosynthesis of cadmium sulphide quantum semiconductor crystallites. Nature, Vol.338, pp. 596-597.

Draine, B.T. & Flatau, P.J. (1994). Discrete-dipole approximation for scattering calculations. J. Opt. Soc. Am. A, Vol.11, pp. 1491-1499.

Droge, W. (2002). Free radicals inthe physiologic control of cell function. Physiol. Rev., Vol.82, pp. 47-95.

Elghanian, R.; Storhoff, J.J.; Mucic, R.C.; Letsinger, R.L. & Mirkin, C.A. (1997). Selective colorimetric detection of polynucleotides based on the distance-dependent optical properties of gold nanoparticles. Science, Vol.277, pp. 1078-1081.

Etchegoin, P.G.; Ru, E.C.L. & Meyer, M. (2006). An analytic model for the optical properties of gold. J Chem Phys, Vol.125, pp. 164705-1-164705-3.

Gerdon, A.E.; Wright, D.W. & Cliffel, D.E. (2005). Quartz Crystal Microbalance Detection of Glutathione-Protected Nanoclusters Using Antibody Recognition. Anal. Chem., Vol.77, pp. 304-310.

Gonzales, A.L. & Noguez, C. (2007). Influence of Morphology on the Optical Properties of Metal Nanoparticles. J Comput Theor Nanos, Vol.4, pp. 231-238.

Graham, I.M.; Daly, L.E.; Refsum, H.M.; Robinson, K.; Brattström, L.E.; Ueland, P.M.; Palma-Reis, R.J.; Boers, G.H.J.; Sheahan, R.G.; Israelsson, B.; Uiterwaal, C.S.; Meleady, R.; McMaster, D.; Verhoef, P.; Witteman, J.; Rubba, P.; Bellet, H.; Wautrecht, J.C.; Valk, H.W.d.; Lúis, A.C.S.; Parrot-Roulaud, F.M.; Tan, K.S.; Higgins, I.; Garcon, D.; Medrano, M.J.; Candito, M.; Evans, A.E. & Andria, G. (1997). Plasma homocysteine as a risk factor for vascular disease: the European concerted action project. JAMA, Vol.277, pp. 1775-1781.

Greene, N.T. & Shimizu, K.D. (2005). Colorimetric Molecularly Imprinted Polymer Sensor Array using Dye Displacement. J. Am. Chem. Soc., Vol.127, pp. 5695-5700.

Hepel, M. (1996). Composite polypyrrole films switchable between the anion-and cation-exchanger states. Electrochim. Acta, Vol.41, pp. 63-76.

Hepel, M. (1999). Electrode-Solution Interface Studied with Electrochemical Quartz Crystal Nanobalance In: Interfacial Electrochemistry. Theory, Experiment and Applications, A. Wieckowski, (Eds), 599-630, Marcel Dekker, Inc., New York.

Hepel, M. & Scendo, M. (2002). Kinetics of CuEtX film formation on copper piezoelectrodes. J. Electroanal. Chem., Vol.538-539, pp. 121-132.

Hepel, M. & Tewksbury, E. (2003). Ion-gating phenomena of self-assembling glutathione films on gold piezoelectrodes. J. Electroanal. Chem., Vol.552, pp. 291-305.

Hepel, M.; Kumarihamy, I. & Zhong, C.J. (2006). Nanoporous TiO_2-supported bimetallic catalysts for methanol oxidation in acidic media. Electrochem. Commun., Vol.8, pp. 1439-1444.

Hepel, M.; Dela, I.; Hepel, T.; Luo, J. & Zhong, C.J. (2007). Novel dynamic effects in electrocatalysis of methanol oxidation on supported nanoporous TiO_2 bimetallic nanocatalysts. Electrochim. Acta, Vol.52, pp. 5529-5547.

Hianik, T.; Ostatna, V.; Sonlajtnerova, M. & Grman, I. (2007). Influence of ionic strength, pH and aptamer configuration for binding affinity to thrombin. Bioelectrochem, Vol.70, pp. 127-133.

Hostetler, M.J.; Wingate, J.E.; Zhong, C.J.; Harris, J.E.; Vachet, R.W.; Clark, M.R.; Londono, J.D.; Green, S.J.; Stokes, J.J.; Wignall, G.D.; Glish, J.L.; Porter, M.D.; Evans, N.D. & Murray, R.W. (1998). Alkanethiolate gold cluster molecules with core diameters from 1.5 to 5.2 nm: core and monolayer properties as a function of core size. Langmuir, Vol.14, pp. 17-30.

Hostetler, M.J.; Templeton, A.C. & Murray, R.W. (1999). Dynamics of place-exchange reactions on monolayer-protected gold cluster molecule. Langmuir, Vol.15, pp. 3782-3789.

Inouhe, M. (2005). Phytochelatins. Braz. J. Plant Physiol., Vol.17, pp. 65-78.

Jacobsen, D.W. (2000). Hyperhomocysteinemia and Oxidative Stress : Time for a Reality Check? Arterioscler. Thromb. Vasc. Biol., Vol.20, pp. 1182-1184.

Jain, P.K.; Lee, K.S.; El-Sayed, I.H. & El-Sayed, M.A. (2006). Calculated Absorption and Scattering Properties of Gold Nanoparticles of Different Size, Shape, and Composition: Applications in Biological Imaging and Biomedicine. J. Phys. Chem. B, Vol.110, pp. 7238-7248.

James, S.J.; Melnyk, S.; Jernigan, S.; Cleves, M.A.; Halsted, C.H.; Wong, D.J.; Cutler, P.; Bock, K.; Boris, M.; Bradstreet, J.J.; Baker, S.M. & Gaylor, D.W. (2006). Metabolic endophenotype and related genotypes are associated with oxidative stress in children with autism. Am J Med Genet B Neuropsychiatr Genet., Vol.141B, pp. 947-956.

Javanbakht, M.; Fard, S.E.; Mohammadi, A.; Abdouss, M.; Ganjali, M.R.; Norouzi, P. & Safaraliee, L. (2008). Molecularly imprinted polymer based potentiometric sensor for the determination of hydroxyzine in tablets and biological fluids. Anal. Chim. Acta, Vol.612, pp. 65-74.

Jenkins, A.L.; Yin, R. & Jensen, J.L. (2001). Molecularly imprinted polymer sensors for pesticide and insecticide detection in water. Analyst, Vol.126, pp. 798-802.

Johnson, P.B. & Christy, R.W. (1972). Optical Constants of the Noble Metals. Phys. Rev. B, Vol.6, pp. 4370-4379.

Kamat, P.V. (2002). Photophysical, photochemical and photocatalytic aspects of metal nanoparticles. J. Phys. Chem. B, Vol.106, pp. 7729-7744.

Kariuki, N.N.; Luo, J.; Han, L.; Maye, M.M.; Moussa, L.; Patterson, M.; Lin, Y.; Engelhard, M.H. & Zhong, C.J. (2004). Nanoparticle-structured ligand framework as electrode interfaces. Electroanalysis, Vol.16, pp. 120-126.

Kelly, K.L.; Coronado, E.; Zhao, L.L. & Schatz, G.C. (2003). The Optical Properties of Metal Nanoparticles: The Influence of Size, Shape, and Dielectric Environment. J. Phys. Chem. B, Vol.107, pp. 668-677.

Kikuchi, M.; Tsuru, N. & Shiratori, S. (2006). Recognition of terpenes using molecular imprinted polymer coated quartz crystal microbalance in air phase Sci Technol Adv Mat, Vol.7, pp. 156–161.

Knoll, N.; Ruhe, C.; Veeriah, S.; Sauer, J.; Glei, M.; Gallagher, E.P. & Pool-Zobel, B.L. (2005). Genotoxicity of 4-hydroxy-2-nonenal in human colon tumor cells is associated with cellular levels of glutathione and the modulation of glutathione S-transferase A4 expression by butyrate. Toxicol Sci, Vol.86, pp. 27-35.

Kohen, R. & Nyska, A. (2002). Oxidation of Biological Systems: Oxidative Stress Phenomena, Antioxidants, Redox Reactions, and Methods for Their Quantification. Toxicol Pathol, Vol.30, pp. 620-650.

Kooij, E.S. & Poelsema, B. (2006). Shape and size effects in the optical properties of metallic nanorods. Phys. Chem. Chem. Phys, Vol.8, pp. 3349-3357.

Kriz, D.; Kempe, M. & Mosbach, K. (1996). Introduction of molecularly imprinted polymers as recognition elements in conductometric chemical sensors. Sensor Actuator B, Vol.33, pp. 178-181.

Kugimiya, A. & Takeuchi, T. (1999). Molecularly Imprinted Polymer-Coated Quartz Crystal Microbalance for Detection of Biological Hormone. Electroanalysis, Vol.11, pp. 1158-1160.

Lee, K.S. & El-Sayed, M.A. (2005). Dependence of the Enhanced Optical Scattering Efficiency Relative to That of Absorption for Gold Metal Nanorods on Aspect Ratio, Size, End-Cap Shape, and Medium Refractive Index. J. Phys. Chem. B, Vol.109, pp. 20331-20338.

Lee, K.S. & El-Sayed, M.A. (2006). Gold and Silver Nanoparticles in Sensing and Imaging: Sensitivity of Plasmon Response to Size, Shape, and Metal Composition. J. Phys. Chem. B, Vol.110, pp. 19220-19225.

Lentz, S.R. & Haynes, W.G. (2004). Homocysteine: Is it a clinically important cardiovascular risk factor? Clev Clin J Med, Vol.71, pp. 729-734.

Levit, N.; Pestov, D. & Tepper, G. (2002). High surface area polymer coatings for SAW-based chemical sensor applications. Sensors and Actuators B, Vol.82, pp. 241-249.

Li, F. & Zu, Y. (2004). Effect of Nonionic Fluorosurfactant on the Electrogenerated Chemiluminescence of the Tris(2,2′-bipyridine)ruthenium(II)/Tri-n-propylamine

System: Lower Oxidation Potential and Higher Emission Intensity. Anal. Chem., Vol.76, pp. 1768-1772.
Liang, C.; Peng, H.; Nie, L. & Yao, S. (2000). Bulk acoustic wave sensor for herbicide assay based on molecularly imprinted polymer Fresenius' J. Anal. Chem, Vol.367, pp. 551-555.
Lim, I.I.S.; Ip, W.; Crew, E.; Njoki, P.N.; Mott, D.; Zhong, C.J.; Pan, Y. & Zhou, S. (2007). Homocysteine-mediated reactivity and assembly of gold nanoparticles. Langmuir, Vol.23, pp. 826-833.
Lim, I.I.S.; Mott, D.; Ip, W.; Njoki, P.N.; Pan, Y.; Zhou, S. & Zhong, C.J. (2008). Interparticle interactions of glutathione mediated assembly of gold nanoparticles. Langmuir, Vol.24, pp. 8857-8863.
Lim, S.I. & Zhong, C.J. (2009). Molelucarly Mediated Processing and Assembly of Nanoparticles: Exploring the Interparticle Interactions and Structures. Accounts of chemical research, Vol.42, pp. 798-808.
Link, S. & El-Sayed, M.A. (1999a). Spectral properties and relaxation dynamics of surface plasmon electronic oscillations in gold and silver nanodots and nanorods. J. Phys. Chem. B, Vol.103, pp. 8410-8426.
Link, S.; Mohamed, M.B. & El-Sayed, M.A. (1999b). Simulation of the Optical Absorption Spectra of Gold Nanorods as a Function of Their Aspect Ratio and the Effect of the Medium Dielectric Constant. J. Phys. Chem. B, Vol.103, pp. 3073-3077.
Mahony, J.O.; Nolan, K.; Smyth, M.R. & Mizaikoff, B. (2005). Molecularly imprinted polymers—potential and challenges in analytical chemistry. Anal Chim Acta, Vol.534, pp. 31-39.
Malinski, T. & Taha, Z. (1992). Nitric oxide release from a single cell measured in situ by a porphyrinic-based microsensor. Nature, Vol.358, pp. 676-678.
Malitesta, C.; Picca, R.A.; Ciccarella, G.; Sgobba, V. & Brattoli, M. (2006). Synthesis of a Molecularly Imprinted Polymer for Dioxin. Sensors, Vol.6, pp. 915-924.
Masque, N.; Marce, R.M. & Borrull, F. (2001). Molecularly imprinted polymers: new tailor-made materials for selective solid-phase extraction. Trends Anal. Chem, Vol.20, pp. 477-486.
Matsuguchi, M. & Uno, T. (2006). Molecular imprinting strategy for solvent molecules and its application for QCM-based VOC vapor sensing. Sensor Actuator B, Vol.113, pp. 94-99.
Maye, M.M.; Lim, I.I.S.; Luo, J.; Rab, Z.; Rabinovich, D.; Liu, T. & Zhong, C.J. (2005). Mediator-Template Assembly of Nanoparticles. J. Am. Chem. Soc., Vol.127, pp. 1519-1529.
Mehra, R.K. & Winge, D.R. (1991). Metal ion resistance in fungi: molecular mechanisms and their regulated expression. J. Cell. Biochem., Vol.45, pp. 30-40.
Mills, J.L.; Scott, J.M.; Kirke, P.N.; McPartlin, J.M.; Conley, M.R.; Weir, D.G.; Molloy, A.M. & Lee, Y.J. (1996). Homocysteine and neural tube defects. J Nutr, Vol.126, pp. 756S-760S.
Mishchenko, M.; Travis, L.D. & Lacis, A.A. (2002). Scattering, Absorption, and Emission of Light by Small Particles, Cambridge.
Moreno-Bondi, M.C.; Benito-Pena, E.; San-Vicente, B.; Navarro-Villoslada, F.; Leon, M.E.d.; Orellana, G.; Aparicio, S.; Molina, J.; Kempe, M. & Fiaccabrino, G.C. (2003). Molecularly imprinted polymers as selective recognition elements for optical

sensors based on fluorescent measurements. Digest of Technical Papers. Transducers '03 Boston, 12th International Conference on Solid-State Sensors, Actuators and Microsystems Vol.2, pp. 975-978.

Noble, M.; Mayer-Proschel, M. & Proschel, C. (2005). Redox Regulation of Precursor Cell Function: Insights and Paradoxes. Antioxid Redox Sign, Vol. 7, pp. 1456-1467

Panasyuk, T.L.; Mirsky, V.M.; Piletsky, S.A. & Wolfbeis, O.S. (1999). Electropolymerized Molecularly Imprinted Polymers as Receptor Layers in Capacitive Chemical Sensors. Anal. Chem., Vol.71, pp. 4609-4613.

Park, S.J.; Taton, T.A. & Mirkin, C.A. (2002). Array-based electrical detection of DNA with nanoparticle probe. Science, Vol.295, pp. 1503-1506

Percival, C.J.; Stanley, S.; Galle, N.; Braihwaite, A.; Newton, M.I.; McHale, G. & Hayes, W. (2001). Molecular-Imprinted, Polymer-Coated Quartz Crystal Microbalances for the Detection of Terpenes. Anal. Chem., Vol.73, pp. 4225-4228.

Perez-Juste, J.; Pastoriza-Santos, I.; Liz-Marzan, L.M. & Mulvaney, P. (2005). Gold nanorods: Synthesis, characterization and applications. Coordin Chem Rev, Vol.249, pp. 1870–1901.

Perez, N.; Whitcombe, M.J. & Vulfson, E.N. (2000). Molecularly imprinted nanoparticles prepared by core-shell emulsion polymerization. J. App. Polym. Sci, Vol.77, pp. 1851-1859.

Piletsky, S.A.; Subrahmanyam, S. & Turner, A.P.F. (2001). Application of molecularly imprinted polymers in sensors for the environment and biotechnology. Sensor Rev, Vol.21, pp. 292 - 296.

Ping, Y.; Hanson, D.; Koslow, I.; Ogitsu, T.; Prendergast, O.; Schwegler, E.; Collins, G. & Ng, A. (2008). Dielectric function of warm dense gold. Phys. Plasmas, Vol.15, pp. 56303-056303-7.

Pohanka, M. & Skládal, P. (2008). Electrochemical biosensors – principles and applications. J. Appl. Biomed., Vol.6, pp. 57-64.

Polidoro, G.; Ilio, C.D.; Arduini, A.; Rovere, G.L. & Federici, G. (1984). Superoxide dismutase, reduced glutathione and TBA-reactive products in erythrocytes of patients with multiple sclerosis. Int. J. Biochem, Vol.16, pp. 505-509.

Prasad, B.B. & Lakshmi, D. (2005). Barbituric Acid Sensor Based on Molecularly Imprinted Polymer- Modified Hanging Mercury Drop Electrode. Electroanalysis, Vol.17, pp. 1260-1268.

Prescott, S.W. & Mulvaney, P. (2006). Gold nanorod extinction spectra. J. Appl. Phys. , Vol.99, pp. 123504.

Priego-Capote, F.; L.Ye; Shakil, S.; Shamsi, S.A. & Nilsson, S. (2008). Monoclonal Behavior of Molecularly Imprinted Polymer Nanoparticles in Capillary Electrochromatography. Anal. Chem., Vol.80, pp. 2881-2887.

Reddy, S. & Bradley, J. (2004). Immunohistochemical Demonstration of Nitrotyrosine, a Biomarker of Oxidative Stress, in Islet Cells of the NOD Mouse. Ann. N. Y. Acad. Sci., Vol.1037, pp. 199-202.

Refsum, H.; Ueland, P.M.; Nygard, O. & Vollset, S.E. (1989). Homocysteine and cardiovascular disease. Annu Rev Med, Vol.49, pp. 31-62.

Repetto, M.; Reides, C.; Carretero, M.L.G.; Costa, M.; Griemberg, G. & Llesuy, S. (1996). Oxidative stress in blood of HIV infected patients. Clin. Chim. Acta, Vol.255, pp. 107-117.

Reynolds, R.A.; Mirkin, C.A. & Letsinger, R.L. (2000). Homogeneous, nanoparticle-based quantitative colorimetric detection of oligonucleotides. J. Am. Chem. Soc., Vol.122, pp. 3795-3796.

Sergeyeva, T.A.; Piletsky, S.A.; Panasyuk, T.L.; El'skaya, A.V.; Brovko, A.A.; Slinchenko, E.A. & Sergeeva, L.M. (1999). Conductimetric sensor for atrazine detection based on molecularly imprinted polymer membranes. Analyst, Vol.124, pp. 331-334.

Seshadri, S.; Beiser, A.; Selhub, J.; Jaques, P.F.; Rosenberg, I.H.; D'Agostino, R.B.; Wilson, P.W. & Wolf, P.A. (2002). Plasma homocysteine as a risk factor for dementia and Alzheimer's disease. NEJM, Vol.346, pp. 476-483.

Sestrem, R.H.; Ferreira, D.C.; Landers, R.; Temperini, M.L.A. & Nascimento, G.M.d. (2010). Synthesis and spectroscopic characterization of polymer and oligomers of ortho-phenylenediamine. Eur Polym J, Vol.46, pp. 484-493.

Skládal, P. (2003). Piezoelectric quartz crystal sensors applied for bioanalytical assays and characterization of affinity interactions. J. Brazil. Chem. Soc., Vol.14, pp. 491-502.

Stephenson, C.J. & Shimizu, K.D. (2007). Colorimetric and fluorometric molecularly imprinted polymer sensors and binding assays. Polym Int, Vol.56, pp. 482-488.

Stobiecka, M.; Deeb, J. & Hepel, M. (2009). Molecularly Templated Polymer Matrix Films for Biorecognition Processes: Sensors for Evaluating Oxidative Stress and Redox Buffering Capacity. ECS Transactions, Vol.19, pp. 15-32.

Stobiecka, M.; Coopersmith, K. & Hepel, M. (2010a). Resonance elastic light scattering (RELS) spectroscopy of fast non-Langmuirian ligand-exchange in glutathione-induced gold nanoparticle assembly. J. Coll. Interf. Sci., Vol.350, pp. 168-177.

Stobiecka, M.; Deeb, J. & Hepel, M. (2010b). Ligand exchange effects in gold nanoparticle assembly induced by oxidative stress biomarkers: Homocysteine and cysteine. Biophys Chem, Vol.146, pp. 98-107.

Stobiecka, M. & Hepel, M. (2011). Effect of buried potential barrier in label-less electrochemical immunodetection of glutathione and glutathione-capped gold nanoparticles. Biosens. Bioelectron., Vol.26, pp. 3524-3530.

Storhoff, J.J.; Elghanian, R.; Mucic, R.C.; Mirkin, C.A. & Letsinger, R.L. (1998). One-pot colorimetric differentiation of polynucleotides with single base imperfections using gold nanoparticle probes. J. Am. Chem. Soc., Vol.120, pp. 1959-1964.

Taton, T.A.; Mucic, R.C.; Mirkin, C.A. & Letsinger, R.L. (2000). The DNA-mediated formation of supramolecular mono- and multilayered nanoparticle structures. J. Am. Chem. Soc., Vol.122, pp. 6305-6306.

Taton, T.A.; Lu, G. & Mirkin, C.A. (2001). Two-color labeling of oligonucleotide arrays via size-selective scattering of nanoparticle probes. J. Am. Chem. Soc., Vol.123, pp. 5164-5165.

Tokareva, I.; Tokarev, I.; Minko, S.; Hutter, E. & Fendle, J.H. (2006). Ultrathin molecularly imprinted polymer sensors employing enhanced transmission surface plasmon resonance spectroscopy. Chem. Commun., pp. 3343-3345

Tombelli, S.; Minunni, M.; Luzi, E. & Mascini, M. (2005). Aptamer-based biosensors for the detection of HIV-1 Tat protein. Bioelectrochemistry Vol.67, pp. 135- 141.

Tsuru, N.; Kikuchi, M.; Kawaguchi, H. & Shiratori, S. (2006). A quartz crystal microbalance sensor coated with MIP for ''Bisphenol A'' and its properties. Thin Solid Films, Vol.499, pp. 380-385.

Ungureanu, C.; Rayavarapu, R.G.; Manohar, S. & Leeuwen, T.G.v. (2009). Discrete dipole approximation simulations of gold nanorod optical properties: Choice of input parameters and comparison with experiment. J. App. Phys., Vol.105, pp. 102032-102032-7.

Upadhya, S.; Upadhya, S.; Mohan, S.K.; Vanajakshamma, K.; Kunder, M. & Mathias, S. (2004). Oxidant-antioxidant status in colorectal cancer patients before and after treatment. Indian J Clin Biochem, Vol.19 pp. 80-83.

Varadarajan, S.; Kanski, J.; Aksenova, M.; Lauderback, C. & Butterfield, D.A. (2001). Different mechanisms of oxidative stress and neurotoxicity for Alzheimer's A*b*(1-42) and A*b*(25-35). J. Am. Chem. Soc., Vol.123, pp. 5625-5631.

Vatamaniuk, O.K.; Mari, S.; Lu, Y.P. & Rea, P.A. (2000). Mechanism of Heavy Metal Ion Activation of Phytochelatin (PC) Synthase.Blocked thiols are sufficient for PC synthase-catalyzed transpeptidation of glutathione and related thiol peptides. J Biol Chem, Vol.275, pp. 31451-31459.

Vatamaniuk, O.K.; Bucher, E.A.; Ward, J.T. & Rea, P.A. (2001). A New Pathway for Heavy Metal Detoxification in Animals. Phytochelatin synthase is required for cadmium tolerance in *Caenorhabditis elegans*. J Biol Chem, Vol.276, pp. 20817-20820.

Welch, G.N. & Loscalzo, J. (1998). Homocysteine and atherothrombosis. NEJM, Vol.338, pp. 1042-1050.

Whitesides, G.M.; Kriebel, J.K. & Love, J.C. (2005). Molecular Engineering of Surfaces using Self-Assembled Monolayers. Sci Prog, Vol.88, pp. 17-48.

Yamamoto, Y. & Yamashita, S. (2002). Ubiquinol/ubiquinone ratio as a marker of oxidative stress, In: Methods in Molecular Biology. Oxidative Stress Biomarkers and Antioxidant Protocols, D. Armstrong, (Eds), 241-246, Totowa, NJ.

Yan, M. & Ramstrom, O. (2005). Molecularly Imprinted Materials. Science and Technology, New York.

Yang, W.H.; Schatz, G.C. & Duyne, R.P.V. (1995). Discrete dipole approximation for calculating extinction and Raman intensities for small particles with arbitrary shapes. J Chem Phys, Vol.103, pp. 869-875.

Ye, L.; Weiss, R. & Mosbach, K. (2000). Synthesis and Characterization of Molecularly Imprinted Microspheres. Macromolecules, Vol.33, pp. 8239-8245.

Yilmaz, E.; Mosbach, K. & Haupt, K. (1999). Influence of functional and cross-linking monomers and the amount of template on the performance of molecularly imprinted polymers in binding assays. Anal. Commun., Vol.36, pp. 167-170.

Yin, G.; Wang, S.Y.; Xu, M. & Chen, L.Y. (2006). Theoretical Calculation of the Optical Properties of Gold Nanoparticles. J Korean Phys Soc, Vol.49, pp. 2108-2111.

Zhang, X.; Li, H.; Jin, H.; Ebin, Z.; Brodsky, S. & Goligorsky, M.S. (2000). Effects of homocysteine on endothelialnitric nitric oxide production. Am. J. Physiol. Renal. Physiol., Vol.279, pp. F671-F678.

Zheng, W.; Maye, M.M.; Leibowitz, F.L. & Zhong, C.J. (2000). Imparting Biomimetic Ion-Gating Recognition Properties to Electrodes with a Hydrogen-Bonding Structured Core-Shell Nanoparticle Network. Anal. Chem., Vol.72, pp. 2190-2199.

18

Portable Bio-Devices: Design of Electrochemical Instruments from Miniaturized to Implantable Devices

Jordi Colomer-Farrarons[1], Pere Ll. Miribel-Català[1],
A. Ivón Rodríguez-Villarreal[1,2] and Josep Samitier[1,2,3]
[1]*Department of Electronics, Bioelectronics and Nanobioengineering Research Group (SIC-BIO), University of Barcelona,*
[2]*IBEC-Institute for Bioengineering of Catalonia,Nanobioengineering group,*
[3]*CIBER-BBN-Biomedical Research Networking Center in Bioengineering, Biomaterials and Nanomedicine,*
Spain

1. Introduction

The integration of biosensors and electronic technologies allows the development of biomedical systems able to diagnose and monitoring pathologies by detecting specific biomarkers.

The chapter presents the main modules involved in the development of such devices, generically represented in Fig. 1, and focuses its attention on the essential components of these systems to address questions such as: how is the device powered? How does it communicate the measured data? What kind of sensors could be used?, and What kinds of electronics are used?

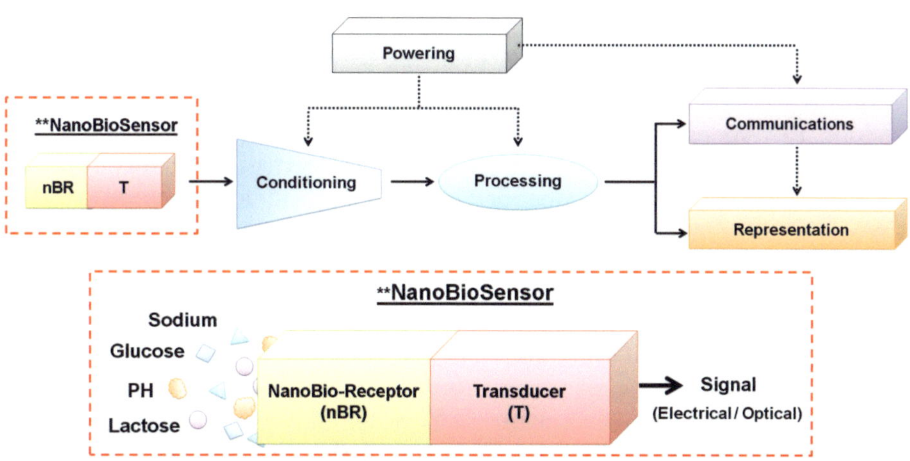

Fig. 1. Generic conception of the portable device specifying the different main components that are described throughout the chapter.

Two main fields of application are observed:
Health: Point of care technologies (POCT) can be defined as immediately actionable healthcare information outside the clinic laboratory in applications from diagnosis, to monitoring and therapy adjustment. A fundamental aspect of POCT versus clinical laboratory is the portability and the capacity to provide results in a shorter time frame. However, the higher costs of performing medical test at the point of care will only be accepted if the patient clinical condition strictly requires immediate results to guarantee more efficient and safer treatments. In the near future, healthcare systems will find a rational equilibrium for clinical laboratory and point of care utilization, where the most efficient technologies and systems will self-impose by factual clinical and economic evidences.
An evolution of these systems is the implantable lab-on-a-chip devices for in vivo continuous monitoring of the patients. In this case, the idea of the miniaturized devices is to integrate several functions in a microchip. The advances in biotechnology take us to the development of microdevices to detect proteins and/or ions suspended in blood/plasma related to specific pathologies or any other alteration of the standard health values. The integration of the detection and self-powered systems in the biological field are the basis of these new technologies. As a consequence, the major challenge of the electronic advances is to develop low powered consumption systems able to work under different environmental and physiological conditions. Besides, the devices should be covered or made with biocompatible and/or bioactive materials to reduce immune responses such as inflammation, thrombosis or any reaction induced by the implementation of the device. On the other hand, heat generated by the electronic devices must be controlled to avoid irreversible protein damage that could alter the measurements and/or necrosis caused by the implanted device.
Environment: The air and water pollutants are affecting the health of living beings (humans, animals, and plants), agriculture, fisheries and physical infrastructures (Cleven et al., 2005; Poyatos et al., 2010; Terbouche et al., 2011). Water pollution is present in all these fields. The hazardous residues of heavy metals, fertilizers, pesticides, toxic chemicals products, oil and other contaminants poured by companies all around the world, and humans waste such plastics; lubricants, etc., are contained in the drinking water, oceans, lakes and food. In the past years, it has become a global concern of associations such the U.S. and Scottish Environmental Protection Agency (EPA), American Water Resource Association (AWRA), the World Water Council, the European Environment Commission and others organizations. In response of the actual necessities, the research in systems designed to detect and monitor pollutants is exponentially increased. Devices able to detect in less time, in the point of care, handled by non-qualified personal and with lower cost in the fabrication process are the main aim of these research groups. In this way it is expected for example the detection of toxic drinking water that could cause health problems and in many cases the dead of living beings.
This chapter will discuss two approaches taking into account the envisaged fields of application: firstly, a discrete small and portable potentiostat amplifier integrated with detection and microfluidic systems result in a cheap and miniaturized device that can be applied for on-site simultaneous measurements of O2 and temperature values in water systems. Dissolved oxygen concentration (DO) is an important index of water quality and the ability to measure the oxygen concentration and temperature, at different positions and water depths, would be an important attribute for environmental analysis.

The second device presented is an approach for an in-vivo biomedical implantable device. The system is conceived to be implanted under the human skin. The powering and communication between this device and an external primary transmitter is based on an inductive link. The presented architecture is oriented for two different approaches defining a True/False alarm system, based on amperometric or impedance biosensors.

Two main problems from the point of view of the electronics, have to be overcome to obtain implantable devices (Colomer et al., 2009a), for true/false alarm, or event detector applications. The first, is how to transfer enough energy to power the devices, and the second, consists in the integration of the necessary instrumentation and communication electronics to control the sensors and to send the information provided by the sensors through human skin, avoiding excessively high levels of locally power dissipation. In this sense, our group works in the field of energy harvesting (Colomer et al., 2008), with experience of different sources (Juanola et al., 2010), which is one of our main interests. One experience is based on the use of an inductive coupling Radio Frequency (RF) power harvesting solution, to transmit energy to the implanted device, replacing the use of batteries or wires. Furthermore, this mechanism permits the establishment of a bidirectional communication between the implanted and the external interface devices.

In particular, the measurement of an electrical signal opens the second main field of interest, which is the instrumentation electronics. Looking for electrochemical instrumentation, the solutions vary from discrete to mixed and full custom-ASICs devices. The definition of the adopted solution is given by the size of the sensor, and the complexity of the system. For electrode areas greater than $1mm^2$, electronics based on low-cost surface mount components alone can be adopted. On the other hand, for the use of smaller and multiplexed solutions, a valid approach is a full custom ASIC solution. If very low current levels are derived from the sensors, an ASIC interface near the electrodes is indicated. Other key indicators for an ASIC solution near the electrodes are not only the degree of miniaturization, but also the fact that EMI can be reduced avoiding external disturbances such as vibrations, moisture, sources of electrical noise, etc.

Experiences with amperometric sensors, calibration voltammetries and amperometric measurements, related to the presentation of the main techniques that can be used with such biosensors, are presented in this chapter, as well as the different results achieved in each case. A prototype to detect O_2 in water for environmental purposes is presented as an example of a discrete disposable (Colomer et al., 2009c). The architecture and implementation of the electronics for an implantable approach is introduced (Colomer et al., 2009b), and comments concerning the implantable devices are included.

2. Conception of a generic bio-portable device

2.1 Powering

From the point of view of an implantable electronic device, the first decision to make is regarding to the power system that should be used to produce the energy necessary for the system. Thereafter, this section summarizes the topic of batteries and fuel cells, and describes particularly the interest in using free available external energy sources for powering small electronic systems knows as energy harvesting. Subsequently, this section will be focused in the description of energy harvesting and the kind of sources available in the environment in order to recover energy, more explicit (or getting into more detail) in the one obtained from the human body.

2.1.1 Batteries and fuel cells

Battery technology has undergone tremendous progress since it was first discovered. This progress has enabled the explosion of a wide-range of new applications such as in mobile devices. However, new trends in technology added to some intrinsic limitations of batteries have motivated research into new energy generation solutions. An emerging generation of ultra-small rechargeable batteries can remain installed for decades if not the entire life of the system, restoring that promise of freedom. Many of these new-generation batteries are solid-state, thin-film lithium cells comparable in size to a large IC package. Now available, these thin-film batteries provide many design options in terms of storage capacity, output voltage, and size. Cymbet's EnerChip CBC3150 is a 9- by 9-mm, 3.3-V battery with 50 μA-H of capacity, figure 27, and its CBC012 provides 12 μA-H at 3.8 V in a 5- by 5-mm package.
Solicore provides the larger 26- by 29-mm Flexion battery with 3-V output and up to 14 mA-H of capacity. Similarly, Infinite Power Solutions is offering its Thinergy batteries which are just entering the product shipment phase. More introductions are likely to be forthcoming from companies that are now licensing thin-film battery technology developed at Oak Ridge Micro Energy.
An interesting field in storage elements is also covered by the micro-fuel cells. A micro fuel cell is a power source for electronic devices that converts chemical into electrical energy. Fuel cells differ from conventional electrochemical cells and batteries. Both technologies involve the conversion of potential chemical energy into electricity. But while a conventional cell or battery employs reactions among metals and electrolytes whose chemical nature changes over time, the fuel cell actually consumes its fuel, leaving nothing but an empty reservoir or cartridge. A fuel cell is replenished merely be refilling its reservoir, or by removing the spent fuel cartridge and replacing it with a fresh one. The micro fuel cells represent power for devices that include a range of PC, handset, PDA, and digital device segments in a variety of industry, military, and health care segments. The research in this field is very important. A popular fuel cell is direct methanol fuel cell. The methanol reacts electrochemically with water at the anode, producing free electrons and protons, with power levels reported as high as $47mW/cm^2$. Specific fuel cells have a particular interest for the development of implantable devices. These devices can be achieved by using bodily fluids as the fuel source, such glucose and oxygen in blood (Sato et al., 2005).

2.1.2 Energy harvesting and ambient energy sources

There is a great interest in harvest the energy to power small electronic systems. We must distinguish between macro and micro energy harvesting scale. Macro harvesting, is related to energy recovery in the range from kilowatts to megawatts, which are fed to the grid. On the other hand, from the micro scale point of view, a limited amount of energy, in the range from nanowatts to milliwats, can be obtained from different types of external ambient sources and energy transducers (Niyato et al., 2007; Paradiso & Staner, 2005; Roundy et al., 2004), like vibrations (Garbuio et al., 2009; Kiziroglou et al., 2009; Le et al., 2006), heat (Carlson et al., 2009; Stark, 2006), and , light (Celik & Kusetogullari, 2010; Nasari et al., 2009), radio waves (Sogorb et al., 2008). Estimates of the energy available per unit area, or volume, for each harvesting source, are reported in Table 1.
These values are strongly dependent on the excitation conditions and the used technologies. From these different types of power sources and harvesting solutions, it is possible to recover peak power of 400μW for mechanical to electrical harvesting based on piezoelectric

Energy Source	Performance	
Ambient Light	· Indoor 10µW/cm² (low illumination) · Typical office 100µW/cm² Outdoor 10mW/cm² Full bright sun 10mW/cm²	· Solar cells (6830 lx 10W/m²) · Indoor solar cells (10lx to 1400 lx)
Vibrational	· 4 µW/cm³ (human motion Hz range) · 800 µW/cm³ (machines-kHz ranges) · These numbers depend heavily on size, excitations, technologies, etc. Typically: Piezoelectric ~ 200µW/cm³ Electrostatic ~ 50-100µW/cm³ Electromagnetic < 1µW/cm³	· Microgenerators 350 µW 22µW 400 µW
Radio Frequency (RF)	· GSM 4 µW/cm² · WiFi 0.001mW/cm² · These numbers strongly depend on operation frequency and distance between the base station and the receiver.	· < 1µW/cm² unless near a transmitter · ≈ 1mW for proximate stations (inductive coils) · @900MHz, 1.1meter @ 24.98dBm (0.315W), ~ 20µW [48] @4MHz, 25mm (subcutaneous powering) >5mW [62]
Temperature Difference	· Human 25 µW/cm²- 60 µW/cm² · Industry 10mW/cm²	· Thermoelectric generators 60 µW/cm² Thermolife® ΔT=5°C. [7][14][48]

Table 1. Energy Harvesting Sources and estimations.

MEMS, operating at 1kHz and generating voltages below 1V (Garbuio et al., 2009) for optimal load conditions, or as in (Le et al., 2006), based on micro-power generators based on a laminate piezoelectric membrane, generating 22µW of power and peak voltages up to 2.45V with no load. Following the objective to design energy-harvesting devices based on MEMS solutions, an electrostatic micro-generator is presented in (Le et al., 2006). In this case, a mechanical to electrical conversion based on an electrostatic solution instead of a piezoelectric or electromagnetic solution, the peak voltage generated can be up to 65V, and discrete electronics are used. In (Li et al., 2010), a piezoelectric cantilever working at lower frequencies of operation (65Hz), generating higher voltages (up to 15V) and in consequence presented a maximum power of 350µW. An interesting point of progress is shown in (Khaligh et al., 2008), where two power sources are combined: a piezoelectric and permanent magnetic energy scavenging. These elements are discrete and the total power theoretically generated is 44mW: 37mW from the electromagnetic source and 6mW from the piezoelectric source. In (Celik&Kusetogullari, 2010), the utilization of indoor cells for extreme low conditions of illumination, and low voltages of operation, is shown for a cell of 55mm x 20mm x 1.1mm with a power of 5µW@10lx to 200µW@1450lx for a voltage drop of 2V. The advances in semiconductor technologies related to the reduction of the transistor's size allow the industry to obtain more interest in the development of new self-powered portable electronic devices that incorporate a great variety of circuitry and functions as is stated in works like (Ferrari et al., 2009; Khaligh et al., 2010).

Energy harvesting, small-format batteries and power management ICs are technologies that will enable commercialization of the next-generation of ultra-low-power electronic devices and systems.

2.1.3 Body harvesting

In the particular case of energy scavenging in human beings, there are two approaches that are defined as passive or active power generation. Passive powering takes place when the user does not have to do any task different to normal tasks associated with the product, which is the main difference with an active generation. Generally speaking, higher amount of power can be generated actively than passively. A nice reference comes from (Paradiso& Starner, 2005), at the MIT.

There are different sources available in the body to harvest energy. The human body is a tremendous storehouse of energy, but some key aspects must be taken into account for its harvest. The first approach is related to the body heat. Since the human body emits energy as heat, it follows naturally to try to harness this energy. However, the efficiency of the Carnot thermodynamic cycle puts an upper limit on how well this waste heat can be recovered. Assuming normal body temperature and a relatively low room temperature (20 °C), the Carnot efficiency is 5.5% at 25 °C which drops to 3.2% in a warmer environment (27 °C). Since the total amount of wasted heat can be turned into a power of 100W, the energy that can be recovered, using the Carnot engine, it is in the range of 2.4W to 4.8W. While a full wetsuit or even a torso body suit is inappropriate for many applications, the neck offers a good location for a tight seal, owing that access to major centres of blood flow, and could be easily removed by the user. The neck is approximately 1/15 of the surface area of the "core" region (those parts that the body tries to keep warm at all times). As a rough estimate, assuming even heat dissipation over the body, a maximum of 0.20-0.32W could be recovered conveniently by a neck brace for instance. There are different approaches to recover this energy thanks to thermoelectric generators. Low power thermoelectrically-driven products have appeared, for example, Applied Digital Solutions' Thermo Life, is a thermoelectric generator that measures 0.5 cm^2 in an area 1.6mm thick. Comprising a dense array of low-temperature thermopiles, it can generate 10 μA at 3 V (6 V open circuit) with only 5° C of temperature difference. In addition, the motion of the body could be also be an option for power harvesting. There are different approaches based on the movement of the human being to recover energy and studies that analyse this energy recovered from some human movements. Table 2 presents some references about the energy recovered from frequent human movements, Table 2.

In (Kazazian&Jansen, 2004) appears the idea of an energy fitness club where people could reload their portable device while getting in shape. They estimated that 10 minutes pedalling on a bicycle could generate 2 W, and therefore reload a mobile phone described by the authors as HUMAN POWERED. Moreover, the MIT Media Lab has developed a full system that harvests parasitic power in shoes employing piezoelectric materials (Shenck&Paradiso, 2001). The low-frequency piezoelectric shoe signals are converted into a continuous electrical energy source. The first system consists on harvesting the energy dissipated in bending the ball of the foot, placing a multilaminar PVDF bimorph under the insole. The second one consists on harvesting the foot strike energy by the curved, pre-stressed spring metal strips laminated with a semi-flexible form of PZT under the heel. Both devices were excited under a 0.9 Hz walking activity.

The e-health monitoring is a significant field in research which is related to the conception and definition of Body-sensor networks in the body, looking for external and internal biosensors implanted in the body. This approach of WBAN ubiquitous health monitoring is exposed in (Jovanov et al., 2005).
IMEC is one of the world leaders in smart textiles using the power harvesting technology. IMEC in Belgium associated with the laboratory of the Ghent University presented their newly developed UTCP (ultra-thin chip package) technology which can be seen as a big boost towards fully integrated, complex electronic into textiles. UTCP allows the integration of complete systems in a conventional low-cost flex substrate. IMEC demonstrated the integration technology with a flexible wireless monitored prototype that measures the heart rate and muscle activity. IMEC at Netherlands has presented the conception of an smart T-shirt, used to monitoring the cardiac activity, powered by body heat (Van Hoof, 2009), figure 2. Besides, IMEC has demonstrated the integration of a wireless autonomous sensor system in clothes. The system is fully autonomous for its entire life and requires no service - like replacing or recharging the battery - from the user. The shirt with integrated electronics can be washed in a regular washing machine. It occupies less than 1.5% of the shirt area and typically generates a power of 0.8–1mW at about 1V at regular sedentary office activity. However, if the user walks indoors, the power increases up to 2.7mW at 22°C due to forced convection. In colder environments where other clothes need to be worn on top of the shirt, the power generation is usually not affected.

Activity	Power generation
Finger (pushing pen)	0.3 W
Legs (cycling 25 km/h)	100 W
Hand and arm (Freeplay)	21 W
Hand (Aladdinpower) 3.6 W	3.6 W

Table 2. Examples of active human power generated by body movements.

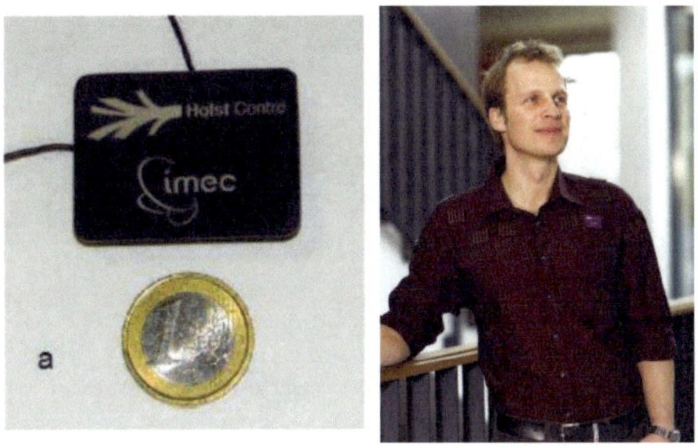

Fig. 2. Smart T-shirt by IMEC-NL.

2.2 Communications

Referring to Fig. 1, communications are one of the last, but not the less important, steps when designing miniaturized equipment for environmental or BioMedical applications.

Basically, two main topologies can be studied, wired or wireless communications. Since wireless architectures are becoming more popular for such devices we will focus on them in more detail. It is well known that wireless communication consists on transmit data (information) over a short (few cm or meters) or long distance (kilometers or more) without the use of wires or electrical conductors. In a miniaturized device, the wireless information transmission process could represent an important part of the power consumption, so it is important to minimize the required power levels (Colomer & Miribel, 2011), with an accurate design of the antennas and associated circuits.
The basic communication scheme uses one antenna (and its associated circuits and modulations) to receive and transmit data (Fig. 3). It is tunned at the desired working frequency, typically one of the standards of the ISM (Industrial, Scientific and Medical radio bands) band for Wireless sensor networks like, Bluetooth or ZigBee for short communications range, or GPRS or WLAN for long ranges. Some low power transceivers are available from all major vendors like, Microchip® or Texas Instruments®.

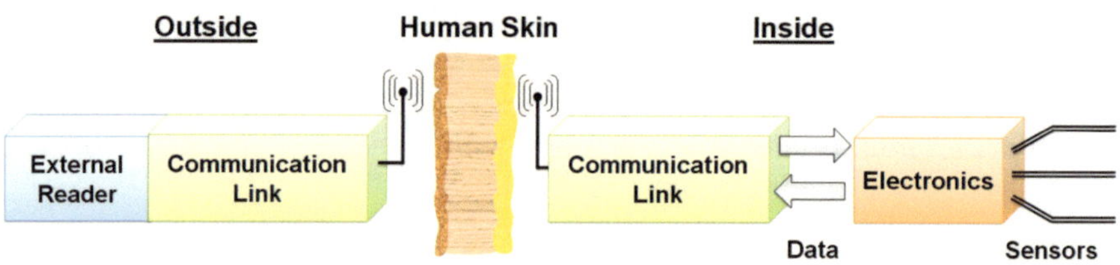

Fig. 3. Basic Communication scheme.

On the other side, if the applications require the design of a full-custom transceiver, some examples can be found in the literature (Roundy et al., 2004). Furthermore, magnetic induction communications based on the inductive coupling of two coils can be used to transmit bidirectional data i.g., Backscattering, with some implanted device (Colomer & Miribel, 2011), at the frequency operation of 1M to 15MHz range. One antenna is located under the skin while the other one is at the external side creating an inductive link used for communications and powering.

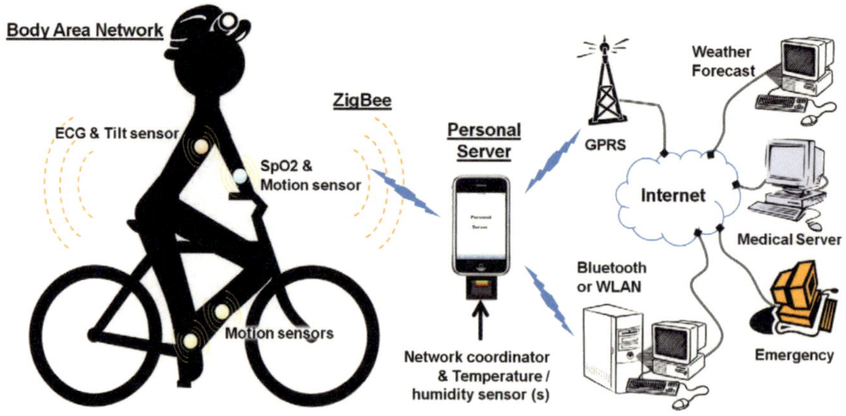

Fig. 4. Example of a distributed sensors networks and Wireless Body Area Networks (WBAN).

The combination of these standards allows the development of distributed sensors networks and Wireless Body Area Networks (WBAN). An example of WBAN is presented in Fig. 4. There, several sensors are distributed around the human body and use different type of protocols to communicate with a Central Control Unit or Personal Server. Then, this CCU module collects the data coming from all the sensors and transmits it to other users.

2.3 Biosensors and measurement techniques

2.3.1 What is a biosensor?

A biosensor is a measurement system for the detection of an analyte that combines a biological component with a physicochemical detector. The general function of a biosensor is to convert binding events between biological receptors and target agents into a signal thanks to a transducer (Fig. 5) which can be based on an optical, a thermal, a gravimetric or an electrochemical detection. This last one has gained increasing attention in the last years. The high sensitivity, low cost and easy miniaturization of the electronic detection taken in conjunction with the wide range of applications, has become these devices a perfect analytical tool in different fields, such as diagnosis of genetic diseases, detection of infectious agents, study of genetic predisposition, development of personalized medicine, detection of differential genetic expression, forensic science, drug screening, food safety and environmental monitoring. In order to develop portable systems, from discrete to integrated solutions for a discrete or continuous monitoring, electrochemical biosensors are the best choice. The generic components of a biosensor are depicted in Fig. 6.

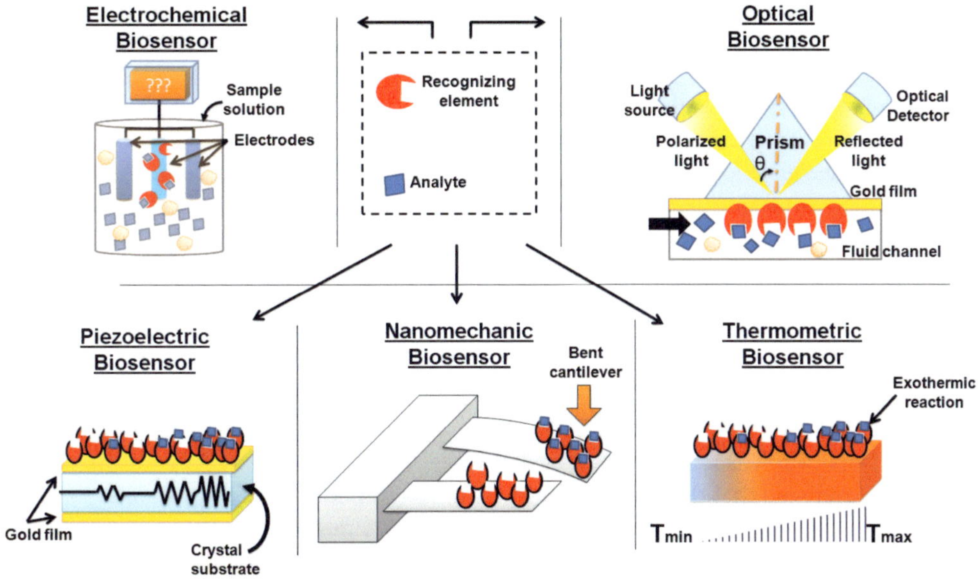

Fig. 5. Generic function of a biosensor is to convert binding events between biological receptors and target agents into a signal.

First we have the sensing element (a). It is where the biological system is immobilized. The agent can be an enzyme, antibody, DNA chains, etc, and is used for the recognition of the analyte. (b) is the transducer, where the biological signal is converted into a signal, which may be; optical, thermal, and electrical signal: current, potential, conductance, impedance, etc. Then, such signal must me amplified and then processed. This amplifier module is the detector stage (c). Thinking in electrical signals, an amplifier stage is used to amplify the biological signal, which is generally very low. Then, (d) is the electronics module which has the role to process such measurements. Finally, (e), the results are presented thanks to a user-friendly interface to visualize the data.

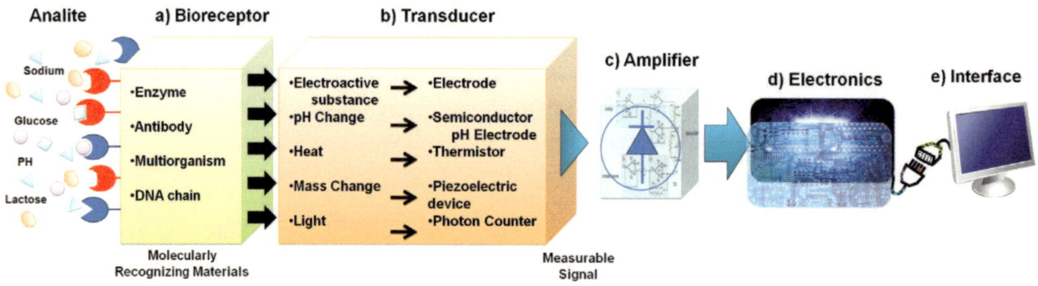

Fig. 6. Generic components of a biosensor.

2.3.2 Electrochemical biosensors

Electrochemical biosensors are the largest group of chemical sensors. All of them are based on fixing some variables of the electrochemical cell and check how the other variables change with the fluctuations of the controlled variables. These biosensors are normally based on enzymatic catalysis of a reaction that produces or consumes electrons (such as enzymes are rightly called redox enzymes). The sensor substrate usually contains three electrodes, a reference, an active or working and a counter or auxiliary electrode. Electrochemical sensors allow three main different configurations: voltammetric, potentiometric and conductrometric measurements. Voltammetric biosensors are those based on the measurement of the current-voltage variations. Voltammetric measurements typically consist of a three-electrode arrangement. Measurement of current occurs at the redox electrode as a function of the electrode potential. The solution must contain electro active species that can undergo electrode reaction. Amperometric biosensors are a particular case of them, where is determined electrical currents associated with a redox process where a fixed voltage in the sensor is applied. In potentiometric biosensors, the electrode and solution are in chemical equilibrium, the current flow is near zero and a voltage is measured relative to a reference electrode. Conductometric biosensors are based on the measurement of the variations of the conductance with the use on an alternating current at a fixed frequency of operation. Special interests, as is stated in more detail in the next section, have Impedance biosensors that determine variations of the impedance of the sensor.

For voltammetry biosensors, and in particular for amperometric biosensors, the most standard measurement method is based on the three-electrode configuration. By applying a proper fixed potential between them, a current is generated, which is related to the concentration of the electro active species in the sample solution. These species are generated by oxidation or reduction in the sample solution. The potentiostat amplifier, presented in 2.4.2, controls the voltage between the working and reference electrodes, and the current through the electrochemical cell formed by the three electrodes of the biosensor and the solution where the reaction takes place is conveyed through the counter electrode. Based on the use of the potentiostat amplifier, there are different kind of electrochemical test that can be carried out in order to analyze the electrochemical cell formed by the biosensor and the solution media, Fig. 8. The most popular electrochemical technique used with electrochemical sensor is the cyclic voltammetry, depicted in Fig. 7.

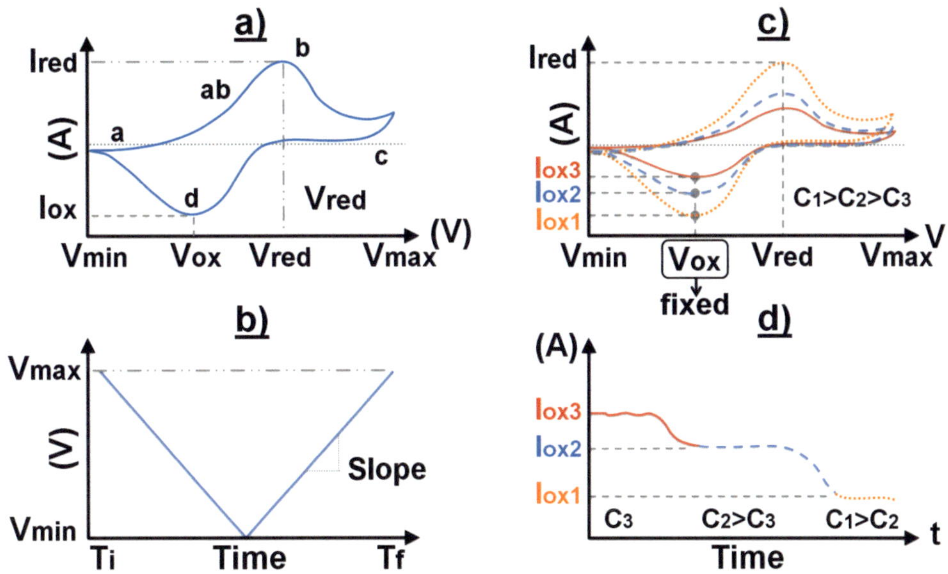

Fig. 7. Cyclic voltammetry.

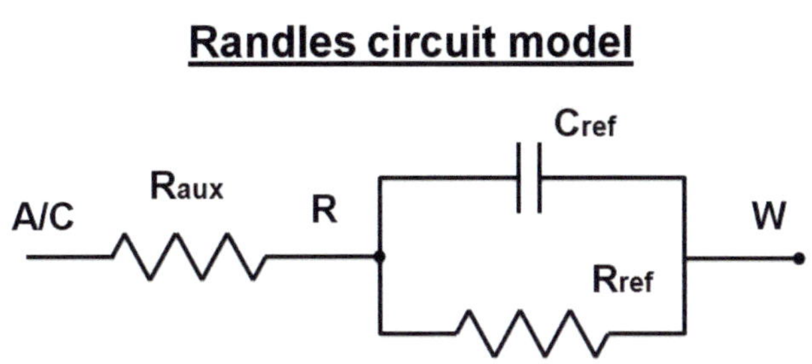

Fig. 8. Randles model.

The voltage applied in b) is fixed by the potentiostat between the working and reference electrodes. In a) is depicted the characteristic cyclic voltammetry, where the path between point (a) and (b) represent the reduction phase, that is, the electrons are derived to the solution from the electrodes. During the path (c) to (d) the oxidation takes place. The chemical species pass electrons to the electrode. Characteristic peaks for the oxidation and reduction are obtained, (d) and (a) respectively. Different voltage ramps define different reactions. Also, for different concentrations of the analytes the peaks of reduction and oxidation change, as depicted in c). Based on this technique the amperometric analysis is introduced. As it was mentioned above, a fixed voltage now is fixed and the current is directly measured. Usually this voltage is fixed at that point where the electrochemical response is maximized. In d) is depicted this situation of the maximum point of oxidation, and for different concentrations. Several other techniques are used for a voltammetric analysis like staircase or sampled DC voltammetry, normal pulse voltammetry, differential pulse voltammetry, square wave voltametry and differential normal pulse voltammetry. All of these techniques are based in a potential that is scanned, defining an initial and final steps of voltage vs. time.

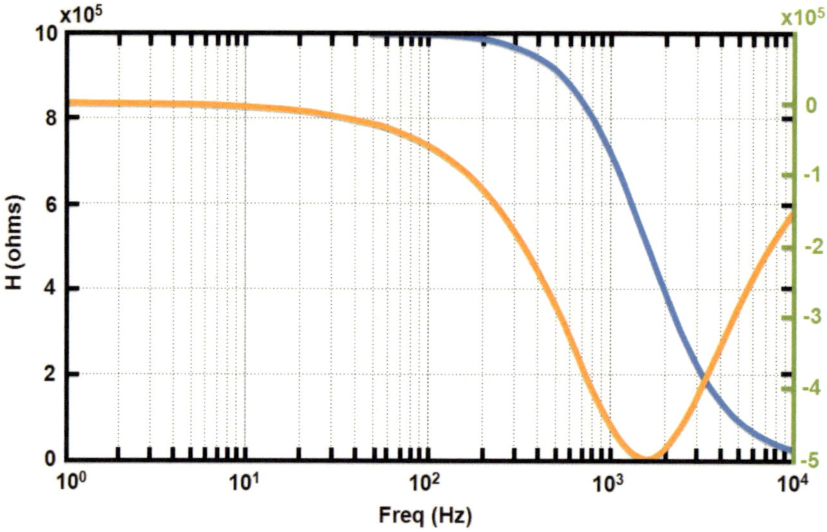

Fig. 9. Plof the Bode Polt for an EIS.

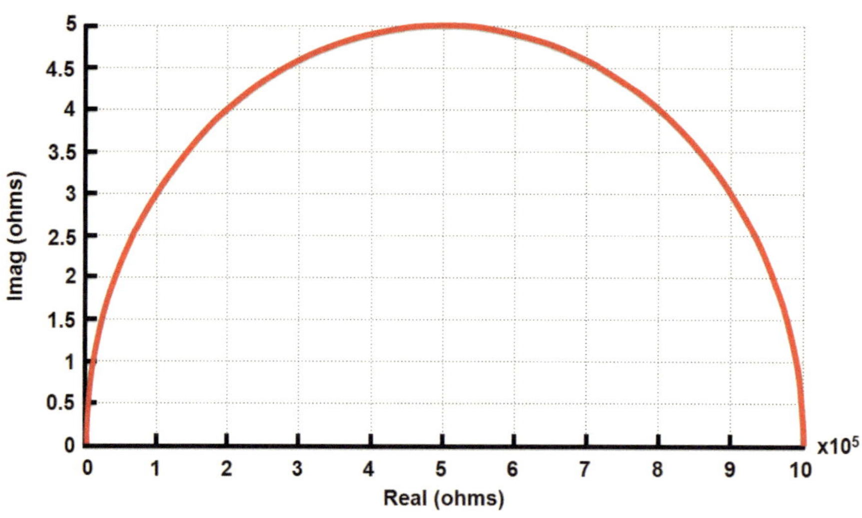

Fig. 10. Plot of the Nyquist Polt for an EIS.

The Electrochemical Impedance Spectroscopy (EIS), is a more effective method to probe the interfacial properties of the modified electrode through measuring the change of electron transfer resistance at the electrode surface, which is caused by the adsorption and desorption of chemical or biological molecules. There are different electrical models that represent the electrochemical cell, and the easiest one is the Randles model, Fig. 8, just defined by three elements: by the double-layer capacitor in parallel with a polarization resistor, which is also described as a charge transfer resistor, and the solution resistor. In an electrochemical cell, electrode kinetics, redox reactions, diffusion phenomena and molecular interactions at the electrode surface can be considered analogous to the above components that impede the flow of electrons in an ac circuit. The measurement of the impedance variation of the cell can be depicted following two different approaches: a) the magnitude and phase of the impedance are depicted as a Bode plot, as depicted in Fig. 9, or b) a Nyquist plot, Fig. 10, where in the complex plane are depicted the real impedance component in the X coordinates, and the imaginary impedance component in the Y coordinates.

2.3.3 Some examples

Most of the biosensors are based on electrochemical transducer method. The clearest example is the blood glucose monitoring marker, based on amperometric enzyme biosensors. Here an enzyme glucose oxidise catalyses the conversion of the analyte to a molecule that can be detected by the transducer. First, it oxidises glucose and uses two electrons to reduce a component of the enzyme, FAD to FADH2, which is also oxidased. The resulting current in the electrode is a measurement of the concentration of glucose. Oxidades oxidize their substrates and they need oxygen as a co-substrate, re-oxidizing the enzyme to the initial state. The hydrogen peroxide produced is again oxidized at the electrode:

$$\text{Glucose} + O_2 \leftrightarrows \text{Gluconolactone} + H_2O_2$$

The glucose oxidase with its prosthetic group FAD

$$\text{Glucose} + \text{FAD} \leftrightarrows \text{Gluconolactone} + \text{FADH}_2$$

$$\text{FADH}_2 + O_2 \leftrightarrows H_2O_2 + \text{FAD}$$

And at the electrode takes place an anodic reaction, on platinum, @ 0.6V vs. Ag/AgCl; 3M.

$$H_2O_2 \leftrightarrows 2H^+ + O_2 + 2e^-$$

Then, the detected current by the potentiostat, which is proportional to the concentration of the analyte in the sample, is:

$$I_d = n \cdot A \cdot F \cdot D_s \cdot c^0 / \delta_N \quad (1)$$

Where A is the area of the electrode, D_S is the diffusion coefficient of the analyte S, c^0 is the bulk solution concentration of the analyte and finally δ_N is the thickness of the stagnant layer.

The glucose biosensor (Fiorito and De Toresi, 2001; Hiller et al., 1996; Kros et al., 2001) is an example of this this applications. The biosensor is based on the electron transfer that occurs during the enzymatic reduction of glucose. Nowadays, there is an increasing interest in the field of glucose biosensors, looking for Glucose Continous Monitoring (GCM). In the last years several works have been published in the field like Patel et al., (2007), where it's presented an electro-enzymatic glucose sensor, (Xi Huang et al., 2009), where it is introduced a capacitive based MEMS affinity sensor for continuous glucose monitoring applications, (Teymoori, Mir Majid et al., 2009) introducing a MEMS for glucose and other generical sensors in medical applications and (Rodrigues et al., 2007) where it's developed a new cell-based biochip dedicated to the real-time monitoring of transient effluxes of glucose and oxygen, using arrays of amperometric microsensors integrated in the inlet and the outlet of a PDMS cell chamber, and complete designs like (Rahman et al., 2009) where is presented the design, microfabrication, packaging, surface functionalization and in vitro testing of a complete electrochemical cell-on-a-chip (ECC) for the continuous amperometric monitoring of glucose, performing cyclic voltammetry, electrical impedance spectroscopy (EIS), and microscopic examination.

Special interest has the development of nanosensors applied in this field. Some examples are reported, like (Usman Ali, S.M et al., 2009), where ZnO Nanowires are used for a GCM application directly connected to the gate of a standard low-threshold MOSFET, (Lee Y.J. et al., 2009), where a flexible enzyme-free glucose micro-sensor with nanoporous platinum working electrode on a bio-compatible PET film was designed, (Goud et al., 2007), where it's presented nanobioelectronic system-on-package (SOP) with integrated glucose sensor based on carbon nanotubes working electrodes, (Jining Xie et al., 2007) where it's studied a platinum nanoparticle-coated carbon nanotubes for amperometric glucose biosensing, or in (Ekanayake, E.M.I et. al., 2007) where it's described fabrication and characterization of a novel nano-porous polypyrrole (PPy) electrode and its application in amperometric biosensors, with enhanced characteristics for glucose sensing.

2.4 Electronics for electrochemical biosensors

2.4.1 Two and three electrodes configurations

Two are the minimum of electrodes that are required in order to control the interface between an electrode and a solution, forming a simple electrochemical cell. One of these electrodes is the working electrode (W), where the reaction of interest takes place. The other electrode is the reference electrode (R) where is fixed a constant potential reference. Generally for a voltammetry experience this approach it is not enough when the potential applied must be controlled owing to the equivalent resistance of the solution. Then, when a current circulates through the solution a voltage drop is generated. Also, when current is present at the reference electrode implies a variation of the voltage interface of it. This situation implies that the voltage difference between the reference and the working electrodes is not well defined. A simple solution is based on the use of a large reference electrode and a small working electrode but sometime this is not possible. The solution to this situation is the use of a three-electrode system, placing an extra electrode which is usually called counter (C) or auxiliary electrode, as is depicted in Fig. 11. The voltage difference is fixed between the (W) and (R) electrodes and the current is injected by the (C) electrode and the potential is well defined at the cell (Vcell). The potentiostat amplifier is the instrumentation that has the role to control this bias and read the current of the cell.

2.4.2 The potentiostat amplifier

The main electronics involved in the design of the instrumentation are defined by the potentiostat amplifier, to drive and control the electrodes, and to measure the output signal and the processing electronics. The potentiostat amplifier is the electrochemical measurement technique to interface the biological elements with the electronics. Electronic measurement of the biochemical analyte concentrations is essential for diseases diagnose and study of biological systems.

Two different ways can be followed: a) the potentiometric configuration, where a fixed current it is applied and the output voltage is measured, or b) the amperometric

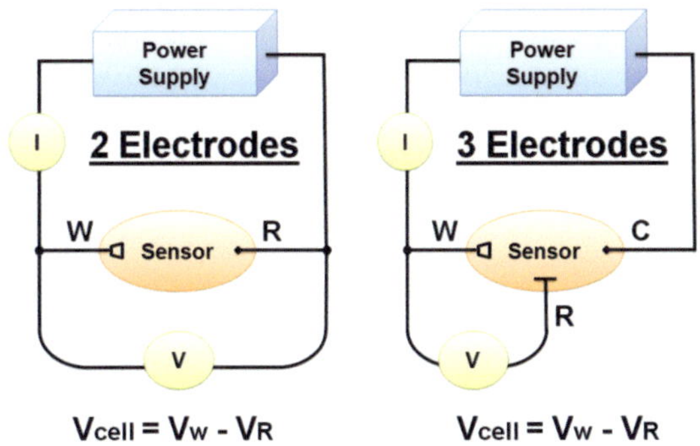

Fig. 11. Two and Three-electrode electrochemical measurement system.

configuration, where a fixed voltage is applied and the output current is read, and converted to a voltage signal by the transimpedance amplifier. If the size of the electrodes is decreased, defining micron-sized electrodes, the current level decreases up to femto-amperes. Some references are described in (Choi Myung-suk et al., 2007), in their work "Implantable Bio system design for displacement measurement of living life", in the work by (K.Kitamori, 2007), where he described micro and nano chemical sensors on-a-chip, and the by (Wen-Yaw Chung et al., 2007), where they present a low power readout circuit with an potentiostat amplifier for amperometric chemical sensors for a Glucose Meter Application. Other interesting biosensors are the piezoelectric immunosensors, like the developed for the rapid diagnosis of M. tuberculosis by (Eric Carnes et al., 2005).

The state of the art of the potentiostat amplifiers has evolved in such a different ways from discrete or integrated solutions. In order to design a portable system for standard electrochemical assays, discrete solutions become an extremely good choice in terms of portability, accuracy and economical cost. But, demands for increased functionality, reduced system size, reduced electrodes size, ultra-low current detection and versatility will force potentiostats to be designed on a system-on-chip (SoC) to be implemented in advanced CMOS processes. The scaled supply voltages in these processes (Kakerow et al., 1995; Kraver et al., 2001; Reay et al., 1994), however, seriously limit the chemical analysis range. The drive voltages of amperometric chemical sensors do not scale with electrode size, but are instead defined by the reduction/oxidation (redox) potentials of the analysis been investigated. In fact, many analysis are undetectable using standard potentiostats in a 0.18μm CMOS process due to its maximum supply voltage of 1.8V (Kissinger et al., 1996). Standard, single-ended (SE) potentiostats force the sensor's electrode to a fixed potential, Fig. 12, while fully differential (FD) potentiostat, employing a FD operational amplifier, dynamically controls the electrode's potential and doubles its voltage swing.

2.4.3 The lock-in amplifier

EIS is an ac method that describes the response of an electrochemical cell to a small amplitude sinusoidal voltage signal as a function of frequency. EIS technique consists on applying an AC voltage to the *R*- *W* electrodes and measure the resulting AC current at the *Working* electrode (Fig. 13). Then, it is possible to represent the impedance of the electrochemical cell. The resulting current sine wave differs in time (phase shift) with respect to the perturbing (voltage) wave, and the ratio V(t)/I(t) is defined as the impedance (Z), that accounts for the combined opposition of all the components within the electrochemical cell (resistors, capacitors, inductors) to the flow of electrons. The variations in the electronic signal are due to the antibody-antigen (Ab-Ag) interactions. The signal processing circuitry has the role to obtain the real and imaginary components of the measurement of the Electrochemical Impedance.

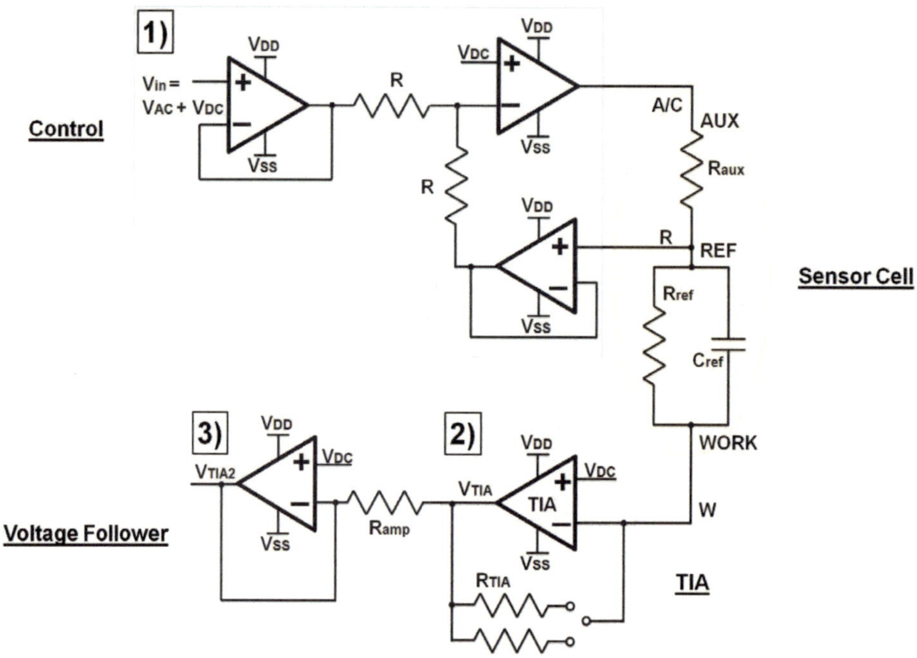

Fig. 12. Potentiostat Amplifier with electrochemical sensor's model.

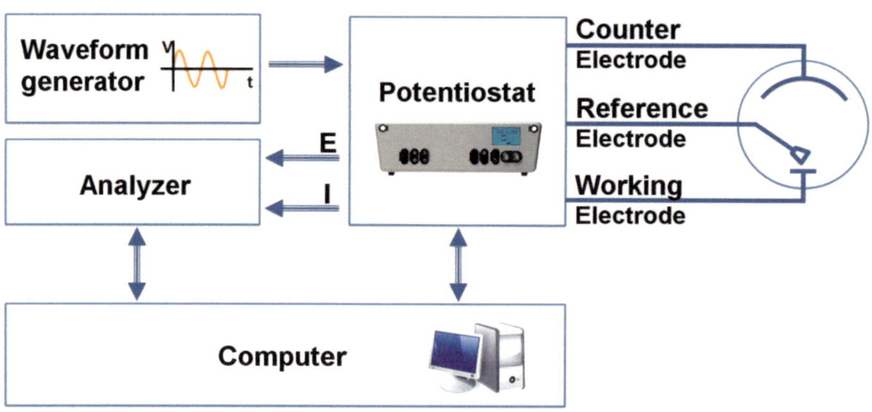

Fig. 13. Generic setup for an EIS experiment.

Based on the nature of the measured signal there are two main approaches: a) the capacitive immunosensors, where the surface of the electrode is completely covered by a dielectric layer and the whole electrode assembly behaves as an insulator. The variation of the capacitance is measured, in frequency ranges up to 100kHz, and b) the faradaic immunosensors, which have the surface of the electrode partially or wholly covered by a non insulating layer or partially covered by an insulating layer, are able to catalyse a redox probe that exists in the measuring solution. In this case, the measured parameter is the charge transfer resistance (the real component of impedance at low frequency values, typically 0.1-1.0 Hz), and Ab-Ag interactions are expected to cause an increase in its value as the faradic reaction becomes increasingly hindered.

In order to proceed with the signal processing, there are mainly two approaches: a) the Fast Fourier Transform (FFT), and b) the Frequency Response Analyzer (FRA). In the case of the FFT, a pulse or step, -the approach to be followed is the ideal Dirac delta function-, is applied to the sample because it contains a wide frequency content. Then, the response of the sample is digitized and processed in a digital processor, for instance a DSP, and using the FFT algorithm, the different frequency components are obtained for their analysis. Also, other possibility that could be followed is the logarithmic sampling in the DFFT calculus, reducing the data that must be required in the process. A simpler solution is based on the FRA approach. In this case, a sine and cosine signals are adopted, and using two multipliers and a filter stage the real an imaginary components of the response are obtained. This measurement must be done for each frequency. Working with just one sensor and in terms of the size of the final product, the FFT option could be adopted, because the response for several frequencies is obtained. The FRA solution is a solution more oriented to multi-sensor approaches but also in the case of single sensors it is a nice option, in terms of the trade-off between complexity and speed, if not too low frequencies must be measured. This lock-in approach is more feasible.

2.5 Integration of lab on a chip devices

The fabrication of lab-on-a-chip devices require the integration of several systems such as microfluidic, detection (BioLED Technology, 2007), power supply (Colomer et al., 2008) and/or communication in a small and portable device.

The aim of the microfluidic system is to transport the fluid into the microcapillaries as well as its preparation for their proper analysis. The preparation step consists in the separation of the fluidic and/or suspended particles (Rodríguez-Villarreal et al., 2010), the mixing of the fluids for cell activation and/or mixing reactants for initiation. It could takes place along the capillaries or inside of created droplets (Xia et al. 2010), which can also be useful to encapsulate biological particles or chemical reagents. In some cases, the sample needs to be focalized (Rodríguez-Trujillo et al., 2008) before it flow through the electrical or optical detection system (Fig. 14) to achieve a better detection signal.

A complete portable lab-on-a-chip device required an integrated power supply for the functionality of the detection and the communications systems. The last one, has the objective to inform by sending the relevant results of the biological analysis.

The integration of all these Microsystems requires sophisticated microfabrication techniques such as photolithography, chemical vapour deposition, dry and wet etching and many more (Chen, 2006; Chinn, 2008) to create a final prototype made of biocompatible materials. The integration of the silicon, polymer or glass devices are the main concerns of research groups. There are two ways of integrating such microdevices, the fabrication of all of them on the same device or the assembly of several microdevices previously fabricated as shown in Fig. 15. A). But up to now, although there are many portable devices, the lab on a chip technology still required of external sources for energy supply and the human-device interface.

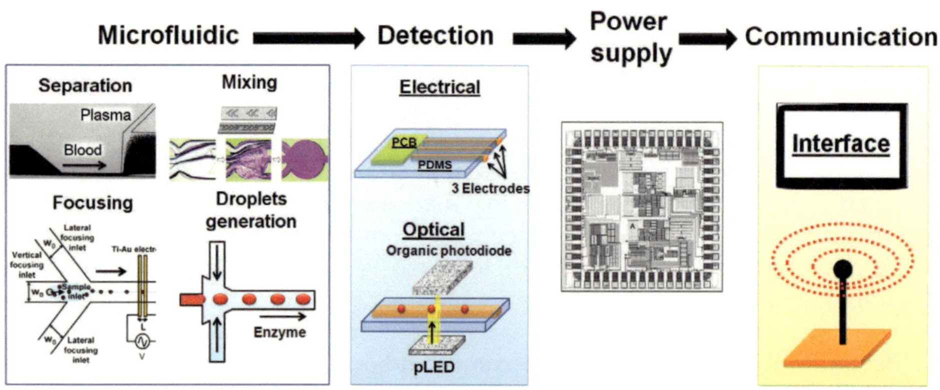

Fig. 14. Microsystems required for a complete Lab-on-chip device.

Different companies of biomedical devices such as Philips, Biosite Inc. and Medimate are developing small devices that integrate some fluidic/detection microsystems with portable power/interface macrosystems to commercialize analytical biomedical devices, Fig 15.B. Besides, the development of a full custom lab-on-a-chip device envisaged for implantable applications, keeps been the objective of the new medical technologies.

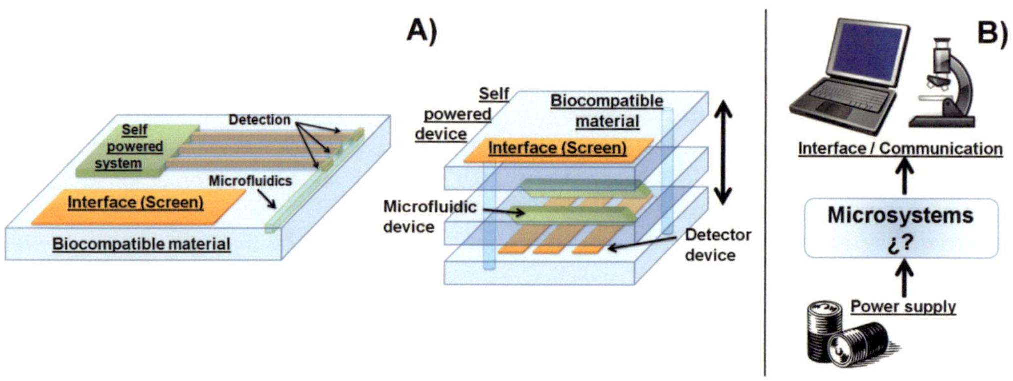

Fig. 15. Scheme of integration of A) full lab-on-a-chip devices and B) portable and microdevices.

3. An example of a miniaturized electrochemical instrument for in- situ O_2 monitoring

The decrease of oxygen concentration in water is a clear indication of water pollution, which is one of the main concerns of the Water Framework directive in the European Union, as the pollution is mainly due to nitrogen-based fertilisers used in agriculture. One of the direct consequences of reduced levels of dissolved oxygen is suffocation especially in acute cases where fish live in well-oxygenated waters which suddenly become oxygen deficient, usually as a result of intervention by man rather than natural changes in oxygen levels (Kramer, 1987). In addition to pollution and biological processes including primary production and respiration, in open water systems, other sources of variation in the dissolved oxygen concentration come into play which includes physical mechanisms such as diffusion as a function of wind and waves (Irigoien et al., 1999). Due to the complexity of these variables, the dissolved oxygen budget can be difficult to estimate requiring continuous and spatial on-line monitoring.

As a first approach a discrete PCB, covered with a hydrophobic polymer, has been designed based on commercial discrete electronics and specific oxygen sensors. The coated electronics (with PDMS), can be immersed in water without affecting its functionality.

This section presents the development of a low power portable potentiostat for In-Situ electrochemical measurements, covered by PDMS. The core of the electronics is defined by a potentiostat amplifier, as the structure presented in 2.4.2, Fig.12. The custom electronics, which includes a small printed circuit board (PCB) of 31mm X 21 mm, has been designed using commercial amplifiers, looking for the best performances, as described in the paper.

Some commercially available oxygen analyzers tend to be large, cumbersome and expensive. Here the electronics and sensors are miniaturized and placed in close proximity to each other and subsequently covered by a hydrophobic material. The size of the contact pads is 5mmX 2.5 mm, in order to have a good soldering area between the contacts and the electrodes, Fig. 16. The power consumption of this implementation is around 350 mW.

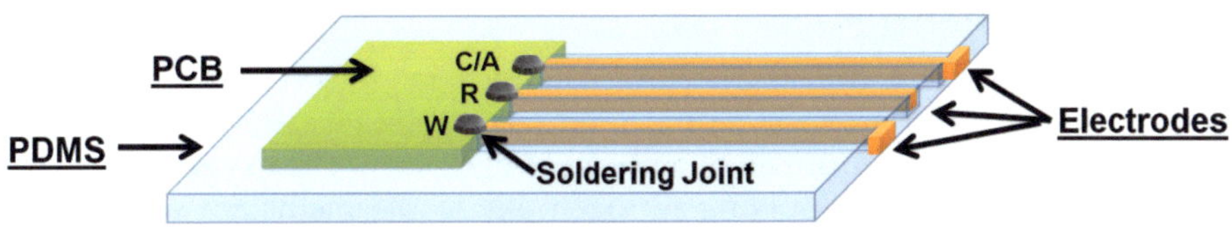

Fig. 16. PCB and connections of the electrodes.

The commercial amplifiers used, were the OPA 656 and the OPA 657 working as the transimpedance amplifier, both from Texas Instrument. These amplifiers were selected for their good characteristics in terms of high input impedance, low bias and offset input currents and voltages. It is important that the reference input has a high impedance in such a way that almost the same current flows between the counter/auxiliary electrode and the working electrode. The oxygen analyzer, coated with PDMS, is depicted in Fig.17. The PCB was tested before and after its introduction into water. Some experiments were carried out to analyze its performances compared with commercial equipment. The used instrument was the CH 1200A from CH Instruments.

Different fixed DC voltages were fixed, and the variation of O2 was measured in a programmed time interval. For testing purposes a three electrode electrochemical sensor (Advent Research Materials, UK), was fabricated using a 200µm platinum wire for the counter electrode, a 200µm silver wire for the pseudo reference electrode and a 75µm gold wire, with 18µm Teflon insulation, for the working electrode. The electrodes were cut into approximately 1cm lengths sections and soldered to the potentiostat. The insulated gold working electrode was cut so that the sensor tip was a 75 µm gold disc electrode. The gold electrode was cut each time with a new scalpel blade and the resulting disc electrode was checked under a microscope. The electrodes were placed approximately 1mm apart from each other during the experimental measurements. For the amperometry test, the gold working electrode was set at -1V where the oxygen was reduced to give a more negative current. Therefore, for high oxygen concentrations the current was more negative than for lower concentrations of oxygen. This was used as the main indicative of oxygen detection in water.

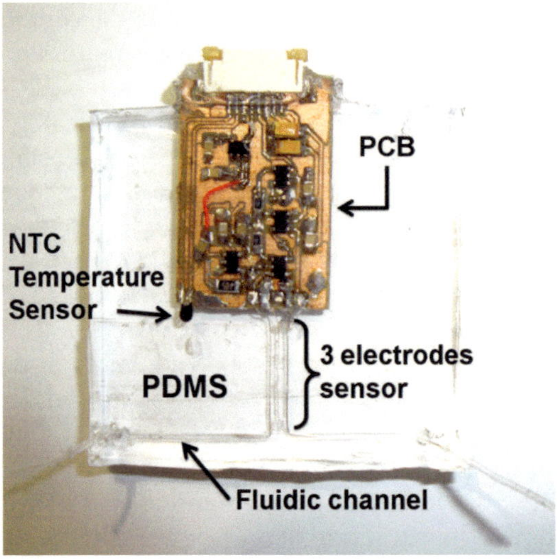

Fig. 17. PCB capture coated with PDMS.

The sensors were tested in different media solutions to detect changes in the oxygen concentration. The different media solutions used were Mili-Q water, TAP Water and 1mM PBS solution. All tests were performed at ambient temperature. The oxygen concentration in the solutions was reduced by applying nitrogen gas to the media for approximately 20 minutes. The measurements obtained are shown below, comparing the performance of the custom potentiostat with the commercial one. Fig. 18.A shows the experimental overlaid voltammograms obtained with tap water (with oxygen) concentration (Region A), and low O_2 concentration (Region B) using the commercial potentiostat and with the electronics coated with PDMS. The more negative peak shown in (A) results from the water sample that has been exposed to ambient air compared to the less negative peak (B) where the water sample has been bubbled with nitrogen to remove the oxygen.

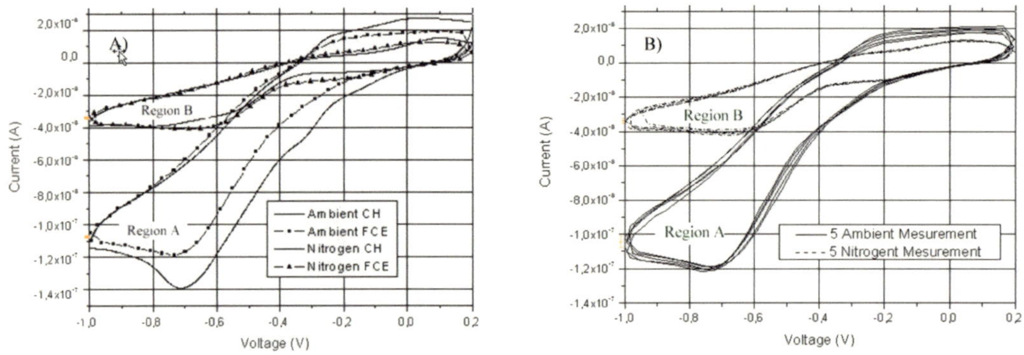

Fig. 18. A) Voltametry with CH Instrument and custom system in Ambient TAP Water and with nitrogen.; B) Custom Cyclic measurements, for different sensors and electronics, with tap water in the case of high and a very low concentration of oxygen.

Measurements with tap water have been carried out in order to characterise the custom potentiostat, as shown in Fig. 18.B) It can be noticed how the measurement of the current level and the minimum operating voltage are very similar. We have measured a variation lower than 4.5% in the case of high level concentration of oxygen, and even a lower variation (2.5%), in the case of low level oxigen concentration.

4. An example of an in-vivo biomedical implantable device

In this section, the conception of a generic CMOS architecture for an implantable device, (Colomer&Miribel, 2011) is presented. Nowadays, special interest in nanobiosensors is increasing in the field of medical diagnosis. From the market point of view, the main opportunity of such sensors is focused on on-line devices and in-vivo or implantable devices. The impact of such devices for each individual being will open the possibility to define a personalized diagnosis, and monitoring each patient. The development of such devices and the derived telemedicine environments has a great market potential. Different approaches should be followed for a discrete, small cm^3 or for an implantable device, and performances, communications capabilities, etc, are very different. The size of this implantable device is envisaged as a capsule of an ideal size less than 4.5 cm long and 2.5 cm in diameter, following the same philosophy like some subcutaneous implantable devices like Norplant®, Jadelle® or Implanon®, as implantable contraceptives. A proposal would be a True/False implantable system, or event detector that works as an alarm. When the analyzed concentration level is out of a range of accepted values, a threshold value activates the alarm, and a mapping could be defined, but sizing the complexity and the required power. The proposed generic implantable architecture is presented in Fig. 19. It is composed by a three electrodes BioSensor, an antenna and the electronic modules.
Such system combines different modules introduced thought the chapter. The antenna and the AC/DC module that is used to supply energy to the device (inductive powering), and the communication set-up (backscattering), as stated in 2.2, defining and AM modulation. Then, an integrated a low-voltage and low-power potentiostat is placed, as described in 2.4.2. Finally, in the modulation/Data Processing module an analog lock-in amplifier can be integrated. In this case an FRA approach is followed. An interesting approach to work with in-vivo biosensors is to sense its impedance variation at one defined frequency, where the sensor is more sensitive to changes in its impedance. Not a full Electrochemical Impedance Spectroscopy is carried out. Just the variation of the impedance or capacitance of the biosensor when the target analyte is captured by the probe is of interest. Looking for this kind of implementations, there is a trade-off between complexity, area, power consumption, with the desired measurements and the electronic implementation. In this sense, a fully integrated DSP solution, as a digital lock-in amplifier, would present a big challenge. The design looks forward to very small power consumption, working at very low power supply. Following this assumption, an analogue lock-in amplifier is derived, Fig. 20, completely integrated and conceived in a commercial technology, as electronic interface with implantable biosensors in low-frequency applications. The integrated lock-in is based on two Synchronous Demodulated Channels. Both channels are used to find two DC components at the same time. These DC levels would be used by other two comparators, defining in the same way an alarm system, or two ADC converters to send its digital words by a backscattering method for monitoring the impedance. From these rectified signals are obtained two DC components, VREout and VIMout, after a low-pass filter placed for each channel. The magnitude and phase of the electrochemical cell are then obtained afterwards using (2) and (3).

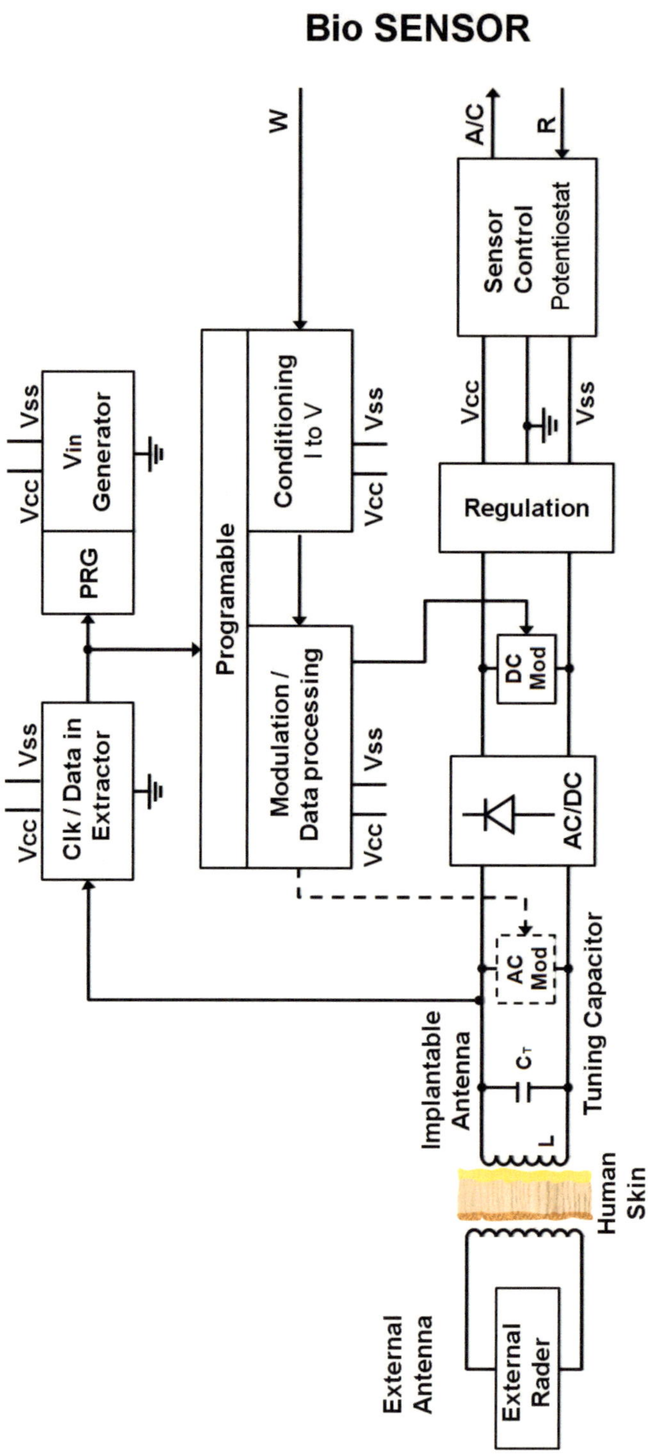

Fig. 19. Proposed generic implantable front-end architecture.

$$Magnitude = \sqrt{VREout^2 + VIMout^2} \tag{2}$$

$$Phase = Tan^{-1}\left(\frac{VIMout}{VREout}\right) \tag{3}$$

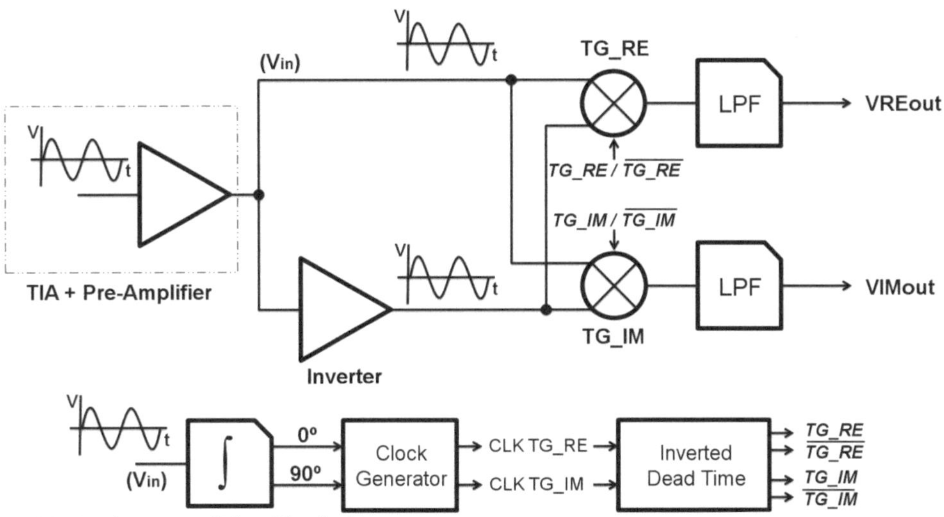

Fig. 20. Lock-in amplifier block diagram.

5. Summary and conclusions

In this chapter, we started with an introduction to the conception of a generic bio-portable device, which can be a miniaturized solution to an envisaged implantable device. This device is based on several components, which are basically represented by: the powering module, the communications module, the biosensors, the bioelectronics and the micro fluidics. These key elements have been introduced regarding the state-of-the-art and the trends involved in the development of such systems. In terms of the power module, special attention has been focused on the energy that can be harvested from ambient sources to body harvesting. A brief introduction to the communications module has been also presented. Biosensors and the needed bioelectronics involved in the design of such system were explained. Different approaches to work with electrochemical sensors, for potential control and measurement were introduced: potentiostat amplifiers and the use of a lock-in amplifier for an electrochemical impedance analysis. Finally, two implementations of electrochemical devices, from a discrete to an integrated approach, were also presented: an O_2 monitoring instrument and an approach for and In-vivo implantable device as an event detector.

6. References

Bender, S., and Sadik, O.A. (1998). Direct electrochemical immunosensor for polychlorinated biphenyls. *Environ. Sci. Technol*, vol. 32, pp. 788–797

BioLED Technology (2007). Internet Journal of emerging medical technologies, Available from http://www.medgadget.com/archives/2007/02/bioled_technolo.html

Carlson, E., Strunz, K., and Otis, B. (2009). 20mV input boost converter for thermoelectric energy harvesting. *Proc. of the 2009 Symposium on VLSI Circuits*, pp.162 - 163.

Carnes, E., and Wilkins, E. (2005). The development of a new, rapid, amperometric immunosensor for the detection of low concentrations of bacteria. *American Journal of Applied Sciences.*

Celik, T., and Kusetogullari, H. (2010). Solar-Powered Automated Road Survillance Systems for Speed Violation Detection. *IEEE Transactions on Industrial Electronics*, vol. 57, no. 9, pp. 3216– 3227.

Chen, Jingkuang. (2006). *Micro-machined medical devices, methods of fabricating microdevices, and medical diagnosis, imaging, stimulation, and treatment.* USPatent11/320921

Chinn, Douglas. (2008). Microfabricatin techniques for biologists: A Primer on Building Micromachines, In: *Microengineering in Biotechnology*. Michael P. Hugehs and Kai F. Hoettges. Springer. Methods in Molecular Biology, vol. 583, pp 1-53, ISBN:978-1-58829-381-7.

Chung, W.Y., Paglinawan, A.C., Wang, Y.H., and Kuo, T.T. (2007). A 600μW Readout Circuit with Potentiostat for Amperometric Chemical Sensors and Glucose Meter Applications. *Proc. of the IEEE Conference on Electron Devices and Solid- State Circuits*, pp. 1087 - 1090.

Cleven, R., Nur, Y., Krystek, P., and Van den Berg, G. (2005). Monitoring Metal Speciation in the Rivers Meuse and Rhine using DGT. *Water, air and Soil Pollution*, vol.165, pp. 249-263.

Colomer-Farrarons, J., Miribel-Catala, P., Saiz-Vela, A., Puig-Vidal, M., & Samitier, J. (2008). Power-Conditioning Circuitry for a Self-Powered System Based on Micro PZT Generators in a 0.13μm Low-Voltage Low-Power Technology. *IEEE Trans. on Industrial Electronics*, vol. 55, no. 9, Sept 2008, pp. 3249-3257.

Colomer-Farrarons, J., Miribel-Català, P., Rodríguez, I., & Samitier, J. (2009).CMOS Front-End Architecture for In-Vivo Biomedical Implantable Devices. *Proc. of the 35th Annual Conference of the IEEE Industrial Electronics*, Nov. 2009, pp.4437-4444.

Colomer, J., Miribel-Catala, P., Saiz-Vela, A., Rodriguez, I, &; Samitier, J. (2009). A low power CMOS biopotentiostat in a low-voltage 0.13 μm digital technology. 52nd IEEE International Midwest Symposium on Circuits and Systems, 2009. MWSCAS '09.

Colomer-Farrarons, J., Miribel-Català, P., Samitier, J., Arundell, M., & Rodríguez, I. (2009). Design of a miniaturized electrochemical instrument for in- situ O2 monitoring. (Proceedings Paper), *VLSI Circuits and Systems IV, Microtechnologies for the New Millennium*, Vol. 7363, Spie'09.

Colomer-Farrarons, J., Miribel-Català. P. (2011). *A CMOS Self-Powred Front-End Architecture for Subcutaneous Event-Detector Devices. Three-Electrodes Amperometric Biosensor Approach.* Springer, ISBN:978-94-007-0685-9, March 2011.

Ekanayake, E.M.I., Preethichandra, D.M.G., Kaneto, K. (2007). Fabrication and characterization of nano-structured conducting polymer electrodes for glucose biosensor applications. *Proc. Of the International Conference on Industrial and Information Systems*, pp. 63 – 66

Farace, G., Lillie, T., Hianik, P., Payne and Vadgama, P. (2002). Reagentless biosensing using electrochemical impedance spectroscopy. *Bioelectrochemistry*, vol. 55 , pp. 1–3.

Fiorito, P.A., and De Torresi, S.I.C. (2001). Glucose amperometric biosensor based on the co-immobilization of glucose oxidase (Gox) and ferrocene in poly(pyrrole) generated from ethanol/water mixtures. *J. Braz. Chem. Soc.*, vol. 12, pp. 729–733.

Garbuio, L., Lallart, M., Guyomar, D., Richard, C., and Audigier, D. (2009). Mechanical Energy Harvester With Ultralow Threshold Rectification Based on SSHI Nonlinear Technique. *IEEE Transactions on Industrial Electronics*, vol. 56, no. 4, pp. 1048 - 1056, April 2009.

Ghafar-Zadeh, E., Sawan, M., and Therriault, D. (2009).CMOS based capacitive sensor laboratory-on-chip: a multidisciplinary approach. *Analog Integrated Circuits and Signal Processing*, vol. 59, issue 1, pp. 1-12

Goud, J.D., Raj, P.M., Jin Liu, Narayan, R., Iyer, M., Tummala, R. (2007). Electrochemical Biosensors and Microfluidics in Organic System-on- Package Technology. *Proc. Of the Electronic Components and Technology Conference, 2007. ECTC '07, pp.* 1550 - 1555.

Hiller, M., Kranz, C., Huber, J., Bauerle, P., and Schuhmann, W. (1996). Amperometric biosensors produced by immobilization of redox enzymes at polythiophene-modified electrode surfaces. *Adv. Mater*, vol.8, pp. 219–222.

Huang, X., Li S., Schultz, J., Wang, Q., and Lin, Q. (2009).A capacitively based MEMS affinity glucose sensor. *Proc. of the International Solid-State Sensors, Actuators and Microsystems Conference*, TRANSDUCERS 2009, 21-25 June 2009, pp. 1457 - 1460.

Irigoien, X., Post, J., Castel, J., Pfeiffer ,K.F., HellmannB. (1999). Nycthemeral variations of the dissolved oxygen concentration in the turbidity maximum of three European estuaries: biological vs. physical processes. *Journal of Marine Systems,* vol. 22 , pp. 173-177.

Jining Xie; Shouyan Wang; Aryasomayajula, L.; Varadan, V.K. (2007).Material and electrochemical studies of platinum nanoparticle-coated carbon nanotubes for biosensing. *Proc. Of the IEEE Conference Nanotechnology*, pp.1077 - 1080

Johannessen, E.A., Wang, L., Cui, L., Tang, T.B., Astaras, A., Ahmadian, M., Cooper, J.M. (2004). Implementation of Multichannel Sensors for Remote Biomedical Measurements in a Microsystems Format. *IEEE Tran. Biomedical Engineering,* vol.51, issue 3, pp. 525-535.

Jovanov, E., Milenkovic, A., Otto, C., de Groen, P. (2005). A wireless body area network of intelligent motion sensors for computer assisted physical rehabilitation. *Journal of NeuroEngineering and* Rehabilitation, March, pp.2-6.

Juanola, E., Miribel-Català, P., Colomer-Fararrons, J., & Samitier, J. (2010). New green market opportunities from novel autonomous low power systems by energy harvesting. XXVII World Conference on Science and Technology Parks, IASP1020,

Kakerow, R., Kappert, H., Spiegel, E., and Manoli, Y. (1995). Low-power single-chip CMOS potentiostat. *Proc. of the International Conference on Solid-State Sensors and Actuators.*

Katz, E., and Willner, I. (2003). Probing biomolecular interactions at conductive and semiconductive surfaces by impedance spectroscopy: routes to impedimetric immunosensors. DNA-sensors, and enzyme biosensors. *Electroanalysis,* vol. 15, pp. 913–947.

Kazazian T., and Jansen, A.J. (2004). Eco-desing and human-powered products. *Proceedings of the Electronics Goes Green* 2004, 6-10 September 2004.

Khaligh, A., Zeng P., Xiaochun, W., and Yang, X. (2008). A hybrid energy scavenging topology for human-powered mobile electronics. *Proc. of the 34th Annual Conference of IEEE Industrial Electronics,* Nov. 2008 pp. 448 - 453.

Khaligh, A., Zheng, P., and Zheng, C. (2010). Kinetic Energy Harvesting Using Piezoelectric and Electromagnetic Technologies-State of the Art. *IEEE Transactions on Industrial Electronics,* vol.57, no. 3, March 2010, pp. 850-860.

Kissinger, P., Preddy, C., et.al. (1996). *Laboratory Techniques in Electroanalytical Chemistry.* Second Edition, P. Kissinger, and W. Heineman Eds., Marcel Dekker, Inc.,ISBN: 0-8247-9445-1, New York.

Kitamori, K. (2007). Micro and Nano Chemical System on Chip. *Proc. of the International Solid-State Sensors, Actuators and Microsystems Conference*, pp. 11 - 16

Kiziroglou, M.E., He, C., and Yeatman, E.M. (2009). Rolling Rod Electrostatic Microgenerator. *IEEE Transactions on Industrial Electronics*, vol. 56, no. 4, pp. 1101 - 1108.

Kramer,D.L. (1987). Dissolved oxygen and fish behavior. Environmental Biology of Fishes, vol.18, pp. 81-92 .

Kraver, K., Guthaus, M., Strong, T., Bird, P., Cha, G., Hold, W., and Brown, R. (2001). A mixed-signal sensor interface microinstrument. *Sensors and Actuators A*, vol. 91, pp. 266-277.

Kros, A., Van Hovell, W.F.M, Sommerdijk, N.A.J.M., and Nolte, R.J.M. (2001). Poly(3, 4-thylenedioxythiophene)-based glucose biosensors. *Adv. Mater*, vol. 13, pp. 1555–1557.

Laureyn, W., Nelis, D., Van Gerwen, P., Baert, K., Hermans, L., Magnee, R., Pireaux, J.J., and Maes, G. (2000). Nanoscaled interdigitated titanium electrodes for impedimetric biosensing. *Sens. Actuators B-Chem*, vol. 68, pp. 360–370

Le, T.T., Han, J., Jouanne, A. Von., Mayaram, K., and Fiez, T.S. (2006). Piezoelectric Micro-Power Generation Interface Circuits. *IEEE Journal of Solid-State Circuits*, vol.41, no.6, pp. 1411-1420, June 2006.

Lee, Y.J., Kim, J.D., Park, J.Y., (2009). Flexible enzyme free glucose micro-sensor for continuous monitoring applications. *Proc. Of the Solid-State Sensors, Actuators and Microsystems Conference, 2009, pp.* 1806 - 1809

Li, W., He, S., and Yu, S. (2010). Improving Power Density of a Cantilever Piezoelectric Power Harvester Through a Curved L-Shape Proof Mass. *IEEE Transactions on Industrial Electronics*, vol.57, no.3, pp. 868-876.

Lillie, G., Payne, P., and Vadgama, P. (2001). Electrochemical impedance spectroscopy as a platform for reagentless bioaffinity sensing. *Sens. Actuators B-Chem, vol.* 78, pp. 249–256.

Liu, Y., Chakrabartty, S., and Alocilja. E.C. (2007). Fundamental building blocks for molecular biowire based forward error-correcting biosensors. *Nanotechnology*, vol. 18, 424017, pp. 1-6.

Mohseni, P., Najafi, K., Eliades, S.J., Xiaoqin Wang, (2005). Wireless multichannel biopotential recording using an integrated FM telemetry circuit. *IEEE Tran. on Neural Systems and Rehabilitation Engineering*, vol. 13, issue 3, pp. 263-271

Murari, K., Sauer, C.M., Stanacevic, M., Cauwenberghs, G., and Thakor, N. (2005). Wireless Multichannel Integrated Potentiostat for Distributed Neurotransmitter Sensing. *Prof. Of the Engineering in Medicine and Biology Conference.*

Myung-suk, C., Sang-won, L., Jong-chul, K., Jun-dong, C., Jin-kwon, K., Hang-sik. S., Myung-ho, L., Un-sun, C., and Jae-seok, K. (2007). Implantable Bio system design for displacement measurement of living life. *Proc. of the International Conference on Advanced Communication Technology*, vol. 1, pp.299 – 304

Nasiri, A., Zabalawi, S.A., and Mandic, G. (2009). Indoor Power Harvesting Using Photovoltaic Cells for Low-Power Applications. *IEEE Transactions on Industrial Electronics*, vol. 56, no. 11, pp. 4502 – 4509.

Niyato, D., Hossain, E., Rashid, M.M., and Bhargava, V.K. (2007).Wireless sensor networks with energy harvesting technologies: a game-theoretic approach to optimal energy management. *IEEE Wireless Communications*, vol.14, no. 4, pp.90-96.

Paradiso, J.A. Starner, T. (2005). Energy scavenging for mobile and wireless electronics. *IEEE Pervasive Computing*, vol.4, Issue 1, pp. 18-27.

Patel, J.N., Kaminska, B., Gray, B., Gates, B.D. (2007). Electro-Enzymatic Glucose Sensor Using Hybrid Polymer Fabrication Process. *Proc. Of IEEE International Conference the Electronics, Circuits and Systems, 2007. ICECS 2007,* pp. 403 - 406

Poyatos, J.M., Muñio, M.M., Almecija, M.C., Toress, J.C., Hontoria, E., and Osorio.F. (2010). Advanced Oxidation Processes for Wastewater Treatment: State of the Art. *Water Air Soil Pollut*, vol.205, pp. 187-204.

Rahman, A.R.A., Justin, G., Guiseppi-Wilson, A., Guiseppi-Elie, A., (2009). Fabrication and Packaging of a Dual Sensing Electrochemical Biotransducer for Glucose and Lactate Useful in Intramuscular Physiologic Status Monitoring. *Sensors Journal*, vol. 9, issue 12, pp. 1856 - 1863

Reay, R., Kounaves, S., and Kovacs, G. (1994). An integrated CMOS potentiostat for miniaturized electroanalytical instrumentation. *Proc. of the IEEE Solid-State Circuits Conf.*

Rodrigues, N.P., Kimura, H., Sakai, Y., Fujii, T. (2007). Cell-Based Microfluidic Biochip for Electrochemical Real-Time Monitoring of Glucose and Oxygen. *Proc. Of the Solid-State Sensors, Actuators and Microsystems Conference*, pp. 843 - 846

Rodríguez-Trujillo, R., Castillo-Fernandez, O., Garrido, M., Arundell, M., Valencia, A., Gomila, G. (2008). High-Speed particle detection in a micro-Coulter counter with two-dimensional adjustable aperture. *Biosensors and Bioelectronics*. vol 24:2, pp. 290-296

Rodríguez-Villarrea, A.I., Arundell, M., Carmona, M., Samitier, J. (2010) -High flow rate microfluidic device for blood plasma separation using a range of temperaturas. *Lab on a Chip*, vol 10, pp. 211-219.

Roundy, S. Steingart,D., Frechette, L., Wright, P., and Rabaey, J. (2004). Power sources for wireless sensors networks. *Proc. of the 1st European Workshop on Wireless Sensors Networks*, Jan.2004, pp. 1-17.

Sato, F., Togo, M., Islam, MK., Matsue, T., Kosuge, J., et al. (2005). Enzymebased glucose fuel cell using Vitamin K-3-immobilized polymer as an electron mediator. *Electrochemistry Communications*, vol.7, no.7, pp. 643-647.

Shenck, N.S., and Paradiso, J. (2001). Energy scavenging with shoe-mounted piezoelectrics. *IEEE Micro*, Vol. 21, No. 3, May-June 2001, pp. 30-42.

Sogorb, T., Llario, J.V., Pelegri, J., Lajara, R., and Alberola, J. (2008).Studying the Feasibility of Energy Harvesting from Broadcast RF Station for WSN. *Proc. of the IEEE Instrumentation and Measurement Technology Conference,* May 2008, pp. 1360 - 1363.

Stark, J. (2006). Thermal Energy Harvesting with Thermo Life. *Proc. of the International Workshop on Wearable and Implantable Body Sensor Networks*, pp.19 - 22.

Teymoori, M.M., Asadollahi, H. (2009). MEMS Based Medical Microsensors. *Proc. Of the Computer and Electrical Engineering International Conference,* vol. 1, pp.158 - 162.

Terbouche, A., Djebbar, S., Benali-Baitich, O., and Hauchard, D. (2011). Complexation Study of Humic Acids Extracted from Sahara Soils with Zuinc (II) and Cadmium (II) by Differential Pulse Anodic Stripping Voltammetry (DPASV) and Conductimetric Methods. Water Air Soil Pollut, vol.216, pp. 679-691.

Thewes, R., Hofmann, F., Frey, A., Holzapfl, B., Schienle, M., Paulus, C., Schindler,P., Eckstein, G., Kassel, C., Stanzel, M., Hintsche, R., Nebling, E., Albers, J., Hassman, J., Schülein, J., Goemann, W., and Gumbrecht, W. (2002). Sensor Arrays for Fully-Electronic DNA Detection on CMOS. *Proc. Of the IEEE International Solid-State Circuits Conference.*

Usman Ali, S.M., Nur, O., Willander, M., Danielsson, B. (2009). Glucose Detection With a Commercial MOSFET Using a ZnO Nanowires Extended Gate. *IEEE Transactions on Nanotechnology*, vol. 8, issue 6, pp. 678 - 683.

Van Hoof, C., Leonov, V., Vullers, R.J.M. (2009). Thermoelectric and Hybrid Generators in Wearable Devices and Clothes. *Sixth International Workshop on Wearable and Implantable Body Sensor Networks*. 3-5 June, pp. 195 - 200.

Part 3

Biosensors for Environment and Biosecurity

19

Carbon Nanotube-based Cholinesterase Biosensors for the Detection of Pesticides

Xiuli Yue and Zhifei Dai
Nanomedicine and Biosensor Laboratory, School of Sciences, State Key Laboratory of Urban Water Resources and Environment, Harbin Institute of Technology, Harbin 150001, China

1. Introduction

Pesticides play an important role in the high productivity achieved in agriculture through the control of pests. However, the presence of pesticide residues and metabolites in food, water and soil currently represents one of the major issues for the environmental chemistry(Ongley, 1996; Smith and Gangolli, 2002; Lintellman et al., 2003). Pesticides are often very persistent with half-lives of decades and are transported over long distances by global circulation, and through run-off, find their way into aquatic systems. They are intentionally toxic, often towards non-target organisms. Three classes of pesticides have been problematic, namely organophosphates, carbamates and organochlorines. Organophosphate(OPs) pesticides obtain their toxicity from their ability to inhibit acetylcholinesterase (AChE), causing neurotoxicity (Fukuto, 1990). The presence of this enzyme in insects, birds, fish and all mammals give this class of pesticides enormous toxicity towards unintended targets. Carbamate pesticides are also cholinesterase inhibitors with a similar mechanism of action as organophosphate pesticides (Fukuto, 1990). An effective strategy for dealing with pesticide contamination in the environment has to commence with an assessment of the extent of the problem. Traditionally, chromatographic methods have been used to analyze the presence of compounds in environmental samples. These techniques are very powerful tools for monitoring toxic pesticides, but, they are expensive, time-consuming (involve extensive preparation steps), are not adapted for in situ and real time detection and require highly trained personnel. They are therefore unsuitable for screening of large volumes of samples, and due to their cost, developing countries do not readily have access to such methods.

Biosensors has attracted intensive research interest as a result of the need for cheap, fast and easy to use analytical tools that are able to provide real-time qualitative and quantitative information about the composition of a sample with minimum sample preparation (Dyk and Pletschke, 2011). Biosensors are analytical devices which utilize the sensitivity and selectivity of a bio-receptor attached onto the surface of a physical transducer. The cholinesterase (ChE) enzymes based biosensors have emerged as an ultrasensitive and selective technique for toxicity monitoring for environmental, agricultural, food or military applications (Silvana and Marty, 2006). These devices are based on the inhibition of ChE by toxicants such as pesticides. The principal motivation for designing ChE biosensors for toxicity monitoring is to provide a reliable alternative to classical methods currently used in chromatographic methods. A successful ChE biosensor for toxicity monitoring should offer comparable or even better analytical performances than the traditional chromatographic systems. Ideally, such sensors should be small, cheap, simple to handle and able to provide reliable information in real-time without or with a minimum sample preparation. The use of the enzyme should also provide increased sensitivity and selectivity for the analyte of interest.

Electrochemical biosensors are currently among the most popular of the various types of biosensors. Carbon nanotubes (CNTs) are promising materials for sensing applications due to fascinating electronic and optoelectronic properties that are distinct from other carbonaceous materials and nanoparticles of other types (Balasubramanian and Burghard, 2006). Particularly, the properties of small dimensions, functional surfaces, good conductivity, excellent biocompatibility, modifiable sidewall, and high reactivity make CNTs have some overwhelming advantages in fabricating electrochemical sensors with high performances (Rivas et al, 2007). Moreover, CNTs have an outstanding ability to mediate fast electron-transfer kinetics for a wide range of electroactive species, such as AChE. CNT chemical functionalization can be used to attach almost any desired chemical species to them, which allows us to enhance the solubility and biocompatibility of the tubes. This has permitted the realization of composite electrodes comprising CNTs well-dispersed in an appropriate polymer matrix(Wang et al, 2003).

Generally, the replacement of ordinary materials by CNTs can effectively improve the redox currents of inorganic molecules, organic compounds, macrobiomolecules or even biological cells. Due to the well-defined structure, the chemistry stability and the electrocatalytic activity toward many substances, CNTs are also extensively used as the carrier platforms for constructing various electrochemical sensors. Herein, we present an overview of significant advances in the research and development of CNT-based ChE biosensors. We will discuss the different configurations and fabrication techniques of CNT-based biosensors with a special emphasis on the low-cost electrochemical biosensors and the approaches used for enzyme immobilization.

2. Inhibitory effect of pesticides on Cholinesterase

Many enzymes used for the detection of pesticides are inhibited by the pesticide and the extent of inhibition is correlated to the concentration of the analyte. Acetylcholinesterases are a class of enzymes that catalyze the hydrolysis of acetylcholine, an ester which is a neurotransmitter (Fukuto, 1990; Stenersen, 2004). The reaction catalyzed by AChE is: acetylcholine+H_2O→choline+acetate. Organophosphate and carbamate pesticides are designed to inhibit AChE and this enzyme has been mostly used in enzymatic detection of these pesticides. The inhibition of AChE by organophosphates takes place as a result of the phosphorylation of the serine residue in the active site of the enzyme. The hydroxyl group on the serine residue acts as an electrophile which attacks the nucleophilic phosphorus. The phosphorylated enzyme is highly stable and the hydrolysis of acetylcholine is blocked. In some cases, depending on the chemical structure of the pesticide, the phosphorylation, and thus the inhibition, may be irreversible (Fukuto, 1990). Where the pesticide is a phosphorothionate ester with a P=S moiety rather that a P=O, these pesticides generally act as poor cholinesterase inhibitors, due to the low reactivity of the compound (Fukuto, 1990). An example of two phosphorothionate ester compounds is malathion or chloropyrifos. It would be expected that these compounds would be poor cholinesterase inhibitors. This can be overcome by chemically oxidizing the phosphorothionate ester compounds into its more active form prior to detection (Lee et al., 2002).

It is helpful for the development of a biosensor based on enzyme inhibition to know the structure of ChE enzyme and the mechanism of inhibition in order to better optimize several parameters which affect the degree of inhibition such as enzyme loading, incubation time, reaction time, concentration of substrate, pH and organic solvent (Arduini, 2010). The principal biological role of AChE is the termination of the nervous impulse transmission at cholinergic synapses by rapid hydrolysis of the neurotransmitter acetylcholine. Early kinetic studies indicated that the active site of AChE contains two sub-sites, the esteratic and anionic sub-sites, corresponding respectively, to the catalytic site and choline-binding pocket (Gordon, 1976). The esteratic site contains a serine residue which reacts with the substrate and, also, with the organophosphates and carbamates. This site is similar in the multiple forms of AChE (Electrophorus, Torpedo, rat and chicken) and it is also located in the butyrylcholinesterase (BChE) enzyme. For this reason, it is possible to use several species of AChE and BChE enzymes to develop a ChE biosensor for insecticides.

The substrate concentration can affect the degree of inhibition. It was found that the inhibition level (%) increases with increasing of the substrate concentration in the case of pesticide inhibition when a saturating substrate concentration was used (Kok et al, 2002). Joshi et al. (2005) have used a concentration of acetylhtiocholine two times higher than the apparent Michaelis-Menten constant (K_m) for the determination of the maximum activity of AChE before and after the inhibition by the paraoxon which was selected as model pesticide. In the case of competitive inhibition, at high substrate concentrations, the inhibition effect is not observed since the substrate competes with the inhibitor. Another enzyme that is related to AChE is BChE which is also termed pseudocholinesterase (Andreescu and Marty, 2006). Both these enzymes have been used for the detection of pesticides in the environment, but use different substrates. AChE and BChE also differ in that AChE is inhibited by excess substrate whereas BChE is not. In the case of irreversible inhibition, the high substrate concentration can be chosen in order to have a higher output signal. For AChE biosensor a concentration of 1 mM acetylthiocholine was adopted (Arduini, 2006). In order to obtain higher sensitivity in the case of biosensor format for insecticides, acetylcholine or acetylthiocholine for AChE biosensor and butyrylcholine or butyrylthiocholine for BChE biosensor is highly suggested (Arkhypova, 2004).

For irreversible inhibition it is possible to achieve lower detection limits using longer incubation times; in fact, usually the degree of the enzyme inhibition increases with the incubation time until reaching a plateau (Kok, 2004). The incubation time is usually chosen as compromise between a sensitive measurement and a measurement carried out in a reasonable time (Dzyadevych, 2005). Usually, the incubation time should be not longer than 1 h because one of the biosensor advantage than i.e. HPLC should be the short time of analysis. In order to increase the sensitivity of the biosensor, it is better varying the enzyme loading than to use the incubation time longer than 1 h. In fact, for irreversible inhibition the degree of inhibition depends of the enzyme concentration.

The pH of the solutions containing substrates can affect the overall enzymatic activity since, like all natural proteins, enzymes have a native tertiary structure that is sensitive to pH;

denaturation of enzymes can occur at extreme pHs. It is well known that the enzyme activity is highly pH dependent and the optimum pH for an enzymatic assay must be determined empirically. It is best to choose a plateau region so that the pH should not have any effect on enzyme activity and will not interfere with the results obtained relative to the inhibition of the enzyme by the inhibitor. The activity of the immobilized acetylcholinesterase as a function of pH was studied between pH 2 and 9 and the activity of approximately 70% decreased at pH 2 in comparison with that at pH 7 (Stoytcheva et al, 2002). For the selection of the pH, it should be considered that certain enzymes have ionic groups on their active site and these groups must be in a suitable form such as the serine group in the catalytic site of ChE enzymes. The optimum pH for the free enzyme is pH=8. The acid pH should be avoided, in fact in the case of insecticide detection during wine fermentation (Suprun, 2005) it is necessary to adjust the pH towards neutral value.
The extraction of pesticides is carried out using organic solvents as reported in the official methods for pesticides detection, so it is important to choose an appropriate organic solvent to reduce the enzyme inactivation. To understand the possibility to use the organic solvents for insecticide detection with biosensor, their effect on ChE activity was investigated. Depending on the nature and the amount of organic solvent involved, the enzyme can be strongly inactivated when experiments are performed in these media. Thus, the choice of organic solvent needs to be considered as part of the method development in order to avoid undesirable effects. The effects of organic solvents have been shown to be quite variable and depend on the configuration in which the enzyme is employed. For example, the influence of acetonitrile, ethanol and DMSO on a cholinesterase sensor was studied using acetylthiocholine as substrate (Montesinos et al, 2001). An increase of the output current was noticed when working in 5% acetonitrile and 10% ethanol, resulting from partial deactivation of the enzyme. Therefore, the choice of an appropriate organic solvent is important to circumvent or minimize the enzyme inactivation.
AChE from different sources may vary in their reactivity to pesticide inhibition and sensitivity (limit of detection). Comparative studies have been performed with various wild-type AChE as well as some genetically modified enzymes. Of the wild-type enzymes, AChE from electric eel was more sensitive than AChE from bovine and human erythrocytes. In addition, greater sensitivity was achieved with the genetically modified AChE from Drosophylla melanogaster.

3. Pretreatment and dispersion of carbon nanotube

3.1 Pretreatment of carbon nanotube

CNTs possess interesting electrochemical properties and the improvement in the electron transfer is due to the curvature of the tubes that originate changes in the energy bands close to the Fermi level (Britto et al, 1999). The presence of pentagonal defects produce regions with charge density higher than those observed in the region of hexagonal graphite, either in planar or in tubular structures (Britto et al, 1999). Usually, CNTs should be pretreated in order to eliminate metallic impurities, and/or to improve the electron transfer properties and/or to allow further functionalization. The protocols are based on the oxidation of CNTs under different conditions. In all cases the ends and side-walls become rich in oxygenated functions, mainly carboxylic groups. Depending on how drastic is the treatment, it is possible not only to increase the density of oxygenated functions but also to break the tubes or even to shorten them(Rivas et al, 2007). Solutions of sulfuric, nitric, and hydrochloric

acids and, either concentrated or diluted, alone or mixed have been extensively used for activation of CNTs. In some cases, the pretreatments were based on a combination of different chemical and electrochemical protocols (Rivas et al, 2007).
Generally, CNTs exist as highly tangled ropes and are insoluble in almost all solvents, thus, greatly hindering their capacity of forming uniform and stable films. Therefore, the major problem on the promising applications of CNTs in electrochemical sensors is the immobilization of activated CNTs on the electrode surface. To overcome this deficiency, CNTs are firstly dispersed or dissolved in various solutions or suspensions and immobilized on the surfaces of various substrates by physical or chemical methods.

3.2 Solvent dispersion of carbon nanotube

The most widely protocols for fabricating CNT-based electrochemical sensors involve the dispersing of CNTs in a certain solvent with sonication after purification and activation pretreatments of CNTs, followed by dropping the resultant suspensions on the electrode surfaces and allowing to dry (i.e., the casting methods). Among the reported solvents, N,N-dimethylformamide (DMF) is the most extensively used polar solvent and more than half of the papers deal with CNT-based electrochemical sensors using DMF as the dispersing solvent (Xu et al, 2004). The other solvents, which have been used to prepare CNT suspensions, include water (Guo et al, 2005), acetone (Wu et al, 2002), ethanol (Qu et al, 2004) and even toluene (Lefrant et al, 2004). Compared with other approaches, the solvent-dispersing methods of CNTs inevitably suffer from some disadvantages, such as low solubility, low stability and low exfoliation efficiency, due to the rather weak interactions between these solvents and CNTs.

3.3 Additives -assisted dispersion of carbon nanotube

The preparation of an electrochemical sensor modified with a CNT-dispersion basically consists of casting the electrode, usually glassy carbon or gold, with a drop of the given dispersion, followed by a drying step under different conditions. To improve the solubility and stability of CNTs in their suspensions, various additives are added into solvents to assist the dispersion of CNTs, such as surfactants, polymers, proteins and cyclodextrins.
Dihexadecyl hydrogen phosphate (DHP) consists of two hydrophobic tails and a dissociable phosphate group. Based on the hydrophobic interactions between the hydrophobic tails of DHP and the sidewall of the nanotubes as well as the possible interactions between the phosphate groups on DHP and the oxygen-containing groups on acid-treated CNTs, MWNTs were able to disperse in the aqueous suspension of DHP with sonication, resulting in the formation of a stable and homogeneous aqueous suspension of DHP and CNTs (Wu et al, 2003 and 2004; Wang et al, 2004). Sodium dodecyl sulphate (SDS) has been widely used to prepare stable suspensions of purified SWNTs in water with the aid of sonication (Abatemarco, 1999). It is suggested that the encapsulation of SWNTs in SDS micelles and the repulsive interactions between negatively charged SDS micelles account for the stable suspension of SWNTs in solution. The suspension of CNTs in cetyltrimethylammonium bromide (CTAB) aqueous solution was also reported (Cai and Chen, 2004). Nafion has been used extensively for the modification of electrode surfaces and for the construction of amperometric biosensors because of the unique ion-exchange, discriminative, and biocompatibility properties (Fortier et al, 1992; Fan et al, 1992). Nafion contains two different regions: the hydrophobic polymer backbone and the ionized hydrophilic sulfonate groups

outside the hydrophobic region. This special amphiphilic structure makes Nafion bear the capacity of combining with CNTs by hydrophobic interactions between the hydrophobic backbone of Nafion and the sidewall of CNTs as well as dispersing them in solutions by the hydrophilic groups.
As a kind of special amphiphilic biomacromolecues, proteins are proved to be capable of dispersing CNTs in water. It was found that SWNTs are naturally protein-affinitive in an aqueous ferritin solution (Lin et al, 2004). The conjugation can be further enhanced and stabilized in the presence of a coupling agent for amidation to promote the formation of covalent linkages.
Cyclodextrins (CDs) are cyclic oligosaccharides and contain a relatively hydrophobic central cavity and hydrophilic outer surface. CDs were able to adsorb onto the surface of nanotubes via van der Waals forces. The soft cutting of SWNTs by CDs was observed, indicating the use of CDs for the chemical manipulation and processing of CNTs (Chen et al, 2001).
Positively charged polyethyleneimine (PEI) has also been extensively employed as an efficient additive for the dispersion of CNTs in aqueous solutions. The resulting PEI-CNT composite was proved to have good stability and biocompatibility. Based on the reactivity of amino groups on PEI, the noncovalent or covalent modification of CNTs by PEI provides a simple approach to the further surface functionalization of CNTs by quantum dots (Shan and Gao, 2006), metal nanoparticles (Hu et al, 2006 and 2007). PEI-functionlized CNTs are a useful nanocomposite in electromistry and electroanalytical chemistry. Similar to PEI, Polylysine is an efficient dispersing agent of MWCNT because of the large amount of amine residues that facilitate the interaction with the MWCNT(Rivas et al, 2007). It was found that the mild sonication of MWNTs in aqueous poly(diallyl dimethyl ammonium) chloride (PDDA) resulted in a significant improvement of CNT dispersibility and enhanced their adhesion to Au and Si substrates (Mamedov et al, 2002).
Chitosan (CHIT) displays excellent film-forming ability, high water permeability, good adhesion, and susceptibility to chemical modifications due to the presence of reactive amino and hydroxyl functional groups. The stable dispersion of CNTs was prepared in the acidic aqueous solutions of CHIT with the help of sonication (Jiang et al, 2004). It was demonstrated that CHIT might be adsorbed onto CNTs and form a special CHIT-CNT system, which can be precipitated from the solutions by the addition of concentrated salts or the adjustment of solution acidity. The selective interaction between CHIT and CNTs also provided a possible approach for separating CNTs from carbonaceous impurities.

4. Modification of CNT-based electrodes by metallic nanoparticles

Transition metals such as gold, platinum, palladium, copper, silver and nickel are well-known for their high catalytic activity. Nanoparticles (NPs) made from these transition nanoparticles have been widely utilized to enhance the performances of electrodes made of carbonaceous materials, and, in particular, to increase their sensitivity towards a specific analyte. Because nanoparticles can provide a larger surface area and be easily modified with a wide range of biomolecules they enable the fabrication of biosensors with a plethora of sensing possibilities.
Both single-walled carbon nanotubes (SWCNTs) and multiwalled carbon nanotubes (MWCNTs) have been modified with different metal nanoparticles via the adsorption of preformed nanoparticles, or via electrodeposition from metal salt solutions. The latter

method is especially attractive since it allows precise control over the degree of modification in a reproducible manner (2004; Day et al, 2005). By controlling the duration and magnitude of the applied potential in conjunction with the concentration of the salt used, different sizes and densities of such particles can be obtained (Day et al, 2005). Among those nanoparticles that have been commonly deposited on carbon nanotubes, gold nanoparticles (GNPs) have been paid much interest. It has been reported that CNTs/GNPs composites could be synthesized through citrate reduction or were electrochemical deposition of GNPs on CNTs via in situ reduction of $HAuCl_4$ by $NaBH_4$ (Xiao et al, 2008). Choi et al. reported that GNPs could be generated on single-walled carbon nanotubes (SWCNTs) through direct redox reactions by immersing SWCNTs in a solution of Au^{3+} ions (Choi et al, 2002). Another reports demonstrated that GNPs was deposited on the side wall of multiwalled carbon nanotubes(MWCNTs) by one-step reaction with $NaBH_4$ as reductant and stabilized with sodium citrate in aqueous solution to form MWCNTs-GNPs nanocomposite(Du et al, 2010). During this synthesis process, GNPs could be self-coated on the MWCNTs to form uniform nanocomposites. The formed MWCNTs-Au nanocomposites offered an extremely hydrophilic surface for biomolecule adhesion, leading to a stable acetylcholinesterase biosensor. Due to the excellent conductivity of the nanocomposites, the immobilized AChE showed favorable affinity to acetylthiocholine (ATCl) and could catalyze the hydrolysis of acetylthiocholine to form thiocholine, which was then oxidized to produce a detectable and fast response. Using malathion as a model compound, the inhibition of malathion was proportional to its concentration ranging from 1.0 to 1000 ng mL^{-1} and from 2 to 15 μgmL^{-1}, with a detection limit 0.6 $ngmL^{-1}$.

5. Immobilization of cholinesterase onto CNT-based electrodes

The selectivity and sensitivity of CNT-modified electrodes can be improved through the immobilization of enzymes. In such electrodes, the CNTs mainly serve as transducers, communicating the signal effectively from the active enzyme centers to the substrate. After the choice of transducer, the enzyme immobilization is an important step in the biosensor design. The development of biosensors based on immobilized enzymes came about to solve several problems such as loss of enzyme (especially if expensive), maintenance of enzyme stability and shelf life of the biosensor, and additionally to reduce the time of the enzymatic response and offer disposable devices which can be easily used in stationary or in flow systems. In order to increase the storage stability in a dry state, which is a key point to commercialize the ChE biosensor, the immobilization should maintain the enzyme activity also in a dry state for several days. To do this, several types of immobilization techniques relying on noncovalent, covalent bonding or covalent cross-linking of the enzyme were investigated in order to obtain sensitive and stable ChE biosensors. The noncovalent approach, which has a negligible effect on the activity of the enzyme, can be subdivided into adsorption, entrapment and microencapsulation techniques. In the first technique, the enzyme is attached with the help of a binder or an ion-exchange resin onto CNT-modified electrodes. Alternatively, the enzyme can be immobilized using surface groups of self-assembled monolayers or Langmuir–Blodgett (LB) films. In the entrapment method, a (electro)polymerization reaction is carried out during which the enzyme is incorporated into the resulting polymer matrix. The encapsulation method makes use of hydrogels or sol-gels to immobilize the enzyme.

5.1 Enzyme adsorption

The physical immobilization such as adsorption is one of the simple procedure to immobilize the biocomponent onto the transducer (Bonnet, 2003). AChE was immobilized by adsorption on screen printed electrodes modified with multiwall carbon nanotubes (MWCNTs). In this way, some µL of AChE solution were dropped on the MWCNT modified electrode surface and allowed to evaporate at room temperature under a current of air. The electrode was then rinsed twice with buffer to remove the loosely adsorbed enzyme molecules on MWCNTs (Joshi, 2005). This was an important step to avoid the leakage of the enzyme during the measurement. One of the most sensitive biosensors was developed by immobilizing AChE via physical adsorption in nanostructured carbon matrix as reported (Sotiropoulou and Chaniotakis, 2005). The obtained biosensor is very stable and has very low detection limit for dichlorvos at picomolar levels. This promising result was attributed to the properties of the activated carbon to preconcentrate the insecticides and the hyperactivity of enzyme within the nanopores. Nevertheless, the immobilization of enzymes via adsorption faces several problems, such as the low quantity of adsorbed enzyme, leaching of the enzyme and so on. Some of these limitations can be overcome by adsorbing enzymes onto CNT-modified electrodes decorated with metallic nanoparticles, such as Pt-NP. By subsequently depositing a Nafion film onto the electrode, it is possible to reduce leaching of the enzyme and to improve the stability of the biosensor.

5.2 Self-assembling immobilization

During the acid treatments of CNTs, the negatively charged carboxyl groups produce, providing two methods for the direct self-assembling immobilization of CNTs on electrode surfaces. In the first method, CNTs are adsorbed onto electrode surfaces via the electrostatic interactions between negatively charged carboxyl groups on CNTs and the positively charged species on the electrode surfaces. The second method is the covalent bonding of CNTs to cysteamine self-assembled monolayer (SAM) modified gold electrodes via the reaction of carboxyl groups on CNTs and amino groups on cysteamine SAM in the presence of coupling reagents (Liu et al, 2000). As-grown nanotubes were first cut into short pipes and thiol-derivatized at the open ends by chemical methods. The ordered assembly of SWNTs was then made by their spontaneous chemical adsorption to gold via Au–S bonds. The nanotubes were found to be organized on gold, forming a self-assembled monolayer structure with a perpendicular orientation.

A recent approach to immobilize AChE was proposed based on the layer-by-layer (LbL) self-assembly of oppositely charged polyelectrolyte and enzyme onto previously functionalized CNT-modified electrode (Liu et al, 2006). In one case, the negative charges were originated onto the surface of carbon nanotubes by adsorbing a pyrene derivative, which serves as platform for further assembling of poly(diallyldimethylammonium) (PDDA) and polystyrene sulfonate (PSS).

For the detection of carbaryl pesticides, an amperometric biosensor is fabricated based on consectively adsorption of the PDDA modified single walled carbon nanotubes (PDDA-SWCNTs) and acetyl cholinestrase onto the surface of glassy carbon electrode(Firdoz et al, 2010). The optical intensity of UV/vis spectra increased with the number of layers, indicating the build up of a multilayer coating on the electrode. The biosensor from $[(PDDA\text{-}SWCNTs)/AchE]_5$ coated glassy carbon electrode showed good sensitivity and stability towards the monitoring of carbaryl pesticides in water with the detection limit of 10^{-12} g.L^{-1} and recovery of 99.8 ±2.7% to 10^{-10} g.L^{-1}.

A highly sensitive flow injection amperometric biosensor is fabricated for the detection of organophosphate pesticides based on self-assembled AChE on a carbon nanotube-modified glassy carbon electrode. The MWCNTs was initially treated with NaOH in order to assume a negative charge and then was dipped into a solution of cationic PDDA which leads to the adsorption of positively charged polycation layer (MWCNTs-PDDA). After the negatively charged AChE was adsorbed on MWCNTs-PDDA to obtain MWCNTs-PDDA-AchE, another PDDA layer was absorbed in order to avoid the leakage of AChE from the electrode surface, resulting in sandwich structure of PDDA/AChE/PDDA(Liu et al, 2006). The unique sandwich-like structure (PDDA/AChE/PDDA) on the MWCNTs surface formed by self-assembling provides a favorable microenvironment to keep the bioactivity of AChE. The electrocatalytic activity of MWCNTs leads to a greatly improved electrochemical detection of the enzymatically generated thiocholine product, including a low oxidation overvoltage (+150 mV), higher sensitivity, and stability. The developed PDDA/AChE/PDDA/ MWCNTs/GC biosensor integrated into a flow injection system was used to monitor organophosphate pesticides and nerve agents, such as paraoxon. Under the optimal conditions, this biosensor allows a low detection limit of paraoxon equal to 0.4×10^{-12} M with a 6-min inhibition time. The biosensor had excellent operational lifetime stability with no decrease in the activity of enzymes for more than 20 repeated measurements over a 1-week period.

5.3 Covalent attachment

The adsorption method normally yields a random distribution of the enzymes on the electrode. However, direct anchoring of the enzymes to the carbon framework becomes feasible if the covalent immobilization approach is used. In addition, it often enables direct electron transfer to the active center of the enzyme. One of the most used types of enzyme immobilization is the chemical immobilization by means of cross-linking with glutaraldeyde. This method confers to the biosensor high working stability even if there is usually a decrease of the enzymatic affinity towards its substrate due to the distortion of the enzyme structure (Arduini et al, 2006 and 2007; Vakurov, 2004). An example of chemical immobilization is based on a non-conducting polymer electrosynthetized onto the electrode after the enzyme was immobilized by crosslinking with glutaraldehyde (Curulli et al, 2001; Suprun et al, 2004). ChE immobilization was able to carry out by cross-linking method with glutaraldehyde vapour (Arkhypova et al, 2003, 2004 and 2008). It was reported a ChE membrane formed on the electrode with ChE, Nafion and glutaraldehyde (Suprun et al, 2005; Ivanov et al, 2003). In this case, it was found that the use of albumin bovine serum at 3% increases the enzyme stability (Arduini et al, 2006; Laschi et al 2007).

5.4 Electropolymerization

The polymerization of various monomers in the presence of dispersed CNTs in solutions by electrochemical methods has been employed for the immobilization of CNTs on the electrode surface. In this process, CNTs were enwrapped in polymers during the electropolymerization process in the form of counter ions or dopants. A marvelous method was proposed for the dispersion and immobilization of CNTs on the electrode surface by water-soluble alizarin red S (Wu et al, 2004). Electropolymerization is also an attractive and well-controlled method for immobilizing enzymes onto electrodes. In this methodology, the enzyme is mixed with a monomer which is electropolymerized at a GCE or a metal electrode, whereupon the enzyme becomes embedded into the polymer matrix. The incorporation of the enzyme into the matrix is often promoted through electrostatic interactions. Numerous enzymes have been incorporated into electropolymerized films(Bartlett and Cooper, 1993). In many cases conductive polypyrrole (PPy) has been used as a polymer matrix. This choice relates to the fact that pyrrole can be electropolymerized at low oxidation potentials in aqueous solutions at neutral pH, which is compatible with a wide range of biological molecules. Polypyrrole has proven effective at electrically wiring the enzymes and CNTs to the underlying electrode. During the fabrication of such biosensors, CNTs bearing carboxylic groups are often used due to their ability to function as an anionic dopant in the matrix.

Recently, a simple method to immobilize AChE on PPy and polyaniline (PAn) copolymer doped with multi-walled carbon nanotubes (MWCNTs) was proposed(Du et al, 2010). The synthesized PAn-PPy-MWCNTs copolymer presented a porous and homogeneous morphology which provided an ideal size to entrap enzyme molecules. The surface hydrophilicity was improved greatly after forming a complex structure instead of a separate layer. It provided an excellent environmental and chemical stability around the enzyme molecule to stabilize its biological activity to a large extent, resulting in a stable AChE biosensor for screening of organophosphates exposure. MWCNTs promoted electron-transfer reactions at a lower potential and catalyzed the electro-oxidation of thiocholine, thus increasing detection sensitivity. Based on the inhibition of OPs on the AChE activity, using malathion as a model compound, the inhibition of malathion was proportional to its concentration ranging from 0.01 to 0.5 μg/mL and from 1 to 25 μg/mL, with a detection limit of 1.0 ng/mL. Advantages of the electropolymerization approach include the good control over the film thickness and the ability to selectively attach biomaterials onto nanoscale electrode surfaces. The developed biosensor exhibited good reproducibility and acceptable stability.

5.5 Encapsulation

The sol-gel and hydrogel have been widely used in recent years to immobilize biomolecules (e.g., enzymes) for constructing electrochemical biosensors because of their easy fabrication, chemical inertness, thermal stability and good biocompatibility. It was reported that the immobilization of ChE by encapsulation in sol-gel prepared by tetramethoxysilane (TMSO) and methyltrimethoxysilane (MTMSOS) showed in both cases a storage stability of several months (Anitha et al, 2004). However, the lack of electrochemical reactivity and the poor conductivity of these materials greatly hinder their promising applications. Therefore, carbon nanotube has been widely incorporated into the sol-gel or hydrogel matrix. A typical procedure for preparing CNT-based hydrogel or sol-gel consists of the dispersion of CNTs in solvents, the mixing of the CNT suspensions with the hydrogel or the sol-gel and finally the casting of the resultant matrix containing the immobilized enzyme on the electrode surfaces. CNT acted as both nanometer conducting wires and catalysts, which can effectively promote electron transfer between enzymes and the electrode surface. The main advantage of the encapsulation process is that the entrapped species often preserves its intrinsic bioactivity. Additionally, such sensors exhibit enhanced sensor response, due to an increase in the surface area as well as an improvement in the electrical communication between the redox centers of the hydrogel or the sol-gel-derived matrix and the electrode. Apart from hydrogels and sol-gels, Nafion has also been found to be useful when fabricating composite electrodes. A broad range of enzymes has been successfully immobilized onto CNT-incorporated redox hydrogels to yield sensitive biosensors (Joshi, 2005). These CNT-based sol-gel electrochemical biosensing platforms were demonstrated to possess both the electrochemical characteristics of CNTs and the role of sol-gel for eliminating byproducts. In contrast to the conventional sol-gel or CNT-based electrochemical sensors, the electrochemical response of these electrodes can be conveniently tuned from that of conventional scale electrodes to that of microelectrodes by just varying the content of MWNTs in the composites. A sensitive and stable amperometric sensor has been devised for rapid determination of triazophos based on efficient immobilization of AChE on silica sol-gel film assembling MWNTs (Du et al, 2007). Under optimum conditions, the inhibition of triazophos was proportional to its concentration from 0.02 μM to 1 μM and from 5 μM to 30 μM, with a detection limit of 0.005 μM.

6. Practical concerns

The detection of pesticides is essential for the protection of water resources and food supplies. The designed biosensor should be sensitive enough to decrease the threshold detection as low as possible (Villatte et al., 1998 and Sotiropoulou et al., 2005). In addition, it should be selective towards the target analyte or class analytes. Before the benefits of enzymatic methods can be transferred from the laboratory to the field, it is important to stress that in the case of real samples the ChE biosensor is not a selective system because organophosphorus and carbamic insecticides and some other compounds have an inhibition effect on ChE. It has been demonstrated that an enzyme such as AChE is inhibited by organophosphate and carbamate pesticides by a similar mechanism of action but with different inhibition degree (Fukuto, 1990). This makes ChE biosensors unable to correctly differentiate and identify particular analytes, so the selectivity for measuring ChE inhibitors is very poor (Schulze et al., 2003 and Luque de Castro and Herrera, 2003). Therefore, ChE biosensors are mainly attractive for measuring the total toxicity of the sample, rather than a specific inhibitor. In fact, this behavior can be a disadvantage because other techniques are required in order to evaluate which inhibitor is present. Therefore, little success has been realized through real practical applications and commercialization of these devices for solving real world problems despite a significant amount of scientific research dedicated to ChE biosensors. Nontheless, this aspect can be also an advantage taking in consideration that this system is a screening method. Biosensors can be very useful tool to understand the presence of possible toxic compounds able to inhibit the ChEs, and only the samples in which the inhibition is observed will be measured by the reference method with a relevant saving in terms of time and cost of analysis (Dzydevych et al, 2002).

Further improvement in sensitivity and selectivity can be obtained with the use of sensitive multienzymes which allow discrimination between the insecticides and other interferences. Enzymes extracted from different sources have different sensitivities and selectivities toward pesticides. For instance, the AChE extracted from the Drosophila melanogaster is 8-fold more sensitive than the AChE from the Electric eel (Tsai and Doog, 2005). Moreover, advances in molecular biology have made possible engineering of more sensitive and selective ChE with individual sensitivity patterns towards a target inhibitor. Recombinant AChEs have been undertaken to increase the sensitivity of AChE to specific organophosphates and carbamates using site-directed mutagenesis and employing the enzyme in different assay formats (Schulze et al, 2003). It was reported that an array of multienzyme biosensors constructed with four immobilized AChEs (wild type and three recombinant mutants) allowed discrimination of malaoxon and parathion in a binary composite mixture and enabled detection of 11 out of 14 organophosphate and carbamate pesticides (Bachmann et al., 2000 and Schulze et al., 2005).

ChE biosensors have great application potentials in environmental and food matrices, public safety and military/antiterrorism. Most ChE biosensors designed for practical applications use immobilized enzyme. However, as applied to inhibitor determination, the practical application of immobilized ChE has a significant limitation. The inhibition results in a decrease of the ChE activity so that repetitive use of the same biosensor without enzyme reloading or reactivation is limited. The solution to this problem is to employ single use disposable electrodes. These are usually prepared by screen-printed technology which allows mass production with significant reduction in the price per electrode.

The most studied pesticides are paraoxon, dichlorvos, diazinon, aldicarb and carbofuran. Paraoxon is commonly used as a model example for ChE inhibition. Some pesticides have nearly no or little inhibitory effect on ChE in their pure form. In this case, detection is still possible by oxidizing them to oxon forms, which are much more toxic. The typical example is the case of parathion, and its corresponding oxon form, paraoxon. In some cases, oxidation and detection of these pesticides has been improved with the use of a genetically modified mutant ChE enzyme (Schulze et al., 2004). Anatoxin-a(s) is a natural organophosphate which irreversibly inhibits AChE, similar to organophosphorus and carbamate pesticides. Due to the difficulty to detect this compound using classical analytical chemistry methodologies, research efforts have been directed toward the use of ChE biosensors, which allow detection of anatoxin-a(s) at very low concentrations (detection limit of 5×10^{-10}M) (Vilatte et al., 2002).

The superior electrocatalytic activity of CNT-based electrodes has sparked an explosive amount of research directed at using CNTs for electrochemical biosensing. In fact, a range of molecules can be easily oxidized at low potentials at CNT-based electrodes. Even if such electrodes are equipped with analyte-specific recognition units such as enzymes, they are still vulnerable to other electroactive compounds that can also be oxidized at these low potentials. Thus, for the assessment of a CNT-based biosensor, it is of utmost importance to carefully consider the interferents involved in the sample under consideration. The optimal composition of the biosensor is a trade-off between the various device parameters. A low amount of immobilized enzyme provides only a limited concentration range where the response is linear, whereas a large amount of enzyme could reduce the electrochemical activity of the CNTs. While direct immobilization of the enzyme without a matrix would be ideal for obtaining sensitive responses, such electrodes are prone to leaching of the enzyme. This loss and the subsequent reduction in sensitivity and reproducibility can be largely avoided by electropolymerized matrices.

In enzymatic detection methods, an initial concentrating step of the target analyte by liquid–liquid or solid-phase extraction methods has not been commonly used for further improvement of the sensitivity of detection. Yet, Marchesini et al. (2005) reported an increase in the limit of detection of 40 times where solid-phase extraction was used, although in this case the biorecognition element was not an enzyme but an antibody. It is expected that such methods could be applied to enzymatic detection to improve sensitivity, but may affect the portability of the method.

7. Conclusion

The most important challenge in the development of ChE biosensors for practical applications is the transfer of these devices from pristine research laboratory conditions to real-life and commercial applications. In this direction, some critical parameters such as enzyme stability, reliability and selectivity still have to be improved. This review highlighted the analytical parameters that should be investigated in order to increase the assay sensitivity using inhibition biosensors. The knowledge of the type of inhibition allows thus to optimize in a fast way the biosensor in order to increase the performance of the system and also to reduce the interferences. CNTs have been demonstrated to be an excellent material for the development of electrochemical biosensors. The incorporation of CNTs within composites offers the advantages of an easy and fast preparation, and represents a very convenient alternative as a platform for further design of biosensors with the improved performance. Considerable progress in genetic engineering allows for the production of more selective and sensitive ChEs. The design of each sensor containing a different immobilized enzyme (wild type and mutants ChEs extracted from different sources) could allow sensitive detection and differentiation of multianalyte mixtures. In addition, automated and continuous systems have been developed for measuring ChE inhibitors in flow conditions by a computer controlled-programmable valve system which allows reproducible pumping of different reagents including buffers, substrate and inhibitor solutions, reactivating agents and real samples. The combination of the unique properties of CNTs with the powerful recognition properties of sensitive multienzymes and the known advantages of the automated and continuous systems represents a very good alternative for the development of compact and portable devices able to address future biosensing challenges in environmental monitoring and security control, among others.

8. Acknowledgment

This research was financially supported by the National Natural Science Foundation of China (No.20977021), Natural Science Foundation of Heilongjiang Province (E-2007-12), Key Project of Science and Technology of Heilongjiang (GC07C104) and the State Key Lab of Urban Water Resource and Environment (2010TS07).

9. References

Abatemarco, T.; Stickel, J.; Belfort, J.; Frank, B. P.; Ajayan, P. M. & Belfort, G. (1999). Fractionation of multiwalled carbon nanotubes by cascade membrane microfiltration. *Journal of Physical Chemistry B*, Vol.103, No.18, pp. 3534–3538.

Andreescu, S. & Marty, J.-L. (2006). Twenty years research in cholinesterase biosensors: From basic research to practical applications. *Biomolecular Engineering*, Vol.23, No.1, pp. 1–15.

Anitha, K.; Venkata Mohan, S. & Jayarama Reddy, S. (2004). Development of acetylcholinesterase silica sol-gel immobilised biosensor-an application towards oxydemeton methyl detection. *Biosensors and Bioelectronics*, Vol.20, No.4, pp. 848–856.

Arduini, F.; Ricci, F.; Tuta, C.S.; Moscone, D.; Amine, A. & Palleschi, G. (2006). Detection of carbammic and organophosphorus pesticides in water samples using cholinesterase biosensor based on Prussian Blue modified screen printed electrode. *Analytica Chimica Acta*, Vol.580, No.2, pp. 155–162.

Arduini, F.; Amine, A.; Moscone, D.; Ricci, F. & Palleschi, G. (2007). Fast, sensitive and cost-effective detection of nerve agents in the gas phase using a portable instrument and an electrochemical biosensor. *Analytical and Bioanalytical Chemistry*, Vol.388, No.5-6, pp. 1049–1057.

Arduini, F.; Amine, A.; Moscone, D. & Palleschi, G.(2010). Biosensors based on cholinesterase inhibition for insecticides, nerve agents and aflatoxin B1 detection. *Microchimica Acta*, Vol.170, No.3-4, pp. 193–214.

Arkhypova, V.N.; Dzyadevych, S.V.; Soldatkin, A.P.; El'skaya, A.V.; Martelet, C. & Jaffrezic-Renault, N. (2003). Development and optimisation of biosensors based on pH-sensitive field effect transistor an cholinesterases for sensitive detection solaneceous glycoalkaloids. *Biosensors and Bioelectronics*, Vol.18, No.8, pp. 1047–1053.

Arkhypova, V.N.; Dzyadevych, S.V.; Jaffrezic-Renault, N.; Martelet, C. & Soldatkin, A.P. (2008). Biosensor for assay of glycoalkaloids in potato tubers. *Applied Biochemistry and Microbiology*, Vol.44, No.3, pp. 314–318.

Balasubramanian, K. & Burghard, M. (2006). Biosensors based on carbon nanotubes. *Analytical and Bioanalytical Chemistry*, Vol.385, No.3, pp. 452–468.

Bartlett, P.N. & Cooper, J.M. (1993). A review of the immobilization of enzymes in electropolymerized films. *Journal of Electroanalytical Chemistry*, Vol. 362, No.1-2, pp. 1–12.

Bonnet, C.; Andreescu, S. & Marty, J.-L. (2003). Adsorption: an easy and efficient immobilisation of acetylcholinesterase on screen-printed electrodes. *Analytica Chimica Acta*, Vol.481, No.2, pp. 209–211.

Britto, P.J.; Santhanam, K.S.V.; Rubio, A.; Alonso, J.A. & Ajayan, P.M. (1999). Improved charge transfer at carbon nanotube electrodes. *Advanced Materials*, Vol.11, No.2, pp. 154-157.

Cai, C. & Chen, J. (2004). Direct electron transfer and bioelectrocatalysis of hemoglobin at a carbon nanotube electrode. *Analytical Biochemistry*, Vol.325, No.2, pp. 285–292.

Chen, J.; Dyer, M. J. & Yu, M.-F. (2001). Cyclodextrin-mediated soft cutting of single-walled carbon nanotubes. *Journal of the American Chemical Society*, Vol.123, No.25, pp. 6201–6202.

Choi, H.C.; Shim, M.; Bangsaruntip, S. & Dai, H.J. (2002). Spontaneous reduction of metal ions on the sidewalls of carbon nanotubes. *Journal of the American Chemical Society*, Vol.124, No.31, pp. 9058–9059.

Curulli, A.; Drugulescu, S.; Cremisini, C. & Palleschi, G. (2001). Bienzyme amperometric probes for choline and choline esters assembled with nonconducting electrosynthesized polymers. *Electroanalysis*, Vol.13, No.3, pp. 236–242.

Day, T.M.; Unwin, P.R.; Wilson, N.R. & Macpherson, J.V. (2005). Electrochemical templating of metal nanoparticles and nanowires on single-walled carbon nanotube networks. *Journal of the American Chemical Society*, Vol.127, No.30, pp. 10639–10647.

Du, D.; Cai, J.; Song, D.; Zhang, A. D. (2007). Rapid determination of triazophos using acetylcholinesterase biosensor based on sol-gel interface assembling multiwall carbon nanotubes. *Journal of Applied Electrochemistry*, Vol. 37, No. 8, pp.893-898.

Du, D.; Wang, M.; Cai, J.; Qin, Y. & Zhang, A. (2010). One-step synthesis of multiwalled carbon nanotubes-gold nanocomposites for fabricating amperometric acetylcholinesterase biosensor. *Sensors and Actuators B: Chemical*, Vol.143, No.2, pp. 524-529.

Du D.; Ye, X. X., Cai, J.; Liu, J. & Zhang, A. (2010). Acetylcholinesterase biosensor design based on carbon nanotube-encapsulated polypyrrole and polyaniline copolymer for amperometric detection of organophosphates, *Biosensors and Bioelectronics*, Vol. 25, pp.2503–2508.

Dzydevych, S.V. & Chovelon, J.-M. (2002). A comparative photodegradation studies of methyl parathion by using Lumistox and conductometric biosensor technique. *Materials Science and Engineering: C*, Vol.21, No.1-2, pp. 55–60.

Dzyadevych, S.V.; Arkhypova, V.N.; Martelet, C.; Jaffrezic-Renault, N.; Chovelon, J.-M., El'skaya, A.V. & Soldatkin, A.P. (2004). Potentiometric biosensor based on ISFETs and immobilised cholinesterases. *Electroanalysis*, Vol.16, No.22, pp. 1873–1882.

Dzyadevych, S.V.; Soldatkin, A.P.; Arkhypova, V.N.; El'skaya, A.V.; Chovelon, J.-M.; Georgiu, C.A.; Martelet, C. & Jaffrezic-Renault, N. (2005). Early-warning electrochemical biosensor system for environmental monitoring based enzyme inhibition. *Sensors and Actuators B: Chemical*, Vol.105, No.1, pp. 81–87.

Fan, Z. & Harrison, D. J. (1992). Permeability of glucose and other neutral species through recast perfluorosulfonated ionomer films. *Analytical Chemistry*, Vol.64, No.11, pp. 1304–1311.

Firdoz, S.; Ma, F.; Yue, X. L.; Dai, Z. F.; Kumar, A. & Jiang, B. (2010). A novel amperometric biosensor based on single walled carbon nanotubes with acetylcholine esterase for the detection of carbaryl pesticide in water. *Talanta*, Vol. 83, pp. 269–273.

Fortier, G.; Vaillancourt, M. & Bélanger, D. (1992). Evaluation of nafion as media for glucose oxidase immobilization for the development of an amperometric glucose biosensor. *Electroanalysis*, Vol.4, No.3, pp. 275–283.

Fukuto, T.R. (1990). Mechanism of action of organophosphorus and carbamate insecticides. *Environmental Health Perspectives*, Vol.87, pp. 245–254.

Gordon, M.A.; Chan, S.L. & Trevor, A.J. (1976). Active-site determinations on forms of mammalian brain and eel acetylcholinesterase. *Biochemistry Journal*, Vol.157, No.1, pp. 69–76.

Guo, M.; Chen, J.; Li, J.; Tao, B. & Yao, S. (2005). Fabrication of polyaniline/carbon nanotube composite modified electrode and its electrocatalytic property to the reduction of nitrite. *Analytica Chimica Acta*, Vol.532, No.1, pp. 71–77.

Hu, X.; Wang, T.; Qu, X. & Dong, S. (2006). In situ synthesis and characterization of multiwalled carbon nanotube/Au nanoparticle composite materials. *The Journal of Physical Chemistry B*, Vol.110, No.2, pp. 853–857.

Hu, X.; Wang, T.; Wang, L.; Guo, S. & Dong, S. (2007). A general route to prepare one- and three-dimensional carbon nanotube/metal nanoparticle composite nanostructures. *Langmuir*, Vol.23, No.11, pp. 6352–6357.

Ivanov, A.; Evtugyn, G.; Budnikov, H.; Ricci, F.; Moscone, D. & Palleschi, G. (2003). Cholinesterase sensors based on screen-printed electrodes for detection of organophosphorus and carbamic pesticides. *Analytical and Bioanalytical Chemistry*, Vol.377, No.4, pp. 624–631.

Jiang, L.; Liu, C.; Jiang, L.; Peng, Z. & Lu, G. (2004). A chitosan-multiwall carbon nanotube modified electrode for simultaneous detection of dopamine and ascorbic acid. *Analytical Sciences*, Vol.20, No.7, pp. 1055–1059.

Joshi, K.A.; Tang, J.; Haddon, R.; Wang, J.; Chen, W. & Mulchandani, A. (2005). A disposaple biosensor for organophosphorus nerve agents based on carbon nanotubes modified thick film strip electrode, *Electroanalysis*, Vol.17, No.1, pp. 54–58.

Joshi, P.P.; Merchant, S.A.; Wang, Y. & Schmidtke, D.W. (2005). Amperometric Biosensors Based on Redox Polymer−Carbon Nanotube−Enzyme Composites. *Analytical Chemistry*, Vol.77, No.10, pp. 3183-3188.

Kok, F.N.; Bozoglu, F. & Hasirci, V. (2002). Construction of an acethylcholinesterase-choline oxidase biosensopr for aldicarb determination. *Biosensors and Bioelectronics*, Vol.17, No.6-7, pp. 531–539.

Kok, F.N. & Hasirci, V. (2004). Determination of binary pesticides mixture by an acetylcholinesterase-choline oxidase biosensor. *Biosensors and Bioelectronics*, Vol.19, No.7, pp. 661–665.

Laschi, S.; Ogończyk, D.; Palchetti, I. & Mascini, M. (2007). Evaluation of pesticides-induced acetylcholinesterase inhibition by means of disposable carbon-modified electrochemical biosensors. *Enzyme and Microbial Technology*, Vol.40, No.3, pp. 485–489.

Lee, H.-S.; Kim, Y.A.; Cho, Y.A. & Lee, Y.T. (2002). Oxidation of organophosphorus pesticides for the sensitive detection by a cholinesterase-based biosensor. *Chemosphere*, Vol.46, No.4, pp. 571–576.

Lefrant, S.; Baibarac, M.; Baltog, I.; Mevellec, J. Y.; Mihut, L. & Chauvet, O. (2004). SERS spectroscopy studies on the electrochemical oxidation of single-walled carbon nanotubes in sulfuric acid solutions. *Synthetic Metals*, Vol.144, No.2, pp. 133–142.

Lintellman, J.; Katayama, A.; Kurihara, N.; Shore, L. & Wenzel, A. (2003). Endocrine disruptors in the environment (IUPAC Technical Report). *Pure and Applied Chemistry*, Vol.75, No.5, pp. 631–681.

Liu, G. & Lin, Y. (2006). Biosensor based on self-assembling acetylcholinesterase on carbon nanotubes for flow injection/amperometric detection of organophosphate pesticides and nerve agents. *Analytical Chemistry*, Vol.78, No.3, pp. 835–843.

Lin, Y.; Allard, L. F. & Sun, Y.-P. (2004). Protein-affinity of single-walled carbon nanotubes in water. *The Journal of Physical Chemistry B*, Vol.108, No.12, pp. 3760–3764.

Liu, Z.; Shen, Z.; Zhu, T.; Hou, S. & Ying, L. (2000). Organizing single-walled carbon nanotubes on gold using a wet chemical self-assembling technique. *Langmuir*, Vol.16, No.8, pp. 3569–3573.

Luque de Castro, M.D. & Herrera, M.C. (2003). Enzyme inhibition biosensors and biosensing systems: questionable analytical devices. *Biosensors and Bioelectronics*, Vol.18, No.2-3, pp. 279–294.

Mamedov, A. A.; Kotov, N. A.; Prato, M.; Guldi, D. M.; Wicksted, J. P. & Hirsch, A. (2002). Molecular design of strong single-wall carbon nanotube/polyelectrolyte multilayer composites. *Nature Materials*, Vol.1, No.3, pp. 190–194.

Montesinos, T.; Pérez-Munguia, S.; Valdez, F. & Marty, J.-L. (2001). Disposable cholinesterase biosensor for the detection of pesticides in water-miscible organic solvents. *Analytica Chimica Acta*, Vol.431, No.2, pp. 231–237.

Qu, J.; Shen, Y.; Qu, X. & Dong, S. (2004). Preparation of hybrid thin film modified carbon nanotubes on glassy carbon electrode and its electrocatalysis for oxygen reduction. *Chemical Communications*, No.1, pp. 34–35.

Rivas, G. A.; Rubianes, M. D.; Rodríguez, M. C.; Ferreyra, N. F.; Luque, G. L.; Pedano, M.L.; Miscoria, S.A. & Parrado, C. (2007). Carbon nanotubes for electrochemical biosensing. *Talanta*, Vol.74, No.3, pp. 291–307.

Schulze, H.; Vorlová, S.; Villatte, F.; Bachmann, T.T. & Schmid, R.D. (2003). Design of acetylcholinesterases for biosensors applications. *Biosensors and Bioelectronics*, Vol.18, No.2-3, pp. 201–209.

Schulze, H.; Schmid, R.D. & Bachmann, T.T. (2004). Activation of phosphorothionate pesticides based on a cytochrome P450 BM-3 (CYP102 A1) mutant for expanded neurotoxin detection in food using acetylcholinesterase biosensors. *Analytical Chemistry*, Vol.76, No.6, pp. 1720–1725.

Shan, Y. & Gao, L. (2006). In situ coating carbon nanotubes with wurtzite ZnS nanocrystals. *Journal of the American Ceramic Society*, Vol.89, No.2, pp. 759–762.

Smith, A.G. & Gangolli, S.D. (2002). Organochlorine chemicals in seafood: occurence and health concerns. *Food and Chemical Toxicology*, Vol.40, No.6, pp. 767–779.

Sotiropoulou, S. & Chaniotakis, N.A. (2005). Lowering the detection limit of the acethylcholinesterase biosensor using a nanoporous carbon matrix. *Analytica Chimica Acta*, Vol.530, No.2, pp. 199–204.

Sotiropoulou, S.; Fournier, D. & Chaniotakis, N.A. (2005). Genetically engineered acetylcholinesterase-based biosensor for attomolar detectrion of dichlorvos. *Biosensors and Bioelectronics*, Vol.20, No.11, pp. 2347–2352.

Stenersen, J. (2004). Chemical Pesticides. *Mode of Action and Toxicology*, CRC Press, Boca Raton.

Stoytcheva, M. (2002). Electrochemical evaluation of the kinetic parameters of a heterogeneous enzyme reaction in presence of metal ions. *Electroanalysis*, Vol.14, No.13, pp. 923–927.

Suprun, E.V.; Budnikov H.C.; Evtugyn, G.A. & Brainina, Kh.Z. (2004). Bi-enzyme sensor based on thick-film carbon electrode modified with electropolymerized tyramine. *Bioelectrochemistry*, Vol.63, No.1-2, pp. 281–284.

Suprun, E.; Evtugyn, G.; Budnikov, H.; Ricci, F.; Moscone, D. & Palleschi, G. (2005). Acetylcholinesterase sensor based on screenprinted carbon electrode modified with prussian blue. *Analytical and Bioanalytical Chemistry*, Vol.383, No.4, pp. 597–604.

Susan Van Dyk, J. & Pletschke, B. (2011). Review on the use of enzymes for the detection of organochlorine, organophosphate and carbamate pesticides in the environment. *Chemosphere*, Vol.82, No.3, pp. 291–307.

Tsai, H. & Doog, R. (2005). Simultaneous determination of pH, urea, acetylcholine and heavy metal using array-based enzymatic optical biosensor. *Biosensors and Bioelectronics*, Vol.20, No.9, pp. 1796–1804.

Vakurov, A.; Simpson, C.E.; Daly, C.L.; Gibson, T.D. & Millner, P.A. (2004). Acetylcholinesterase-based biosensor electrodes for organophosphate pesticides detection: 1.Modification of carbon surface for immobilization of acetylcholinesterase. *Biosensors and Bioelectronics*, Vol.20, No.6, pp. 1118–1125.

Vilatte, F.; Schulze, H.; Schmid, R.D. & Bachmann, T.T. (2002). A disposable acetylcholinesterase-based electrode biosensor to detect anatoxin-a(s) in water. *Analytical and Bioanalytical Chemistry*, Vol.372, No.2, pp. 322–326.

Villatte, F.; Marcel, V.; Estrada-Mondaca, S. & Fournier, D. (1998). Engineering sensitive acetylcholinesterase for detection of organophosphate and carbamate insecticides. *Biosensors and Bioelectronics*, Vol.13, No.2, pp. 157–164.

Wang, F.; Fei, J. & Hu, S. (2004). The influence of cetyltrimethyl ammonium bromide on electrochemical properties of thyroxine reduction at carbon nanotubes modified electrode. *Colloids and Surfaces B*, Vol.39, No.1-2, pp. 95–101.

Wang, J.; Musameh, M. & Lin, Y. (2003). Solubilization of Carbon Nanotubes by Nafion toward the Preparation of Amperometric Biosensors. *Journal of the American Chemical Society*, Vol.125, No.9, pp. 2408–2409.

Wu, F.H.; Zhao, G.C. & Wei, X.W. (2002). Electrocatalytic oxidation of nitric oxide at multi-walled carbon nanotubes modified electrode. *Electrochemistry Communications*, Vol.4, No.9, pp. 690–694.

Wu, K.; Sun, Y. & Hu, S. (2003). Development of an amperometric indole-3-acetic acid sensor based on carbon nanotubes film coated glassy carbon electrode. *Sensors and Actuators B*, Vol.96, No.3, pp. 658–662.

Wu, K. & Hu, S. (2004). Deposition of a thin film of carbon nanotubes onto a glassy carbon electrode by electropolymerization. *Carbon*, Vol.42, No.15, pp. 3237–3242.

Wu, K.; Ji, X.; Fei, J. & Hu, S. (2004). The fabrication of a carbon nanotube film on a glassy carbon electrode and its application to determining thyroxine. *Nanotechnology*, Vol.15, No.3, pp. 287–291.

Xiao, L.; Wildgoose, G.G. & Compton, R.G. (2008). Sensitive electrochemical detection of arsenic (III) using gold nanoparticle modified carbon nanotubes via anodic stripping voltammetry. *Analytica Chimica Acta*, Vol.620, No.1-2, pp. 44–49.

Xu, Z.; Chen, X.; Qu, X.; Jia, J. & Dong, S. (2004). Single-wall carbon nanotube-based voltammetric sensor and biosensor. *Biosensors and Bioelectronics*, Vol.20, No.3, pp. 579–584.

20

Sensor Enhancement Using Nanomaterials to Detect Pharmaceutical Residue: Nanointegration Using Phenol as Environmental Pollutant

Chandra S. Padidem[1], Sajid Bashir[2] and Jingbo Liu[1,3]
[1]*Nanotech and Cleantech Group, Texas A&M University-Kingsville,*
[2]*Chemical Biological Group, Texas A&M University-Kingsville*
[3]*Department of Chemistry, Texas A&M University*
United States of America

1. Introduction

Phenol is an aromatic compound, with a wide variety of uses both medical and industrial. During its production, emissions of even low amounts have been demonstrated to be toxic at submicrogram/liter levels. Phenol is also a good model compound to assess environmental impact of its emission particularly in wastewater. However, the current approach, methodologies and application described herein can also be applied to other organic environmental / pharmaceutical pollutants. Phenol has been removed from wastewater through a number of different approaches and monitored using spectroscopy and chromatography. In the field the most common method is detection through electrochemical or colorimetric sensors, which are described in this study.

1.1 Source and properties of phenol

Phenol is an organic compound, which can be generated from petroleum by-products like tar (reviewed by Gerberding, 2002) or from the metabolism of benzene or organic matter containing appropriate motifs (Martus *et al.*, 2003). Phenol also occurs in thyme oil, oil of wintergreen and methyl salicylate and has been generated as a by-product in various industrial processes, such as coke production, in the manufacturer of wood preservatives, fungicides and as a synthetic precursor in the synthesis of organic compounds used in pesticide, dye and pharmaceutical synthesis (Akai *et al.*, 1998) and in disinfection (Chick, 1908). In the production of epoxy resins and nylon, phenol is required for synthesis of caprolactam and bisphenol A, which are carcinogenic intermediate molecules (Jones, 1981). The disinfectant properties of phenol have applications in over-the-counter medicines such as mouthwash, disinfectants, or fungicides, which have traces of phenol, and in throat lozenges. The approximate usage of phenol varies by industry, but is in the millions of kilograms per year range (Gilman *et al.*, 1988). Phenols (or phenolic resins) if directly released into environment (air, soil or water) are toxic (reviewed by Gogate, 2008). The release is not common but can occur as a result of its widespread use, for example in the

automotive, construction, plywood, and appliance industries (Zhang *et al.*, 2006) and in the manufacture of plastics as a plasticizer or antioxidant (reviewed by Xanthos, 1969). The type and degree of substitution would dictate the stability and reactivity of the phenol derivative (reviewed by Babich & Davis, 1981; Salkinoja-Salone, 1981).
The ease of removing hydrogen ion at the hydroxy-position can give information on acidity/basicity, as a general rule more electronegative groups such as nitro led to stronger acids than the parent alone (reviewed by Kozak *et al.*, 1979). Once phenol is synthesized, it can be converted to the end-product through the appropriate synthetic routes, for example if chlorophenol or trichlorophenol isomers are required, they can be synthesized through the Boehringer Process with iron salt as the catalyst, under low, similarly for the synthesis of pentachlorobenzene, or chlorobenzene, or hexachlorobenzene isomers, the appropriate precursor is hydrolyzed under alkaline conditions (reviewed by Buehler & Pearson, 1970; McKillop *et al.*, 1974), noting that phenol can also be readily oxidized.

1.2 Toxicological effects of phenol

Phenol can induce skin cancer as documented in dermal studies of cutaneous application of phenol and can act as a tumor promoter or a weak skin carcinogen in mice (USDA, 1980a; Kreijl & Slooff, 1983). Teratogenic effects of phenol have also been reported in animal studies. With nasal and cutaneous exposure, the results are irritation of the skin, eyes and mucus membranes. Cutaneous application of phenol results in dermal inflammation and necrosis. Dermatological disorders including discoloration of the skin (Deichmann & Keplinger, 1962; reviewed by Bruce *et al.*, 1987). Different derivatives have different toxicities (with the toxicity being related to acidity and persistence being related to degree of solubility in fats and lipids), with nitrophenol being the most toxic followed by chlorophenols which in turn are more toxic than phenol alone, however, chlorophenols are more difficult to biodegrade, therefore pose more of a problem than phenol in terms of toxicity and persistence (reviewed by Crosby, 1982; Folke, 1985).

1.3 Sampling and cleanup

Procedures have been developed to monitor the different species of phenol generated such that they are below toxic levels in a variety of matrices (Fichnolz *et al.*, 1965; West *et al.*, 1966; Chau & Coburn, 1974). Generally, the sample which is thought to contain phenol has its pH changed to non-neutral pH values to minimize microbial degradation and stored in brown glass vials to decrease the loss to adsorption and photodecomposition, respectively (Afghan *et al.*, 1974). The extraction of phenol from the matrices as varied as water, fish, air, soil or plants has relied on organic solvents such as petroleum ether, benzene, or chloroform for polysubstituted phenols and butyl acetate or isomayl acetate for (monosubstituted) phenol (Taras *et al.*, 1971; Afghan *et al.*, 1974; Greminger *et al.*, 1982). Liquid-liquid partitioning can be used to separate phenol from other organic compounds found in the matrices, or column chromatography, silica gel chromatography have been used to achieve separation (reviewed by Rao *et al.*, 1978; EPA 1980; USDA 1980b; Renberg & Björseth, 1983; reviewed by Busca *et al.*, 2008).

1.4 Sensor overview

With the advancement of science and technology sensor can change the data into a digital reading or some other form for easy perception of results (reviewed by Karube *et al.*, 1995 and Rogers, 1995). Actual sensor design and manufacturing for environmental (reviewed by Hart & Wring, 1997) monitoring or sensor architecture (reviewed by Lynch & Loh, 2006) for monitoring ands reporting are beyond the scope of this chapter. The generic approaches and applications will be discussed with emphasis on environmental monitoring or chemical detection particularly for phenol. Since the development of a blood sugar monitoring sensor, the miniaturization of sensors has been advanced dramatically in detection of other molecules of interest (Kadish & Hall, 1965). In environmental and medical applications sensors have been used in the monitoring of phenol, the widespread use of sensors is due to their small size, operational suitability (e.g. good linear range, selectivity and sensitivity for the target molecule), robustness, ease of operation and the ability for micro-fabrication and auto-control (reviewed by Wang, 1997; Yu *et al.*, 2003).

Sensors can be fabricated under ambient conditions with excellent pressure and temperature stability coupled to negligible expansion or swelling in protic /aprotic solutions (i.e. chemical inertness, Yu *et al.*, 2003). These favourable operation parameters have led to their widespread adaptability for various applications. Most methods of analysis require site identification, collection, storage and shipment of the samples for further processing at the laboratory equipped to do the chemical / biological analysis. Poor handling during this sample acquisition process can led to high statistical variability of the measured values (Chau & Coburn, 1974; Klein, 1988; Shammala, 1999). Due to their size and portability, sensors have been evaluated more in instant field testing of analytes as opposed to lengthy laboratory testing of analytes (reviewed by Rodriguez-Mozaz *et al.*, 2005) where a quick determination is required. Sensors may be in the form of microchips, electrodes or thin films. The most common methods for sensor fabrication are sensors with amperometric detection (Hanrahan *et al.*, 2004), although gas-chromatography and colorimetric sensors have also been used (Saby *et al.*, 1997). The colorimetric method relies on the formation of a colored complex either as the final product or as stable intermediate (Martin, 1949). Common colorimetric tests include use of tretracyanoethylene or tetracyanoethylene ($(NC)_2C{=}C(CN)_2$, Smith *et al.*, 1963a), diamine ($(C_2H_5)_2NC_6H_4NH_2$, Houghton & Pelly, 1937; Eksperiandova et al, 1999) leading to the formation of indophenol (Ettinger & Ruchhoft, 1948; Smith *et al.*, 1963b; Gupta, 2006), which is measured through titration extracted with carbon tetrachloride as summarised by Hill (Hill & Herndon, 1952; Benvenue & Beckman, 1967; Regnier & Watson, 1971; NRCC-18578, 1982). In addition, derivatization with 4-aminoantipyrine ($C_{11}H_{13}N_3O$) followed by ultraviolet (UV) spectrophotometric / spectrofluorometric detection, usually at 254 (or 280) nm can be used with a limit of detection (LOD) in the sub microgram / liter range (Lykken *et al.*, 1946; Dannis , 1951; Afghan *et al.*, 1974; Norwitz et al, 1979; Realini, 1980; Farino et al, 1981). Other methods utilize gas chromatography (Renberg, 1981; Giger & Schaffner, 1983) coupled with flame ionization detection (FID) for derivatized phenol (e.g. acetylated, or heptafluorobutyl, or pentafluorobenzyl ether phenol) to increase volatility of phenol to enable GC-based analysis, (Corcia, 1973; Renberg, 1982, 1983) or liquid chromatography (LC) methods such as reverse phase (RP) with UV or electrochemical (EC) detection (ECD, Bhatia, 1973; Churatek & Houpek, 1975; Bidlingmeyer, 1980; Ogan & Katz, 1980). The RPLC method can give ultrahigh sensitivity in the parts-per-billion (ppb) range (Hoffsommer *et al.*, 1980; Wegman & Wammes, 1983; Lee *et al.*, 1984a, 1984b). Other chromatographic methods (Armentrout *et al.*, 1979) include ion-pair chromatography (Tomlinson *et al.*, 1978) followed by RP separation have been reported with a LOD in the (< 0.1 - 30) microgram / liter range (Goulden *et al.*, 1973; Chau & Coburn, 1974; Kuehl & Dougherty, 1980; Mathew & Elzerman, 1981; Ribick *et al.*, 1981; Lindinger *et al.*, 1998).

Lastly, chemical / electron ionization and fast atom bombardment in positive-ion mode, have been applied in the analysis of phenol (reviewed by Lisk, 1970; and C. Staples *et al.*, 1998; Santana *et al.*, 2009). Over the last decade, there has been a shift from analysis by analytical biochemists to analysis by technicians. This has necessitated a re-design of sensors to be portable, rugged, with low manufacturing costs, the desired selectivity and sensitivity, and ease of interpretation of results. Colorimetric-based readouts (Folin & Denis, 1915; Rakestraw, 1923; Box, 1983) have inherent advantages over other EC sensors, in terms of cost, robustness and ease of operation. The sensor must consist of a : (i) trapping element in which the target molecule is selectively bound and held in place; and (ii) sensing or detecting element, which interacts with the target molecule leading to a quantified chemical reaction, as the output parameter for detection and quantification. In this regards, a colorimetric sensor based on Gibbs reagent as the sensing element and cyclodextrin and / or gold nanoparticles as the trapping elements were designed with the aim of detecting organic pollutants exemplified by phenol.

1.4.1 Gibbs-based sensor

Dihalogen-substituted quinonechloroimides (such as 2,6-dichloroquinone-4-chloroimide and 2,6-dibromoquinone-4-chloroimide, also known as Gibbs reagent) give the most stable indophenols. The test employing the 2,6-dichloroquinone-4-chloroimide, has a sensitivity of at least 1 part of phenol in $20x10^6$. The indophenol formation can be measured quantitatively by means of the spectrophotometer. The maximum absorption for 2,6-dichloroquinoneimine was 280.5 nm with a change at 275 nm (at pH 8.5, Svobodová et al, 1977a) where indophenol formation was measured at 610 nm in the spectrophotometer. Subsequently, it was proposed to use 2,6-dichloroquinone-4-chloroimide as the standard Gibbs' reagent for the detection and determination of uric acid (Raybin, 1945). The quinonechloroimides do not react with all phenols and the primary requisite is that the position para to the hydroxyl must be unsubstituted (Gibbs, 1927a, 1927b). Different indophenol formations require different pH, but all are formed in the alkaline region (Gibbs, 1927a). Phenols substituted in the 2- and 6-positions (2,6-di-tertbutyl- and 2-tert-butyl-6-methyl-4-methoxyphenol) tended to give a typical magenta color (absorption region 565-575 nm, Dacrel, 1971). For photometric purposes, acetone, dioxan, methanol and ethanol are required for preparation of stock solutions. Sensitivity is hampered by reagent instability, which can be minimised through careful preparation against changes in temperature, light and moisture (Svobodová & Gasparič, 1971; Svobodová *et al.*, 1977a, 1977b).

1.4.2 Gold modified Gibbs sensor

Nanoparticles (NPs) as the sensing element can be synthesized in solution and operated at ambient temperature. Gold NPs (Au-NPs) provide facile route toward synthesis, precise control of formulation and low cost of synthesis and application (Kim *et al.*, 2005). Noble metals have desirable properties for use in sensors such as chemical resistance to oxidation, chemical inertness in the bulk form, which is lost in the nanoform, leading to enhanced catalytically. These properties are due to the nanosurfaces intrinsic properties, and ultrahigh surface area, leading to excellent electrical response of the sensor at the nanoscale (Kim *et al.*; 2005).

An additional advantage in consideration of Au is its optical properties, for example, surface plasmon resonance (SPR) of Au-NPs has widely been used in sensing bio-molecules (Nath &

Chilkoti, 2002; reviewed by Aslan *et al.*, 2004). Au-NPs display wide variation in optical properties including variation in the dielectric in part due to the nanoscale size and in part due to the microenvironment (e.g. solvent) via surface plasmon resonance (SPR, Liz-Marzan, 2004; Hornyak *et al.*, 1997; reviewed by Link & El-Sayed, 2003) effects. This property can enable the fabrication of tuneable colorimetric sensor for detection of different environment pollutants, such as phenol which was used in our study. These fabricated Au-NPs / Au-NRs can therefore have wavelengths which vary at least by an order of magnitude from infra-red to visible spectrum of light. Likewise, Au nanoclusters can be fabricated with precise size and absorption / emission properties ('tunability') through formulation of surfaces of defined size (Aslan *et al.*, 2004). This tunability can be achieved in the fabrication process through judicious use of solvents, dispersing agents and synthesis parameters to finely control surface size, layering and dimensionality. One application of Au-NP-based sensors is detection of alterations in SPR, due to changes in the local environment (via changes in the dielectric constant). The measured changes may be due to Au-NP-analyte (e.g. phenol) interactions due to surface adsorption, or nanocluster formation or aggregation due to analyte effects (J. Liu & Lu, 2004). The most common approach to tap into SPR changes is through functionalization of the Au-NPs, for example, through incorporation of gum Arabic (GA) or other long chain macromolecules, which have detergent-like properties aiding in Au-NP size selection (Bashir & Liu, 2009) in aqueous-based devices..Au-NPs increase the specificity of sensor by binding of the sensing element to the sol-gel and increasing electron tunneling to Gibbs reagent (as detecting agent) for detection of phenol.

1.4.3 Cyclodextrin as trapping agent

Cyclodextrins (CDs) are oligomers of D-glucose, which are linked through the 1→4 position. The oligomers can have from six (α-CD) to eight (γ-CD) residues linked end-to-end in cyclic fashion. In this manner, CDs can form 3D like 'bucket' structures, which can facilitate CD (host) and analyte (guest) interactions, including formation of non-covalent complexes, particularly with alkali metal cations (Kutner & Doblhofer, 1992; Bashir et al, 2003). These host-guest interactions can be exploited towards construction of trapping elements with in-built selectivity (due to ring size) for certain sensor applications, with the most common CD being β-CD. CDs exhibit two distinct 'faces' including an 'inner' and 'outer' face. The primarily face has a narrower entrance than the secondary face with the narrower/wider sides being associated with primary/secondary hydroxyl groups, respectively. This size difference can thus be exploited in group modification or decoration.

Decoration and end-capping of CDs, particularly β-CDs has led to their application as selective agents in chromatography, as tagging agents in pharmaceutics and also as host-guest probes (reviewed by Gattuso *et al.*, 1998, and Khan *et al.*, 1998, and Engeldinger *et al.*, 2003) in biomedicine. The degree of bonding or interaction between the host-guest is determined by hydrophobicity and van der Waals forces. CDs bind to the Gibbs reagent by intermolecular forces, such as dipole–dipole forces. Other factors include expulsion of water molecules from the core, hydrophobic interactions, van der Waals forces and hydrogen bonding (Salústio *et al.*, 2009). As such CDs have been used as separation surfaces or chromatography media for the separation of drugs, or as encapsulation matrices for enzymes or drugs (Sahoo *et al.*, 2008) for drug interaction, catalytic reactions to occur under normal or photoactive conditions (reviewed by Mallick *et al.*, 2007) in addition to enhancement of transport of molecules such as phenol in animal models.

1.5 Evaluation of sensor performance

Sensors should be a part of the environmental monitoring system and can provide early-warning about build-up or release of pollutants or molecules of interest. Colorimetric sensors meet the pre-requisites (of reliability and dynamic response), in addition to appropriate operational parameters and as such have been utilised in studies for evaluation of xenobiotic / environmental pollutants or chemicals of interest (Smyth *et al.*, 2008) in which a change in color upon interaction with the target substrate allow for substrate determination, either quantitative or qualitative. In our study, indophenol, (the colored complex), is formed from phenol reacting with 2,6-dichloro-*p*-quinone-4-chloroimide or 2,6-dibromo-*p*-quinone-4-chloroimide. The sensor is evaluated for its performance, the detection of phenol, reproducibility and stability at different known concentrations of this analyte.

1.6 Nanotechnology: definition, fabrication and characterization techniques

The design of an optimal sensor necessitates material characterization at the nanoscale level, using nantechniological tools and resources. Nanotechnology revolves around fabrication of materials of dimensions of less than 100 nm which are used in designing, constructing and utilizing functional structures. Nanomaterials are synthesized or fabricated by top-down and bottom-up processes. Common top-down processes of operation are to grind materials into extremely fine powder, or via ball milling and lithographic processes. Bottom-up methods of fabricating nanomaterials commonly employed include epitaxial deposition of thin films and sol-gel fabrication. In this study, a bottom-up approach was used to prepare the sensing element.

Most commonly used instruments for characterization of nanomaterials are 'nano' microscopy related techniques, such as scanning electron microscopy (SEM), transmission electron microscopy (TEM), atomic force microscopy (AFM) or spectroscopy based techniques, such as X-ray powered diffraction (XRD), single-crystal X-ray diffraction (SCD), or energy dispersive spectroscopy (EDX). With the advancement of technology, electron microscopy has become primary tool for characterization of nanomaterials. In this study, all of the above except SCD were used for nanostructural analyses of the phenol sensor.

Another important feature to evaluate the sensing element stability is measurement of the electrokinetic potential (also known as zetapotential, ζ). ζ is the difference in potential between the fluid in the stationary and continuous phase respectively attached to the dispersion phase. ζ arises due to dissociation of atoms capable of producing ions, such as an electrolyte on the surface of the nanoparticle and solvent ions at the surface. The net change in charge on the nanoparticle will influence the distribution of ions in the local microenvironment, for examples by either increasing the concentration of anions (if the surface is positive) near the nanoparticle surface.

As a consequence of this counter charge (between the ions) an electrical double layer is created near the nanoparticle surface micro-environment or interface. ζ exists for colloidal systems and indicates the stability of the colloidal suspension. Lower ζ values, indicate that the attractive cohesive forces dominate, leading to aggregation, whereas higher (±) values indicate the contrary, leading to dispersion and nanoparticle stabilization. Colloid suspensions with ζ values from ±30 to ±40 (mV) are moderately stable with values of ±40 to ±60 (mV) exhibiting good stability. Electrophoretic mobility is often used as a starting pointing in theoretical calculations to compare with ζ values, which in turn are based upon electroacoustics (Lyklema, 1995) measurements. Au-NPs (of diameter of 30-40 nm) are suspended as a dispersion phase and the measurement of ζ is a valuable method of determining the stability of sol for the preparation of sensor.

2. Experimental approach

In this chapter, we are designing a nanoscaled sensor to overcome the shortcomings of phenol sensor designs, limited detection resolution, and slow response time. The overall experiments are carried out for the construction of phenol film sensor derived by sol method. The structural characterization of the phenol sensor is by optical and nanomicroscopy and colorimetric evaluation of sensor performance. Importantly, as previously indicated in the introduction, this approach can also be applied to the detection of other organic environmental / pharmaceutical pollutants, along the same principles as described in the following sections.

All chemicals used are of analytical grade and were obtained from various vendors as listed. 2,6-dichloroquinomine-4-chlorimide (Fluka, St Louis, MO), gold (III) chloride trihydrate (Sigma–Aldrich, St Louis, MO), α-cyclodextrin hydrate (Alfa Aesar, Ward Hill, MA), L-ascorbic acid (Fisher, Thermo scientific, Pittsburgh, PA), gum Arabica (M.P. Biomedicals, Morgan Irvine, CA) were used without modification.

α-CD interacts with the Gibbs reagents as the trapping element through a color change. This color change is due to transfer of electrons from the Gibbs molecule to the phenol molecules. In this research, the Gibbs reagent (also known as the 'detecting/sensing agent') and CD (as the 'trapping agent') are used to detect for phenol. The detecting agent coupled to the trapping agent, which is embedded in a sol-type matrix. Other biological sensing elements (such as gold with trapping element such as: cyclodextrins (Janshoff *et al.*, 2000), laccase, (Y. Liu *et al.*, 2006), dendrimers, (Manna *et al.*, 2001) gold-nanotubes-chitosan, (Y. Liu *et al.*, 2006) or C_{60}–sugar composites (reviewed by Pumera *et al.*, 2007) with gold nanoparticles for building a biosensor can also be utilized. In our case, we utilized cyclodextrin-Gibbs as the trapping/detecting elements with Au-NPs. Separately, Au-NPs and Gibbs (with Arabica Gum as the dispersing agent to minimise aggregation of the Au-NPs) towards enhanced detection of phenol was also used in our specific case, although other general approaches (e.g. Au-laccase-Gibbs) summarized above could have also been used.

2.1 Experimental procedure

Colorimetric studies have been implemented toward study of agents (Lante *et al.*, 2000), as potential detecting or sensing elements related to alterations in color upon interaction with the target molecule. In our study, indophenol complex was formed from phenol reacting with Gibbs reagent. The sensor was involved in a number of fabrication parameters (described in § 2.2), which were extensively characterized using microscopy to determine the nanostructure of the catalytic surface (described in § 2.3) and dynamic light scattering to determine electrokinetic behavior of the colloidal suspensions (described in § 2.4). Once the sensor was optimized in terms of limit of detection (LOD) of phenol through a trial-and-error approach, its performance was evaluated through colorimetric measurement of relative optical densities (described in § 2.5). The workflow of the nanofabrication and performance evaluation of phenol sensor is summarized in Figure 1A.

2.2 Fabrication of sensor

The experimental workflow for construction of phenol sensor is shown in Figure 1B. Briefly, the phenol sensor was created by dissolving different concentrations of Gibbs reagent in the mixture of water and methanol (1:1 volume ratio, solution A). Solution A was mixed continuously with a magnetic stirrer for 30 min. Gum Arabica (GA, as a surfactant) was added (2 % by mass) to solution A to improve the uniformity of the resulting film and to control the particle size of the sensing elements. To solution A, an aqueous solution of gold (III) chloride trihydrate ($HAuCl_4 \cdot 3H_2O$) and seperately an aqueous solution of ascorbic acid ($C_6H_8O_6$) at different concentrations were simutaneuously injected. The molar ratio of Au^{3+} to ascorbic acid in solution A was controlled at 1:2 to produce 16 formulations with Gibbs concentration ranging from 0.025-0.25 μM, phenol concentration from 6-50 Vol %, Au-NPs concentration from 0.01-0.04 M to form the gold modified Gibbs hybrid (GGH) composite to extend the detection range of the sensor (*cf.* Table 1, § 3.6). The precursor sols were heated between 60 and 80 (C for 2 hrs to increase the sol viscosity, through evaporation of methanol.

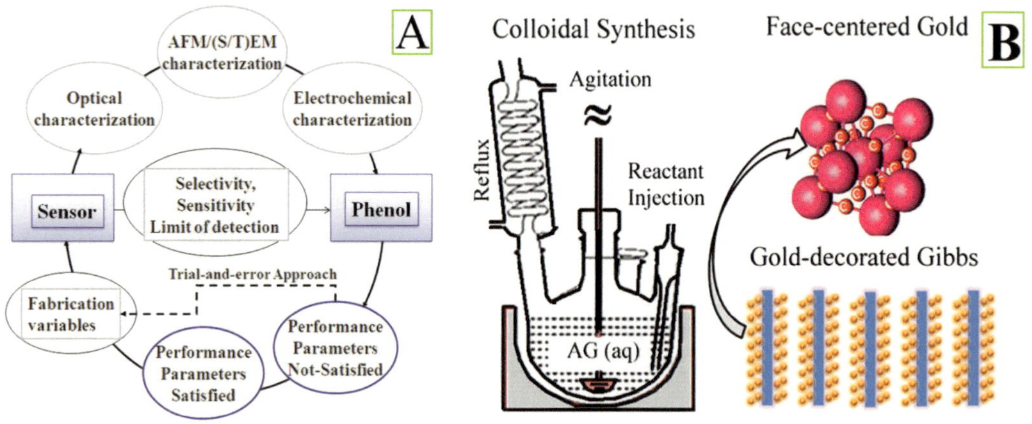

Fig. 1. The workflow employed in the fabrication and characterization of the sensor (A) and schematic of the synthesis procedure and likely nanostructure (B).

2.3 Structural characterization

Advanced instrumentation techniques provide higher magnification for analyzing elemental composition and particle size distribution of the sensing elements and structural changes with addition of phenol. A phase contrast optical microscope (M 021, Olympus, Olympus America Incorporation, Irving, TX) was used to determine the texture of the GGH sensor and textural changes on interactions of the phenol substrate onto the surface of the sensor.

A field emission SEM (JSM-6701F, JEOL Ltd, Peabody, MA) was used to determine the thickness and surface morphology of the sensor surface sol-derived phenol sensor. An accelerating voltage of 10 kV, current of 5 μA and a high vacuum of 10^{-5} Pa for specimen chamber were employed to obtain the optimal resolution. An air-dried GGH phenol sensor films were mechanically fractured using a diamond blade before mounting to the aluminum (Al) stubs. A thin layer of Au was sputtered using Denton Vacuum LLC Desk IV Sputter, (Moorestown, NJ) operating at a vacuum of 50 mTorr. Au coating was applied to improve surface conductivity and prevent charging by the electron beam with high energy.

A TEM (Tecnai G^2 F20, FEI Company, Hillsboro, OH) was used to determine the fine structure of the sol-derived GGH phenol sensor. Tungsten (W) crystal field emission gun with extraction voltage of 4 kV was the source of electrons and electrons were accelerated in the vacuum chamber to 200 kV and a high vacuum of 0.39 mbar was employed to obtain optimal resolution. Samples were diluted and sonicated for 10 minutes for uniform distribution of the particles and deposited onto carbon coated copper (Cu) grids. The crystal

structure was studied with electron diffraction resulting from either single crystal units or polycrystals of the sensing elements. As a complementary approach of crystalline phase identification, an Ultima III XRD with Cu diffractometer and visual XRD Jade 7 software (Rigaku Americas Incorporation, Houston, TX) was used to determine the phase structure. The operating voltage and current were controlled at 40 kV and 44 mA, respectively.
An AFM (Nanoscope III, Veeco Cooperation, Santa Barbara, CA) was used to determine the topography, surface uniformity and three-dimension (3D) surface image of the GGH sensor. Samples for analysis were greatly diluted diluted and loaded on to the surface of the mica film. Point probe cantilevers (monolithic silicon AFM probe) were used for analysis in tapping mode of operation. A drive frequency of 362.99 kHz and drive amplitude of 144.1 mV was applied for topographic analysis of the sensor surface.

2.4 Electrokinetic behavior of GGH colloidal suspension

ZetaPALS™ (Brookhaven Instrument Corporation, (BIC), New York City, NY) was utilized for particle size analysis and colloidal stability of sol prepared. Diluted samples of the GGH were analyzed for particle distribution and zetapotential measurement. The instrument was operated at room temperature and the samples were analyzed for 8 runs and each run for 15 sec to give the best results. The angle of incidence light was 90° and wavelength of operation was 659.0 nm. Results were analyzed with BIC particle sizing software and BIC zetapotential analyzer.

2.5 Evaluation of sensor performance

In order to evaluate the sensor performance, a colorimetric study was undertaken to determine the limit of detection (LOD), response time, and sensitivity of the sensor. Formation of the indophenols with significant color changes was the key principle for the colorimetric studies. Studies were conducted in a ceramic watch plate with 12 wells, each well with a surface area of approximately 3.14 cm^2. Various volumes and concentration of Gibbs reagent and phenol buffer were added to observe the color changes (Table 1, also *cf.* § 3.6). At intervals of 15 minutes, a photograph of the sample was collected with computer assisted camera, and the whole experiment was conducted over 24 hr. The collected samples were re-imaged after two weeks and the initial and two-week intensities were compared. No difference was found, indicating that the samples are at least stable up to two weeks. The significance of the background and maximum values were to enable normalization of the different colors in grey-scale mode with background substraction. In this manner, different intenties due to differences in background color could be compensated for and different formulations directly compared. The grey-scale calibration tablet provided 'internal' calibration allowing changes due to actual phenol to be determined.

3. Results and discussion

The optical properties of the GGH sensor will be discussed first (described in § 3.1), followed by electron and atomic microscopy morphological analysis (described in § 3.2-3.4). The electrokinetic properties will be discussed next (described in § 3.5) followed by actual sensor performance with literature comparison (described in § 2.4) and a conclusion on sensor testing to close the chapter (described in § 4.0).

Sl. No	Parameter 1: Gibbs conc. (μM)	Parameter 2: Au NPs conc. (M)	Parameter 3: Phenol Conc. (Vol %)	R.O.D = 1/O.D
1	0.025	0.01	6.67	50.21
2	0.025	0.02	7.69	48.41
3	0.025	0.04	8.33	51.37
4	0.05	0.01	15.38	58.06
5	0.05	0.02	10.00	56.51
6	0.05	0.04	12.50	53.84
7	0.10	0.01	14.28	59.85
8	0.10	0.02	25.00	63.98
9	0.10	0.04	14.28	62.72
10	0.15	0.01	20.00	54.50
11	0.15	0.02	25.00	56.80
12	0.15	0.04	40.00	64.31
13	0.20	0.01	16.67	44.31
14	0.20	0.02	25.00	44.25
15	0.20	0.04	33.33	41.56
16	0.25	0.01	50.00	39.62

Average back ground-174.02 Maximum value-255

Table 1. The measurement of relative optical density as function of fabrication variable.

3.1 Optical microscopic study on GGH phenol sensor

Optical microscopic images showing the morphological structures of the Gibbs reagent were captured with and without the addition of the phenol. Figure 2A (100×) micrographs show cylindrical and linear nature of the Gibbs reagent (without AgNPs) which were sparsely distributed. The cylindrical properties of these compounds increase the surface area for exposure to phenol for better sensitivity. Figure 2B (400×) indicates that the Gibbs reagent is impregnated with Au-NP clusters. Au-NPs show uniformity in size and shape increase the sensitivity of the sensor due to SPR and the rapid reaction rate between the two ((Gibbs) and target molecule (phenol)) elements. Figure 2C (400×) also shows the morphological changes to the trapping element upon addition of buffered phenol, for the enhanced GGH sensor. These morphological changes were recognized as loss of linear cylindrical structure of Gibbs reagent polymer and of the indophenol complex, whereas Au-NPs remain intact, which provides conspicuous color changes and consequently improves the LOD of phenol.. It can be surmized that Au-NPs act as heterogeneous catalysts to increase the reaction rate between phenol and Gibbs via lowering the activation energy and creating a new pathway. The indopenol complex with various color schemes serves as a delicate indicator to display the sensor performance.

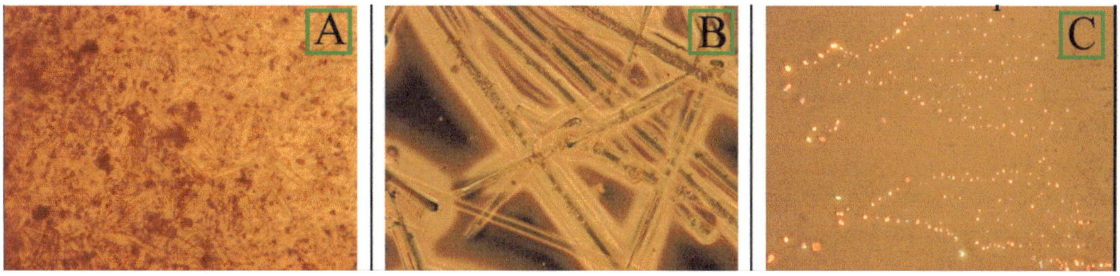

Fig. 2. Optical microscopic photographs of gold-modified Gibbs hybrid sensing element and sensing mechanism, A: the sensor image at 100 ×; B: the sensor image at 400 ×; C: the sensor image at 400 × after addition of buffered phenol analyte.

3.2 Scanning electron microscopic study on GGH phenol sensor

SEM micrographs also exhibit the linear cylindrical nature of the Gibbs reagent (Figure 3A) coated with the spherical Au-NPs (before addition of phenol) and GHH sensing element forms mesh-like network, upon addition. Au-NPs display near-spherical shape and their particle sizes vary from approximately 30-40 nm in diameter. Although Au-NPs aggregate and form several large-size clusters, it was determined that evenness of the GGH sensor increased with electrical activity and resulted in improved sensitivity of Gibbs reagent. Figure 3B is an SEM image of GGH sensing element which interacts with the phenol compound when the buffered phenol analytes with various concentrations were introduced. With the addition of phenol to the surface of the GGH sensor, morphological changes of dissolution of porous nature of Gibbs was seen with the formation of the indophenol (colored complex) and loss of mesh work was characterized. Therefore, the formation of the indophenol becomes a delicate indicator to display the regional differentials in color and morphology of the GGH sensor. In turn, this will enhance the sensor sensitivity and its LOD, which is classified by colorimetric values.

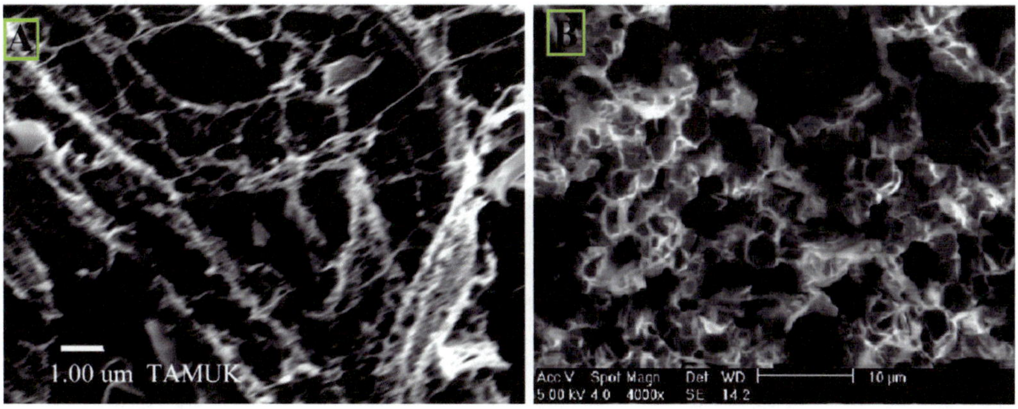

Fig. 3. The SEM top view morphological analyses of sensor, A: the GGH morphology before addition of phenol and B: the GGH morphology after addition of phenol.

3.3 Transmission electron microscopic study on GGH phenol sensor

TEM images also depict the inner structural morphology with high spatial resolution of the film as indicated by SEM. TEM images (Figure 4A-D) of GGH depict linear and cylindrical nature of Gibbs reagent with uniform Au-NP coating. Linear nature of the polymer synthesized in sol method possess better sensitivity for the detection of phenol because large area of contact for electron exchange and consequently for the indophenol complex formation (Figure 4A). Loss of network structure of GGH sensing element was observed upon substrate inclusion via a chemical reaction of the substrate phenol and detecting element, the Gibbs reagent (Figure 4B). These changes were in consistent with the optical and SEM characterization techniques. The significant morphological changes enhanced the limit of detection of the GGH sensor, which allows us to develop sensor with high performance. Figure 4B also depicts the size and shape of Au-NPs of 10-15 nm in diameter. Au-NPs were agglomerating slightly and possess surface plasma resonance. The lattice fringe (Figure 4C) indicates ultrafine Au-NPs were otained. The ring pattern of Ag-NPs (Figure 4D) results from polycrystals, suggesting high degree of crystallinity was acheived. The indexing of ring pattern suggests that the face-center cubic Au (PDF 00-004-0784, a 0.408 nm, α = 90 °) was obtained. This observation is confirmed by XRD analysis (Figure 4E-insert). However, the Gibbs reagent was vaporized under high energy beam of electrons, which is the reason why no ring pattern or electron diffraction was observed. The XRD pattern indicated that the Gibbs reagent (Figure 4E) is well-aligned with the standard 2,6-dichloro-*p*-benzoquinone-4-chlorimine ($C_6H_2Cl_3NO$, PDF 25-1917) using lower energy.

3.4 Atomic force microscopic study on GGH phenol sensor

AFM images depicted the surface morphology and measured the size of the Au-NPs. Figure 5A showed the sparse distribution of the Au-NPs and figure 5B represents the topography of sensor film active surface at nano-range. Size of coated Au-NP cluster in this study was measured as approximately 30-40 nm in diameter. The Au-NPs was coated on the surface by Gibbs reagent. Since AFM studies the top surface layer of sensor film, it depicts the actual layer which is in contact with phenol but it cannot reveal the inner composition and build up of sensor. Au-NPs were measured to have an effective diameter of 12 nm for Au by itself. With the addition of gum Arabic (GA) to the Au-NPs, increase in the size of NPs was observed with an average cluster dimension of 169.6 nm and polydiversity of 0.267 (dimensionless) for the cluster of coated particles. Analysis shows the mean particle size of GGH was 485 nm and the distribution of (up to 20) particles (polydiversity of 0.05), which was consistent with the SEM findings.

3.5 Electrokinetic behavior of GGH colloidal suspension

The measured zetapotentials (ζ, with ZetaPALS™) of GGH colloidal suspension were averaged at -23.0 mV. The negative sign indicates repulsive forces between Au-NPs and GGH preventing flocculation and aggregation of particles and the numerical value indicates samples had colloidal stability (Figure 6). ζ results indicate that the GGH colloid is stable and agglomeration is successfully prevented using GA as the surfactant. The electrokinetic study also confirms that nano-dispersion of Au with size of 10-15 nm (also found by TEM, see Figure 5B) has been achieved. Fluctuations in the measured value of ζ during the experiment were not observed; therefore the measurements were time independent in the present study, which confirms the stability of GGH colloid. Bottom up (sol-gel) green synthesis of Au-NPs modified Gibbs reagent has been developed to prevent the aggregation of the particles during synthesis. To synthesised nanoparticles exhibited high degree of stability (due to the high measured ζ, i.e. steric effects > van der Waals forces). The GA

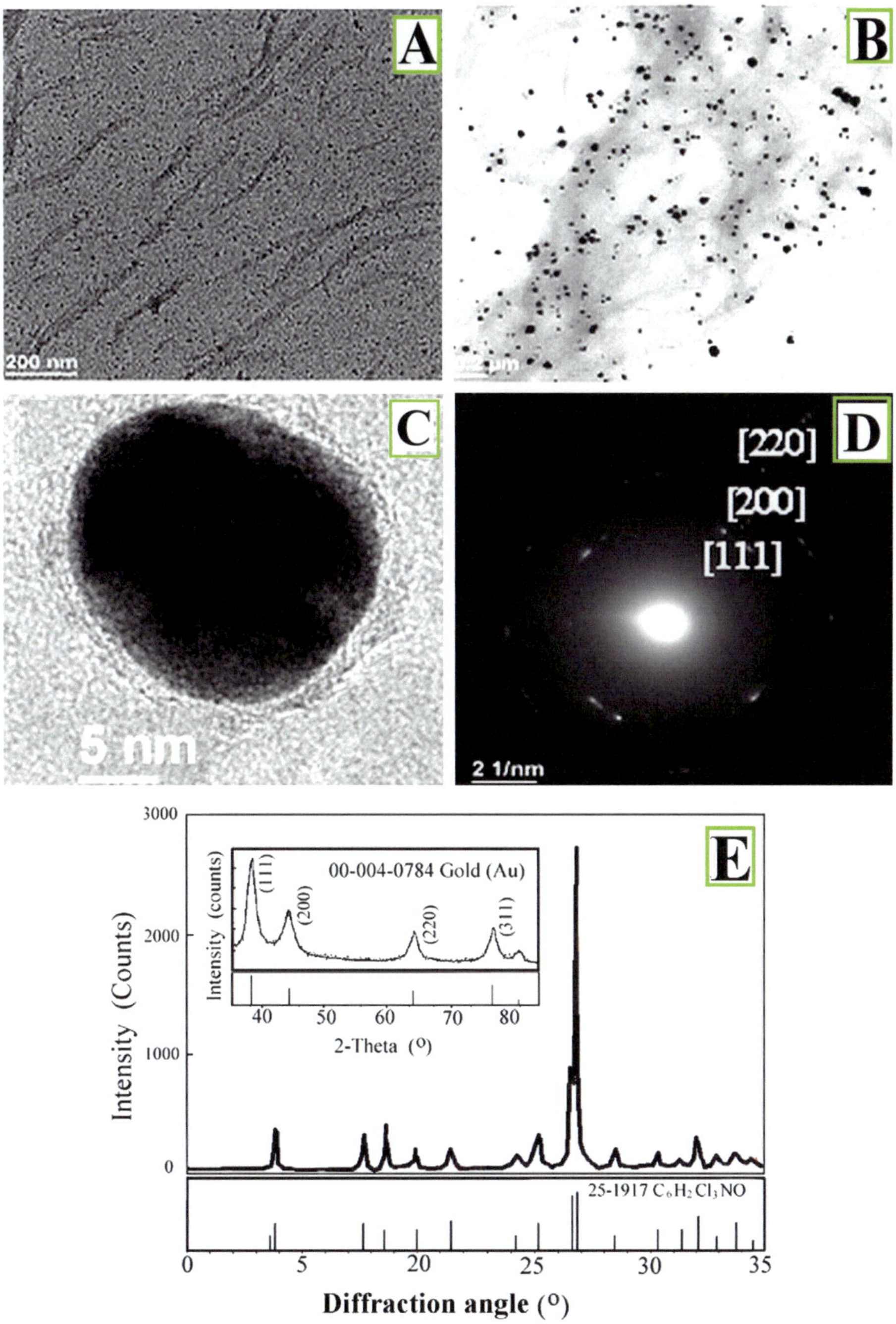

Fig. 4. TEM images of sensing elements, A: morphology of gold-modified Gibbs hybrid sensing element; B: morphology of gold-modified Gibbs hybrid sensing element after addition of buffered phenol analyte; C: lattice fringe of gold-modified Gibbs hybrid sensing element; D: TEM ring pattern of nanogold; E: corresponding X-ray diffraction (XRD) pattern of gold-modified Gibbs hybrid sensing element with standards for gold and Gibbs.

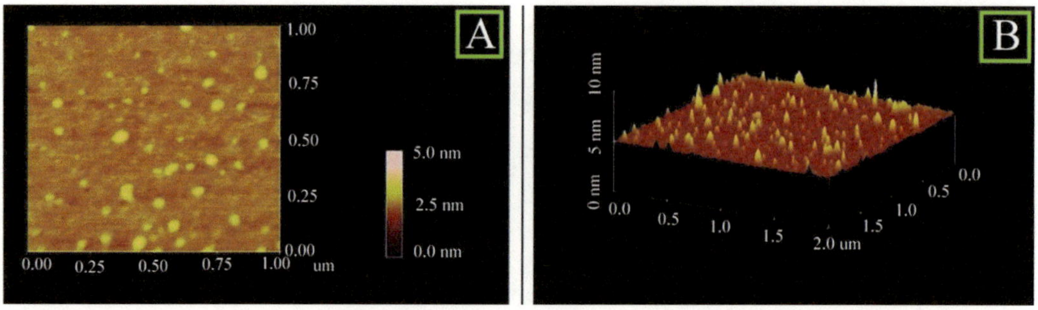

Fig. 5. AFM Images of sensor topology, A: the forward scan of surface 2D topology of gold-modified Gibbs hybrid sensing element; B: the 3D image of gold-modified Gibbs hybrid sensing element to determine the sensor thickness.

polymers are adsorbed onto the particle surface and cause van der Waals forces weakening. Significant steric repulsion prevents Au-NPs from being adhered and the particle surfaces are separated as a result.

The main goal during the synthesis phase was to control the particle size and its structure, followed by nanocharacterization of the nanoparticles. These particles were synthesised using a bottom-up colloidal chemistry approach. Au-NP size was controlled through incorporation of GA as the dispersing agent, which also aids wetting of the metal salt and distribution of the surface of the GGH composed of a continuous Au layer which was then deposited onto the Gibbs cluster successively.

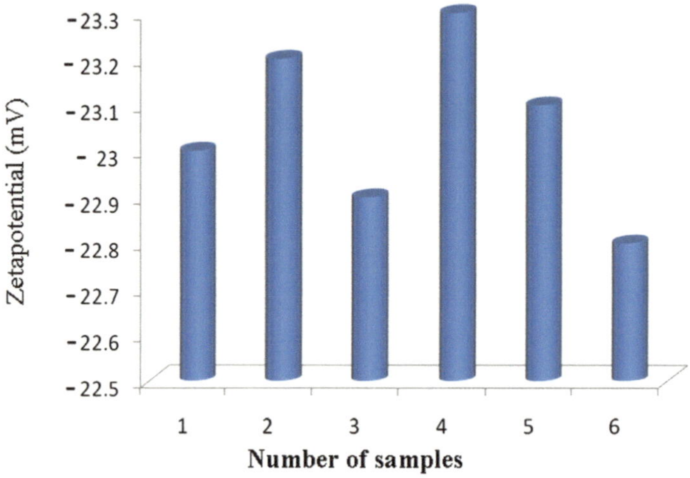

Fig. 6. Zetapotential of gold-modified Gibbs hybrid colloidal suspension, of a number of replicates (n=1-6).

3.6 Evaluation of GGH sensor performance

Colorimetric evaluation of the phenol sensor reagent was performed and color changes of different concentrations of phenol and Gibbs reagent in different dilutions at different intervals of time were captured (images not shown). Initial color was developed within one hour and changes in intensity of color were different in all wells with the passage of time.

Using the calibration grey-scale tablet, the minimum intensity value was set to zero and the maximum optical density set to 255, from which the optical density (OD) was calculated as:

$$OD = \log[(255-p)/(255-x)]$$

where 'p' stands for average background correction for the well-plate(s), 'x' for mean intensity of color converted to grey-scale. The measurements were recorded as relative optical density (ROD) values, where

$$ROD = 1/OD$$

ROD of the 12 wells (numbered 1-12) at various intervals was calculated based upon the intensity of color development of each well, converted to grey-scale. Measured intensties from wells 13 to 16 were used for background correction and average background determination to calculate the p-value. Evaluation of the ROD from the different formulations at different intervals was examined, indicating that the variable which influenced the measured ROD the most was phenol concentration. The observed color change was almost instantaneous (~ 1 sec, various parameters are summarized in Table 1, including color intensity recorded every five minutes from zero minutes to twenty-four hours (data not shown)) was standaridized to one hour. The calibration plot at one hour for different sensor formulations is shown in figure 7. It was found that optimal parameters were having an incubation time of five minutes for phenol to Gibbs reagent, at a molar ratio of 4:1 between Gibbs reagent to phenol and 1:1 molar ratio between Gibbs reagent and Au. Using various volumes of buffered phenol, the LOD was measured in terms of concentration as 0.1 μM, while the variation in measured ROD was 36%. The ROD values (determined as the (minimum measured intensity value / maximum intensity value) x 100)

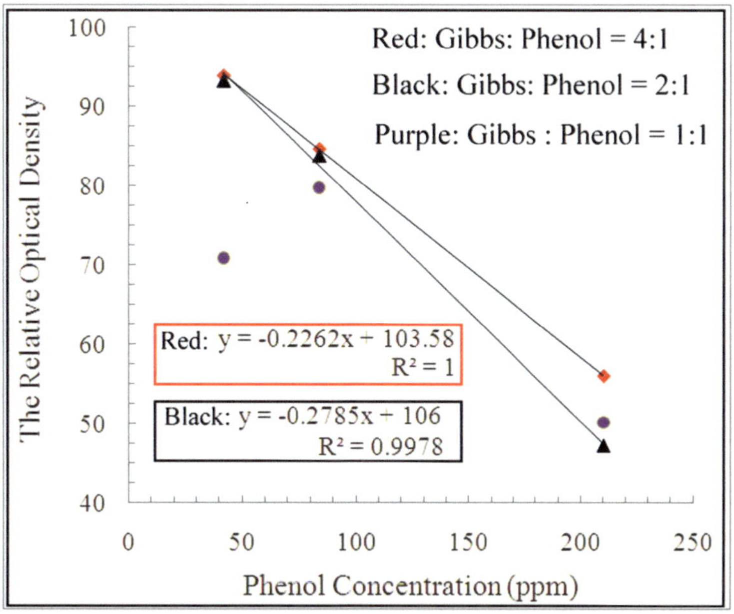

Fig. 7. The sensitivity study using various concentration ratios of Gibbs vs phenols, noting three formulations were selected to demonstrate the linearity of sensitivity.

indicate degree of sensitivity to subtle changes in color, after a fixed time period (optimised to either 5 or 60 min). The mode of sensor operation is schematically illustrated in figure 8.

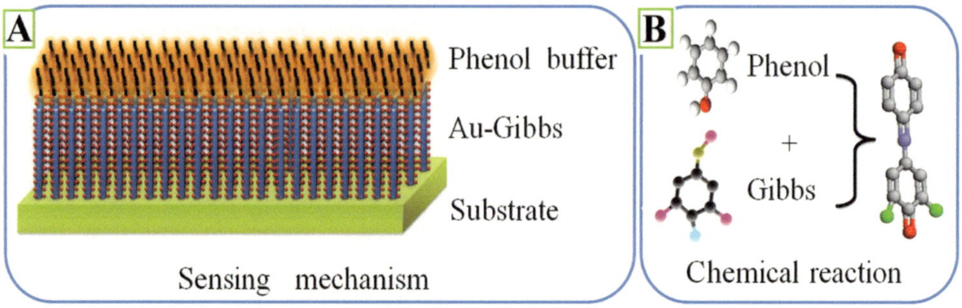

Fig. 8. A: Schematic of likely operation of sensor and B: likely intermediate.

Accurate quantification of phenol is important because of its well documented health side effects such as stress to the kidneys, liver, heart, respiratory tract, mucous membranes and central nervous system upon acute exposure (Diz *et al.*, 2006). In comparison to sol-gel derived Au-NPs, other investigations in the analysis of phenol (Metzger *et al.*, 1998) or its derivatives (Neujahr, 1982) have been based on enzymes (Orupold *et al.*, 1995) from species such as *Trichosporon sporotrichoides.* (Rella *et al.*, 1996) *Pseudomonas putida* (Skládal *et al.*, 2002) and *Bacillus stearothermophilus* (Buswell, 1975) coupled to Clark-type oxygen electrode (reviewed by Patel, 2002) for detection of phenol.

Procedures in preparing a sensor require advanced techniques of immobilization of bacteria (or substrate enzyme) to increase the stability of the final biosensor (reviewed by Warsinke *et al.*, 1999). The roles of enzymes (derived from various plant tissues, spores or bacteria) are as substrate-specific biocatalysts (Wollenberger *et al.*, 1999). Where phenol, is the substrate this involves electron transfer between the enzyme and substrate (phenol + 10 O_2 + $2H^+ \rightarrow$ catechol + tyrosinase + 10 $O_2 \rightarrow$ phthalate quinine) and generation of current, which in turn is related to consumption of oxygen during the oxidation process in a Clark-type electrode (reviewed by Scheller *et al.*, 1988). Thus amperometric tyrosinase-modified imprinted or carbon electrode sensors have been extensively tested in determination of dissolved oxygen and indirectly phenol inculding some derivatives of phenol (reviewed by Riedel *et al.*, 2002). This can be exploited by utilization of enzymes from microorganisms which utilise phenol as a fuel source (such as laccase, Y. Liu *et al.*, 2006) or enzymes, which can accept electrons to generate energy directly such as with *Shewanella oneidensis* via extracellular electron transfer mechanisms (H. Liu *et al.*, 2010) have wider applications in biofuels and energy generation using biocatalysts (reviewed by Ragauskas *et al.*, 2006). In our study, a colorimetric system was used toward detection of phenol (and not generation of energy) by using Gibbs reagent as the detecting/sensing element; because of its high detection limit and formation of indophenol colored complex when in contact with phenol (Raybin, 1945). Sol-based GGH sensors have overcome the problems of enzymatic or bacterial sensors because of their ease of preparation, low cost, high sensitivity, stability and operation under wide temperature, pH ranges. The 0.1 μM LOD compares favorably with other designs and is summarized in Table 2.

Type	LOD (μM)	Linear range (μM)	Response time (s)	Notes or Reference
Resonance-enhanced multiphoton ionization (REMPI) time-of-flight (ToF) mass spectrometry	1 ng L^{-1}	0.1 μg L^{-1} -10 mg L^{-1}	-	Alimpiev *et al.*, 1995
Electrode with enzyme	< 0.1 mg/L	0.1-1.0 mg/L	< 300	Rainina *et al.* 1996
Amperometric biosensor	1.2	-	-	Table 1 of Lindgren *et al.*, 1997
Electrode with enzyme *	0.015 **	0.03 - 100	-	Table 3 of Nistor *et al.*, 1999
Electrode with enzyme	0.2 nM	1.5×10^{-9} - 3.5×10^{-4} mol/L	< 4	Z. Liu *et al.*, 2000
Enzyme-based calorimetric sensor	1 mM	-	< 300	Wolf *et al.*, 2000
Amperometric biosensor	6.1 nM	4- 48	< 5	S. Liu *et al.*, 2003
Gas Chromatography-Mass Spectrometry	10 pg	1 -12 ng	8 - 10	E. Staples, 2004
Amperometric biosensor	0.05	0 - 1	50 - 250	Tingry *et al.*, 2006
Amperometric biosensor	0.36 nM	3.6×10^{-9} - 4×10^{-5} M	-	Han *et al.*, 2007
Amperometric biosensor	1-10	0.005 - 10	10 - 480	Table 3 of Bashir & J. Liu, 2009
Amperometric / colorimetric biosensor	1	2.6 - 5.2	< 5	Bashir & J. Liu, 2009
Electrode with enzyme	0.005 -0.410	-	-	Table 1 of Alarcón *et al.*, 2010
Screen printed electrode (SPE) with enzyme	0.14	0.05 - 1	~ 15	Alarcón *et al.*, 2010

(*) The likely reaction is: phenol+ enzyme → catechol; catechol + tyrosinase → oquinone + H_2O; o-quinone + $2H^+$ + 2ē→ catechol (at electrode surface) (Yu et al, 2003), noting that phenol oxidized to o-quinone and is reduced to catechol (O_2→ $2H_2O$) (Renedo *et al.*, 2007)
(**) as catechol equivalents

Table 2. Literature review of sensors, their limit of detection (LOD in μM), the detection range (Linear range in μM) and the response time (in seconds), unless otherwise stated..

4. Conclusion

A GGH based sensor for the colorimetric detection of phenol was fabricated and evaluated. The sensor was successfully optimized using a trial-and-error approach of 16 formulations, involving a trapping and detecting element with AuNPs to enhance the SPR with phenol incubated at different times. The detector was based upon sol-gel technology utilizing trapping/detecting elements, which can be extended to other environmental pollutants or pharmaceutical organics, if sensor selectivity and sensitivity can be achieved.

Characterization revealed the nanostructure of the gold and GGH complex as spherical Au-NPs with size range of 10-15 nm, for individual NPs or 30-40 nm for metal clusters which were fabricated as linear cylindrical polymers of Gibbs reagents coated with clusters of Au-NPs (optimal molar ratio was 1:1 and 4:1 for Gibbs:phenol respectively). The stability of the sol sensor was measured in terms of zetapotential was shown to be - 23.0 mV indicating stability of the sensor. Colorimetric based detecting elements were incorporated to bench test the performance of the sensor. The results indicate that once the intermediate color is formed was stable for at least for two weeks (the length of the study). The LOD for phenol (at room temperature) was 0.1 μM, with sensor sensitivity to small changes in color being 36% including a fast response time (< 1 sec, although the ROD values are based upon 60 minute incubation) as measured using colorimetric technique. The strategy outlined in the current chapter, although applied specifically to the detection of phenol, can similarly be applied to the detection of other environmental organic pollutants providing an appropriate detecting / sensing element can be found.

5. Acknowledgements

The authors are grateful to Texas A&M University-Kingsville (TAMUK), the College of Arts and Sciences Research and Development Fund and Robert A. Welch Departmental Grant, (AC-0006) for funding this research activity. The technical support from the National Science Foundation, Major Research Instrumentation program is duly acknowledged to allow the use of Rigaku Ultima III X-ray powder diffraction (TAMU-Corpus Christi) and JEOL JSM-6701F field emission scanning electron microscopy (TAMUK, CBET-0821370). The Microscope and Imaging Center and the Center of Materials Characterization Facility at TAMU-College Station are also duly acknowledged for technical support and access to the advanced instrumentation, respectively. Last but not least, the authors wish to thank Dr. Maribel Gonzaléz-Garcia from Texas A&M University-Kingsville (TAMUK) for access to the optical microscopic and Dr. Thomas Hays for copy-editing the book chapter respetively.

6. Author contributions

C. Padidem conducted the synthesis, electrokinetic study and optical characterization of the sensor and co-wrote the first draft. S. Bashir and J. Liu conceived the concept and experiment design and co-supervised C. Padidem. In addition, he did the calibration of the optical study, some of the data analyses and generation of certain graphs, plots and schemes. J. Liu completed the rest of the experimental procedure (except where acknowledged elsewhere). She co-wrote the first draft, and completed the re-writing and editing. J. Liu also supervised the entire study, coordinated with the other investigators and in liaison with (e.g. Dr. Luo at) the Materials Characterization Facility and Microscopy Imaging Center at Texas A&M University-College Station, obtained the AFM and TEM images (see acknowledgment section) and oversaw the entire submission process.

7. References

Afghan, B. K.; Belliveau, P. E.; Larose R. H. & Ryan, J. F. (1974). An Improved Method For Determination of Trace Quantities of Phenols In Natural Waters, *Analytica Chimica Acta*, Vol. 71, No. 2 (August, 1974), pp. 355-366, ISSN 0003-2670

Akai, S. & Kita, Y. (1998). Recent Progress In The Synthesis of P-Quinones and P-Dihydro-Quinones Through Oxidation of Phenol Derivative. *A Review Organic Preparations and Procedures International* Vol. 30, No. 20, (May 1998) pp.603-605, ISSN 0030-4948

Alarcon, G.; Guix, M.; Ambrosi, A.; Silva, M. T. R.; Pardave, M. E. P. & Merkoc, A. (2010). Stable and sensitive flow-through monitoring of phenol using a carbon nanotube based screen printed biosensor. *Nanotechnology*, Vol. 21, No. 24, (June), 245502 pp. 1-to-9, ISSN 1361-6528

Alimpiev, S.S. Mlynski, V. V.; Belov, M.E. & Nikiforov, S. M. (1995). Selective Detection of Phenol Impurities in Water. *Analytical Chemistry*, Vol. 67 , No. 1, (January, 1995), pp. 181–186, ISSN 1306-3057

Armentrout, D. N.; McLean, J. D. & Long, M. W. (1979). Trace determination of phenolic compounds in water by reversed phase liquid chromatography with electrochemical detection using a carbon-polyethylene tubular anode. *Analytical Chemistry, Vol.* 51, No. 7, (June, 1979), pp. 1039–1045, ISSN 13063057

Aslan, K.; Zhang, J.; Lakowicz, J.R. & Geddes, C.D. (2004). Saccharide Sensing Using Gold and SilverNanoparticles-A Review. *Journal of Fluorescence, Vol.* 14, No. 4, (July, 2004), pp. 391–400, ISSN 1053-0509

Babich H. & Davis, D. L. (1981). Phenol: A Review of Environmental and Health Risks, Regulatory. *Regulatory Toxicology and Pharmacology*, Vol.1, No.1, (January 1981), pp. 90-109, ISSN 0273-2300

Bashir, S.; Derrick, P.J.; Critchley, P.; Gates, P.J.& Staunton, J. (2003). Matrix-assisted laser desorption/ionization time-of-flight mass spectrometry of dextran and dextrin derivatives. *European Journal of Mass Spectrometry* , Vol. 9, No. 1, (January,2003), pp.61-70, ISSN 1469-0667

Bashir, S. & Liu, J. L. (2009). Construction and characterization of phenol-based sensor derived from colloidal chemistry. *Sensors and Actuators B*, Vol. 139, No. 2, (June, 2009), pp. 584–591, ISSN 0925-4005

Benvenue, A.& Beckman, H. (1967). Pentachlorophenol: A Discussion of Its Properties and Its Occurrence As A Residue In Human and Animal Tissues, In: *Residue Reviews*, Gunther, F.A. (Eds.), Volume 19, pp. 83-134, Springer, ISSN 0080-181X, New York, USA.

Bhatia, K. (1973). Determination of trace phenol in aqueous solution by aqueous liquid chromatography.*Analytical Chemistry, Vol.* 45, No. 8, (July, 1973), pp. 1344–1347, ISSN 1306-3057

Bidlingmeyer, B.A. (1980). Separation of Ionic Compounds by Reversed-Phase Liquid Chromatography An Update of Ion-Pairing Techniques. *Journal of Chromatographic Science*, Vol. 18, No. 10, (October, 1980), pp. 525-539, ISSN 0021-9665

Box, J.D. (1983). Investigation of the Folin-Ciocalteau phenol reagent for the determination of polyphenolic substances in natural waters. *Water Research*, Vol.17, No. 5, (May 1983), pp. 511-525, ISSN 0043-1354

Bruce, R. M.; Santodonato, J. & Neal, M. W. (1987). Summary Review of The Health Effects Associated With Phenol. *Toxicology and Industrial Health, Vol.* 3, No. 4, (April, 1987), pp. 535-568, ISSN 1477-0393

Buehler C. A & Pearson D. E. (1970). *Survey of Organic Synthesis*, pp. 285–382, Wiley-Interscience, ISBN 9780894644085, New York, USA

Busca, G.; Berardinelli, S.; Resini, C.; Arrighi, L. (2008). Technologies for the removal of phenol from fluid streams: A short review of recent developments. *Journal of Hazardous Materials*, Vol. 160, No. 1 (March, 2008), pp. 265-88, ISSN 0304-3894

Buswell, J.A. (1975). Metabolism of phenol and cresols by *Bacillus stearothermophilus*. *Journal of Bacteriology*, Vol. 124, No. 3, (December, 1975), pp. 1077–1083, ISSN 0021-9193

Chau A. S. Y. & Coburn, J. A. (1974). Determination of Pentachlorophenol In Natural and Waste Waters. *Journal of the Association of Official Analytical Chemists (JAOAC)*, Vol. 57, No. 2 (March, 1974), pp. 389-93, ISSN 0004-5756

Chick, H. (1908). An Investigation of The Laws of Disinfection. *Journal of Hygiene* Vol. 8, No.1, (August 1908), pp. 92-158, ISSN 0022-1724

Churatek, J. & Houpek, J. (1975). Phenols In: *Liquid Column Chromatography A Survey of Modem Techniques and Applications*, Deyl, Z.; Macek, K. & Janák, J. (Eds.), pp. 441-449, Elsevier, New York, USA, ISBN 9780444411563 (Also See *Journal of Chromatography Library, Vol.* 3, No.1, (March, 1975), ISSN 0301-4770)

Crosby, D. G. (1982). Environmental Chemistry: An Overview. *Environmental Toxicological Chemistry*, Vol. 1, No.1, (January , 1982), pp. 1–8, ISSN 0730-7268

Dacre, J.C. (1971). Nonspecificity of the Gibbs reaction. *Analytical Chemistry, Vol.* 43, No. 4, (April, 1971), pp. 589-591, ISSN 1306-3057

Dannis, M. (1951). Determination of Phenols by the Aminoantipyrine Method. *Sewage and Industrial Wastes*, Vol. 23, No. 12, (December, 1951), pp. 1516-1522, ISSN 0096-364X

Deichmann, W.B. & Keplinger, M.L. (1962). Phenols and phenolic compounds. In: *Industrial Hygiene and Toxicology*, Patty, F.A., (Ed.), Interscience, pp. 1363–1375, ISBN , New York, ISBN 0471160466

Di Corcia, A. (1973). Analysis of Phenols by Gas—Liquid—Solid Chromatography. *Journal of Chromatography A, Vol.* 80, No. 1, (June, 1973), pp. 69-74, ISSN 0021-9673

Diz, V.; Cassanello, D. & Negri, R.M. (2006). Detection and discrimination of phenol and primary alcohols in water using electronic noses. *Environmental Science & Technology*, Vol. 40, No. 19, (September, 2006), pp. 6058-6063, ISSN 0013-936X

Eksperiandova, L. P.; Fokina,I. I.; Blank, A. B.; Ivkova, T. I. & Soukhomlinov, B. P.(1999). Determination of small quantities of phenol in water. *Analytica Chimica Acta*, Vol. 396, No. 2-3, (September, 1999), pp.317-320, ISSN 0003-2670

Engeldinger, E.; Armspach, D. & Matt, D. (2003). Capped cyclodextrins. *Chemical Reviews*, Vol 103, No. 11, (November, 2003), pp. 4147-4173, ISSN 0009-2665

Ettinger, M. B. & Ruchhoft, C. C. (1948). Determination of Phenol and Structurally Related Compounds by Gibbs Method. *Analytical Chemistry, Vol.* 20, No. X, (1948), pp.1191-1196, ISSN 1306-3057

Farino, J.; Norwitz, G.; Boyko, W.J. & Keliher, P.N. (1981).Study of the behaviour of various phenolic compounds in the 4-aminoantipyrine and ultraviolet-ratio spectrophotometric methods without and with distillation. *Talanta*, Vol. 28, No. 9, (September, 1981), pp. 705-708, ISSN 0039-9140

Fichnolz, G. G. ; Nagel A. E.& Hughes, R. H. (1965). Adsorption of Ions Dilute Aqueous Solutions On Glass and Plastic Surfaces. *Analytical Chemistry, Vol.* 37, No.7 (June, 1965), pp. 863-868, ISSN 1306-3057

Folin, O.& Denis, W. (1915). A colorimetric method for the determination of phenols (and phenol derivatives) in urine. *Journal of Biological Chemistry*, Vol. 22, No. 2 (September, 1914), pp. 305-320, ISSN 0021-9258

Folke, J. (1985). Environmental Impact Assessment for Aquatic Ecosystems of Industrial Effluents, *Toxicological and Environmental Chemistry*, Vol. 10, No.3, (February , 1985), pp. 201-224, ISSN: 1029-0486

Gattuso, G.;. Nepogodiev, S.A. & Stoddart, J.F. (1998). Synthetic cyclic oligosaccharides. *Chemical Reviews*, Vol. 98, No. 5, (July, 1998), pp. 1919-1958, ISSN 0009-2665

Gerberding, J. L. (Ed.). (2002). *Toxicological Profile For Wood Creosote, Coal Tar Creosote, Coal Tar, Coal Tar Pitch and Coal Tar Pitch Volatiles*, U. S. Department of Health and Human Services, ISBN 978-1-4200-6188-8, Washington D.C, USA

Gibbs, H.D. (1927a). Phenol tests. II. Nitrous acid tests. The Millon and similar tests. Spectrophotometric investigations. *Journal of Biological Chemistry*, Vol. 71, No. 2, (January, 1927), pp. 455-459, ISSN 0021-9258

Gibbs, H.D. (1927b). Phenol Tests. IV. A Study of the Velocity of Indophenol Formation 2,6-Dibromobenzenoneindophenol. *Journal of Physical Chemistry*, Vol. 31, No. 7, (January, 1927), pp. 1053-1081, ISSN 1089-5647

Giger, W. & Schaffner, C. (1981). Determination of Phenolic Water Pollutants By Glass Capillary Gas Chromatography, In: *Advances In The Identification and Analysis of Organic Pollutants In Water*, Keith, L.H. (Ed.), pp. 141–154, Vol. 1, Ann Arbor Science, ISBN 0250403978, Ann Arbor, Michigan, USA

Gilman, A. P. , Douglas, V. M.; Newhook, T. E. Arbuckle, R. C. (Eds.). (1988). *Chlorophenols and Their Impurities: A Health Hazard Evaluation*, Health and Welfare Canada, Document No. H46-2/88-110E, ISBN: 0662173678

Gogate, P. R. (2008). Treatment of Wastewater Streams Containing Phenolic Compounds Using Hybrid Techniques Based On Cavitation: A Review of The Current Status and The Way Forward. *Ultrasonics Sonochemistry, Vol.* 15, No 1, (January 2008), pp. 1-15, ISSN 1350-4177

Goulden, P. D.; Brooksbank, P. & Day, M.B. (1973). Determination of submicrogram levels of phenol in water. *Analytical Chemistry*, Vol. 45, No. 14, (January, 1973), pp. 2430–2433, ISSN 1306-3057

Greminger, D. C.; Burns, G. P.; Lynn, S.; Hanson, D. N.; King, C. J. (1982). Solvent extraction of phenols from water, *Industrial & Engineering Chemistry Process Design and Development*, Vol. 21, No.1 (January, 1982), pp. 51–54, ISSN 0196-4305

Gupta, V.D. (2006).Quantitative Determination of Resorcinol in Presence of Phenol. *Journal of Pharmaceutical Sciences*, Vol. 65, N.1, (September, 2006), pp. 144-145, ISSN 0022-3549

Han, E.; Shan, D.; Xue, H. & Cosnier, S. (2007). Hybrid Material Based on Chitosan and Layered Double Hydroxides: Characterization and Application to the Design of Amperometric Phenol Biosensor. *Biomacromolecules*, Vol. 8, No. 3, (January, 2007), pp. 971–975, ISSN 1525-7797

Hanrahan, G.; Patil, D. G. & Wang, J. (2004). Electrochemical sensors for environmental monitoring: design, development and applications. *Journal of Environmental Monitoring, Vol.* 6, No.8, (August, 2004), pp. 657-664, ISSN 1464-0325

Hart, J. P. & Wring, S. A. (1997). Recent developments in the design and application of screen-printed electrochemical sensors for biomedical, environmental and industrial analyses. *Trends in Analytical Chemistry*, Vol. 16, No. 2, (February, 1997), pp. 89-103, ISSN 0167-2940

Hill, R.H. & Herndon, L.K. (1952).Determination of Phenols by the p-Nitro-Sodimethylaniline Method. *Sewage and Industrial Wastes*, Vol. 24, No. 11, (November, 1952), pp. 1389-1396, ISSN 0096-364X

Hoffsommer, J. C.; Glover D. J. & Hazzard, C. Y. (1980). Quantitative analkysis of polynitrophenols in water in the micro- to nanogram range by reversed-phase ion-pair liquid chromatography. *Journal of Chromatography A, Vol.* 195, No. 3, (July,1980), pp. 435-440, ISSN 0021-9673

Hornyak, G.L.; Patrissi, C.J.; Oberhauser, E.B.; Martin, C.R.; Valmalette, J-C.; Lemaire, L. ; Dutta J. & Hofmann, H. (1997). Effective medium theory characterization of Au/Ag nanoalloy-porous alumina composites. *Nanostructured Materials, Vol.* 9, No. 1-8, (January, 1997), pp. 571–574, ISSN 0965-9773
Houghton G. U. & Pelly R. G. (1937). A colorimetric method for the determination of traces of phenol in water. *The Analyst*, Vol. 62, No. 731, (feburary, 1937), pp. 117-120, ISSN 0003-2654

Janshoff, A.; Steinem,C.; Michalke, A.; Henke, C. & Galla, H.-J. (2000).Monofunctionalized β-cyclodextrins as sensor elements for the detection of small molecules. *Sensors and Actuators B: Chemical*, Vol. 70, No. 1-3, (November, 2000), pp. 243-253 , ISSN 0925-4005

Jones, P.A. (Ed.). (1981). *Chlorophenols, and Their Impurities In The Canadian Environment*, Environmental Impact Control Directorate, Environment Canda, Report EPS 3-EC-81-2, (March 1981), ISBN: 0662114825, Toronto, Canada; Also See The 1983 Supplement, Report 3-EP-84-3 (March 1984) ISBN 0662131592

Kadish, A. H & Hall, D. A. (1965). A New Method for the Continuous Monitoring of Blood Glucose by Measurement of Dissolved Oxygen. *Clinical Chemistry*, Vol. 11, No. 9 (September, 1965), pp. 869-875, ISSN 1434-6621

Karube, I.; Nomura, Y. & Arikawa, Y. (1995). Biosensors for environmental control. *Trends in Analytical Chemistry*, Vol. 14, No. 1, (January, 1995), pp. 295-299, ISSN 0167-2940

Khan, A.R.; Forgo, P.; Stine, K.J. & De Souza, V.T. (1998).Methods for selective modifications of Cyclodextrins. *Chemical Reviews,* Vol. 98, No. 5, (July, 1998), pp. 1977-1996, ISSN 0009-2665

Kim, Y.J., Cho, S.M., Pyo, H-B. & Choi, C. A. (2005). Sub-ppm detection of gold nanoparticle transducer toward carboxylfunctionality. Institute of Electrical and Electronics Engineers (*IEEE) Sensors*, Vol. 6, No. 10-11, (October, 2005), pp. 845-848, ISSN 1530-437X

Klein, L. C. (Ed.). (1988). *Sol-Gel Technology For Thin Films, Fibers, Preforms, Electronics and Specialty Shapes*, Noyes Publications, ISBN 0-8155-1154-X, Berkshire, UK

Kozak, V. P.; Simsiman, G. V. ; Chesters, G.; Stensby D. &. Harkin, J. (Eds.). (1979). *Reviews of The Environmental Effluents of Pollutants: X. Chlorophenols*, United States Environmental Protection Agency (US EPA), EPA-600/1-79-012, Washington, DC, USA, ISBN/OCLC 06950053

Kuehl, D.W. & Dougherty, R. C. (1980). Pentachlorophenol in the environment. Evidence for its origin from commercial pentachlorophenol by negative chemical ionization mass spectrometry. *Environmental Science & Technology, Vol.* 14, No. 4, (April, 1980), pp.447–449, ISSN 0013-936X

Kutner W. & Doblhofer K. (1992). Simultaneous cyclic voltammetry and electrochemical quartz-crystal microbalance study at the polymer film modified electrodes of molecular inclusion of ferrocene by the β-cyclo-dextrin polymer film and carboxymethylated β-cyclodextrin polymers as well as ferrocenecarboxylic acid by the β-cyclodextrin polymer. *Journal of Electroanalytical Chemistry*, Vol. 326, No. 1-2, (May, 1992), pp. 139-160, ISSN 0022-0728

Lante, A.; Crapisi, A.; Krastanov, A. & Spettoli, P. (2000). Biodegradation of phenols by laccase immobilized in a membrane reactor. *Process Biochemistry, Vol.* 36, No. 1-2, (September, 2000), pp. 51-58, ISSN 0032-9592

Lee, H.B.; Weng, L. D. & Chau, A. S. Y. (1984a). Chemical derivatization analysis of pesticide residues. IX. Analysis of phenol and 21 chlorinated phenols in natural waters by formation of pentafluorobenzyl ether derivatives. *Journal of the Association of Official Analytical Chemists, Vol.* 67, No. 6, (November, 1984), pp. 1086-1091, ISSN 0004-5756

Lee, H.B.; Weng, L. D. & Chau, A.S.Y. (1984b). Chemical derivatization analysis of pesticide residues. VIII: Analysis of 15 chlorophenols in natural water by *in situ* acetylation. *Journal of the Association of Official Analytical Chemists, Vol.* 67, No. 4, (July, 1984), pp. 789-794, ISSN 0004-5756

Lindgren, A.; Emneus, J.; Ruzgas, T.; Gorton, L. & Marko-Varga, G. (1997). Amperometric detection of phenols using peroxidase-modified graphite electrodes. *Analytica Chlmica Acta*, Vol. 347, No. 1-2, (May, 1997), pp. 51-62, ISSN 0003-2670

Lindinger, W.; Hansel A. & Jordan, A. (1998). On-line monitoring of volatile organic compounds at pptv levels by means of proton-transfer-reaction mass spectrometry (PTR-MS) medical applications, food control and environmental research. *International Journal of Mass Spectrometry and Ion Processes*, Vol. 173, No.3, (February, 1998), pp. 191-241, ISSN 0168-1176

Link, S. & El-Sayed, M.A. (2003). Optical Properties and Ultrafast Dynamics of Metallic Nanocrystals. *Annual Revision of Physical Chemistry, Vol.* 54, No. 1, (January, 2003), pp. 331–366, ISSN 0066-426X

Lisk, D.J. (1970). The Analysis of Pesticide Residues: New Problems and Methods. *Science*, Vol. 170, No. 958, (November, 1970), pp. 589-593, ISSN 0036-8075

Liu, J. & Lu, Y. (2004). Colorimetric biosensors based on DNAzyme-assembled gold nanoparticles. *Journal of Fluorescence, Vol.* 14, No. 4, (July, 2004), pp. 343–354, ISSN 1053-0509

Liu, H.; Matsuda, S.; Kato, S.; Hashimoto, K. & Nakanishi, S. (2010). Redox-Responsive Switching in bacterial Respiratory Pathways involving Extracellular Electron Transfer. *ChemSusChem*, Vol. 3, No. 1, (March, 2010), pp. 1253-1256, ISSN 1864-5631

Liu, S.; Yu, J. & Ju, H. (2003). Renewable phenol biosensor based on a tyrosinase-colloidal gold modified carbon paste electrode. *Journal of Electroanalytical Chemistry*, Vol. 540, No. 1, (January 2003), pp. 61-67, ISSN 0022-0728

Liu, Y.; Qu, X.; Guo, H.;Chen, H.; Liu, B. & Dong, S. (2006). Facile preparation of amperometric laccase biosensor with multifunction based on the matrix of carbon nanotubes–chitosan composite. *Biosensors and Bioelectronics*, Vol 21, No. 2, (June, 2006), pp. 2195-2201, ISSN 0956-5663

Liu, Z.; Liu, B.; Kong, J. & Deng, J. (2000). Probing Trace Phenols Based on Mediator-Free Alumina Sol−Gel-Derived Tyrosinase Biosensor. *Analytical Chemistry*, Vol. 72, No. 19, (August, 2000), pp. 4707–4712, 1306-3057

Liz-Marzan, L.M. (2004). Nanometals: formation and color. *Materials Today*,Vol. 7, No. 2, (February , 2004), pp. 26-31, ISSN 1369-7021

Lykken, L. ; Treseder, R.S. & Zahn, V. (1946). Colorimetric Determination of Phenols. Application to Petroleum and Allied Products. *Industrial & Engineering Chemistry Research*, Vol. 18, No. 2 (February , 1946), pp. 103–109, ISSN 1520-5045

Lyklema. J. (1995). *Fundamentals of Colloid and Interface Science*, Academic Press, ISBN 0124605249, London, U.K.

Lynch, J.P. & Loh, K. J. (2006). A Summary Review of Wireless Sensors and Sensor Networks for Structural Health Monitoring. *The Shock and Vibration Digest*, Vol. 38, No. 91, (March, 2006), pp. 91-128, ISSN 0583-1024

Mallick, A. Purkayastha, P. & Chattopadhyay, N. (2007). Photoprocesses Of Excited Molecules In Confined Liquid Environments: An Overview. *Journal Of Photochemistry And Photobiology C-Photochemistry Reviews, Vol.* 8, No. 3 (November, 2007), pp. 109-127, ISSN 1389-5567

Manna, A.; Imae,T.; Aoi, K.; Okada, M. & Yogo, T. (2001). Synthesis of Dendrimer-Passivated Noble Metal Nanoparticles in a Polar Medium: Comparison of Size between Silver and Gold Particles. *Chemistry of Materials*, Vol. 13, No. 5, (April, 2001), pp. 1674–1681, ISSN 0897-4756

Martin, R. W. (1949). Rapid Colorimetric Estimation of Phenol,. *Analytical Chemistry*, Vol. 21, No. 11, (November, 1949), pp. 1419–1420, ISSN 1306-3057

Martus, P. & Puttmann, W. (2003). Formation of Alkylated Aromatic Acids In Groundwater By Anaerobic Degradation of Alkylbenzenes. *The Science of The Total Environment, Vol.*307, No.(1-3), (May 2003), pp. 19-33, ISSN 0048-9697

Mathew, J. & Elzerman, A. W. (1981). Gas-Liquid Chromatographic Determination of Some Chloro- and Nitrophenols by Direct Acetylation in Aqueous Solution. *Analytical Letters, Vol.* 14, No. (1981), pp. 1351–1361, ISSN 0003-2719

McKillop, A.; Fiaud, J.-C & Hug, R. P. (1974). The Use of Phase-Transfer Catalysis For The Synthesis of Phenol Ethers. *Tetrahedron* , Vol.30, No. 11 (June, 1974), 1379-1382, ISSN 0040-4020

Metzger, J.; Reiss, M. & Hartmeier, W. (1998). Amperometric phenol biosensor based on a thermostable phenol hydroxylase, *Biosensors and Bioelectronics*, Vol. 13, No. 10, (November, 1998) 1077-1082, ISSN 0956-5663

Nath, N. & Chilkoti, A. (2002). A Colorimetric Gold Nanoparticle Sensor To Interrogate Biomolecular Interactions in Real Time on a Surface. *Analytical Chemistry, Vol.* 74, No. 4, (December, 2002), pp. 504–509, ISSN 1306-3057

National Research Council of Canada (NRCC). (1982). *Chlorinated Phenols: Criteria For Environmental Quality*, NRCC, NRCC No. 18578, ISBN/OCLC 13059308, Ottawa, Ontario, Canada

Neujahr, H.Y. (1982). Determination of phenol and catechol concentrations with oxygen probes coated with immobilized enzymes or immobilized cells. *Applied Biochemistry and Biotechnology*, Vol. 7, No. 1-2, (January, 1982) 107-111, ISSN 0273-2289

Nistor, C.; Emnéus, J.; Gorton, L. & Ciucu, A. (1999). Improved stability and altered selectivity of tyrosinase based graphite electrodes for detection of phenolic compounds. *Analytica Chimica Acta*, Vol. 387, No. 3, (April, 1999), pp. 309-326, ISSN 0003-2670

Norwitz, G.;Farino, J. & Keliher, P.N. (1979). Interference of oxidants in the determination of phenol by the 4-aminoantipyrine and ultraviolet ratio spectrophotometric methods. *Analytical Chemistry*, Vol. 51, No. 11, (September, 1979), ISSN 0003-2700

Ogan K.L. & Katz, E.D. (1980). Retention characteristics of several bonded-phase liquid chromatography columns for some polycyclic aromatic hydrocarbons, *Journal of Chromatography A*, Vol. 188, No. 1, (January, 1980), pp. 115-127, ISSN 0021-9673

Orupold, K.; Mashirin, A. & Tenno, T. (1995). Amperometric phenol sensor with immobilized bacteria. *Electroanalysis, Vol.* 7, No. 9. (September, 1995) 904-906, ISSN 1521-4109

Patel, P.D. (2002) (Bio) sensors for measurement of analytes implicated in food safety: a review. *Trends in Analytical Chemistry*, Vol. 21 , No. 2, (February ,2002), pp. 96-115, ISSN 0167-2940

Pumera,M.;Sánchez, S.; Ichinose, I. & Jie Tang. (2007). Electrochemical nanobiosensors. *Sensors and Actuators B: Chemical*, Vol. 123, No. 2, (May, 2007), pp. 1195-1205, ISSN 0925-4005

Ragauskas, A.J.; Williams, C. K.; Davison, B.H.; Britovsek, G.; Cairney, J.; Eckert, C.A.; Frederick, Jr W.J.; Hallett, J.P.; Leak, D.J.; Liotta, C.L.; Mielenz, J.R.; Murphy, R.; Templer, R. & Tschaplinski, T. (2006). The Path Forward for Biofuels and Biomaterials. *Science*, Vol. 311, No.5760, (January, 2006),pp.484-489, ISSN 0036-8075

Rainina, E. I.; Badalian, I. E.; Ignatov, O. V.; Fedorov, A. Y.; Simonian, A. L. & Varfolomeyev, S. D. (1996). Cell biosensor for detection of phenol in aqueous solution. *Applied Biochemistry and Biotechnology*, Vol.56, No. 2, (February , 1996), pp. 117-127, ISSN 0273-2289

Rakestraw, N.W. (1923). A Quantitative method for the Determination of Phenols in Blood. *Journal of Biological Chemistry*, Vol. 56, No. 1 (May, 1923), pp. 109-119, ISSN 0021-9258

Rao, K.R. (Ed.). (1978). *Pentachlorophenol: Chemistry, Pharmacology and Environmental Toxicology*, Plenum Press, ISBN, New York, USA

Raybin, H.W. (1945). Reaction of Theophylline with Gibbs' Reagent. *Journal of the American Chemical Society*, Vol. 67, No. 9, (September, 1945) pp. 1621-1623, ISSN 0002-7863

Realini, P.A. (1980). Determination of priority pollutant phenols in water by HPLC. *Journal of Chromatographic Science*, Vol. 19, No. 3, (March, 1980), pp. 124-129, ISSN 0021-9665

Regnier Z. & Watson, A. E. P. (1971). The Development of Colorimetric and Fluorometric Automated Methods For Trace Phenol Estimation In: *Natural Waters,* Regnier Z. & Watson, A. E. P. (Eds.), pp. 23-115, Water Quality Division Research Report, Department of The Environment, Ottawa Canada

Rella, R.; Ferrara, G.; Barison, G. & Doretti, L. (1996). High-temperature operating biosensor for the determination of phenol and related compounds. *Biotechnology and Applied Biochemistry, Vol.* 24, No. 1, (1996), pp. 83-88, ISSN 0885-4513

Renberg, L. & Björseth, A. (Eds.). (1983). *Determination of Phenols In Water, A Brief Summary of Current Knowledge and Proposed Analytical Methods*, Commission of The European Communities, COST 64b Bis, Report of The Working Party 8, Specific Analytical Problems OMP/38/83, Hague Holland

Renberg, L. (1981). Gas Chromatographic Determination of Chlorophenols In Water, as their pentafluorobenzoyl derivatives. *Chemosphere*, Vol. 10, No. 7, pp. 767-773, (July 1981), ISSN 0045-6535

Renberg, L. (Ed.). (1982). *Phenolic Compounds - Analytical Methods In Relation To Environmental Aspects*, Commission of The European Communities, COST 64b Bis, Report of The Workshop of The Working Party 8, Specific Analytical Problems, OMP/33/82, Dübendorf, Switzerland

Renedo,O. D.; Alonso-Lomillo, M.A.& Martínez, M.J.A. (2007). Recent developments in the field of screen-printed electrodes and their related applications. Talanta, Vol. 73, No. 2, (September, 2007), pp. 202-219, ISSN 0039-9140

Ribick, M.A.; Smith, L.M.; Dubay, G.R. & Stalling, D.L. (1981). Applications and Results of Analytical Methods Used in Monitoring Environmental Contaminants, In: *Aquatic Toxicology and Hazard Assessment*, Branson D.R. &. Dickson, K.L. (Eds.), pp. 23-45, American Society for testing of Materials (ASTM), ISBN 9789993664383, Philadelphia, USA.

Riedel, K.; Kunze, G. & König, A. (2002). Microbial Sensors on a Respiratory Basis for Wastewater Monitoring In: *History and Trends in Bioprocessing and Biotransformation:* Advances in Biochemical Engineering/Biotechnology, Scheper, E. (Ed.), vol. 75, pp. 81-118 (December, 2002), Springer-Verlag, ISBN 9783540423713, Berlin, Germany

Rodriguez-Mozaz, S.; de Alda, M. J. L.; Marco, M.-P. & Barceló, D. (2005). Biosensors for environmental monitoring: A global perspective, *Talanta, Vol.* 65, No. 2 (January, 2005), pp.291-297, ISSN 0039-9140

Rogers, K. R. (1995). Biosensors for environmental applications, *Biosensors and Bioelectronics.* Vol. 10, No. 6-7 (May-June, 1995), pp. 533-541, ISSN 0956-5663
Saby, C.; Male, K. B. & Luong, J. H. T. (1997). A Combined Chemical and Electrochemical Approach Using Bis(trifluoroacetoxy)iodobenzene and Glucose Oxidase for the Detection of Chlorinated Phenols. *Analytical Chemistry, Vol.* 69, No. 21, (November, 1997), pp. 4324–4330, ISSN 1306-3057

Sahoo, S.K.; Diinawaz, F. & Kumar, S.K. (2008). Nanotechnology In Ocular Drug Delivery. *Drug Discovery Today,* Vol. 13, No. 3-4, (February , 2008), pp. 144-151, ISSN 1359-6446

Salkinoja-Salone, M.; Saxelin, M. -L.; Pere, J.; Jaakkola, T.; Saarikoski, J.; Hakulinen R.& Koistinen, O. (1981). Analysis of Toxicity and Biodegradability of Organochlorine Compounds Released Into The Environment In Bleaching Effluents of Kraft Pulping. In: *Advances In The Identification and Analysis of Organic Pollutants In Water,* Keith, L.H. (Ed.), pp. 1131-1164, Ann Arbor Science, ISBN 0250403986 Ann Arbor, Michigan, USA

Salústio, P.J.; Feio, G.;Figueirinhas, J.L.;Pinto, J.F. & Cabral Marques, H.M. (2009). The influence of the preparation methods on the inclusion of model drugs in a beta-cyclodextrin cavity. European Journal of Pharmaceutics and Biopharmaceutics, Vol.71, No. 2, (February, 2009), pp. 377-386 , ISSN 0939-6411

Scheller, F. W.; Pfeiffer, D.; Lisdat, F.; Bauer, C. & Gajovic, N. (1988). Enzyme Biosensors Based on Oxygen Detection, In: *Enzyme and Microbial Biosensors: Methods in Biotechnology,* Mulchandani, A. & Rogers, K. R. (Eds.), Vol. 6, pp. 51-65, Springer-Verlag, ISBN 0896034100, Berlin, Germany

Shammala, F.A. (1999). Effect of Surfactant Loading on the Extraction Properties of C-18 Bonded Silica used for Solid-Phase Extraction of Phenols. *Analytical Letters,* Vol.32, No.15, (October, 1999), pp. 3083-3110, ISSN 0003-2719

Skládal, P.;Morozova, N.O.& Reshetilov, A.N. (2002). Amperometric biosensors for detection of phenol using chemically modified electrodes containing immobilized bacteria. *Biosensors and Bioelectronics, Vol.* 17, No. 10, (October, 2002), pp. 867-873, ISSN 0956-5663

Smith, B. & Persmark, U. (1963b). Characterization of Certain Ortho Substituted Phenols Using Tetracyanoethylene. *Acta Chemica Scandinavica*, Vol. 17, No. 3, (March, 1963), pp. 651-656, ISSN 0001-5393

Smith, B.; Persmark, U. & Edman, E. (1963a). The Use of Tetracyanoethylene for the Qualitative Analysis of Phenols. *Acta Chemica Scandinavica*, Vol. 17, No.3 (March, 1963), pp. 709-722, ISSN 0001-5393

Smyth, C.; Lau, K. T.; Shepherd, R. L.; Diamond, D.; Wu, Y.; Spinks, G. M. & Wallace, G.G. (2008). Self-maintained colorimetric acid/base sensor using polypyrrole actuator. *Sensors and Actuators B: Chemical, Vol.* 129, No. 2, (February , 2008), pp. 518-524 ISSN 0925-4005

Staples, C. A.; Dome, P. B. & Klecka, G. M. (1998). Sondra T. Oblock, L. R. Harrie, A review of the environmental fate, effects, and exposures of bisphenol A. *Chemosphere*, Vol. 36, No. 10, (April, 1998) 2149-2173, ISSN 0045-6535

Staples, E. J. (2004). Detection of Phenol in Water and Air Using the zNose™. Electronic Sensor Techniology Techncial Report

Svobodová, D.; Kenek, P.,Fraenkl, M. & Gaspari, J. (1977a). Colour Reaction Of Phenols With The Gibbs Reagent. The Reaction Mechanism And Decomposition And Stabilisation Of The Reagent. *Microchimica Acta, Vol.* 67, No. 3-4, (March, 1977), pp. 251-264, ISSN 0026-3672

Svobodová, D.; Křenek, P.; Fraenkl, M. & Gasparič, J. (1977b). Colour reaction of phenols with the gibbs reagent. The reaction mechanism and decomposition and stabilisation of the reagent. *Microchimica Acta*, Vol. 67, No. 3-4, (March, 1971), pp. 251-264, ISSN 0026-3672

Svobodová, D. & Gasparič, J. (1971). Investigation of the colour reaction of phenols with 4-aminoantipyrine. *Microchimica Acta*, Vol. 59, No. 2, (February, 1971), pp. 384-390, ISSN 0026-3672

Taras, M.J.; Greenberg, A.E. & Hoak, R.D. (Eds.). (1971). *Standard Methods For The Examination of Water and Wastewater, American*, Public Health Association, American Water Works Association, & Water Pollution Control Federation, ISBN 0875530605, Washington, D.C

Tingry, S.; Innocent, C.; Touil, S.; Deratani, A. & Seta, P. (2006). Carbon paste biosensor for phenol detection of impregnated tissue: modification of selectivity by using β-cyclodextrin-containing PVA membrane. *Materials Science and Engineering: C*, Vol. 26, No. 2-3, (March 2006), pp. 222-226, ISSN 0928-4931

Tomlinson, E.; Jefferies, T.M. &. Riley, C.M. (1978). Ion-pair high-performance liquid chromatography. *Journal of Chromatography A, Vol.* 159, No. 3, (October, 1978), pp. 315-358, ISSN 0021-9673

United States Department of Agriculture (USDA). (1980a). *The Biological and Economic Assessment of Pentachlorophenol, Inorganic Arsenicals, and Creosote.* USDA, Technical Bulletin No. 1658-1, ISBN/OCLC 48112299, Washington, DC, USA

United States Department of Agriculture (USDA). (1980b). *The Biological and Economic Assessment of Pentachlorophenol, Inorganic Arsenicals, and Creosote,* USDA, TB1658, ISBN/OCLC 21621465, Washington, DC, USA

United States Environmental Protection Agency (US EPA). (1980). *Ambient Water Quality Criteria For Chlorinated Phenols,* USDA,EPA 440/5-80-032, ISBN/OCLC 06998602, Washington, DC: USA

Van Kreijl C. F. & Slooff, W. (Eds.). (1983). *Biological Effects of Phenolic Compounds*, Report of The Workshop of The Working Party 8, Specific Analytical Problems, COST 64b Bis, March 2-4 OMP/37/83, Commission of The European Communities, Hague Holland

Warsinke, A.; Benkert, A. & Scheller, F. W. (1999). Electrochemical immunoassays. *Fresenius' Journal of Analytical Chemistry*, Vol. 366, No. 6-7, (June, 1999), pp. 622-634,ISSN 0937-0633

Wang, J. (1997). Remote electrochemical sensors for monitoring inorganic and organic pollutants. *Trends in Analytical Chemistry*, Vol. 16, No. 2, (February , 1997), pp. 84-88, ISSN 0167-2940

Wegman, R.C.C. &. Wammes, J.I.J. (1983). Determination of nitrophenols in water and sediment samples by high-performance liquid chromatography. *Mededelingen van de Faculteit Landbouw- wetenschappen Rijksuniversiteit Gent*, Vol. 48, pp. 961-969, ISSN 0368-9697

West F. K.; West, P. W. & Iddings, F. A. (1966). Adsorption of Traces of Silver on Container Surfaces. *Analytical Chemistry*, Vol. 38, No. 11, (October, 1966), pp. 1566-1570, ISSN 1306-3057

Wolf, A.; Hüttl, R.& Wolf, G. (2000). Enzymatic Reactions For The Calorimetric Detection Of Phenolic Compounds. *Journal of Thermal Analysis and Calorimetry*, Vol. 61, No. 1, (January, 2000), pp. 37-44, ISSN 1418-2874

Wollenberger, U.; Neumann, B.; Riedel, K. & Scheller, F. W. (1994). Enzyme and microbial sensors for phosphate, phenols, pesticides and peroxides. *Fresenius' Journal of Analytical Chemistry*, Vol. 348, No. 8-9, (August, 1994), pp. 563-566,ISSN 0937-0633

Xanthos, M. (1969). Plastics Processing, In: *Encyclopedia of Polymer Science and Technology*, Mark, H. F. & Gaylord, N. (Eds.), pp. 120-141, Wiley-Interscience, ISBN 0471275077, New York, USA

Yu, J.; Liu, S. & Ju, H. (2003). Mediator-Free Phenol Sensor Based On Titania Sol-Gel Encapsulation Matrix For Immobilization of Tyrosinase By A Vapor Deposition Method. *Biosensors and Bioelectronics*, Vol. 19, No. 5, (December, 2003), pp. 509-514, ISSN 0956-5663

Zhang, X.; Li, A. ; Jiang, Z. & Zhang, Q. (2006). Adsorption of Dyes and Phenol From Water On Resin Adsorbents: Effect of Adsorbate Size and Pore Size Distribution. *Journal of Hazardous Materials* Vol.137, No. 2 (September 2006), pp. 1115-1122, ISSN 0304-3894